Principles of Human Physiology

for Courses in Nursing and Allied Health Sciences

Courses in Allied Health Sciences

- Anesthesiologist assistant
- Anesthesia technician
- Psychotherapist
- Sports / athletics trainer
- Autotransfusionist
- Audiologist
- Cardiovascular technologist
- Medical coder
- Clinical psychologist
- Dental hygienist
- Radiographer
- Dietitian/Nutritionist
- Electrocardiogram technician
- Emergency medical technician
- Environmental health officer
- Exercise physiologist
- Medical assistant
- Medical laboratory technician
- Medical radiation technician
- Neurophysiology technician
- Occupational therapist
- Operation theatre technician
- Orthoptist
- Orthotist / Prosthetist
- Perfusionist
- Phlebotomist
- Podiatrist
- Public health epidemiologist
- Physiotherapist
- Radiotherapist/radiation therapist
- Radiographer, angiographer, mammographer, sonographer
- Rehabilitation counselor
- Renal dialysis technician
- Respiratory therapist
- Medical social worker (employed in hospitals/medical establishments/institutions)
- Speech and language pathologist
- Surgical technologist

Principles of Human Physiology

for Courses in Nursing and Allied Health Sciences

Surrinder H Singh
MBBS, MD, FIMSA, MAMS, FIMA-MS

Ex-Professor of Physiology
Lady Hardinge Medical College
New Delhi

Visiting Faculty and Consultant
Pt Deendayal Upadhyaya Institute for
Physically Handicapped
New Delhi

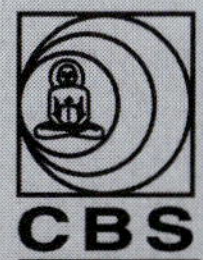

CBS Publishers & Distributors Pvt Ltd

New Delhi • Bengaluru • Chennai • Kochi • Kolkata • Mumbai

Bhopal • Bhubaneswar • Hyderabad • Jharkhand • Nagpur • Patna • Pune • Uttarakhand • Dhaka (Bangladesh) • Kathmandu (Nepal)

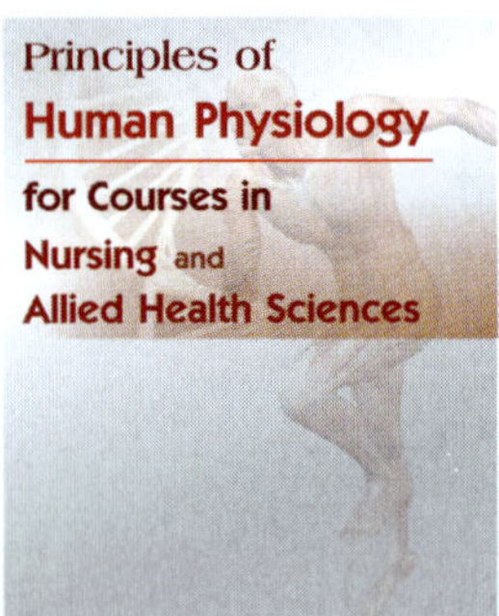

ISBN: 978-93-86217-60-8

First Edition: 2017
Reprint: 2018, 2020

Published by Satish Kumar Jain and produced by Varun Jain for
CBS Publishers & Distributors Pvt Ltd
4819/XI Prahlad Street, 24 Ansari Road, Daryaganj, New Delhi 110 002, India.
Ph: 23289259, 23266861, 23266867 Fax: 011-23243014 Website: www.cbspd.com
e-mail: delhi@cbspd.com; cbspubs@airtelmail.in.
Corporate Office: 204 FIE, Industrial Area, Patparganj, Delhi 110 092
Ph: 4934 4934 Fax: 4934 4935 e-mail: publishing@cbspd.com; publicity@cbspd.com

Branches

- **Bengaluru:** Seema House 2975, 17th Cross, K.R. Road, Banasankari 2nd Stage, Bengaluru 560 070, Karnataka
  Ph: +91-80-26771678/79 Fax: +91-80-26771680 e-mail: bangalore@cbspd.com
- **Chennai:** 7, Subbaraya Street, Shenoy Nagar, Chennai 600 030, Tamil Nadu
  Ph: +91-44-26680620, 26681266 Fax: +91-44-42032115 e-mail: chennai@cbspd.com
- **Kochi:** 42/1325, 1326, Power House Road, Opposite KSEB Power House, Ernakulam 682 018, Kochi, Kerala
  Ph: +91-484-4059061-65 Fax: +91-484-4059065 e-mail: kochi@cbspd.com
- **Kolkata:** 6/B, Ground Floor, Rameswar Shaw Road, Kolkata 700 014, West Bengal
  Ph: +91-33-22891126, 22891127, 22891128 e-mail: kolkata@cbspd.com
- **Mumbai:** 83-C, Dr E Moses Road, Worli, Mumbai 400018, Maharashtra
  Ph: +91-22-24902340/41 Fax: +91-22-24902342 e-mail: mumbai@cbspd.com

Representatives

- **Bhopal** 0-8319310552
- **Bhubaneswar** 0-9911037372
- **Hyderabad** 0-9885175004
- **Jharkhand** 0-9811541605
- **Nagpur** 0-9421945513
- **Patna** 0-9334159340
- **Pune** 0-9623451994
- **Uttarakhand** 0-9716462459
- **Dhaka (Bangladesh)** 01912-003485
- **Kathmandu (Nepal)** 977-9818742655

Printed At : Goyal Offset Works (P) Limited

to

---

the fond memory of my late father
Mr Trilochan Singh

Parents have an important role in guiding
the personalities of their children. Tremendous affection and
care with understanding of the nature of his children
that I received from my father built my personality
to love all children

This book is an effort to be useful to them

Preface

As my first book *Anatomy and Physiology for Nurses and Allied Health Sciences* was published and distributed, it was suggested that the book would be mainly useful for undergraduate courses of Nursing (BSc Nursing) and MSc Nursing. Keeping that in view, this has been written with revisions and additions made to the text in an effort to make it especially useful for the advanced courses in nursing. A large number of illustrations has been provided to facilitate understanding of the subject. Text and illustrations have been made in color to enhance visual impact and cognition. Effort has been made to be brief so as not to burden the students with too many details. However, complete curriculum has been covered leaving no topic of physiology untouched. The common disease conditions encountered by nurses in the hospital have been mentioned. Physiological derangements have been coordinated with the disease conditions.

With complete coverage of topics in physiology, the teachers/tutors will also find the book useful to refer to the topics.

In addition, the book is intended to be useful for courses in allied health sciences as well as those courses in which human physiology is taught as a core subject. Coverage of physiology could make their understanding of the encountered clinical conditions easier and help them in handling these conditions.

A book published in India can be easily available and is economical for purchase in the country and in the neighboring nations as well.

Surrinder H Singh

Acknowledgments

My interest in physiology is as old as my first year of joining a medical college, Lady Hardinge Medical College, New Delhi, when I was taught physiology by Prof (Dr) BK Anand who has been a physiologist of international recognition. His lectures delivered were so clear that it made the subject of physiology very interesting. He had returned from the USA after his MD and research. Further, as I joined Department of Physiology after my graduation in my own college, I was guided by my professor, Dr V Dutt Mullick. I completed my MD from Delhi University remaining in the department at Lady Hardinge Medical College and continued with teaching of physiology till I retired as professor and head of the department.

As the teaching and the subject of physiology has been my keen interest, I have taken to working on books in physiology. The opportunity was provided to me by CBS Publishers & Distributors and I thank Mr SK Jain (CMD) and Mr Varun Jain (Director). Mr YN Arjuna (Senior Vice-President Publishing, Editorial and Publicity) has been providing me with suggestions and help. The atmosphere is very pleasant at their office that helped in my work. Mrs Ritu Chawla (AGM Production) has been very helpful. Mr Ram Murti and Mr Sanjay Chauhan have taken pains to make illustrations; typesetting work has been carefully done by Ms Sunita Rautela; and Mr Vikrant Sharma did a meticulous job of pagination and correction, my special thanks to him. They have a pleasant mannerism and I express my thanks to all of them at CBS.

My colleagues have been very encouraging — to mention some Dr Asha Gandhi, Professor of Physiology; Dr Sunita Mondal, Professor of Physiology, LHMC; Dr Anita Sharma, Head, Physiology Department, Jamia Millia Islamia; Dr Usha Panjwani at DEPAS; Dr Puneet at BOT and BPT teaching at Pt Deen Dayal Upadhyaya Institute for Physically Handicapped, New Delhi, and Ms Resham and Ms Pooja, students of this Institute, have taken keen interest in the book.

Lastly, the affection of my children, extended family and friends, keeps me going for the work: I thank them all.

Surrinder H Singh

Contents

Yoga and Wellness

DEFINITION

The word 'Yoga' is derived from Sanskrit word 'Yug' which means to 'join' or 'to yoke', yoga to the joining of the individual soul to the universal sole. The union of spirit with God. The methods way vary but the goal is one.

Review of literature from both Indian and foreign authors is available on Yoga and meditation. In the 3rd century BC Patanjali the father of modern concept of yoga accurately and precisely defined it as a mystery of mind and emotions. Further it has been claimed that through yoga voluntary control over involuntary activities of the body can be a achieved. Swami Vivekanand (1914) quoted that there is not a single muscle in the body over what man can not establish perfect control by practice, even heart can be made to stop or go on at yogis binding.

Prof (Dr) BK Anand at all India Institute of Medical Sciences, New Delhi, with his colleagues proposed in 1961 that any voluntary control over the metabolic and or autonomic functions of the body if scientifically demonstrated would established the conditioning of the limbic system by yogic practices. A number of scientific studies were carried out on yoga at the Institute.

Yogic centers are now spread all over our country (India) and abroad. People are attending these for either physical or spiritual gains. Various physical yogic exercises are believed to condition the mind and exercises are believed to involve physical and psychic components. Literature from Indian and foreign authors is available on yoga and meditation. Studies were further conducted for any beneficial effects in diseased conditions.

Main Branches of Yoga

Satchinanda (1970) has described the branches of yoga as:

- *Hatha Yoga:* This includes bodily postures ('asanas'), deep relaxation, breath control ('Pranayama'), cleansing process ('Kriyas') and mental concentration.
- *Karma Yoga:* The path of action through selfless service.
- *Bhakti Yoga:* The path of love and devotion to God or a spiritual teacher.
- *Raja Yoga:* This is the path of meditation and control of the mind.
- *Japa Yoga:* This is a part of Raja Yoga; Japa means repetitin of a 'mantra' which is a divine word or phrase.
- *Jnana Yoga:* This is the path of wisdom, self analysis and awareness.

Meditation

There are several types of meditation. Some involve inward concentration and enhanced awareness of bodily sensation (Beaumont, 1988). Meditation often involves concentration on a single point to exclude all thoughts that are associated with everyday life (Eliade, 1950).

Meditation may be active or passive. The former involves effort to direct attention at a point of focus, whereas in the latter type, attention is left free (Naranjo and Ornstein, 1971). Adoption of the appropriate posture is said to be important to enhance concentration (Benson et al, 1974).

Four common elements integral to various practices of meditation are necessary to evoke the relaxation response. These are quiet environment, decreased muscle tone, a mental device (a sound, word or phrase) and a passive attitude (Beary and Benson, 1974).

Sahaja Yoga

The word 'Sahaja' means born with you or inborn. Whatever is inborn would manifest without any effort Sahaja Yoga, a system of 'Kundalini' awakening was introduced by Her Holiness Mataji Nirmala Devi in 1970. Sahaja Yoga is simple to practice. There is no complicated posture to be adopted. It may be practised by any age group. It does not interfere with any religious beliefs.

Kundalini is believed to be the dormant divine energy lying in three and a half coils at the sacrum bone. References to the Kundalini occur in several ancient religious texts.

Physiological processes include tissue growth, and repair or replacement even in an adult. Physiological processes are **synchronized** to promote orderly growth and development of the child.

The fertilization of the ovum by sperm is also governed by normal physiological mechanisms.

The deranged physiology of the systems is called pathology, which results in disease.

A few examples of physiological variables maintained within normal range:

- Body temperature
- ECF (extracellular fluid) osmolality
- Plasma concentration of electrolytes: Na^+, K^+, Ca^{++}
- Blood pH
- Plasma glucose level
- Arterial blood oxygen and carbon dioxide partial pressures
- Arterial blood pressure

Homeostasis is maintained by the operation of *control systems*, which *detect* and *respond* to the changes in the internal environment, i.e. when in between meals the blood glucose level tends to fall, hormonal regulation tends to maintain it; similarly after meals when it tends to rise the hormone with opposing action, i.e. insulin tends to store the glucose to maintain the blood glucose level. The levels are *sensed* by the endocrine glands and the *response* is their secretion.

Similarly the body temperature is maintained despite changing environmental temperature: when the environmental temperature is high, the receptors in the skin detect the change, hypothalamus which is the center regulating the body temperature responds and appropriate mechanisms are brought into action to maintain the temperature, e.g. vasodilatation of skin vessels and sweating; when the external temperature is low, vasoconstriction of skin vessels and increased muscle activity tends to maintain it, the regulation is by hypothalamus.

Many of these regulatory mechanisms operate on the principal of **negative feedback:** change is detected by a sensor; signals from the sensor reach a controlling center; the center activates compensatory changes that continue until the set point is reached again. Thus there is involvement of a *sensing mechanism*, a *center* responsible for setting a level and *efferent mechanisms* that are brought into action to maintain homeostasis.

As every cell of the body is in contact with the ECF and is dependent upon the composition of that fluid for its well being; even slight changes could cause permanent damage, and any change is therefore regulated by the body, through one or more of its many control mechanisms; *this is the description of homeostasis.*

A fall in plasma Ca^{++} level would causes increased excitability of muscle and nervous tissue resulting in tetany (spasmodic muscle contractions). There are normal body mechanisms to raise the plasma calcium level when it falls, if these mechanisms are unable to deal, tetany would result.

The external environment surrounds the body from where the oxygen and nutrients required by the cells of the body are to be derived. Waste products of cellular activity are in the end excreted into the external environment.

The skin provides a barrier between external environment and the watery environment of body cells.

BODY FLUIDS

In an average adult male 18% body weight is protein and related sustances, 7% is mineral, 15% fat and 60% water.

In an average adult the water forms 60% of the body weight. Of this about two-thirds of water, i.e. 40% of body weight is inside the cells, intracellular, forms intracellular fluid (ICF).

The rest of the water, i.e. 20% of the body weight is outside the cells, i.e. forms extracellular fluid (ECF). Of this extracellular fluid about one-fourth, i.e. 5% of the body weight is plasma, the rest is interstitial fluid (tissue fluid) which surrounds the tissue cells (Fig. 1.1).

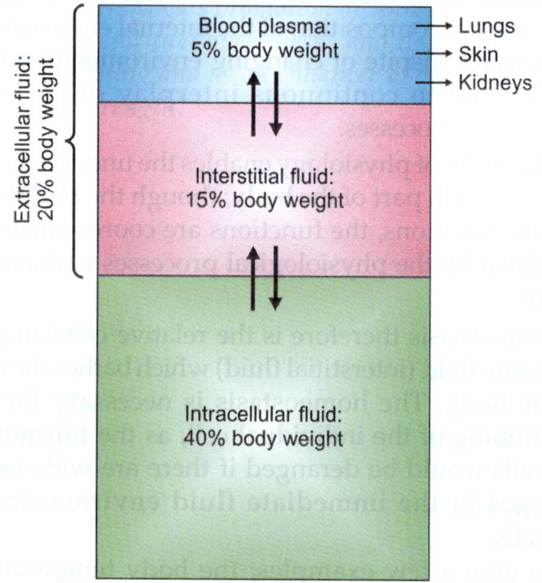

Fig. 1.1: Body fluid compartments. Arrows represent fluid movement

A small portion of ECF is in CSF and in lymph. Dissolved in the water of the ICF and ECF are oxygen, nutrients and variety of ions. The regulatory mechanisms maintain the composition of the ECF for the proper functioning of the body cells (Table 1.1).

The exchange of materials between blood and tissue fluid takes place at the level of the blood capillaries, the blood vessels which have thin walls.

The movement in both directions across capillary wall provides nutrition and oxygen into the tissue fluid for the needs of the cells and removal of waste products from tissue fluid (which are discharged into the tissue fluid from the cells, being products of metabolism).

There are differences in the ionic composition of ECF and ICF. The **ECF** has higher, about 10 times the concentration of Na^+ than that of ICF and has low concentration of the K^+.

INTRACELLULAR FLUID

The composition of intracellular fluid (ICF) is largely controlled by the cell itself, because of selective uptake and discharge mechanisms present in the cell membrane.

The composition of ICF can therefore be very different from ECF. Thus sodium levels are nearly ten times higher in the ECF than in the ICF. This concentration difference is maintained because although sodium diffuses into the cell through the cell membrane, down its concentration gradient there is a pump in the membrane which selectively pumps it back into the ECF. The diffusion is also limited as explained later in text. This concentration gradient is essential for the functions of excitable cells (mainly nerve and muscle). Conversely, many substances are found inside the cell in significantly higher amounts than outside, e.g. ATP, protein and potassium.

Table 1.1: Important constituents of ECF

	Normal value	*Normal range*	*Units*
Oxygen (PO_2)	40	35–45	mmHg
Carbon dioxide (PCO_2)	40	35–45	mmHg
Sodium ion	142	138–146	mmol/L
Potassium ion	4.2	3.8–5.0	mmol/L
Calcium ion	1.2	1.0–1.3	mmol/L
Total calcium concentration is 8.5 to 10.5 mg/dL of which 50% is ionized Ca^{++}			
Chloride ion	108	103–112	mmol/L
Bicarbonate ion	28	24–32	mmol/L
Glucose	80	70–110	mg/dL
Body temperature	98.4 (37.0)	98–98.8 (37.0)	°F (°C)
Acid-base	7.4	7.35–7.45	pH

Cells are the smallest independent units of living matter and there are millions in the body. They are too small to be seen with the naked eyes, but can be seen under the microscope; different types with their sizes and shapes.

Cells are surrounded by the ***cell membrane***, which due to its structural properties is semipermeable, i.e. provides a selective barrier to substances entering or leaving. It prevents movement of large molecules, e.g. protein molecules between the cell and the interstitial fluid. Small particles can usually pass through the membranes, some more readily than others; the **ionic permeability** is regulated by the presence of *channels in the membrane*, some specific for the ions; which may open or close depending upon certain *voltage* or *hormonal factors*; and therefore the chemical composition of the fluid inside is different from that outside the cell (Fig. 1.2).

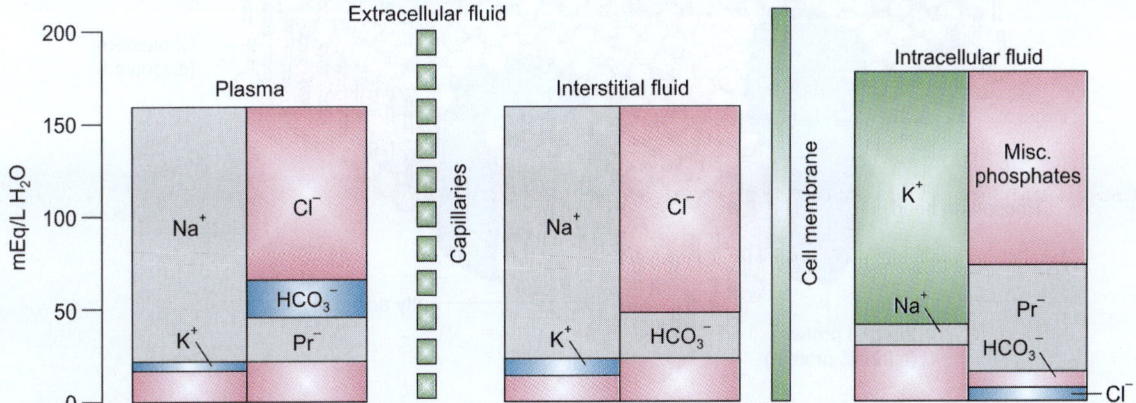

Fig. 1.2: Electrolyte composition of human body fluids. The values are in mEq/L of water, Proteins almost absent in interstitial fluid

CELL STRUCTURE AND ORGANELLES

Cells are the smallest functional unit of the body. They are grouped together to form tissues. Specialization of cells in various organs is very great and so no cell is typical of all the cells in the body. But a number of structures, the organelles are common to most cells.

A cell consists of plasma membrane inside which there are a number of organelles floating in a watery fluid called cytosol or cytoplasm.

The plasma membrane

Proteins and phospholipids are the most abundant constituents of cellular membranes. A phospholipid molecule has a polar head group; contains phosphate portion relatively soluble in water (hydrophilic, polar) and two nonpolar hydrophobic fatty acyl chains.

In the plasma membrane phospholipids form bilayer in which the hydrophilic heads are aligned on the outer surfaces of the membrane and hydrophobic tails form a central water-repelling layer (Fig. 1.3).

The protein molecules are embedded in these lipid layers. Some of the protein molecules are attached to the outside or inside of the membrane; others extend all the way through the membrane, and many of these provide channels that allow the passage of electrolytes and nonlipid soluble substances.

The proteins in the membrane serve several functions as:

- Enzymes
- Receptors for hormones and other chemical messengers
- Cell adhesion molecules that attach cells to adjacent ones or to basal laminas
- Pumps that actively transport ions across the membrane
- Carriers facilitating diffusion of certain substances
- Ion channels

Carbohydrate molecules attached to the outside of some membrane protein molecules give the immunological identity (distinguish self from nonself), i.e. function as antigens; even receptors.

Cholesterol is a major component of plasma membranes present in the nonpolar region.

Organelles are small structures with highly specialized functions, many of which are contained within a membrane or are formed of membrane. They include the nucleus, mitochondria, ribosomes, endoplasmic reticulum, Golgi apparatus, lysosomes, microfilaments and microtubules (Fig. 1.4).

MITOCHONDRIA

Each mitochondrion is a sausage shaped structure (Fig. 1.4). It is made-up of outer membrane and inner membrane, each membrane is lipid bilayer. The inner membrane is folded to form shelves. The mitochondria are the power generating units of the cell (called "**power house**" of the cell) and are most plentiful where energy requiring processes take place.

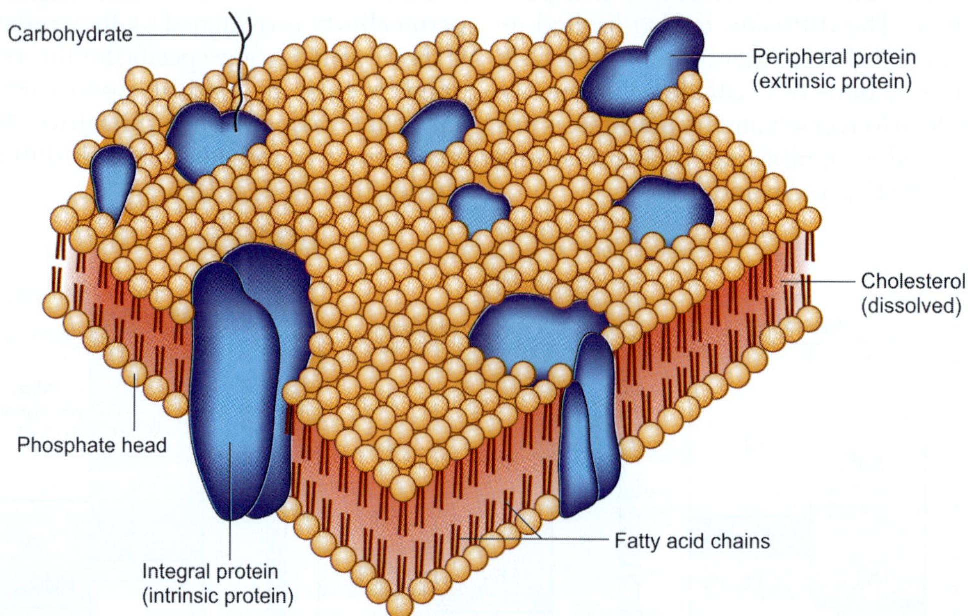

Fig. 1.3: Biologic membrane. The phospholipid molecules have two fatty acid chains attached to a phosphate head (open circle). Proteins are integral proteins, which extend through the membrane, but peripheral proteins are attached to the inside (not shown) and outside of the membrane, are shown as colored globules

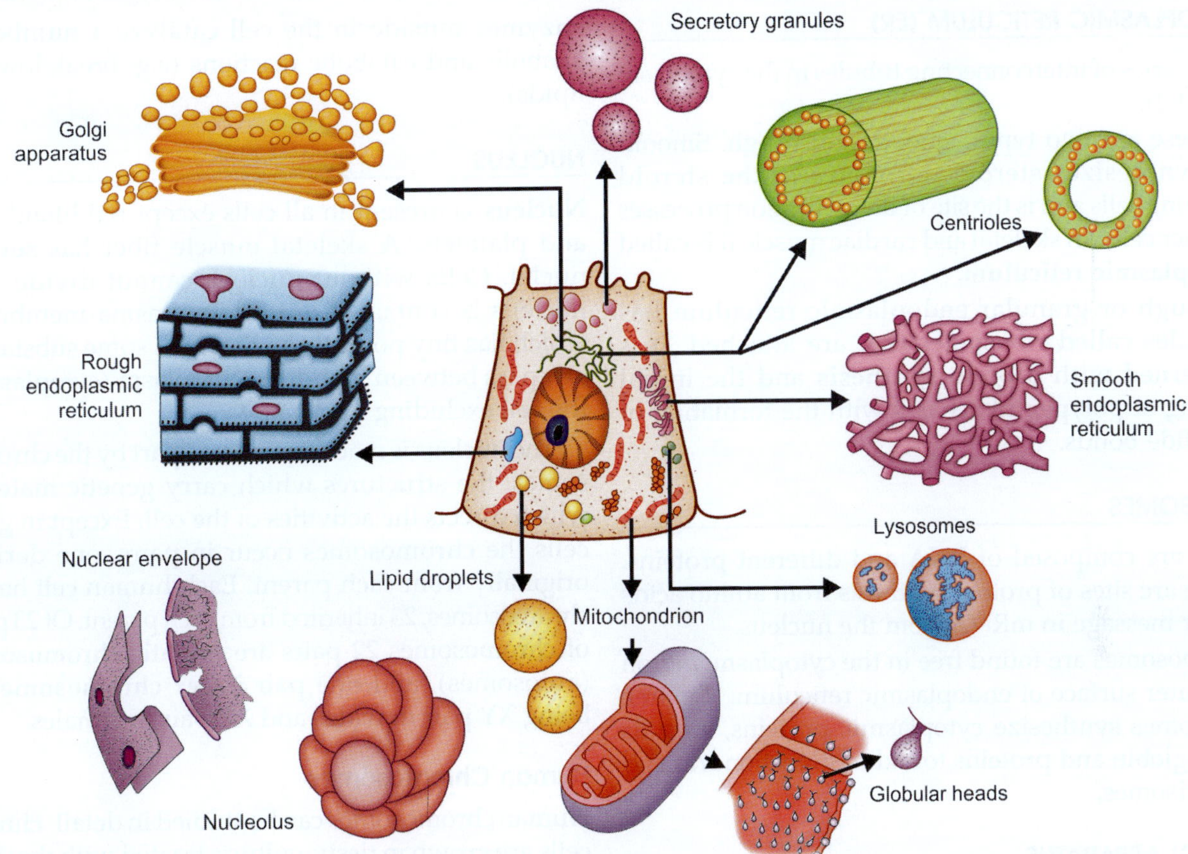

Fig. 1.4: Diagram showing a hypothetical cell in the center, as seen with the light microscope. Various organelles of the cell are shown

The outer membrane of the mitochondrion is studded with enzymes concerned with biological oxidations, providing raw materials for the reactions occurring inside the mitochondrion. In the interior, enzymes that convert the product of carbohydrate, protein, and fat metabolism to CO_2 and water are located on the inner membrane. **The coupling of oxidation with the formation of ATP in the mitochondria is called oxidative phosphorylation.**

The substances from which cells extract energy are oxygen with one or more food stuffs: carbohydrates, fats or proteins. In the human body all the carbohydrates are converted into glucose before they reach the cell metabolism, the proteins are converted into amino acids and the fats are converted into fatty acids.

Inside the cell these food stuffs react chemically with enzymes, forming CO_2 and water, the liberated energy is used to synthesize a high energy substance called adenosine triphosphate (ATP) (For details refer to chapter on metabolism).

Almost all these **oxidative** reactions occur inside the mitochondria and the energy released is used to form mainly ATP. Then the ATP is transported out of the mitochondrion to release its energy whenever needed for cellular reactions.

ATP and not the original foodstuffs themselves are used throughout the cell to energize almost all the intracellular reactions.

Without mitochondria the cell would be unable to extract significant amount of energy from nutrients and oxygen and all cellular functions would cease.

Mitochondria contain own DNA similar to that found in nucleus although less DNA. Sperms contribute no mitochondria to the zygote, mitochondria come from the ovum and inheritance is maternal. 99% of proteins in mitochodria are products of nuclear DNA yet mitochondial DNA is responsible for necessary components of oxidative phosphorylation.

There is no effective DNA repair system in the mitochondria and mutation rate for mitochondrial DNA is over ten times the rate of nuclear DNA. A large number of relatively rare diseases have been traced to mutations in mitochondrial DNA. These include disorders of tissues with high metabolic rate in which energy production is defective as a result of abnormalities in the production of ATP.

ENDOPLASMIC RETICULUM (ER)

It is a series of interconnecting tubules in the cytoplasm (Fig. 1.4).

These are two types: smooth and rough. Smooth ER synthesizes steroid hormones in the steroid secreting cells and is the site of detoxification processes in other cells. In skeletal and cardiac muscle it is called **sarcoplasmic reticulum.**

Rough or granular endoplasmic reticulum has granules called ribosomes that are attached. It is concerned with **protein synthesis** and the initial folding of polypeptide chains with the formation of disulfide bonds.

RIBOSOMES

They are composed of RNA and different proteins. These are sites of protein synthesis from amino acids as per message in mRNA from the nucleus.

Ribosomes are found free in the cytoplasm and on the outer surface of endoplasmic reticulum. The free ribosomes synthesize cytoplasmic proteins, such as hemoglobin and proteins found in mitochondria and peroxisomes.

GOLGI APPARATUS

It (Fig. 1.4) is present in all cells. It is involved in processing proteins formed in the ribosome into secretory granules, vesicles and endosomes. In the protein synthesis and secretion, the proteins move from the endoplasmic reticulum to the Golgi apparatus where they are packed into membrane bound vesicles called secretory granules.

The vesicles are stored and when needed move to the plasma membrane through which proteins are extruded.

LYSOSOMES

They (Fig. 1.4) are one type of secretory vesicles formed by the Golgi apparatus. They contain enzymes involved in breakdown of frameworks of organelles and large molecules (e.g. RNA, DNA, carbohydrates, proteins) inside the cell into smaller particles that are recycled or extruded from the cells. Lysosomes in WBC contain enzymes that digest bacteria.

PEROXISOMES

Surrounded by a membrane and contain enzymes producing H_2O_2 (oxidases) or its breakdown (catalases). Membrane contains specific proteins with which substances move in or out into the cell. The matrix contains enzymes that in conjunction with enzymes outside in the cell catalyze a number of anabolic and catabolic reactions (e.g. breakdown of lipids).

NUCLEUS

Nucleus is present in all cells except red blood cells and platelets. A skeletal muscle fiber has several nuclei. Cells without nucleus cannot divide. The nucleus is contained within its plasma membrane, which has tiny pores through which some substances can pass between it and the cytoplasm (cytoplasm is the cell excluding nucleus).

The nucleus is made-up in large part by the chromosomes, the structures which carry genetic material, which directs the activities of the cell. Except in germ cells the chromosomes occur in pairs, one derived originally from each parent. Each human cell has 46 chromosomes, 23 inherited from each parent. Of 23 pairs of chromosomes 22 pairs are **somatic chromosomes** (autosomes), and one pair is **sex chromosomes**, it being XY pair in males and XX pair in females.

Human Chromosomes

Human chromosomes can be studied in detail. Human cells are grown in tissue culture; treated with the drug which arrests mitosis at the metaphase. Staining techniques make it possible to identify the individual chromosome (Fig. 1.5). The individual autosome pairs are identified by the numbers 1–22 on the basis of their morphological characteristics.

Each chromosome is made-up of a giant molecule of deoxyribonucleic acid (DNA) and proteins called histone. DNA is coiled around a core of histone proteins to form a nucleosome (Fig. 1.6). The structure of chromosome is linked to a string of beads. The beads are nucleosomes and string is linker DNA, together they form chromatin. DNA the component of the chromosomes carries the genetic message; the blue print for all the heritable characteristics of the cell and its descendents.

The nucleus of the cell contains nucleolus (Fig. 1.4), a patch work of granules rich in ribonucleic acid. In growing cells they are more numerous. They are the sites of synthesis of ribosomes, the structures in the cytoplasm in which proteins are synthesized.

Messenger RNA

The genetic message is transferred from DNA in the nucleus to the ribosomes (the sites of protein synthesis) in the cytoplasm by mRNA, a single stranded structure. The proteins formed from DNA blue print

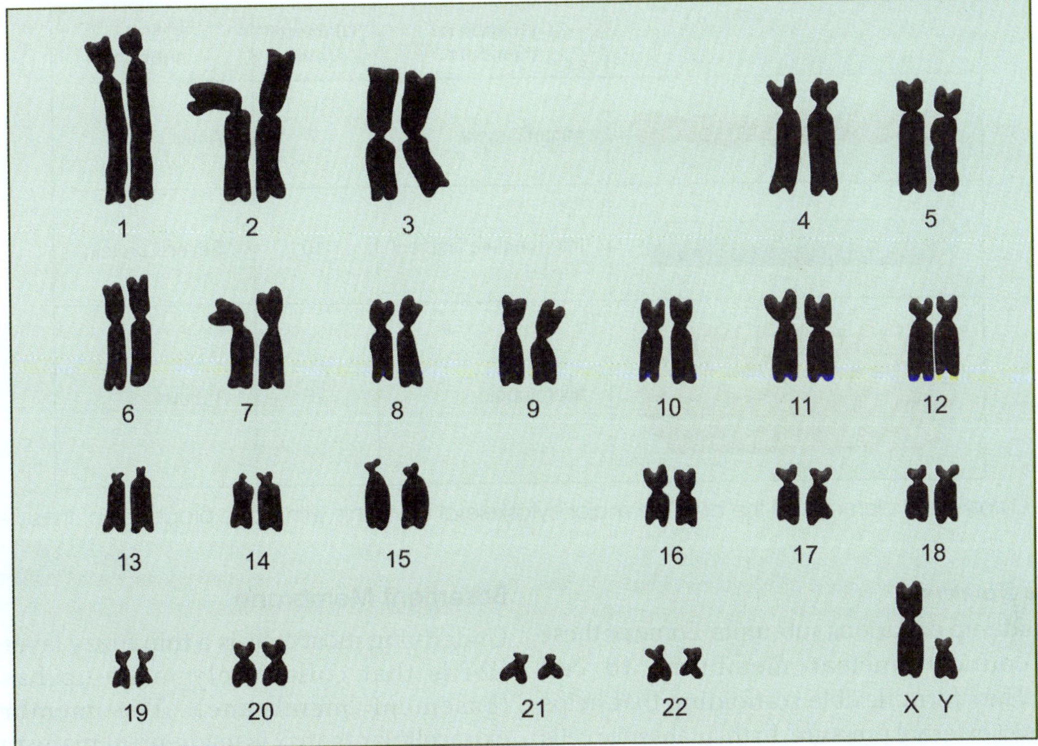

Fig. 1.5: Karyotype of chromosomes from a normal male. The chromosomes have been stained

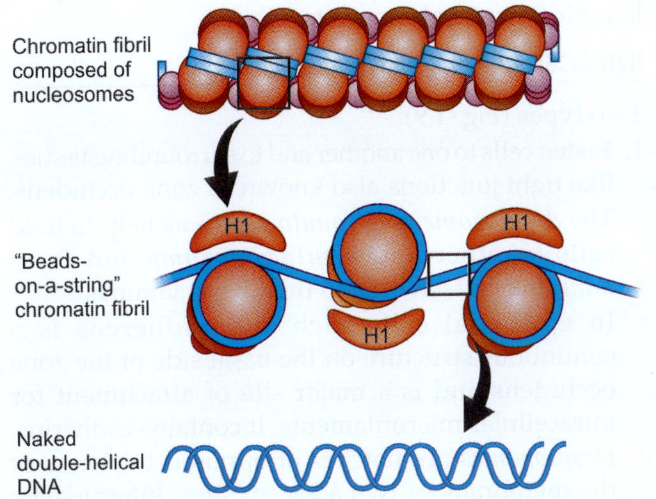

Fig. 1.6: Structure of a part of chromosome. H-Histone

include all the enzymes which in turn control the metabolism of the cell.

CYTOSKELETON

All cells have a cytoskeleton (Fig. 1.7) made-up of microtubules, intermediate filaments and microfilaments along with proteins that anchor them and tie them together.

These maintain the structure of the cell; permit changes in shape and movement.

Microfilaments

Are tiny strands of protein **actin** that provide *structural support* and *maintain the shape of the cell*. Also in the muscle cell filaments are organized into special contractile machinery that is the basis of *muscle contraction*. They are made-up of actin, the protein that by its interaction with myosin brings about contraction of muscle.

Microfilaments in the enterocytes in intestinal villi reach to the tip of microvilli on the epithelial cells of the intestinal mucosa. They are also abundant in the lamellipodia that cell put out when they crawl along surfaces. The actin filaments interact with integrin receptors and form **focal adhesion complexes** which serve as points of traction with surface over which the cells pulls itself.

Microtubules

These are protein structures in the cytoplasm which form tract for *transport of organelles* within the cell, they also *form spindle* which moves chromosomes in mitosis. Microtubules can transport in both directions. They are dynamic portion of cell skeleton; assembly and dissembly talking place. The **centrioles** (Fig. 1.4) and **mitotic spindle** of the mitosing cell are both composed of stiff microtubules.

	Cytoskeletal filaments	Diameter (nm)	Protein subunit
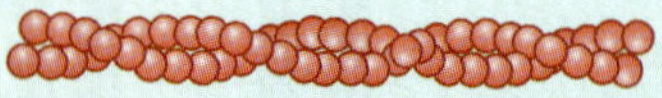	Microfilament	7	Actin
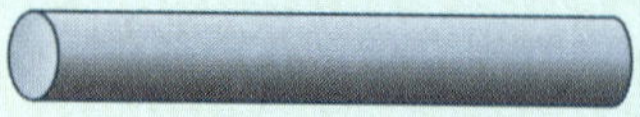	Intermediate filament	10	Several protein
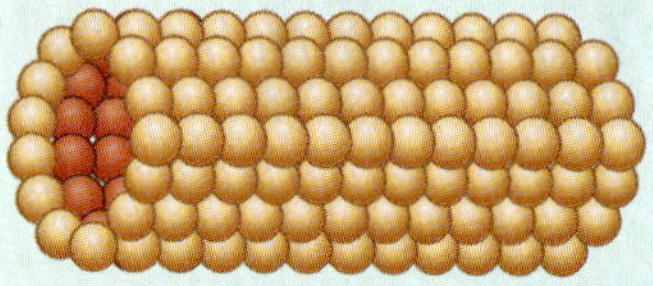	Microtubule	25	Tubulin

Fig. 1.7: Cytoskeletal elements of the cell. The major cytoskeletal elements with basic properties of these elements

Intermediate filaments:

These are made-up of various sub-units. Some of these filaments connect nuclear membrane to cell membrane. They form flexible scaffolding that helps the cell to resist external pressure. In their absence cells rapture easily.

When they are abnormal cell blistering is common. Proteins of intermediate filaments are cell type specific, e.g. vimentin is major protein in fibroblasts; cytokeratin is present in epithelial cells.

MOLECULAR MOTORS

The molecular motors *move proteins, organelles* and other *cells parts* (called cargo) to all parts of the cell; attach to **cargo** at one end of molecule and to *microtubules or actin polymers at the other end* (called the **head**). They convert the *energy of ATP* into movement along the cytoskeleton and take cargo along them (Fig. 1.8). There are three super families; **kinesin, dynein** and **myosin.**

CILIA

Cilia are specialized cellular projections used by multicellular organisms to propell mucus and other substances over surface of epithelial cells. Cilia are functionally indistinct from flagella of sperm cells.

Within the cilium there is axoneme containing arrangement of microtubules. Along this cytoskeleton there is axonal dynein and coordinated movements of these two are responsible ciliary and sperm movement.

Basement Membrane

Underlying most cells is a thin fuzzy layer with some fibrils that collectively make-up basal lamina (basement membrane). The membrane with extracellular matrix is made-up of many proteins that hold cells together, regulate their development and determine their growth. These include collagens, laminins, proteoglycans, etc.

INTERCELLULAR CONNECTIONS

Two types (Fig. 1.9):

1. **Fasten cells** to one another and to surrounding tissues, like tight junctions also known as zona occludens. The ***desmosome*** and ***zonula adherens*** help to hold cells together and ***hemidesmosome*** and ***focal adhesions*** attach cells to their basal laminas.

   In epithelial cells each zona adherens is a continuous structure on the basal side of the zona occludens and is a major site of attachment for intracellular microfilaments. It contains cadherins.

   Desmosomes are patches of opposed thickness of the membrane of two adjacent sites. Intermediate filaments are attached. Between the two membrane thickening the space contains filamentous material that includes cadherins and extracellular portions of other transmembrane proteins.

   Hemidesmosomes are half desmosomes that attach cells to the basal lamina and are connected to intracellular intermediate filaments. But, they contain integrins rather that cadherins.

   Focal adhesions also attach cells to their basal laminas, they are labile structures associated with actin filaments inside the cell and are involved in cell movement.

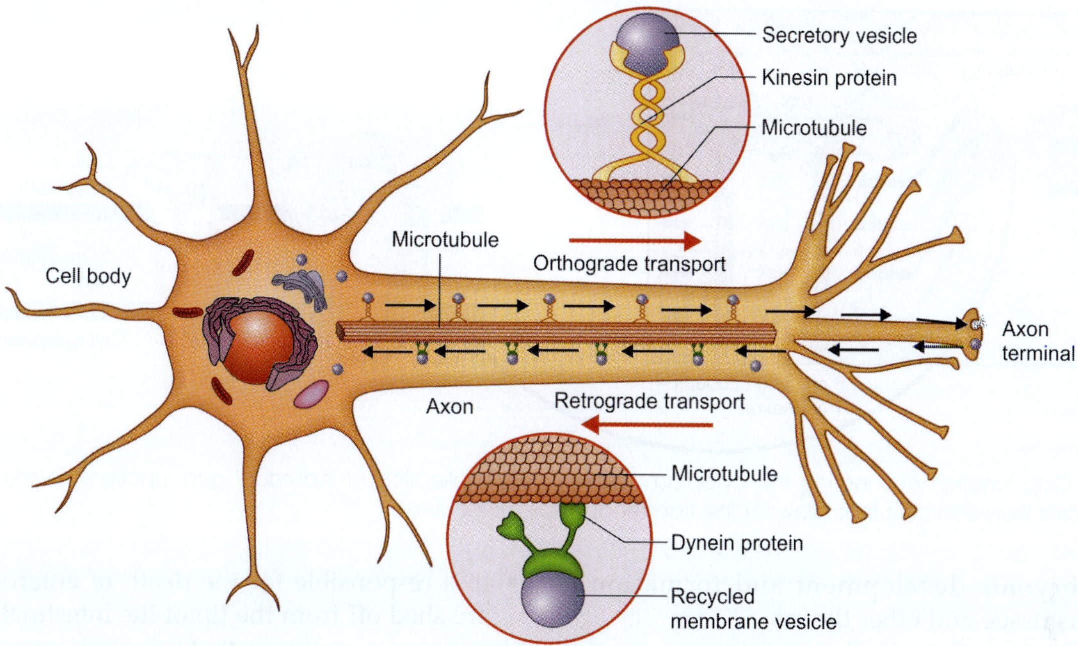

Fig. 1.8: Axonal transport along microtubules by dynein and kinesin: Fast (400 mm/day) and slow (0.5–10 mm/day) axonal transport occurs along microtubules that run along the length of the axon from the cell body to the terminal. Retrograde transport (200 mm/day) occurs from the terminal to the cell body

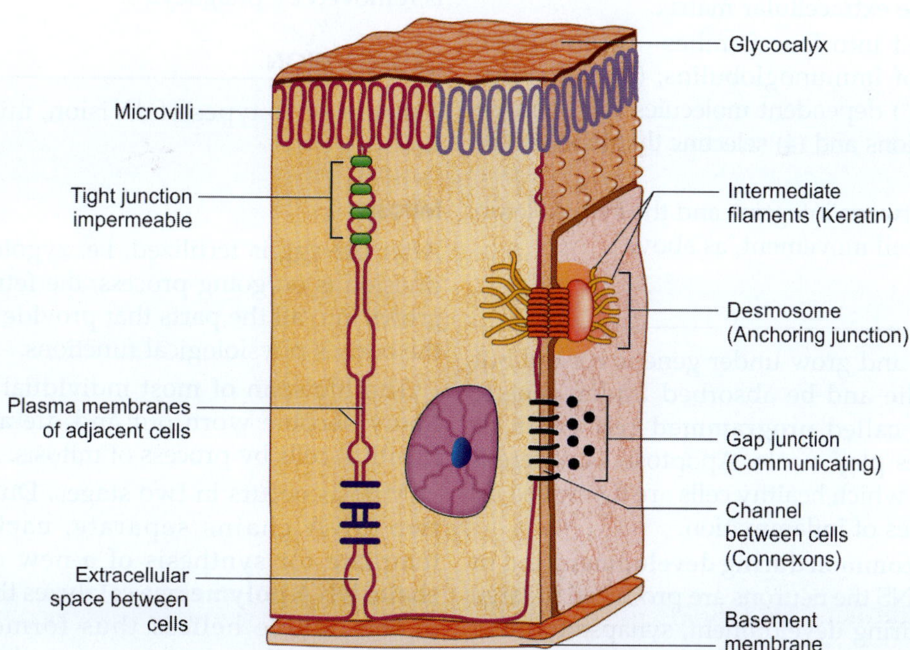

Fig. 1.9: Intercellular connections

2. **Gap junctions:** Form a cytoplasmic tunnel for diffusion of ions or small molecules between two neighboring cells (Fig. 1.10). Junctions permit transfer of ions or molecules from cell to cell without entering extracellular space.

CELL ADHESION MOLECULES (CAMS)

Cells are attached to basal lamina and to each other by CAM which are parts of intercellular connections. These have unique *signaling functions*. They are found to be important:

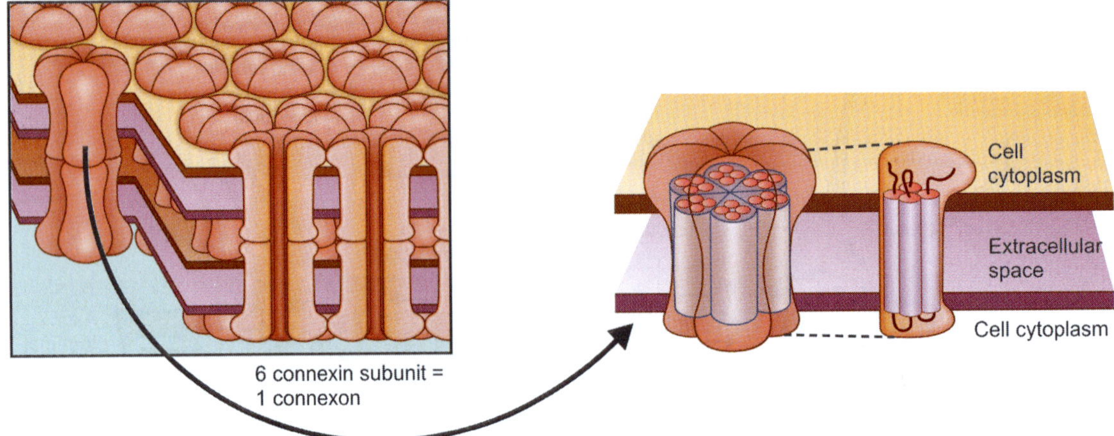

Fig. 1.10: Gap junction connecting the cytoplasm of two cells: Collection of individual gap junctions, is shown to form multiple pores between cells that allow for the transfer of small molecules

- in embryonic development and formation of nervous tissue and other tissues
- in holding together of cells in adults
- in inflammation and wound healing
- in metastasis of tumors

Many pass through the cell membrane and are attached to the cytoskeleton inside the cell. Many bind to laminins in the extracellular matrix.

CAMs divided into four families—(1) integrins; (2) IgG family of immunoglobulins; (3) cadherins, calcium ion (Ca^{2+}) dependent molecules that mediate cell to cell adhesions and (4) selectins that bind carbohydrates.

Interaction between integrins and the cytoskeleton are involved in cell movement, as above.

APOPTOSIS

The cells divide and grow under genetic control but cells can also die and be absorbed under genetic control. This is called **programmed cell death** or **apoptosis.** Genes play a role. Apoptosis is different from necrosis in which healthy cells are destroyed by external processes of inflammation.

Apoptosis is common during development and in adulthood: In CNS the neurons are produced in large numbers and during development, synapse forming and remodelling the neurons die also:

- Apoptosis gets rid of inappropriate clones of immunocytes in the immune system.
- In adulthood apoptosis is the processes that leads to cyclic breakdown of the menstruational endometrium.
- The epithelial cells that lose their connections with the basal lamina or neighboring cells undergo apoptosis.
- It is responsible for the death of enterocytes that are shed off from the tip of the intestinal mucosa.

A common pathway that brings about apoptosis is activation of a group of cysteine proteases (capases), which exist in cells in inactive state and get activated to cause fragmentation of DNA, cytoplasmic and chromatin condensation. The cell breaks up and debris is removed by phagocytes.

CELL DIVISION

There are two types of division, mitosis and meiosis.

Mitosis

After the egg is fertilized, i.e. zygote is formed; cell division is on going process; the fetus develops and grows into all the parts that provide the sum total of the body's physiological functions.

The life span of most individual cells is limited. Many become worn out and die and replaced by identical cells by process of mitosis.

Mitosis occurs in two stages. During mitosis the two DNA chains separate, each serving as a template for synthesis of a new complementary chain. **DNA polymerase** catalyzes this reaction. One of the double helices thus formed goes to one daughter cell and one goes to the other, so that amount of DNA in each daughter cell is the same as in the parent cell.

Chromosomes duplicate themselves and divide in such a way that each daughter cell receives a full complement of chromosomes.

When the cell **splits into two cells** the process is called **mitosis.**

Cell cycle

Initiation of mitosis and normal cell division depends on the orderly occurrence of events called cell cycle.

The stages in the **cell cycle** (Fig. 1.11) are described as:

Interphase interval between mitosis.

The interphase itself has three phases—(1) the first growth phase; (2) synthesis phase and (3) the second growth phase.

1. **First growth phase (G_1):** RNA and proteins are synthesised, the volume of cytoplasm increases. Mitochondria divide. In late G_1 phase, cells must follow one of the two paths. They may either withdraw from the cell cycle and enter a resting phase (R or G_0) or start preparing for the next division by entering the next synthesis phase (S).
2. **Synthesis phase (S):** DNA is synthesised, the chromosomes are duplicated.
3. **Second growth phase (G_2):** This is a shorter growth phase, in which RNA and proteins necessary for cell division continue to be synthesised. Now the cell is ready to start cell division, i.e. mitosis.

The first event takes place in the cytoplasm, occurring during later part of interphase in or around small structures called centrioles. Two pair of centrioles begin to move apart from each other, the mitotic tubules growing between them and pushing them part, at the same time tubules grow radially away from each of the centriole pairs forming a spiny star called the **aster**, in each end of the cell.

The complex of microtubules is called spindle. The mitotic spindle and two pairs of centrioles together are called **mitotic apparatus.**

The stages in mitosis (Fig. 1.12) *are described as:*

Prophase: While the spindle is forming, chromosomes of the nucleus which in interphase consist of loosely coiled strand become condensed into well defined chromosomes.

Prometaphase: The nuclear envelope fragments.

Metaphase: The two asters of mitotic apparatus are pushed further apart by further growth of mitotic spindle and chromatids are pulled to the center of the cell.

Anaphase: The two chromatids of each chromosome are pulled apart.

Telophase: The two sets of chromosomes are pulled completely apart, mitotic apparatus disappears and a new membrane appears around each set of chromosomes. The cell divides into two cells midway between two nuclei.

When DNA is damaged entry into mitosis is inhibited, giving the cell time to repair the DNA; failure to repair could leads to cancer.

The cell cycle is regulated by proteins called **cyclins** and cyclin dependent *protein kinases*. The different cells in the body have life cycle periods that vary from short periods for stimulated bone marrow cells to an entire life time of the human body for nerve and striated muscle cells. Certain cells grow rapidly all the time, the cells of the bone marrow that form blood cells, the cells of the germinal layer of the skin and the intestinal epithelium. On the other hand smooth muscle cells may not reproduce for years. Neurons and most striated muscle cells do not reproduce during the entire life cycle of the individual. In some tissues insufficiency of some types of cells causes them to grow very rapidly until appropriate numbers are again available, e.g. if large part of liver is removed surgically the cells divide until the cell mass again returns to normal.

The **genes** and their **regulatory mechanisms** determine the growth characteristics of the cells and whether these cells divide to form new cells. In this

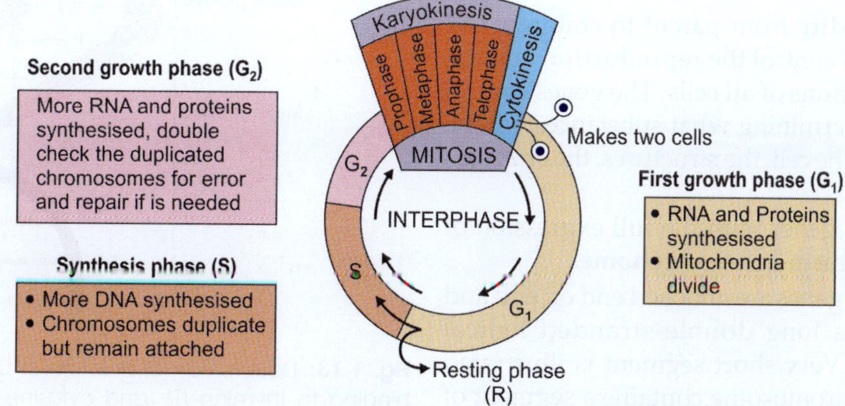

Fig. 1.11: Cell cycle

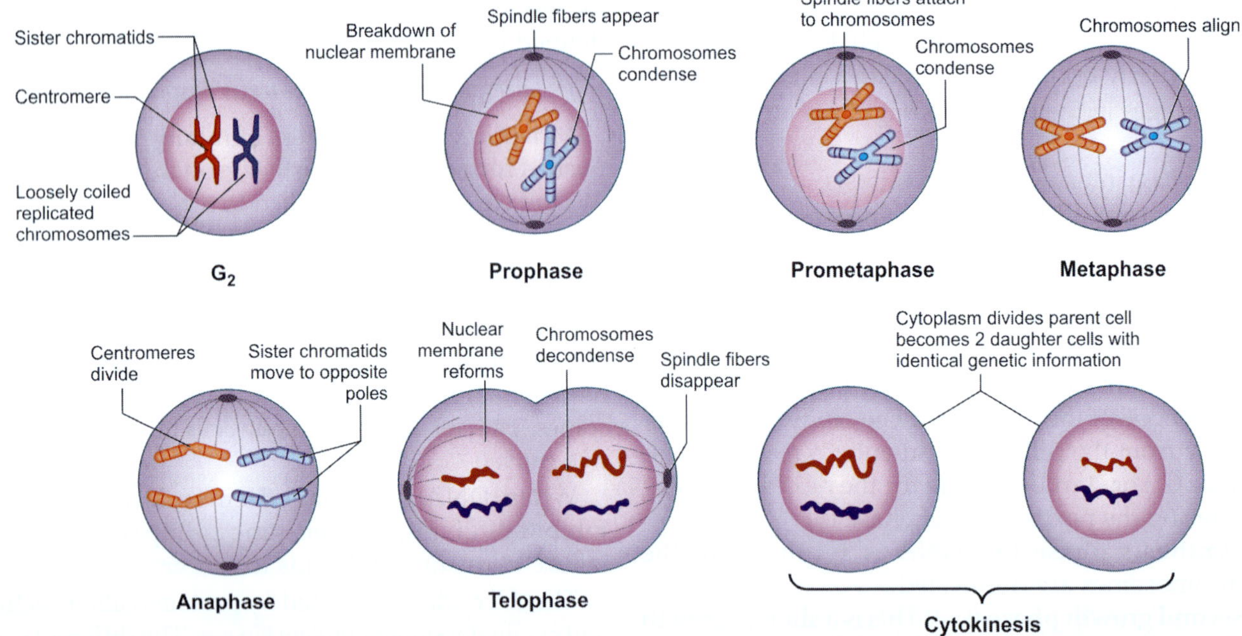

Fig. 1.12: Stages in the reproduction of the cell prophase, prometaphase, metaphase, anaphase, telophase and cytokinesis

way the genetic system controls each stage in the development of human beings from the single cell fertilized ovum to whole functioning body.

Telomeres

Cell replication involves not only DNA polymerase but a special reverse transcriptase that synthesises the short repeats of DNA that are the ends (telomeres) of chromosomes. Without the transcriptase and related enzymes called telomerase, somatic cells lose DNA as they divide for 40–60 times and then become old and undergo apoptosis. On the contrary with high activity of these, the cells keep multiplying indefinitely. This fact is of interest in aging and cancer.

THE GENES

Genes control **heredity** from parent to children, but also the same genes control the **reproduction** and are for **day to day functions** of all cells. The genes control cell function by determining what substances will be synthesised within the cell, the structures, the enzymes and the chemicals.

The collection of genes with the full expression of DNA from an organism is called **genome.**

Large number of genes are attached end on end and are contained in a long double-stranded helical molecule of DNA. Very short segment is illustrated in Fig. 1.13. Each chromosome contains a segment of the DNA double helix which is made-up of two extremely long nucleotide chains containing the bases adenine (A), guanine (G), thymine (T) and cytosine (C). The two chains are bond together by hydrogen binding between bases, with adenine binding to thymine, and guanine to cystosine.

Each Gene is a nucleic acid and is called deoxyribonucleic acid (DNA) that controls automatically the formation of another nucleic acid (RNA) which spreads throughout the cell cytoplasm and controls formation of specific proteins. Some proteins are structural proteins, which are in association with various lipids and carbohydrates for the structure, majority are enzymes that catalyze different chemical reactions in the cells.

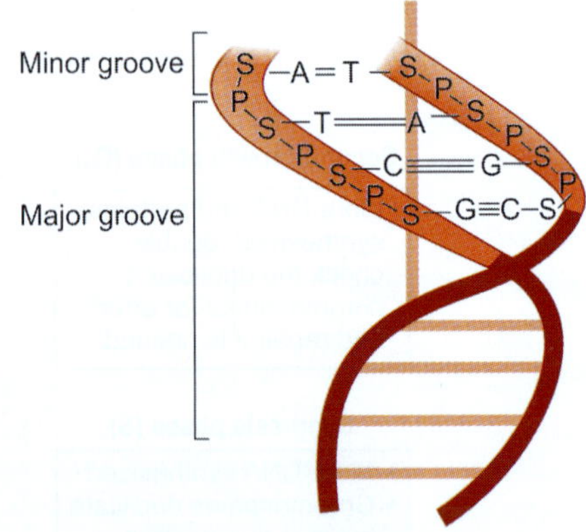

Fig. 1.13: Double-helical structure of DNA, with adenine (A), binding to thymine (T), and cytosine (C), to guanine (G), Phosphoric acid (P), Sugar (S)

For the formation of each of cellular protein there is usually a single gene ***pair*** in each cell.

A gene is used to define, as the amount of information necessary to specify a single protein molecule. But proteins encoded by a single gene may be subsequently divided into several different physiologically active proteins. Each cell contains the total complement of genes required to synthesis all the proteins in the body but the cells in different tissues synthesise only the enzymes required for their function using only a part of genetic code.

The first stage in the formation of DNA is combination of one molecule of phosphoric acid, one molecule of deoxyribose and one of the four bases to form nucleotide. Four separate nucleolides are thus formed, one for each of the four bases, adenine, guanine, cystosine, thymine.

A number of nucleotides are bound together to form DNA. These are combined in such a way that the bases are bound together by very loose hydrogen bonding.

THE GENETIC CODE

The importance of DNA lies in its ability to control the formation of other substances in the cell. When the two strands of DNA are split apart, this exposes the purine and pyrimidine bases projecting to the side of each strand. It is those projecting bases that form the code.

The genetic code consists of successive **triplets of bases,** i.e. each three successive bases is a code word. The successive triplets control the sequence of amino acids in a protein.

Each **DNA strand** in each chromosome is a large molecule that carries code for **numerous genes**. The protein coding genes **(exons)** make-up only 3% of human genome, the remaining is made-up of introns and other DNA; this 97% is called **junk DNA.** A characteristic of human DNA is its structural variability from one individual to another. Most of the variations occur in the noncoding regions, but they can also occur in the coding regions.

DNA fingerprinting is of value in investigating crimes and determining paternity, but reliable techniques must be used.

RNA AND THE PROCESS OF TRANSCRIPTION

The chemical reactions in the cytoplasm are controlled by mRNA the formation of which is controlled by DNA of the nucleus. mRNA diffuses from the nuclear pores into the cytoplasm to control protein synthesis. RNA strand is single strand unlike DNA.

During synthesis of mRNA itself, two strands of DNA molecule separate temporarily, one of these strands is then used as template for synthesis of mRNA, the code triplets (called **codons**) in the mRNA. The same substances are used for formation of mRNA as those for DNA except that sugar deoxyribose is replaced by ribose in the formation of RNA. The same bases are used except for thymine in DNA which is replaced by uracil in mRNA. These codons in turn control the sequence of amino acids in a protein to be synthesised in the cytoplasm. The process of formation of mRNA from DNA is called **transcription** (Fig. 1.14).

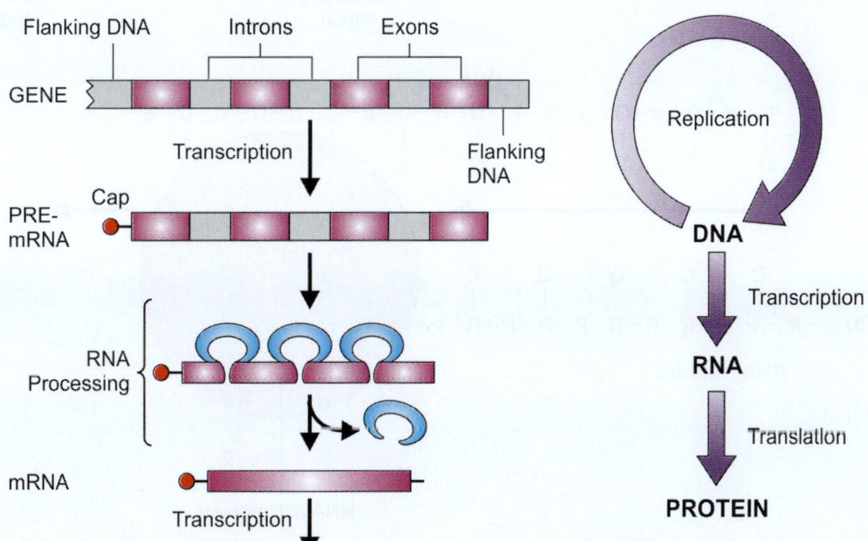

Fig. 1.14: Formation of mRNA from DNA

The formation of mRNA molecule is under the influence of RNA polymerase. In the DNA strand immediately ahead of the initial gene there is a sequence of nucleotides called the promoter. The RNA polymerase attaches to the **promoter** and causes unwinding of about two turns of the DNA helix and separation of the two unwound portion of the strands, this continues successively. Code triplets in DNA cause formation of complementary code triplets the **codons** in the mRNA (Fig. 1.15B); these codons in turn control the sequence of amino acids in the protein to be synthesised later in the cytoplasm.

Types of RNA

There are also other types of RNA. There are three separate types of RNA, each of which plays a role in protein formation. These are:

- *Messenger RNA,* which carries genetic code from DNA to the cytoplasm for controlling the formation of proteins.
- *Transfer RNA,* in the cytoplasm which transports activated amino acids to the ribosomes to be used in assembling protein molecules.
- *Ribosomal RNA,* which along with other different proteins forms the ribosomes, the structures on which protein molecules are assembled.

The ribosomes are physical structures in the cytoplasm in which protein molecules are synthesised (Fig. 1.4).

The synthesis of enzymes, formed in the ribosomes promote the formation of lipids, glycogen, purines and pyrimidines and many other substances in the cell.

Genetic Regulation

A segment of DNA strand is called **promoter** (Fig. 1.15A). This is a series of nucleotides that has special affinity for RNA polymerase. The polymerase must bind with this promoter before it can travel along DNA strand to synthesise mRNA. Therefore the promoter is the essential element.

Formation of all the enzymes needed for the synthetic process is often controlled by a sequence of genes located in series one after the other on the same chromosomal DNA strand. This area of DNA strand is called an **operon.**

Repressor Operator

In the middle of the promoter is an additional band of nucleotides. This area is called **repressor operator** because a regulatory protein can bind here and prevent attachment of RNA polymerase to the promoter, timely blocking transcription of genes. Such regulatory protein is called **repressor protein.**

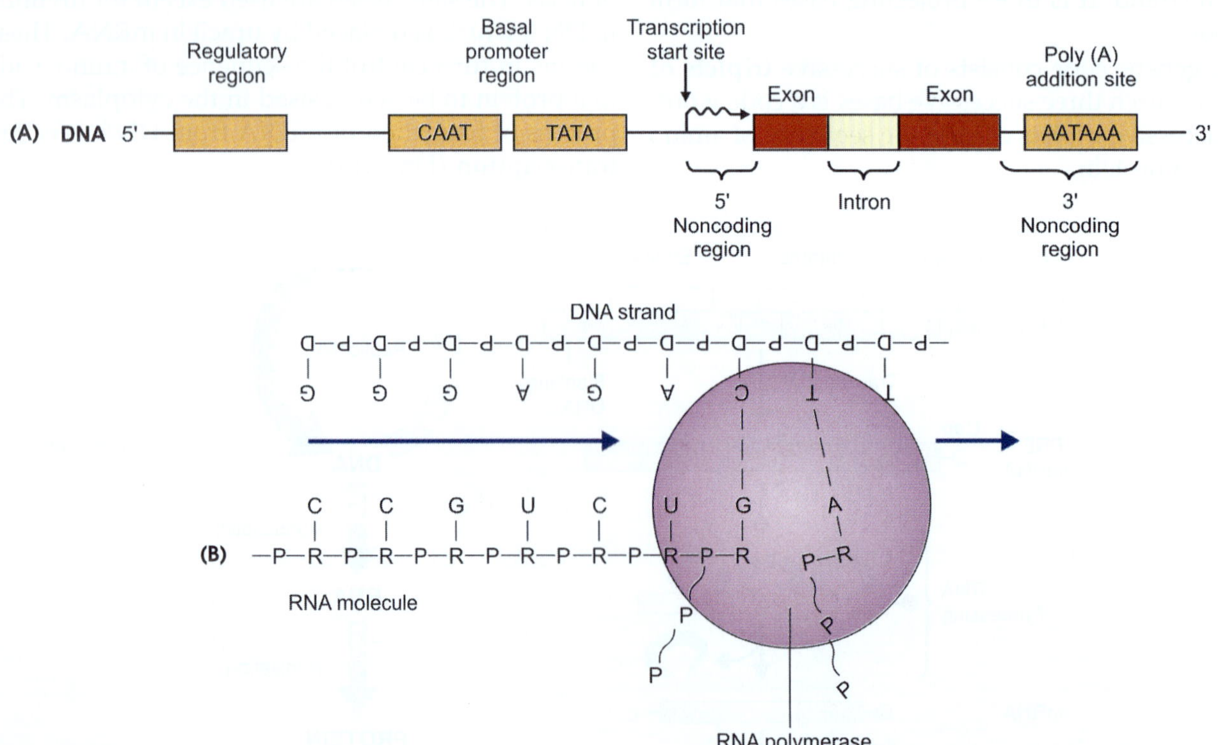

Figs 1.15A and B: (A) A strand of DNA to form a molecule of ribonucleic acid (RNA) that carries the DNA code from the gene to the cytoplasm. (B) The RNA polymerase moves along the DNA strand and builds the RNA molecule

Meiosis

In germ cells reduction division (meiosis) takes place during maturation. The net result is that one of each pair of chromosomes ends up in each mature germ cell; consequently each mature germ cell contains half the amount of chromosomal material found in somatic cells. The chromosomes also undergo recombination which mixes maternal and paternal genes.

Therefore when the sperm unites with an ovum the resulting zygote has the full complement of DNA, half of which is from the father and half from the mother.

Meiosis consists of two cell divisions, during which the number of chromosomes is reduced by half. Meiotic division results in the formation of 4 daughter cells (Fig. 1.16). In males four spermatozoa are functional. In female only one daughter cell, the ovum is functional, remaining three are nonfunctional polar bodies.

Meiosis produces reduction division after two cell divisions called **Meiosis I** and **Meiosis II**. This type of division only occurs in gametes. The stages in each division are the same as in mitosis. The main difference is that during Prophase I the chromosomes arrange into homologous pairs, and at this time maternal and paternal chromosomes swap segments of DNA in the process called crossing over and recombination. In metaphase I centrioles attach spindles to only one of the two in sets of chromosome to be ready to be separated during anaphase I. Hence, at the end of telophase I each of two cells has half the number of chromosomes, but each chromosome consists of a pair of sister chromatids. Meiosis II then in metaphase II and following anaphase II separates out the two sister chromatids. Hence, four gametes with haploid number of chromosomes are formed, i.e. single copy of each chromosome (Figs 1.16A to L).

Mutation

Cells are said to mutate when genetic make-up is altered in anyway. Mutation may occur by X-rays, cosmic rays or other mutagenic agents. Mutation may cause:

- No significant change in cell function
- Physiological abnormality like inborn errors of metabolism
- Cell death

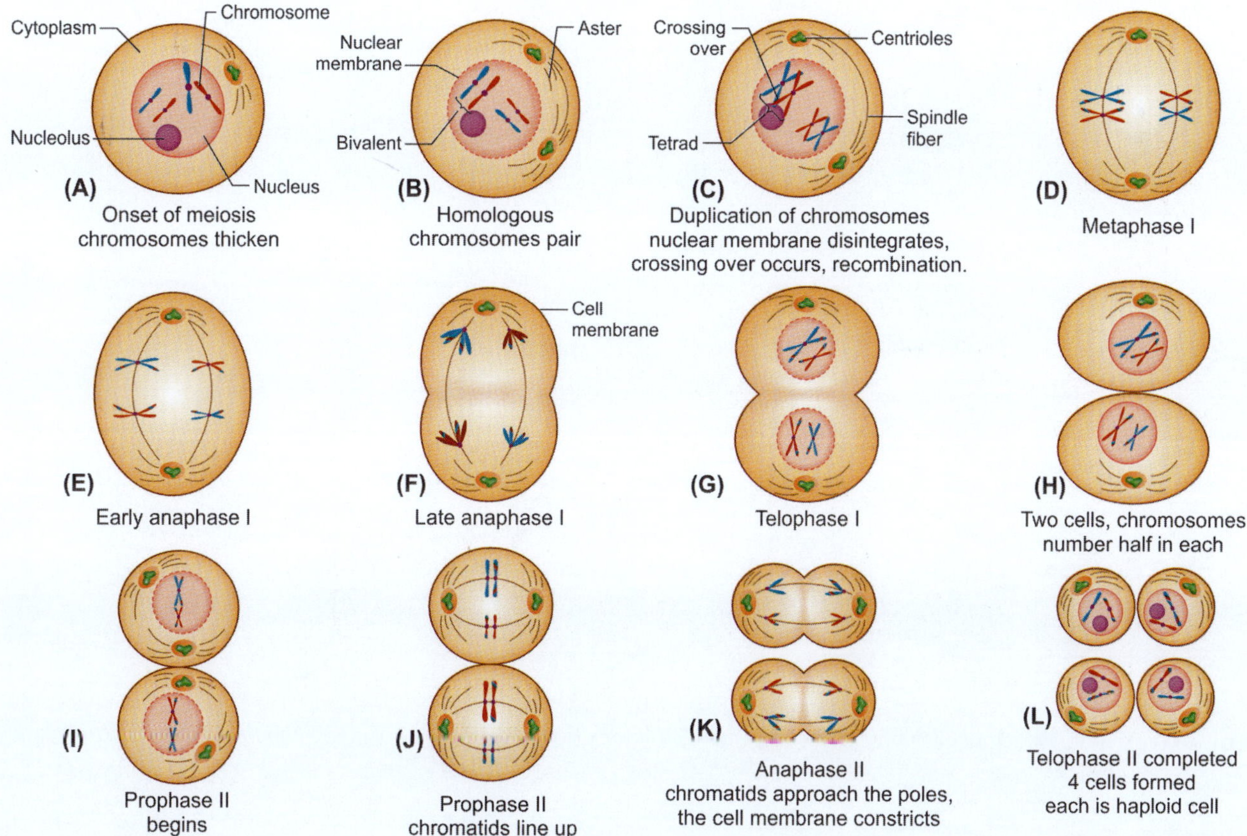

Figs 1.16A to L: Stages in meiosis

Cancer

Cancer is caused by **mutation** or by **abnormal activation** of cellular genes that control cell growth and cell mitosis. The abnormal genes are called **oncogenes.** Only a small fraction of cells that mutate in the body may lead to cancer. The reasons being that mutated cells have less survival capacity than normal cells and so die; secondly the cells that do survive lose the normal feedback control that prevents excessive growth; and third factor is that those cells that are potentially cancerous are often destroyed by body's immune system.

Yet the probability of mutation is increased many fold when a person is exposed to certain chemical, physical or biological factors (e.g. viruses). **Ionizing radiations**, like **X-rays**, gamma rays and radiations from **radioactive** substances and even **ultraviolet** light can predispose to cancer.

A disregulation of the cell cycle components may lead to tumor formation. When some genes like cell cycle inhibitors, RB, p53 mutate they may cause the cell to multiply uncontrollably, forming tumor. In cancer therapy the cells that are actively undergoing cell cycle are targeted. DNA is exposed during cell division and hence susceptible to damage by drugs or radiation. Radiation or chemotherapy kills the cells that have newly entered the cell cycle. In general cells are most sensitive in late M and G_2 phases and most resistant in late S.

The pattern of resistance and sensitively correlates with level of sulfhydryl compounds in the cells, these protect the cells from radiation and tend to be highest in S and lowest in mitosis.

IMPLICATIONS AND APPLICATIONS

- Understand that all body organs contribute to homeostasis. Disease affecting function of anyone of body organs affect the internal environment of the cells that leads to disturbed function of the cells, usually resulting in disease.
- Understand that mitosis is a form of cell division that produces two daughter cells with same genetic material as parent cell.
- Meiosis produces gametes which are haploid cells with a single copy of each chromosome and during the process crossover of genetic material between chromosome pairs takes place.

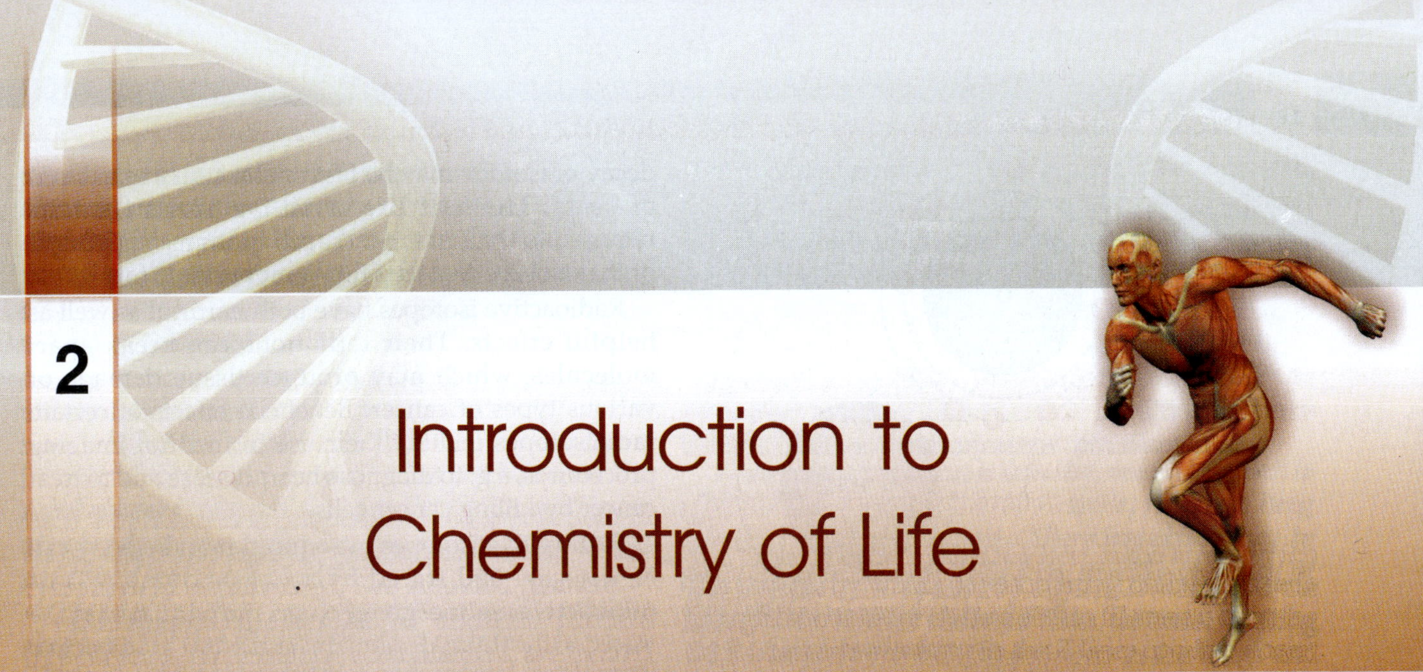

2 Introduction to Chemistry of Life

The atom is the smallest particle of an element which can exist as a stable unit. An element is a chemical substance whose atoms are all of the same type, e.g. sodium contains only sodium atoms; compounds contain more than one type of atom; e.g. water is a compound containing both hydrogen and oxygen atoms.

There are 92 naturally occurring elements. Body is made-up mainly of four elements; carbon, hydrogen, oxygen and nitrogen and small amounts of mineral salts.

ATOMIC STRUCTURE

Atoms are made-up of three main types of particles; protons, neutrons and electrons:

- Protons are particles in the central part, called the nucleus of the atom. Each proton has one unit positive electrical charge and one atomic mass unit.
- Neutrons are also found in the nucleus of the atom. They have no electrical charge, each has one atomic mass unit.
- Electrons are particles which revolve in the orbit around the nucleus of the atom at a distance from it; like the planets revolving around the sun. Each electron carries one unit of negative electrical charge and the mass is so small that it can be disregarded when compared with the mass of other particles (Table 2.1).

In all atoms the number of positively charged protons in the nucleus is equal to the number of negatively charged electrons in the orbit around the nucleus and the atom is electrically neutral.

Table 2.1: Characteristics of subatomic particles

Particle	*Mass*	*Electric charge*
Proton	1 unit	1 positive
Neutron	1 unit	Neutral
Electron	Negligible	1 negative

Atomic Number and Atomic Weight

The number of protons in the nucleus in an atom differ in different atoms, e.g. hydrogen has one and oxygen has eight. The **number of protons in the nucleus is called the *atomic number*** of the atom and hence, different atoms have different atomic numbers, e.g. hydrogen has one and oxygen has eight.

The *atomic weight* of an element is the sum of protons and neutrons in the nucleus of the atom.

As specific groups of electrons are likely to move about within certain regions around the nucleus; regions are called electron shells, to be in concentric rings around the nucleus as in Fig. 2.1. The shells represents the energy levels of the electrons in relation to the nucleus not their physical positions.

The first energy level can hold only two electrons and is filled first. The second energy level can hold only eight electrons and is filled next, the third shell can hold maximum of 18 electrons. Subsequent energy levels hold increasing number of electrons each containing more than preceding level. The electrons configuration denotes the distribution of the electrons in each element, e.g. sodium 281 (first shell has 2, second has 8 and third has 1 electron).

When the outermost shell does not have a stable number of electrons the atom is reactive and will

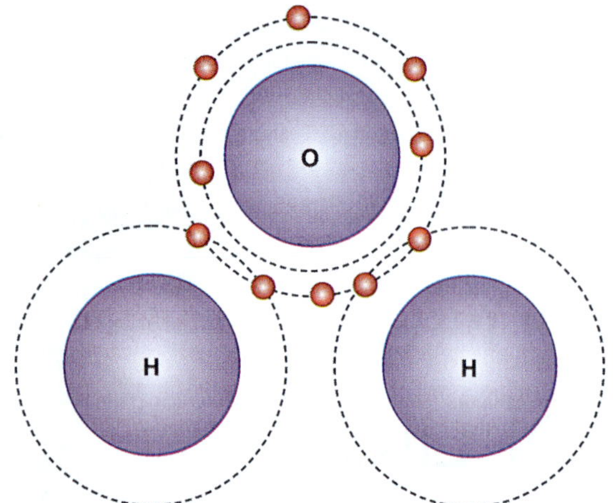

Fig. 2.1: A water molecule, showing the covalent bonds between hydrogen and oxygen

combine with other reactive atoms, forming the complex molecules of life.

This is described further in discussing molecules and compounds.

ISOTOPES

All atoms of an element have same number of protons; they may have different number of neutrons and thus different mass numbers. Isotopes of an atom are, when the numbers of neutrons present in the nucleus differs for the same atom, therefore have different mass numbers. This results in **atoms having different atomic weights** but the electrical activity is not affected as neutrons do not carry any charge, e.g. isotopes of hydrogen. The most common form of hydrogen atom is with one proton in the nucleus and one electron around it. Another isotope is with one proton and one neutron in the nucleus with one electron in the orbit; still another isotope has two neutrons and one proton in the nucleus and one electron in the orbit around.

Taking into account the isotopes of hydrogen, and the proportion in which they are found, the atomic weight of hydrogen is 1.008 though it is usually taken as 1.

Most isotopes are stable, i.e. their nuclear structure does not change overtime. The stable isotopes of oxygen are designated O-16, O-17 and O-18.

Certain isotopes called radioactive isotopes are unstable; their nuclei decay (spontaneous change), into a stable configuration, e.g. the radioactive isotopes are H-3, C-14, O-15; as they decay these atoms emit radiations; either subatomic particles or packets of energy and in the process often change into different element, e.g. radioactive C-12 decays into N-14. The decay of isotope may be fast or slow, taking millions of years. **The half life of an isotope** is the time required for half of the radioactive atoms in a sample of that isotope to decay into a more stable form.

Radioactive isotopes have both harmful as well as helpful effects. Their radiations can break apart molecules, which may produce tissue damage or various types of cancer. Beneficial effects of certain radioisotopes include their use in medical imaging procedures, e.g. to diagnose heart disease and to treat cancer by killing cancer cells.

Radioactive isotopes introduced into the body can be detected and traced by a Geiger counter. Thus radioactive iodine given to an individual may be traced to the thyroid gland. In larger doses radioactive isotopes, e.g. radium, may be used to destroy the abnormal cells which occur in cancer.

The following table lists elements present in the body and their respective symbols.

Carbon (C)	Chlorine (Cl)
Hydrogen (H)	Iodine (I)
Nitrogen (N)	Sodium (Na)
Sulphur (S)	Potassium (K)
Phosphours (P)	Magnesium (Mg)
Calcium (Ca)	
Iron (Fe)	

Many other elements are present in only minute amounts and are known as trace elements. Some of these are essential to life; example are cobalt, copper, manganese, molybdenum and possibly selenium. Chromium may protect arteries from atherosclerosis. Some trace elements serve no useful purpose in the body but are contaminants.

Molecules and Compounds

When the number of electrons in the outer shell of an element is optimum number, the element is inert or chemically unreactive, i.e. it will not easily combine with other elements to form compounds.

These *elements are the inert gases*, e.g. helium, neon, argon, krypton, xenon and radon.

Molecules consist of *two or more atoms which are chemically combined. The atoms may be of same element*, e.g. O_2 consists of two oxygen atoms.

Most molecules contain *two or more different elements*, e.g. H_2O (water), where there are two hydrogen atoms and an oxygen atom. *When two or more elements combine*, the resulting molecule can be referred to as **compound**.

Compounds which contain the element **carbon** are called **organic** and others are inorganic. Both are present in the body.

Covalent and Ionic Bonds

When atoms are joined together they form a chemical bond which is generally one of the two types; covalent or ionic.

Covalent bonds are formed when atoms share their electrons with each other. Most atoms use this type of bond; it forms a strong and stable link. A water molecule is built using covalent bonds (Fig. 2.1). Hydrogen has one electron, but the optimum number is two for this shell. Oxygen has six electrons in outer shell but optimum number for this shell is eight. Therefore if two hydrogen and one oxygen atom combine, each hydrogen atom will share its electron with oxygen atom forming a total of eight electrons in outer shell and so a stable compound.

Ionic bonds are weaker than covalent bonds and are formed when electrons are transferred from one atom to another. The example of sodium chloride, the atom of sodium has eleven electrons and that of chlorine seventeen, in effecting the combination to form a compound. When sodium combines with chlorine to form **sodium chloride** there is a transfer of the only electron in the outer shell of the sodium atom to the outer shell of the chlorine atom. This leaves the sodium atom of the compound with eight electrons in the outer shell and is stable number (Fig. 2.2).

The electron number has changed in the atoms in this type of reaction. There is no change in the number of protons in either atom but chloride atom now has 18 electrons, with 18 negative charges, and protons

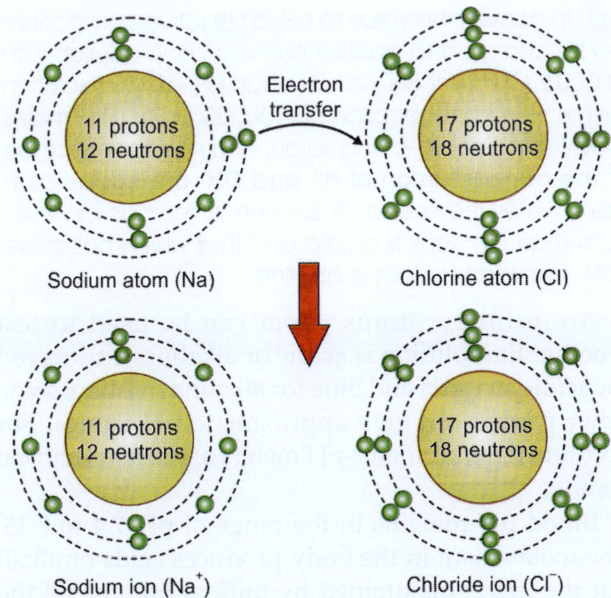

Fig. 2.2: Formation of the ionic compound, sodium chloride

with 17 positive charges. The sodium has lost one electron, leaving 10 electrons with 11 protons. When sodium chloride is dissolved in water the two atoms separate, i.e. they ionize, with formation of sodium with a positive charge it is a cation written as Na^+, and chloride is an anion, written Cl^-. By convention the number of electrical charges is indicated by superscript plus or minus signs.

Electrolytes

An ionic compound, e.g. sodium chloride in solution in water is called **electrolyte** because it can **conduct electricity**. Electrolytes are important body constituents because:

- Some conduct electricity, essential for muscle and nerve function
- Some exert osmotic pressure keeping body fluids in their own compartments
- Some function in acid-base balance

There are other electrolytes in the body. These may enter the body in the form of compounds, such as sodium bicarbonate, they exist in ionic form, i.e. sodium ion and bicarbonate ion.

Acids contain hydrogen combined with another element, or with a group of elements called a radical which acts as a single element. Hydrogen reacts with chlorine to form HCl and with phosphate to form phosphoric acid. When these acids ionize these produce

$$HCl = H^+ \; Cl^-$$

$$H_3PO_4 = 3H^+ \; PO_4^{3-}$$

In the second case each H atom has lost one electron, all of which have been taken up by one unit phosphate radical, making a phosphate ion with three negative charges.

A large number of compounds in the body are not ionic therefore have no electrical properties if dissolved in water, e.g. carbohydrates.

Molecular Weight

Molecular weight of molecule is the sum of the atomic weight of the elements which form the molecule, e.g.

Water (HOH) = 1 + 16 + 1 = 18

Sodium bicarbonate

$NaHCO_3$ = 23 + 1 + 12 + 16 + 16 + 16 = 84

(no units are attached)

Molar Concentration

Mole is the molecular weight in gram of the substance, e.g. one mole of sodium bicarbonate is 84 gm, one mole of calcium chloride (molecular weight 111) is 111 gm of calcium chloride, one mole of glucose (molecular weight 180) contains 180 gm of glucose. A molar solution of a substance is the solution in which 1 mole of a substance is dissolved in 1 liter of solvent. In human body the solvent is water or fat. A molar solution of sodium bicarbonate contains 84 grams of sodium bicarbonate dissolved in 1 liter of solvent.

In physiology this has the advantage, of being a measure of number of particles (molecules, atoms, ions) of substance present because molar solutions of substances contain the same number of particles.

It has advantage over milli-equivalents per liter because it can be used for nonelectrolytes, for any substance with known molecular weight. For substances present in the body in small amounts millimoles per liter or micromoles per liter is used.

For substances with unknown molecular weight, e.g. insulin the expression is in international units per milliliter.

Milliequivalents Per Liter (mEq/l)

Concentration is expressed in mEq/L = mg per L/molecular weight, multiplied by number of electrical charges. A mole of solution with a valency of v is equal to v equivalents of solute. For example:1 mol of Na^+ (valency 1) is equal to 1 eq of Na^+; 1 mole of $CaCl_2$ (total valence 4), is equal to 4 eq of $CaCl_2$; one mol of albumin (valency 18) is equal to 18 eq of albumin. As body fluids are dilute the units meq/liter are used. Solute concentrations expressed in mmol/liter can be converted to meq/liter as follows:

$$\text{meq/liter} = \text{mmol/liter} \times \text{valence}$$

Osmoles

The movement of water in different body compartments is related to the concentration of solute particles or osmotically active particles, regardless of their size or valence. Thus for movement of water, solute concentrations are best expressed in osmoles per liter or osmoles per kg of water. A mole of solute that dissociates into n discrete particles in solution is equal to n osmoles of solute, e.g. 1 mole of Na^+ is equal to 1 osmol of Na^+; 1 mole of $CaCl_2$ is equal to 3 osmol of calcium chloride (since it dissociates into three discrete solute particles); one mol of glucose is equal to 1 osmol of glucose; 1 mol of albumin is equal to one osmol of albumin. The units for osmol/liter and osmol/kg H_2O are respectively called osmolarity and osmolality. For most physiological applications osmolality is preferred unit as it is independent of the temperature of the solution and volume occupied by the solutes in the solution. As the body fluids are dilute the units used are mosmol/kg of water.

Acids, Alkalis and pH

The number of hydrogen ions present in a solution is measure of the acidity of the solution. The maintenance of the normal hydrogen ion concentration $[H^+]$ within the body fluids is an important factor and essential to life.

Expressing hydrogen ion concentration in terms of actual concentration is a cumbersome procedure. Therefore, the symbol pH has come into usage for expressing the concentration; **pH is related to actual hydrogen ion concentration.**

$$\text{pH} = \log 1/\text{H}^+ \text{ conc} = -\log \text{H}^+ \text{ conc}$$

The pH of water at 25°C in which H^+ and OH^- are present in equal numbers is 7.0. For each one unit pH less than 7 the $[H^+]$ is increased ten fold, for each pH unit above 7.0 it is decreased tenfold. The hydrogen ion concentration is measure of the amount of dissociated acid (ionized acid) rather than the total amount of acid present. **Low pH** corresponds to ***high hydrogen ion concentration*** which is called acidosis and a **high pH** corresponds to a ***low hydrogen ion concentration***, which is called alkalosis.

The normal pH of arterial blood is 7.4 and that of venous blood is 7.35 (due to extra quantity of CO_2 in the venous blood).

A solution's acidity or alkalinity is expressed on the pH scale which extends from 0–14. The scale is based on the concentration of H^+ in moles per liter. A pH 7 means that a solution contains 0.0000001 of a mole of hydrogen ion per liter. The number 0.0000001 is written as 1×10^{-7} in scientific notation, which indicates that number is 1 with decimal moved seven places to the left. To convert this value to pH, a negative component (–7) is changed to positive number (7). A solution with 0.0001 (10^{-4}) moles per liter has pH of 4, a solution with H^+ ion concentration of 0.000000001 (10^{-9}) moles per liter has pH of 9; and so on. At a midpoint of **scale 7 the concentration of H^+ and OH^- are equal**, as in pure water, it is neutral. A solution which has more H^+ ions than OH^- ions is acidic and that which has more OH^- ions than H^+ ions is alkaline.

An ordinary litmus paper can be used to test whether the solution is acidic or alkaline, it turns red for acidic solution and blue for alkaline solution, some other papers can give approximate pH values. For accurate measurements pH meters are used in clinical testing.

Blood pH remains in the range of **pH 7.4 to 7.35**. The metabolism in the body produces acids or alkali but the pH is maintained by buffers present till the acid or alkali substances are excreted.

Buffers

Intracellular and extracellular pH are generally maintained at very constant levels, e.g. pH of extracellular fluid is 7.40 and in health this value usually varies less than ± 0.05 pH units. Body pH is stabilized by the buffering capacity of the fluids.

A **buffer** is a substance that has the **ability to bind or release H+ in solution**, thus **keeping the pH of the solution relatively constant** despite addition of considerable quantities of acid or base.

The variation of up to 0.05 pH unit act without untoward effects, though **acidosis is present** whenever arterial **pH is below 7.40** and **alkalosis** is present whenever **it is above 7.40**. Homeostatic mechanisms maintain the pH of blood between 7.35 and 7.45, which is slightly more basic than pure water. Kidneys remove excess acid from the body and therefore urine is usually acidic.

Intracellular H^+ concentration is different from extra cellular pH and is regulated by a variety of intracellular processes. But it is sensitive to changes in ECF, H^+ concentration.

Metabolism of sulfur-containing amino acids produce H_2SO_4 and the metabolism of phosphorylated amino acids, such as phosphoserine produce H_3PO_4.

These strong acids enter the circulation and present a major load to the buffers in the ECF. The H^+ load from amino acid metabolism is about 50 meq/day.

The CO_2 formed by metabolism in the tissues is in large part hydrated to H_2CO_3 and the total H^+ load from this source is about 12,500 meq/day.

Most of the CO_2 is excreted in the lungs and only small quantities of H^+ remain to be excreted by the kidney. Fruits are the main dietary source of alkali.

Even though strong acids and bases are continually taken into and formed by the body, the pH of fluids remains almost constant. Important reason is the presence of buffer systems, which convert strong acids or bases into weak acids or bases. Strong acids (or bases) ionize easily and contribute many H^+ (or OH^-) ions to a solution. Therefore they can change pH drastically, which can disrupt body's metabolism. Weak acids (or bases) do not ionize as much and contribute fewer H^+ (or OH^-). Hence, they have less effect on pH. The chemical compounds that can convert strong acids or bases into weak acids or bases are called **buffers**.

One important buffer system in the body is the **carbonic acid-bicarbonate buffer** system. Carbonic acid (H_2CO_3) can act as weak acid and bicarbonate ion (HCO_3^-) as weak base. Hence, the system can compensate for either excess or shortage of H^+ ion.

If there is excess of H^+ ion, HCO_3^- can remove, as $H^+ + HCO_3^- = H_2CO_3 = CO_2 + H_2O$.

If there is shortage of H^+ ions,

$H_2CO_3 = H^+ + HCO_3^-$

providing extra H^+ ions.

Other buffers present in the blood are **hemoglobin** and **plasma proteins**, of which hemoglobin is a stronger buffer.

Hence, when strong acid is added to the blood levels of three buffer anions Hb^- (haemoglobin) prot– (protein), and HCO_3^- drop.

The buffer system maintain homeostasis by preventing dramatic changes in the pH values of the blood but can only function effectively if there is some means by which excess acid or alkali can be excreted from the body. The organs involved in this are lungs and kidney.

The lungs are important regulators of blood pH since they excrete carbon dioxide. Kidneys eliminate the extra acid and restore the supply of buffer anions to normal concentration.

Acidosis and Alkalosis

The lungs are important regulators of blood pH because they excrete carbon dioxide (CO_2). CO_2 increases $[H^+]$ in body fluids because it combines with water to form carbonic acid, which then dissociates into bicarbonate ion and hydrogen ion.

$CO_2 + H_2O = H_2CO_3 = H^+ + HCO_3^-$

The brain detects the rising $[H^+]$ in the blood and stimulates breathing, causing increased CO_2 loss and a fall in $[H^+]$. In alkalosis the brain by inhibitory effect on respiration decrease the elimination of CO_2.

The kidneys have the ability to excrete H^+ by the mechanisms to be described in the later chapters. In alkalosis the urine becomes alkaline with excretion of bicarbonate ions.

The **buffers, respiratory, and excretory** systems of the body together maintain the acid-base balance so that pH range of the blood remains within normal limits.

Acidosis occurs when extra acid load is presented that the body is not able to deal, as in diabetes, or due to ingestion of acidifying salts, such as NH_4Cl and $CaCl_2$, which in effect add HCl to the body. Failure of the diseased kidney to excrete normal amounts of acid is also a cause of acidosis. **Alkalosis** may result when $NaHCO_3$ and other alkalinizing salts are sometimes ingested in large amounts but more common cause of alkalosis is loss of acid from the body, as a result of vomiting of gastric juice rich in HCl. This is equivalent to adding alkali to the body.

The pH range *compatible with life* is 7.00 to 7.8.

TRANSPORT OF SUBSTANCES ACROSS CELL MEMBRANES

The plasma membrane (i.e. cell membrane) serves as a diffusion barrier enabling the cell to maintain cytoplasmic concentration of many substances that differ markedly from their extracellular concentrations.

The plasma membrane has a lipoid character and compounds that are soluble in nonpolar solvents enter the cells more readily than do water soluble substances of similar molecular weight.

Permeability of Water-Soluble Molecules

Very small *uncharged* water-soluble molecules pass through the cell membrane much more readily than predicted by lipid solubility, e.g. water permeates the cell membrane readily.

As the size of the uncharged, water-soluble molecules increases the membrane permeability decreases. Most plasma membranes are essentially impermeable to water-soluble molecules whose molecular weights are greater than 200.

Because of their charge ions are relatively insoluble in lipid solvents and therefore lipid membranes have low permeability to most ions. Ionic diffusion across the membranes occurs through protein "channels" in the membrane. Some channels are highly specific with respect to ions that can pass. But others allow the passage of all ions below certain size. Some **ions channels** are controlled by the voltage difference across the membrane, whereas others are regulated by neurotransmitters or certain other molecules (Fig. 2.3).

Certain water-soluble molecules such as sugars and amino acids, essential for cellular metabolism do not cross the plasma membrane at appreciable rates by simple diffusion. Plasma membranes have specific proteins (**carrier proteins**) that allow the transfer of into or out of the cell.

Osmosis

Osmosis is the flow of water; across a membrane permeable to water but impermeable to solutes; from a compartment in which the solute concentration is lower to one in which solute concentration is higher.

Osmotically active substances in the body are dissolved in water and osmolal concentrations can be expressed as osmoles per liter of water. Hence osmolal rather then osmolar concentrations are very often expressed as osmoles per liter of water; osmolality is expressed in milliosmoles per liter for body fluids.

NaCl would dissociate into Na^+ and Cl^- so that each mol in solution would dissociate into 2 osm. Thus one mmol of NaCl per liter in body fluids contributes somewhat about 2 mosm of osmotically active particles per liter. The actively being slightly less then two due to it being reduced due to interaction between ions.

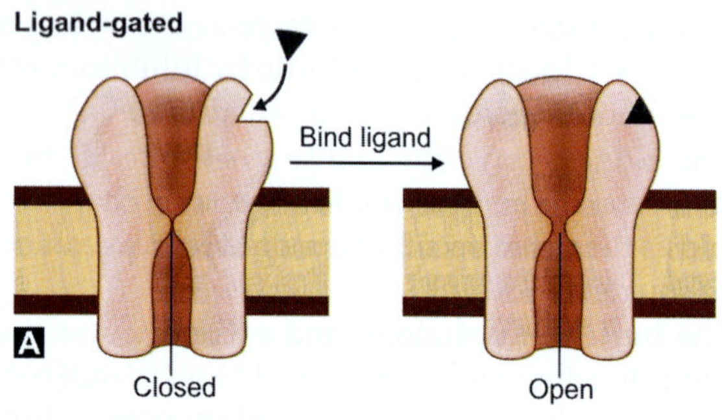

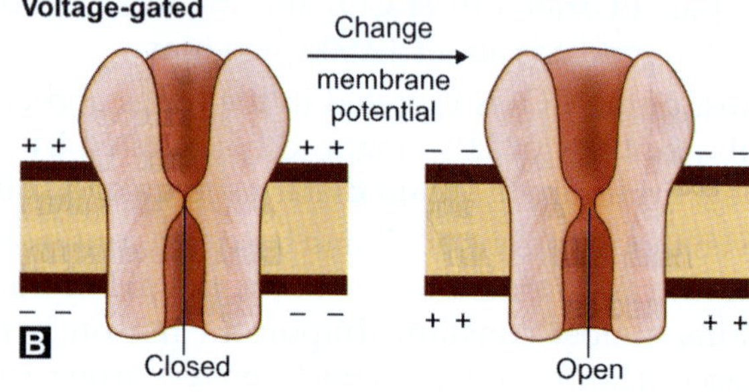

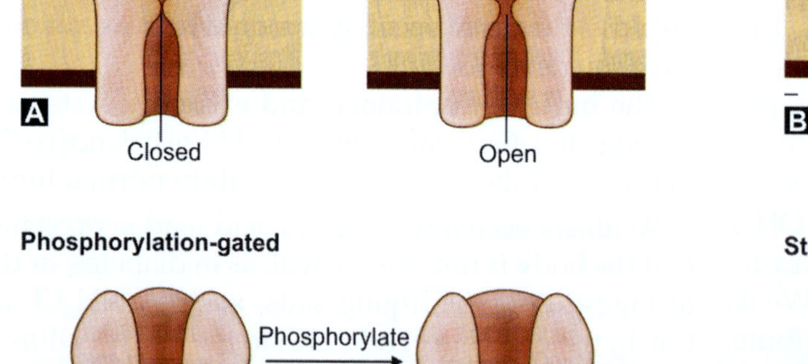

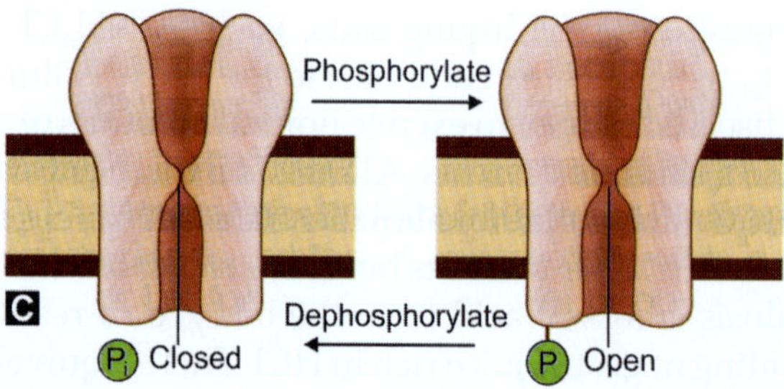

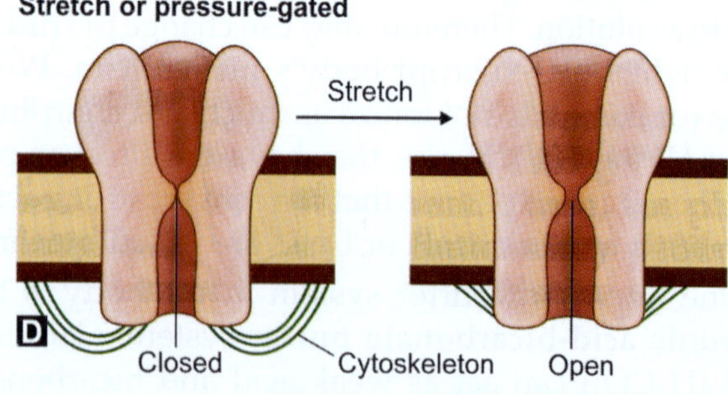

Figs 2.3A to D: Ionic channels. Ligand-gated channels open with specific ligand attachment. Voltage geted open with change of voltage in the membrane. Stretch opens another type

Osmolar Concentration of Plasma

The osmolal concentration of plasma is about 290 mosm/L. All body fluid compartments are in or nearly in osmotic equilibrium. The term tonicity is used to describe the osmolal concentration of a solution relative to plasma.

Solutions that have the *same osmolal concentration as plasma* are said to be ***isotonic,*** those with greater as hypertonic, and those with lesser as hypotonic.

A 0.9% saline solution is isotonic to plasma and remains so because there is no net movement of the osmotically active particles in the solution into cells (and the particles are not metabolized).

But a 5% glucose solution is isotonic to plasma when initially infused intravenously, but glucose is metabolized so that the net effect is that of infusing a hypotonic solution.

The relative contribution of various plasma components to the osmolality of plasma, is that *except* for about 20 out of the 290 mosm/L, all the rest are contributed by *Na^+ and its accompanying anions (Cl^- and HCO_3^- mainly).*

The major nonelectrolytes of plasma are glucose and urea, which in steady state are in equilibrium with cells. Their contribution to osmolality are about 5 mosm/L each but becomes quite large in hyperglycemia or uremia.

Other cations and anions make a relatively small contribution. Although the concentration of plasma proteins is large when expressed in grams per dl; they normally contribute less than 2 mosm/L to this pressure because of their high molecular weights **(but the osmotic pressure exerted by them called the colloidal osmotic pressure, is important in governing fluid exchange across capillaries as explained in CVS chapter).**

The total plasma osmolality is important in assessing dehydration, overhydration and other fluid and electrolyte abnormalities. Hyperosmolality can cause coma.

Regulation of Cell Volume

Cell membranes are **flexible**. Therefore, with extracellular fluid hypotonicity water enters the cell and the cells swell, in hypertonicity of extracellular fluid some water is lost from the cells and they shrink.

The plasma membranes of most of the cells of the body are relatively impermeable to many of the solutes of the interstitial fluid but are highly permeable to water. Therefore when the osmotic pressure of the interstitial fluid is increased water leaves the cells by osmosis. The cells shrink and cellular solutes become more concentrated until effective osmotic pressure of the cytoplasm is again equal to that of interstitial fluid.

Conversely if the osmotic pressure of the extracellular fluid is decreased water enters the cells and the cells swell until the extracellular and intracellular osmotic pressures are equal.

TRANSPORT MECHANISMS ACROSS CELL MEMBRANES

Passive Transport

It occurs when substances can cross plasma *membranes* and move *down a gradient* (downhill) ***without using energy.***

Diffusion of small substances takes place down the concentration gradient crossing membranes by:

- dissolving in the lipid part of the membrane, e.g. lipid soluble substances, fatty acids, steroids, gases oxygen and carbon dioxide.
- passing through channels or pores in the membranes, e.g. small water-soluble substances, i.e. sodium, potassium and calcium.
- osmosis as described above.

Facilitated Diffusion

Larger molecular weight substances are unable to diffuse through the cell membrane unaided, e.g. glucose and amino acids can diffuse aided by specific **carrier proteins** in the cell membrane, which bind these substances. The carrier then changes its shape and deposits the substance on the other side of the membrane. The ***carrier sites are specific*** and can be used only *for one substance*. As the substances are transported along the concentration gradient (or electrochemical potential) ***no energy is used*** and the process is called **facilitated transport** or facilitated diffusion.

Active Transport

Substances are also transported by the carrier proteins **against their concentration gradient** (or ***chemical gradient or electrical potential gradient***), i.e. **from lower to higher gradient**. But this process requires the **use of energy in the form of ATP by the carrier proteins** and ***it cannot take place without use of energy.***

The Sodium Pump Na^+, K^+ ATPase (Fig. 2.4)

It uses energy by hydrolysis of ATP to ADP (adenosine diphosphate). It extrudes three Na^+ from the cell and takes two K^+ into the cell against concentration gradients and uses one ATP.

It **maintains** concentration of Na^+ **low** in the cell.

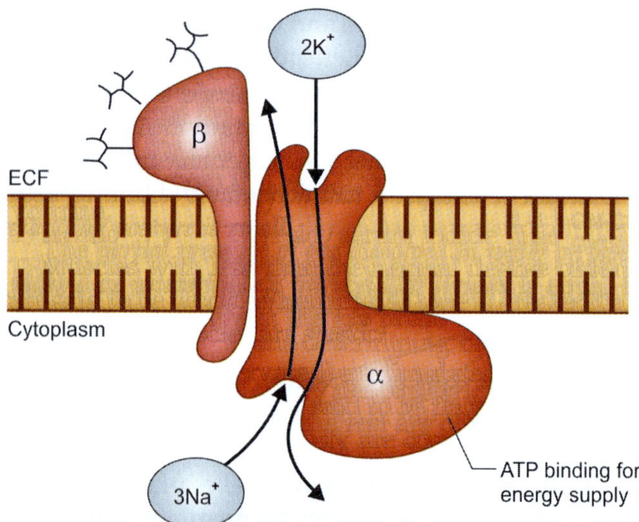

Fig. 2.4: Na^+-K^+ ATPase. The intracellular portion subunit has a Na^+-binding site, and an ATP-binding site, the extracellular portion has a K^+-binding site

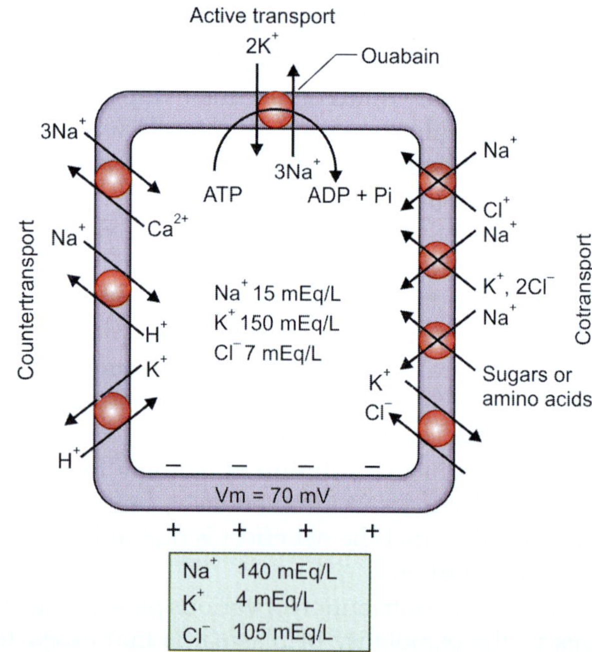

Fig. 2.5: The active transport of Na^+ by Na^+ K^+ ATPase; converts the chemical energy of ATP hydrolysis into maintenance of an inward gradient for Na^+. The energy of the gradients is for countertransport, cotransport, and maintenance of the membrane potential. Concentration gradients for ions across membrane are shown

As it utilizes energy, it is responsible for 30% of the energy used by the body under resting conditions.

Another example of active transport is Ca^{2+} ATPase which pumps out Ca^{2+} from cardiac muscle (after the contraction) against the concentration gradient using energy of ATP.

The carrier sites are specific and can be used only by one substance. The rate at which a substance is transported depends upon the number of active such sites available, e.g. for Na^+ K^+ ATPase; Ca^{2+} ATPase.

Secondary Active Transport

In many sites the active transport of Na^+ is coupled with transport of other substances by a carrier protein called **symport**. The transport of glucose in the intestinal lumen is by a symport, a transporter that combines with glucose and Na^+ *both transported* across the membrane due to ***low*** Na^+ ***concentration inside*** *the intestinal cell*. The transport is dependent on low concentration of Na^+ in the cell. This process is not active by itself but is dependent on low concentration of Na^+ maintained by active process by Na^+, K^+ ATPase at another site at cell membrane. Hence, not being an active process but **dependent on another active process** it is **secondary active process.**

Various other transport mechanisms exist in the cell membrane for transport by carrier proteins which act as antiport (transport one substance in one direction and another coupled with it in the opposite direct) or symport that transport two substances in the same direction (Fig. 2.5).

Transport across but not through the membrane. Transport of substances, too large to cross cell membrane occurs by phagocytosis or pinocytosis. The particles are engulfed by extension of cytoplasm which encloses them, forming a membrane around them (Fig. 2.6). By phagocytosis cell fragments, foreign material or microbes can be taken into cell. Pinocytosis is passage of liquid material across cell membrane.

Clathrin-mediated endocytosis occurs at membrane indentations where protein clathrin accumulates. These are called **coated pits.**

Extrusion of waste material by the reverse processes through the plasma membrane is called **exocytosis.** Secretory granules formed in the Golgi apparatus usually leave the cell by this way as also the ingested residues of substances taken up due to phagocytosis (Fig. 2.7).

Specialized Transport Across Capillary Wall

The transport process here is filtration and it is the pressure difference that is responsible for the fluid to pass through the capillary wall.

The structure of the capillary wall is variable from one vascular bed to another. In skeletal muscle and

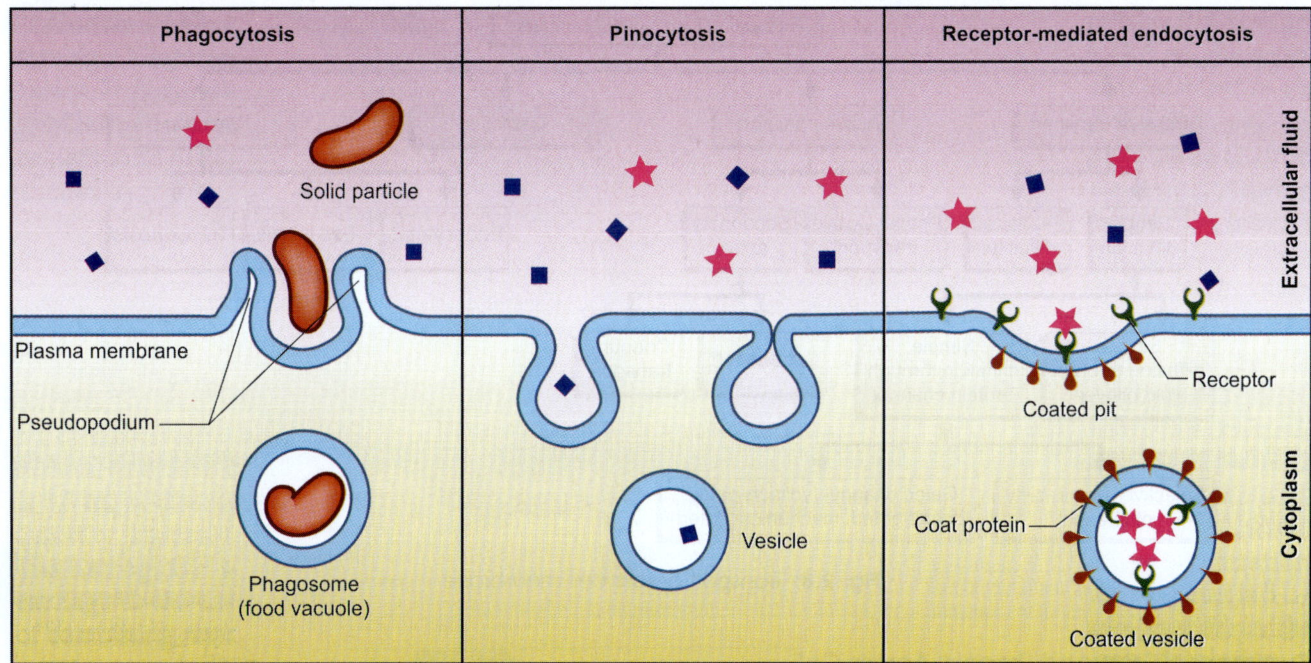

Summary of transport processes across cell membrane

Fig. 2.6: Endocytosis, pinocytosis, coated pits endocytosis

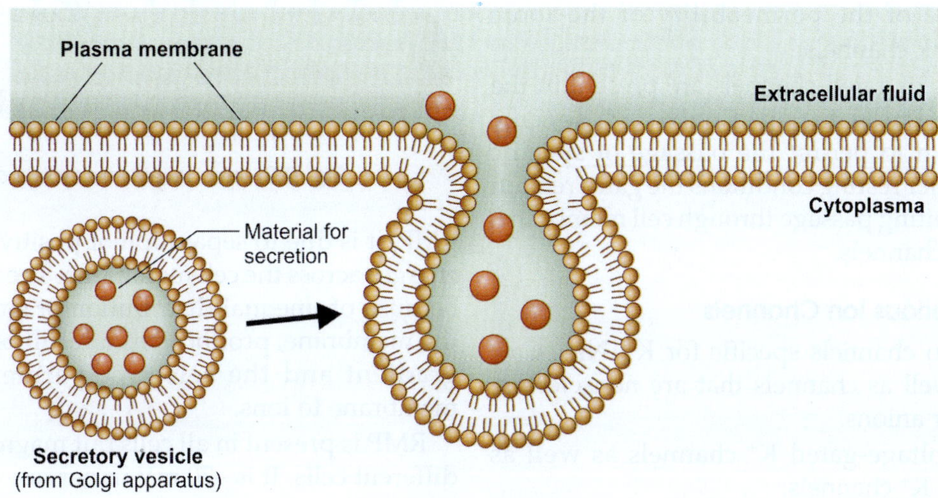

Fig. 2.7: Exocytosis

many other organs water and small solutes are the only substances that cross the wall with ease. The pores in between endothelial cells are too small to permit proteins and other colloids to pass across. Colloids have high molecular weight and are present in large amounts but only small amounts pass across capillary wall by vesicular transport. Hence, colloids exert an osmotic pressure of about **25 mm of Hg** in the plasma called the **oncotic pressure**. This pressure opposes filtration by hydrostatic pressure, i.e. blood pressure in the capillaries. The balance between the **hydrostatic** and **oncotic pressure** determines exchange across capillaries.

Transcytosis

Small amounts of protein are transported out of capillaries across the endothelial cells by endocytosis on the capillary side end by exocytosis on the interstitial side of endothelial cells. The process is called transcytosis, or vesicular transport.

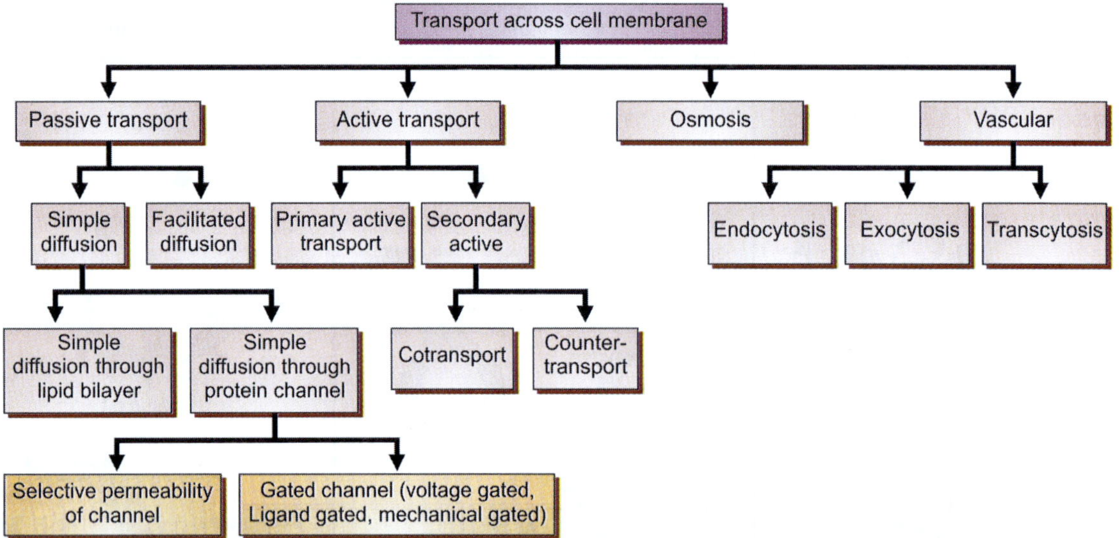

Fig. 2.8: Transport across cell membrane

Summary of Transport Process Across Cell Membranes (Fig. 2.8)

Ionic Channels in Cell Membranes

The ***resting membrane*** is more permeable to K^+ than to Na^+ because of the permeability of the ionic channels the leak channels.

Several types of gated channels are present in the cell membrane, the gates open only with specific stimuli for them to permit the passage of specific substances. Under resting conditions the gates remain closed not permiting passage through cell membrane, e.g. Na^+ gated channels.

Summary of Various Ion Channels

- There are ion channels specific for K^+, Na^+, Ca^{2+} and Cl^- as well as channels that are nonselective for cations or anions.
- There are voltage-gated K^+ channels as well as ligand-gated K^+ channels.
- Aquaporins are channels for water molecules.
- ENaCs are called epithelial Na^+ channels. These channels in the kidney play an important role in the regulation of ECF volume by aldosterone.
- Humans have several types of Cl^- channels. GABA and glycine receptors in CNS are Cl^- channels.

Resting Membrane Potential (RMP)

When two electrodes are placed on outer surface of a nerve and connected through an amplifier no potential difference is recorded. But when one electrode is inserted into the nerve a potential difference with negativity inside is recorded (Fig. 2.9). This is called RMP, it is due to separation of positive and negative charges across the cell membrane. The potential exists because of unequal distribution of some ions across the membrane, produced as a result of concentration gradient and the selective permeability of the membrane to ions.

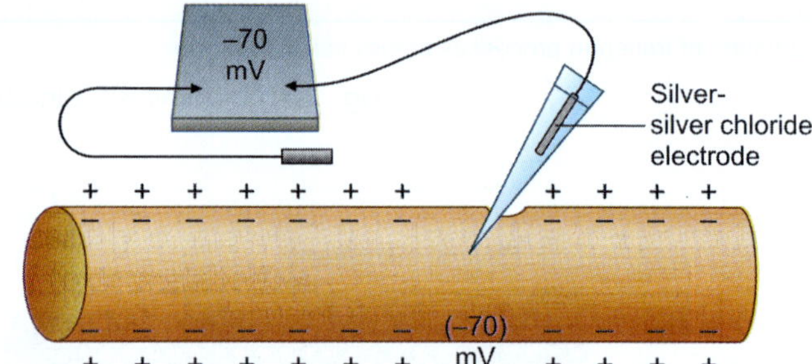

Fig. 2.9: Intracellular recording of RMP

RMP is present in all cells but magnitude differs in different cells. It is –70 mV in nerves.

IONIC BASIS OF MEMBRANE POTENTIALS

Membrane potentials caused by diffusion: *The diffusion potentials is caused by concentration difference on two sides of the membrane:* Potassium concentration is greater inside the cell than outside. As the membrane is permeable to potassium ions (K^+) but much less to sodium ions (Na^+) (due to selective permeability of the membrane to ions) in the resting state the ions distribute according to their concentration gradient.

Hence, there is tendency for K^+ to leave the cell, carry positive charge outside the membrane creating electronegativity inside the membrane and the negative anions (proteins and phosphate anions) inside are too large to pass through the membrane to accompany. The potential created, diffusion potential becomes great enough to block further diffusion of K^+ because of the electrical gradient it created. The magnitude of the membrane potential can be calculated from Nernst equation.

The Nernst Potential. The diffusion potential level across a membrane that opposes the net diffusion of a particular ion through the membrane is called Nernst potential for that ion. The magnitude of the Nernst potential (equilibrium potential) is determined by the ratio of the concentration of that specific ion on the two sides of the membrane. The greater the ratio, the greater the tendency for the ion to diffuse and hence, greater the equilibrium potential to prevent more diffusion.

The Nernst equation for calculation of equilibrium potential at a normal body temperature of 37°C is as:

$$\text{EMF (millivolts)} = \pm 61 \log \frac{\text{Concentration inside}}{\text{Concentration outside}}$$

The sign of the potential is negative if the ion diffusing from inside to outside is positive and it is positive of the ion diffusing from inside to outside is negative. Hence, when the concentration of K^+ on the inside is 10 times than that of outside the log of 10 is 1 so that equilibrium potential by Nernst equation calculates to –60 millivolts inside the membrane.

Goldman Equation for Membrane Potential

When a membrane is permeable to several different ions, the net diffusion potential that develops depends upon three factors:

1. The polarity of each ion, negative or positive
2. The permeability (P) of each ion through membrane
3. Concentration (C) of each of ion on the inside and outside the membrane.

Goldman equation gives the value of the electrical charge when membrane is permeable to several ions, takes into account the above three factors for each ion. The equation is as:

$$\text{EMF (millivolts)} = 61 \log \frac{C_{Na^+_i} P_{Na^+} + C_{K^+_i} P_{K^+} + C_{Cl^-_o} P_{Cl^-}}{C_{Na^+_o} P_{Na^+} + C_{K^+_o} P_{K^+} + C_{Cl^-_i} P_{Cl^-}}$$

o = outside, i = inside (the membrane)

The following features of the Goldman equation are:

- Sodium, potassium and chloride ions are most importantly involved in the development of membrane potentials in the nerve and muscle fibers.
- The degree of importance of each ion in determining to voltage is proportional to the membrane permeability for that particular ion.
- A positive ion concentration gradient from inside the membrane to the outside causes electronegativity inside the membrane.

The concentration gradient for Cl^- which is negatively charged ion is from outside to inside and it contributes a negative potential with diffusion.

During resting conditions the membrane is more permeable to K^+ then to Na^+ and membrane potential is mainly dependent upon concentration gradient for K^+. Hence, the equation gives nearly the same value of membrane potential as calculated from the Nernst equation for K^+ concentration.

Origin of Normal Resting Membrane Potential (RMP)

Contribution of Potassium Diffusion Potential

The diffusion of ***K⁺ across the membrane*** contributes *mainly in the resting membrane potential.* The permeability to Na^+ is low in the membrane. In the resting state the Na^+ channels are closed and only small amount of Na^+ leaks to the inside of the cell despite the concentration of Na^+ being low inside.

Contribution of Na^+ K^+ Pump

It provides additional contribution to the RMP. As it pumps out three Na^+ and pumps in two K^+, results in more positive ions being pumped out and it adds to the RMP value.

In summary the diffusion potentials alone caused by potassium ion would give membrane potential value of about –86 mV almost all being caused by K^+ diffusion. An additional –4 mV is contributed by Na^+ K^+ pump that gives a net potential of –90 mV in excitable tissues.

The Nernst equation is often used for deriving the value of the resting membrane potential, in different tissues.

ACTION POTENTIAL (AP)

The action potential is rapid change the membrane potential, the membrane potential overshoots to become positive followed by a return to the resting membrane potential (Fig. 2.10).

Action Potential (AP)

If an electrical stimulus is given to an excitable tissue, which produces depolarization of the membrane, it opens the voltage gated Na^+ channels and causes

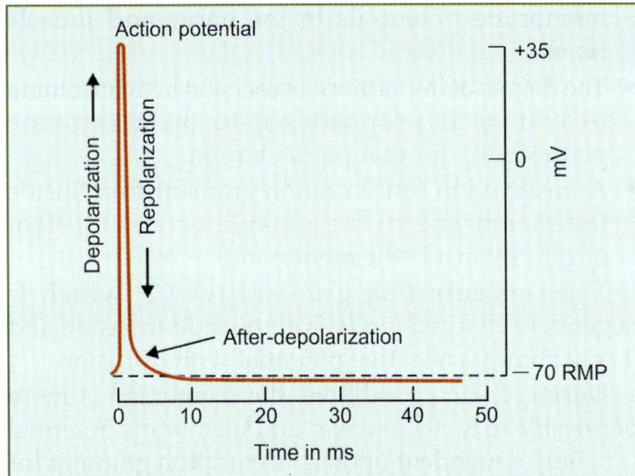

Fig. 2.10: Action potential in a nerve

sudden increase in permeability of membrane to Na^+. Sudden influx of Na^+ takes a place because both the electrical and the concentration gradients for it favour in this direction. The influx of positive ions makes the inside of the membrane positive; when it reaches +35 mV, the inactivation of sodium channels occurs resulting in sudden decrease in the sodium permeability. **Slow voltage gated K^+** channels now open and repolarization brings membrane potential back to resting level. The events fast depolarization and rapid repolarization are described as action potential. In an excitable tissue, nerve or muscle or neuron action potential are produced.

The size and shape of action potential differ from one excitable tissue to another. The properties of AP are:

- an action potential is propogated with the same shape and size along the whole of nerve or muscle cell membrane.
- the action potential is the basis of carrying signals in nerves and in muscle cell membrane.

The voltage dependent ion channel proteins in the plasma membrane are responsible for production and propagation action potential.

Nerve Action Potential

Nerve signals are transmitted by action potentials.

To conduct a **nerve signal** the action potential moves along the nerve until it comes to the end (details in nervous system).

AGING

It is a process which is poorly understood. One theory holds that it is a result of *random mutations in DNA* of somatic cells that produce *cumulative abnormalities*.

Other theory is that cumulative abnormalities are produced as a result of *increased cross linkage of collagen and other proteins* possibly as a result of nonenzymatic combination of glucose with amino acids on these proteins.

Third theory is that it is produced as a result cumulative *damage to tissues caused by free radicals* (free radicals are waste products produced as a result of body metabolism).

Caloric restriction chronically in experimental animals has shown to prolong life and this could be true for human beings.

Intercellular Communications

Cells communicate with one another via chemical messengers:

- Some messenger move through gap junctions without passing through ECF.
- Neuronal communication at synapses is mostly chemical.
- Endocrine communication, hormones and growth factors reach via blood or lymph circulation.
- Paracrine communication of cell products via ECF to the neighbouring cells.
- Autocrine communication the messenger binds to receptors on the same cell.

Receptors for Chemical Messengers

The recognition of chemical messenger by cell is by interaction with receptor on the cell, which are proteins on the cell. When the transmitter is present in excess the active receptors generally decrease (down-regulation); in deficiency of messenger there is increase in the number of active receptors (up-regulation). Exceptions are like action of angiotensin on adrenal cortex where there is increase in the number of receptors on adrenal cortex with increase in concentration of angiotensin.

Mechanisms by Which Chemical Messengers Act

Receptor-ligand interaction is the initial action which is followed by secondary response within the cell that can be any of the types:

- ion channel activation
- G-protein activation
- activation of enzyme activity in the cell membrane
- direct activation of transcription

Many ligands in the ECF bind to receptors on the surface of cells and cause release of intracellular mediator, such as cAMP, IP_3 and DAG that initiate changes in cell function and the mediators are called second messengers whereas the extracellular ligand is called first messenger.

Intracellular Ca^{2+} as a Second Messenger

Ca^{2+} regulates a number of physiological processes like proliferation, neural signaling learning, contraction, secretion. For these **free Ca^{2+}** concentration in the **cytoplasm** becomes important. There are intracellular Ca^{++} stores with high concentration in endoplasmic reticulum and other organelles, and Ca^{++} can be mobilized to increase free Ca^{2+} in the cytoplasm. The increased Ca^{2+} binds to calcium-binding proteins which have biological action. These actions will be described in relevant chapters.

Cyclic AMP

It is an important second messenger (cAMP). It is formed from ATP by the action of enzyme adenylyl cyclase. It is converted into physiologically inactive 5′ AMP by the action of phosphodiesterase.

Growth Factors

These are polypeptides and proteins that are divided into 3 groups.

One group is made-up of agents that stimulate the multiplication or development of various types of cells, e.g. NGF, insulin-like growth factor I (IGF-I), activins and inhibins and epidermal growth factor (EGF).

Second group is **cytokines** produced by lymphocytes, macarophages and some other cells and are important in regulation of immune system. More than 20 have been described.

Third group is colony stimulating factors that regulate proliferation and maturation of red and white blood cells.

IMPLICATIONS AND APPLICATIONS

The knowledge of composition of an atom; helps in understanding the normal function of free radicals and the role of antioxidants, that protect the harmful effects of free radicals.

Antioxidants are vitamin C, vitamin E, beta-carotene.

The normality (N) of a solution is the number of gram equivalent in 1 L. A solution of hydrochloric acid contains both H+ 1 g and Cl– 35.5 g, equivalent = (1 + 35.5 g) L = 36.5 g/L.

Channelopathies (abnormal ionic channels) include a wide range of diseases that can affect both excitable (e.g. neurons and muscle) and nonexcitable cells. In myasthenia, acetylcholine receptor ligand gated nonspecific cation channel is affected. In Myotonia a type of K+ channel is affected; long QT interval syndrome both Na+ and K+ channels are affected. Other diseases classified as channelopathies include cystic fibrosis Bartter syndrome.

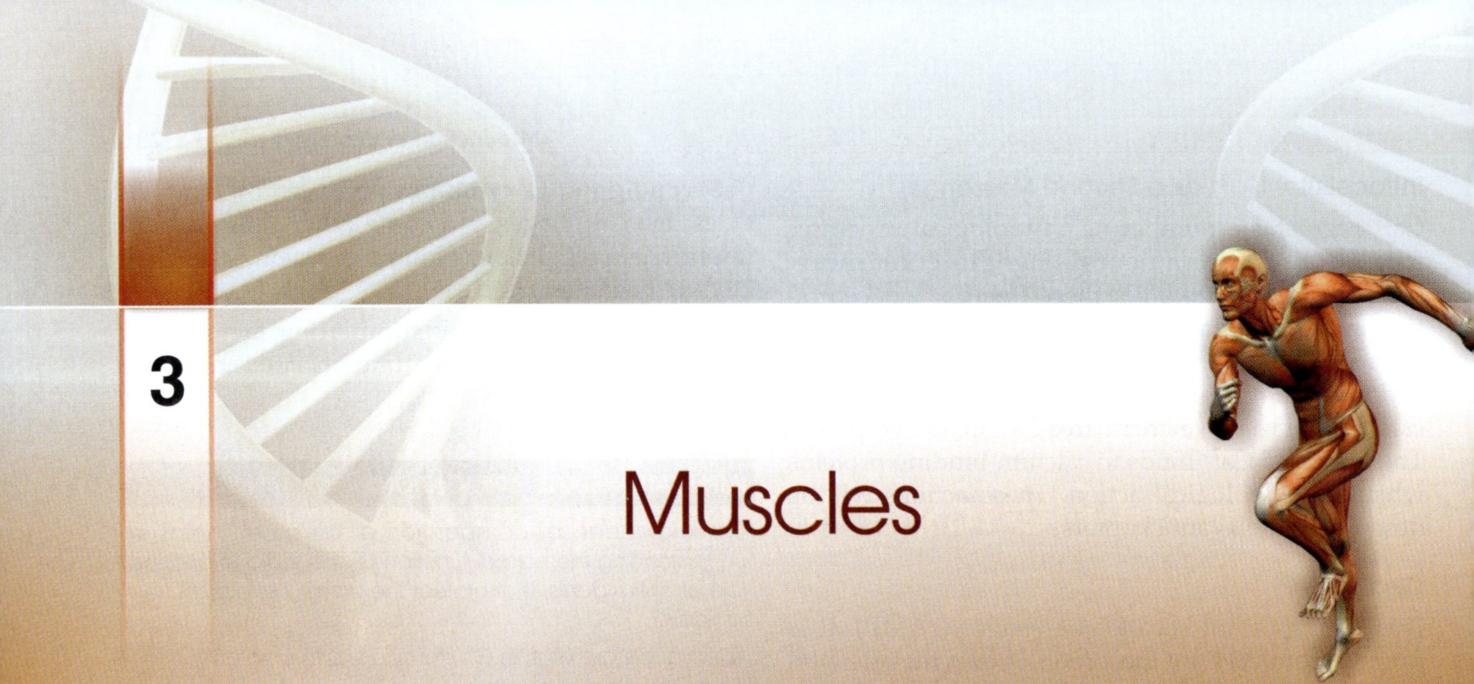

3 Muscles

MUSCLES

There are three types of muscles in the body. These have some common properties but differ in other ways. The types are:

- **Skeletal muscle**
- **Smooth muscle**
- **Cardiac muscle**

Skeletal muscle: Movements result from contraction of muscles. Those movements which are under **our control,** such movements are produced by skeletal muscles attached to bones. These muscles under the microscope show alternate light and dark bands and hence are called *striated muscles* (Fig. 3.1).

Smooth muscle: Movements also occur in the *gastrointestinal tract* due to muscle in layers, and these movements are responsible for **propulsion of food** through the tract so that it can be: digested by different enzymes of the system; useful substances are absorbed; and the residue from food is expelled. The movements here are **not under voluntary control,** but produced under the activity of some **irregular pacemakers** and *local stimuli play a role* in the movements. These movements which are not under our control are produced by *involuntary muscles* which under the ***microscope*** do not show alternating dark and light bands; hence are called *smooth muscles*. Such smooth muscles are present in the **respiratory system**

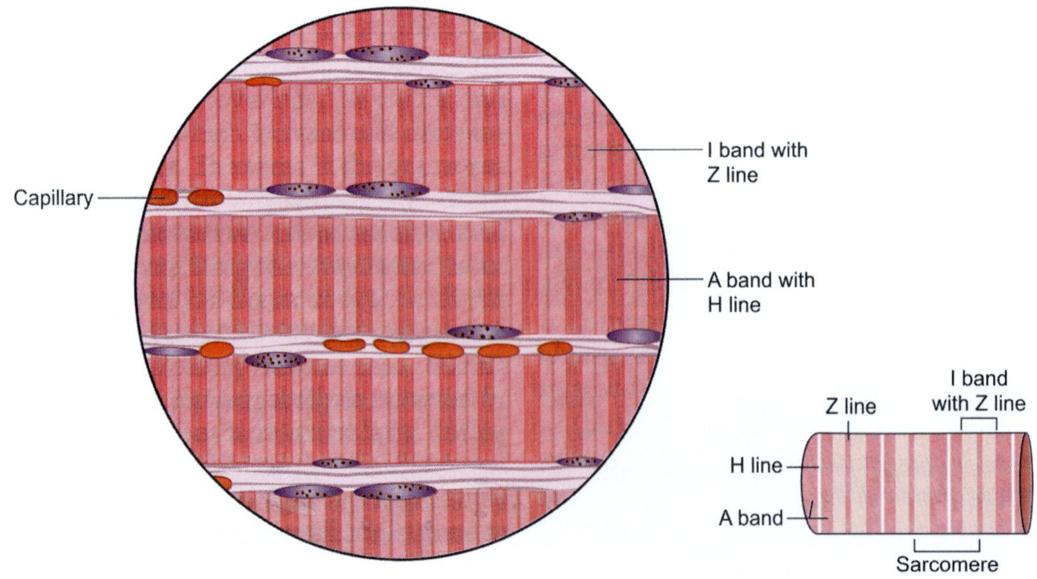

Fig. 3.1: Electron micrograph of human gastrocnemius muscle. The various bands and lines are marked

in the airways, where they influence the *diameter of the airways*. Smooth muscles are also present in **organs like bladder**. **Autonomic nerves** innervate the muscles.

Cardiac muscle: Cardiac muscle is *striated* but **not under voluntary control** and **contracts regularly** due to impulses from its **pacemaker**, present in the heart itself. **Autonomic nerves** supply the cardiac muscle and influence the pacemaker activity. But heart continues to beat regularly even if its nerve supply is cut off. *It beats from womb to tomb.*

SKELETAL MUSCLE

It is called ***skeletal*** or ***voluntary*** muscle; voluntary because there is conscious control over contractions; skeletal as the muscles are attached to skeleton.

Muscle Fibers

Muscle (Fig. 3.2A) is made-up of numerous cells called muscle fibers. Most of the muscles begin and end in tendons and the muscle **fibers are arranged in parallel** between the ends, so that the force of contraction is additive, i.e. more the **number of fibers** that contract the greater is the force of contraction.

Each muscle fiber is a single cell that is *multinucleated, long, cylindrical* and surrounded by cell membrane called the **sarcolemma** (Fig. 3.2B)

Each muscle fiber contracts in response to impulse from its nerve.

Muscle Cell—The Muscle Fiber

Each muscle cell surrounded by sarcolemma is made-up of a number of **myofibrils** present in the cytoplasm **(sarcoplasm)** of the cell. **Each myofibril** is further made-up of **myofilaments,** which are the contractile proteins. Each myofibril shows cross striation and the cross striations in all myofibrils in one muscle cell are in register with each other and so the whole muscle cell shows alternating pattern of cross striations under the microscope. The pattern arises from two sets of filaments in each myofibril. The dark striations are a region containing a number of thick filaments the myosin filaments. This region of myofibril is termed

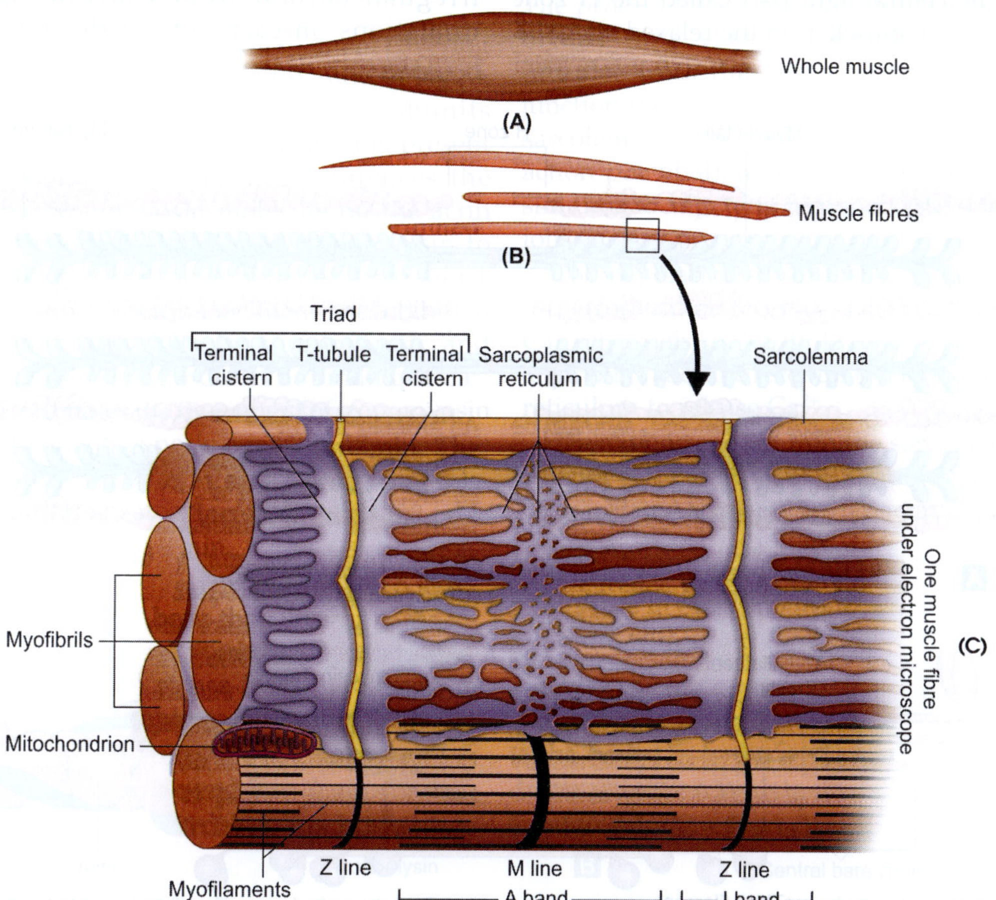

Figs 3.2A to C: (A) Whole muscle, (B) one muscle fibre and (C) One muscle fibre under electron microscope showing relationships between membrane elements and the myofilaments

where myosin head can bind to actin filaments (Fig. 3.7). This binding results in sliding movement of actin filaments towards thick filament; shortening the sarcomere; opposing Z lines coming closer together (Fig. 3.6). The movement requires energy derived from ATP, the myosin head has ATPase activity.

The width of A bands remains constant but Z lines move closer together when the muscle contracts and are further apart when the muscle relaxes. Sliding during muscle contraction occurs because the myosin heads bind firmly to actin, bend at the junction of head with the neck and then detach. This is power stroke and depends on hydrolysis of ATP to provide energy. As long as the Ca^{2+} level in sarcoplasm remains elevated and sufficient ATP is available the cycle repeats with myosin head binding to the next site. Many myosin heads cycle at or near the same time producing gross muscle contraction.

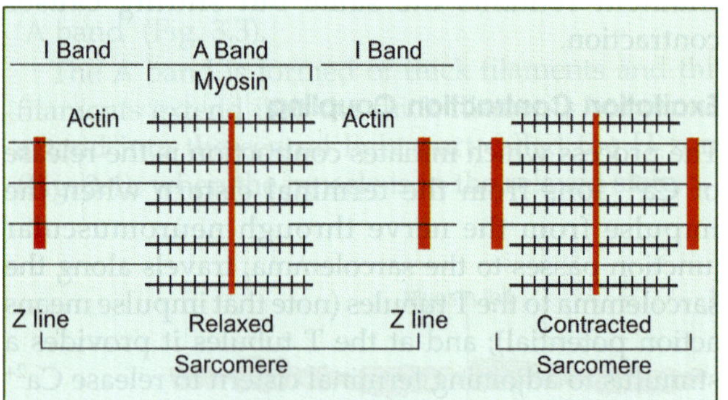

Fig. 3.6: Muscle relaxed and when contracted the actin filament slide and extend towards the center of A band with shortening of the sarcomere

Muscle Relaxation

Shortly after releasing Ca^{2+} the sarcoplasmic reticulum begins to re-accumulate Ca^{2+} using Ca^{2+} pump and energy derived from ATP; into the longitudinal portion of the reticulum from where the Ca^{2+} diffuses into the terminal cisterns to be stored. As the calcium concentration in the cytoplasm is lowered; Ca^{2+} is released from troponin C; chemical interaction between myosin and actin ceases and muscle relaxes. *Hence, both contraction and relaxation of muscle require energy and are active processes.* If the energy is not available to transport Ca^{2+} back into sarcoplasmic reticulum, muscle remains in the state of contraction; such sustained contraction is called **contracture.**

CONTRACTILE RESPONSES

Electrical and mechanical events occur in skeletal muscle (Fig. 3.8). The electrical response leads to contraction. Muscle membrane depolarization (action potential) starts at the motor end plate (which is specialized structure under the motor nerve ending). The action potential is transmitted along the sarcolemma of muscle fiber and initiates the contractile response with release of Ca^{2+}.

Types of Muscle Contractions

Muscular contraction involves shortening of contractile elements but there are elastic and viscous elements in series with the contractile elements. Hence, when the *contraction takes place without the change in the length of the whole muscle the tension in the muscle*

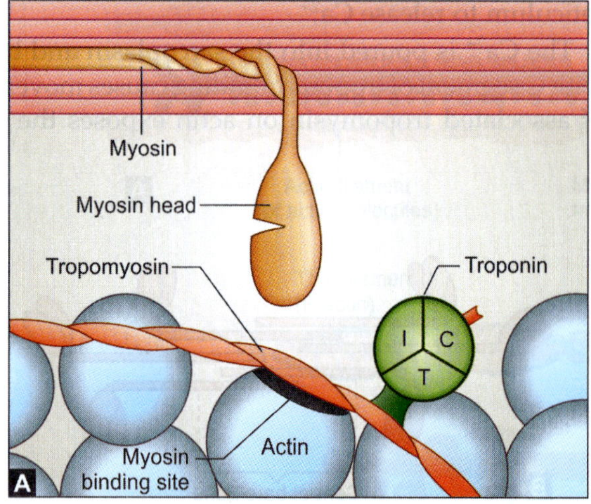

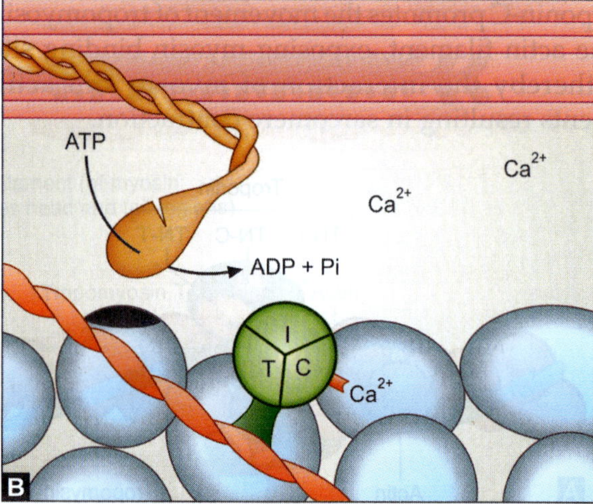

Figs 3.7A and B: (A) Myosin binding region (dark area) on actin is covered by tropomyosin and (B) Initiation of muscle contraction by Ca^{2+}, Ca^{2+} binds to troponin C, tropomyosin is displaced laterally, exposing the binding site. Binding of myosin to the site, using energy from ATP causes sliding movement of actin over myosin, shortening the sarcomere

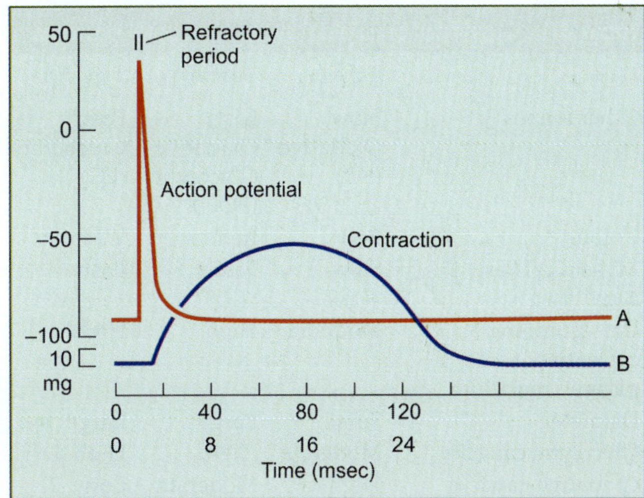

Fig. 3.8: Electrical (A) and mechanical (B) responses of a fast-twitch skeletal muscle fiber. Because the refractory period of the action potential is over before the mechanical response of the fibre even begins, skeletal muscle can be tetanized by rapid stimulation

increases, such a contraction is described as ***isometric contraction*** (there is no change in the length of the muscle but there is increase in the tension in the muscle).

On the other hand when *contraction occurs with shortening in the length of the muscle and no change in the tension in the muscle it is described as* ***isotonic contraction***.

Body posture is maintained by isometric contraction. Majority of the muscles can contract both isometrically and isotonically and many physical activities as such walking or running involve both type of contractions.

The Muscle Twitch

A single impulse (action potential) to the muscle causes a brief contraction followed by relaxation. This response is called muscle twitch (Fig. 3.8). The duration of the twitch varies with the type of muscle fiber. **Fast muscle fibers** produce *brief twitches* whereas **slow fibers produce** long twitches and they are concerned with *strong, gross sustained contraction* (as in the **maintenance of posture**) as opposed to the ***fast fibers*** which are concerned with *fine, rapid and accurate movements* (as described later).

Summation of Contractions and Tetanus

If another stimulus is given to the muscle before there is relaxation from the previous contraction, the responses add up resulting in stronger contraction which is called summation of contractions. If stimuli are repeatedly given, so that activation of the contractile mechanism occurs repeatedly before relaxation has occurred and the individual contractions fuse into a continuous contraction, this response is called tetanus (Fig. 3.9).

It is complete tetanus if there is no relaxation between contractions; incomplete tetanus when there are periods of incomplete relaxation between the responses.

Relation between Muscle Length, Tension and Velocity of Contraction

If length of muscle is increased the tension developed increases up to a length after which it decreases as recorded in experiments.

The length of the muscle at which active tension is maximal is called the resting length (Fig. 3.10). It is believed to be the length (of the muscle) in the body.

The **velocity** of muscle contraction varies inversely with load on the muscle.

At a given load, the **velocity** of contraction is maximal at the resting length and declines if the muscle is shorter or longer than this length.

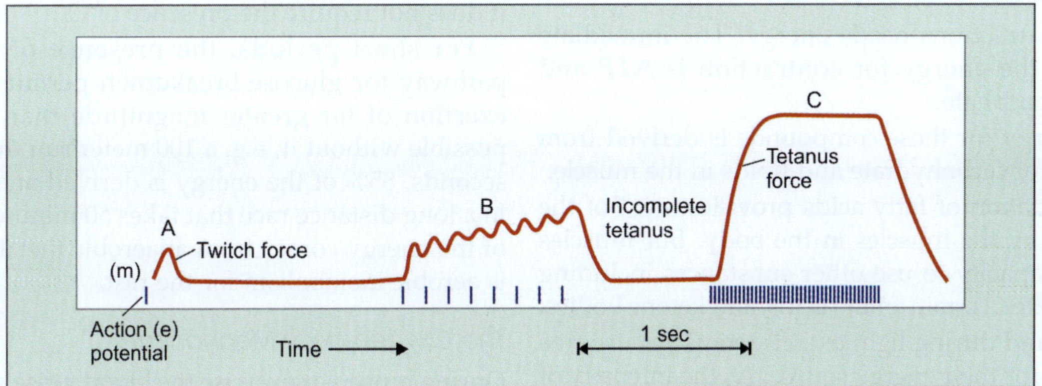

Fig. 3.9: (A) Single stimulus and contraction in response to it; (B) Incomplete tetanus; (C) Complete tetanus (e) electrical stimulus; (m) mechanical response

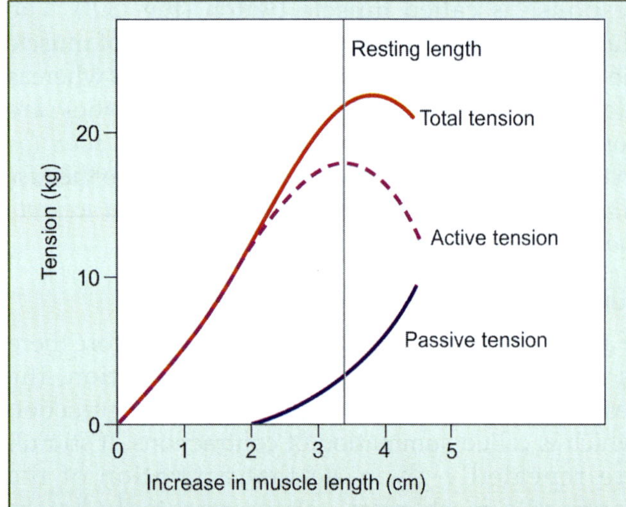

Fig. 3.10: Length-tension relationship for the human muscle. The passive tension curve measures the tension exerted by muscle at each length when it is not stimulated. The total tension curve represents the tension developed when the muscle contracts isometrically in response to a maximal stimulus. The active tension is the difference between the two

Table 3.1: Classification of fiber types in skeletal muscles

	Type I	*Type IIA*	*Type IIB*
Other names	Slow, Oxidative (SO)	Fast, Oxidative Glycolytic (FOG)	Fast, Glycolytic (FG)
Colour	Red	Red	White
Myosin ATPase activity	Slow	Fast	Fast
Ca^{2+}-pumping capacity of sarcoplasmic reticulum	Moderate	High	High
Diameter	Small	Large	Large
Glycolytic capacity	Moderate	High	High
Oxidative capacity	High	Moderate	Low
Associated motor unit type	Slow (S)	Fast Resistant to Fatigue (FR)	Fast Fatigable (FF)
Resting Membrane potential = – 90 mv			

Fiber types

The skeletal muscle fibers differ in some ways from one another. The fibers are roughly divided into two, type I and type II.

The muscles containing many type I fibers are called **red muscles**, because they are darker than other muscles. *They respond slowly and are adapted for slow posture maintaining contractions*. The long muscles of the back are red muscles. **White muscles** contain mostly type II fibers, have short twitch durations and are specialized for fine, skilled movements. The extraocular muscles and some hand muscles contain many type II fibers and are classified as white muscles. Table 3.1 shows different characteristics of fiber types.

Energy Sources and Metabolism

Muscle contractions needs energy. The immediate source of the energy for contraction is ATP and creatine phosphate.

The energy for these compounds is derived from *metabolism* of carbohydrate and lipids in the muscle.

The oxidation of fatty acids provides most of the ATP used by the muscles in the body. But muscles have the capacity to use other substances including carbohydrates, certain amino acids, and ketone bodies.

At rest and during light exercise, muscles use free fatty acids for their energy source. As the intensity of exercise increases, lipids alone cannot supply energy fast enough and utilization of carbohydrates become predominant source. Glucose from bloodstream enters the muscle cells and is degraded through series of reactions to pyruvate; another source of pyruvate is glycogen in the muscle (Fig. 3.11A).

Metabolism: When adequate O_2 is present, pyruvate enters the citric acid cycle in mitrochondria and is metabolized to CO_2 and H_2O. This is ***aerobic glycolysis*** and large amounts of ATP are formed from ADP, during this whole process which started from glucose or glycogen in the muscle or from free fatty acids (Fig. 3.11B).

If O_2 supplies are insufficient the pyruvate formed from glucose does not enter the tricarboxylic acid cycle but is reduced to lactate. This process of ***anaerobic glycolysis*** is associated with net production of much smaller quantities of energy rich phosphate bonds, but it does not require the presence of O_2.

For short periods, the presence of anaerobic pathway for glucose breakdown permits muscular exertion of far greater magnitude than would be possible without it, e.g. a 100 meter run that takes 10 seconds, 85% of the energy is derived anaerobically; in a long distance race that takes 60 minutes, only 5% of the energy comes from anaerobic metabolism and is aerobic metabolism for the rest.

The Oxygen debt Mechanism

During muscular exercise the blood vessels dilate, the oxygen supply is increased and the oxygen consumption is increased; up to a point all the needs

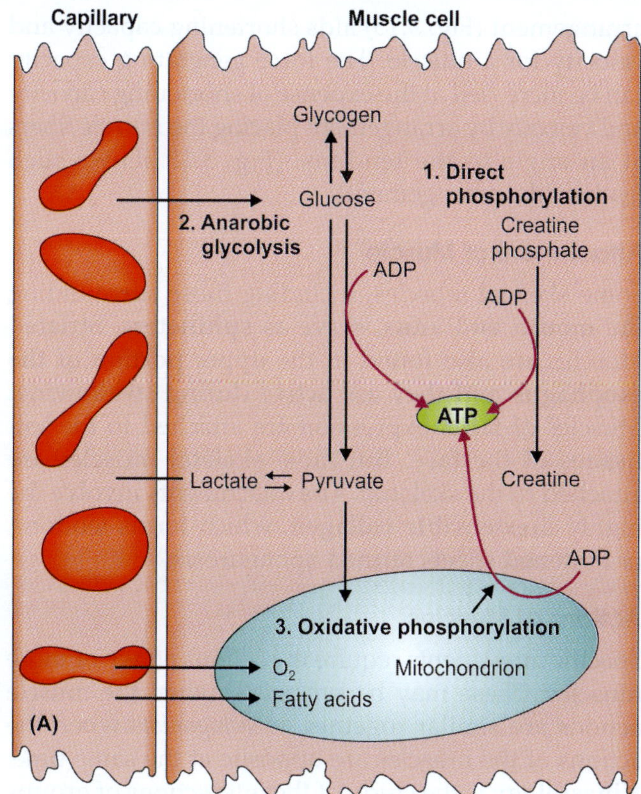

$$ATP + H_2O \longrightarrow ADP + H_3PO_4 + 7.3 \text{ kcal}$$

$$\text{Phosphorylcreatine} + ADP \rightleftharpoons \text{Creatine} + ATP$$

$$\text{Glucose} + 2\ ATP \text{ (or glycogen + 1 ATP)} \xrightarrow{\text{Anaerobic}} 2 \text{ Lactic acid} + 4\ ATP$$

$$\text{Glucose} + 2\ ATP \text{ (or glycogen + 1 ATP)} \xrightarrow{\text{Oxygen}} 6\ CO_2 + 6\ H_2O + 40\ ATP$$

$$FFA \xrightarrow{\text{Oxygen}} CO_2 + H_2O + ATP$$

(B)

Figs 3.11A and B: (A) Metabolic pathways in muscle. ATP is supplied via direct phosphorylation of ADP (1), glycolysis (2) and oxidative phosphorylation (3), (B) Comparison of number of ATP units formed from glucose under anaerobic and aerobic conditions. The amount of ATP formed per mole of free fatty acid (FFA) oxidized is large but varies with the size of the FFA. For example, complete oxidation of 1 mol of palmitic acid generates 140 mol of ATP.

are met with aerobic processes. But when muscular exertion is very great the energy stores cannot keep pace with their utilization.

Creatine phosphate is still used to re-synthesize ATP; it can only supply this energy for short periods; when the *oxygen supply is inadequate* anaerobic glycolysis takes place; it is rapid process and readily meets the ATP demands, even of very fast muscles. Hence, ***anaerobic glycolysis*** is important in these fast muscles and in all muscle cells when oxygen supply is inadequate; but the use of the anaerobic pathway is self-limiting because even with rapid diffusion of lactate into the bloodstream (Fig. 3.11A), enough accumulates in the muscle to ultimately exceed the capacity of the tissue buffers; resulting in the creation of an enzyme inhibiting decline in pH in the cell.

For ***long periods*** of **less intense aerobic exercise** oxidation is required for which necessary substrates are added from circulation to muscle glycogen for the production of necessary energy. With exercise of longer duration gluconeogeneses becomes increasingly important, amino acids are released by muscle and uptake by liver is increased.

Slow type I fibers can meet relatively low metabolic demands with oxidative phosphorylation. Molecules associated with oxygen binding (e.g. myoglobin, cytochromes) contain iron are red. Therefore, the red color of the oxidative muscle cell or a tissue containing mostly type I fibers has led to the classification of such types as red fibers. Myoglobin releases oxygen when oxygen tension falls very low in the cell.

Oxygen Debt

Muscle blood flow and oxygen uptake remain elevated for sometime after exercise; oxygen debt is the excess amount of oxygen consumed over that required for the resting metabolism when energy is not being used by the contractile system. The extra oxygen is consumed to remove the excess lactate, replenish the ATP and creatine phosphate stores and replace the small amounts of oxygen that have come from myoglobin. The debt is incured during exercise.

The amount of oxygen debt may be six times the basal O_2 consumption. The maximal debt can be incurred rapidly or slowly; violent exertion is possible for only short periods, whereas less strenuous exercise can be carried on for longer periods.

Rigor

When muscles are completely **depleted of ATP** and **creatine phosphate** they develop a **state of rigidity** called **Rigor**. When this occurs ***after death***, the condition is called **rigor mortis**. In rigor, almost all of the myosin heads attach to actin, but in abnormally fixed and resistant way.

Musculoskeletal Relationships

Individual muscle cells are enclosed in connective tissue layer called **endomysium.** Groups of muscle cells are bound by the **perimysium**. These are grouped together into the muscle which is covered by the **epimysium**. *These three connective tissue layers are composed of* **elastin** *and* **collagen** *fibrils.*

The muscles exert specific movements via tendons which are attached to the skeleton in most cases.

The output of the muscle depends on the size of the muscle cells and their anatomical arrangement. Increasing the diameter of a fiber by synthesis of new myofibrils **(hypertrophy)** will increase the force generating capacity of the cell.

The differentiated skeletal muscle has only a limited capacity to form new cells.

The force generating capacity is unchanged if the length of the cells is increased by adding more sacromeres in series without increasing the cross-sectional area of the cells; but the velocity of contraction and the total shortening capacity of the cell increase with the addition of more sacrcomeres (Fig. 3.12).

The output of muscle depends also in the orientation of the cells within the tissue. Parallel arrangement (Fig. 3.13) aids shortening capacity and velocity for a muscle. The force generating capacity can be increased at the expense of shortening capacity and velocity by arrangement placing the muscle fibers at an angle to the tendons. (Fig. 3.13 shows such feather like arrangement).

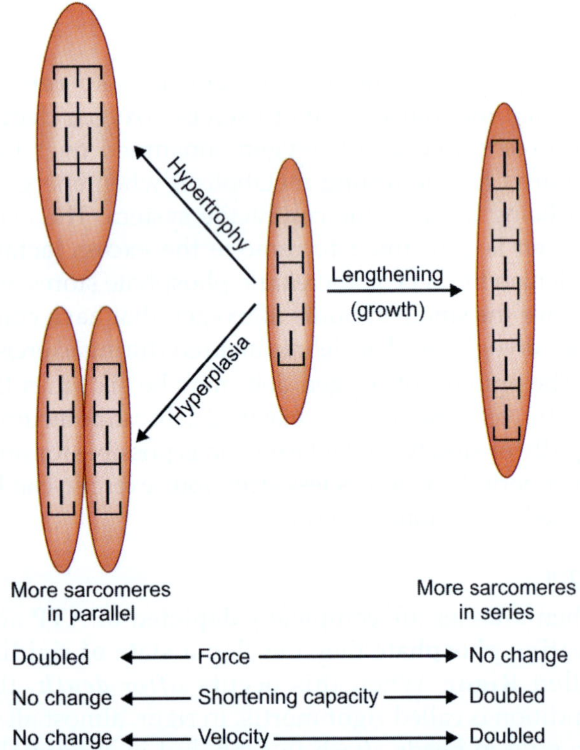

Fig. 3.12: Effects of growth on the muscle cell. Growth may be hypertrophy, i.e. adding of new myofibrils within a cell, hyperplasia, i.e. formation of new cells or adding more sarcomeres in series when the muscle cells lengthen along with skeletal growth. The effects of the cell growth on the force, shortening capacity and velocity of contraction are summarized

Attachment of Muscle

Some skeletal muscles, including those surrounding the **mouth and anus**, serve as **sphincters**. Striated muscles are also found in the **upper portion of the esophagus** and they are active during swallowing. Muscles of facial expression are attached to the soft tissues of the face. But most skeletal muscles are attached to the skeleton. The attachments involve the highly **inextensible collagen,** which forms tendons, or flattened sheets termed aponeurosis.

Actions of Muscles

Specific movements require the actions of two or more muscles. These may be *synergists*, when the muscle actions are similar together or *antagonists* when the actions of the muscles are opposite at the same time. **Kinesiology** is the study of the interactions of groups of muscles. Interactions of the muscles serve not only

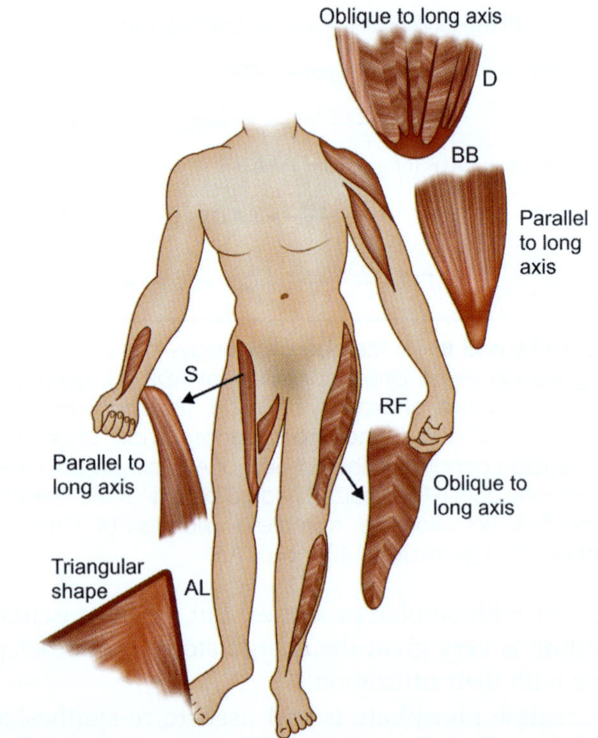

Fig. 3.13: The form and distribution of several varieties of striated skeletal muscle; the multipennate, deltoid (D); fusiform, biceps brachi (BB), bipennate, rectus femoris (RF) triangular adductor longus (AL) and strap-like sartorius (S)

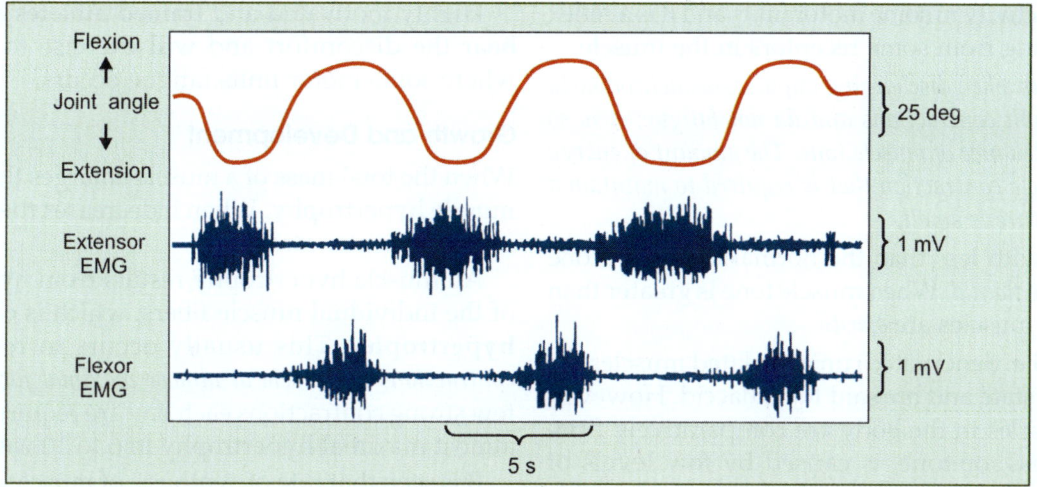

Fig. 3.14: EMG record

to move a specific bone but also to fix or stabilize another bone or joint.

The skeleton also acts as a lever system with mechanical advantages, large movements can occur with little shortening.

Large forces can be placed on tendons by large muscles, such as gastrocnemius. This can lead to rupture of the tendon.

Electromyography

Summed electrical activity of a muscle (Fig. 3.14) is detected from the electrodes placed over the skin. Also a technique can detect the activity of a single cell with needle electrodes inserted into the muscle.

MOTOR UNIT

Axons of spinal ***motor neurons*** supply the muscle fibers. Each axon on reaching the muscle divides into a number of branches and each one branch supplies one single muscle fiber. *One motor neuron and all the muscle fibers it supplies are called a* **motor unit** (Fig. 3.15). It is the smallest unit which contracts, i.e. the impulse originating from one motor neuron and traveling via its axons stimulates all the muscle fibers that this nerve fiber supplies; resulting in their contraction and so the *smallest unit of contraction is not a single fiber but one motor unit. The strength of contraction increases as more motor units are recruited.*

The number of muscle fibers in each motor unit varies. The muscles, such as those of hand and those concerned with motion of the eye, i.e. *muscle concerned with fine graded precise movements have few muscle fibers in one motor unit. The large muscles of the back have large numbers of muscle fibers in one motor unit.*

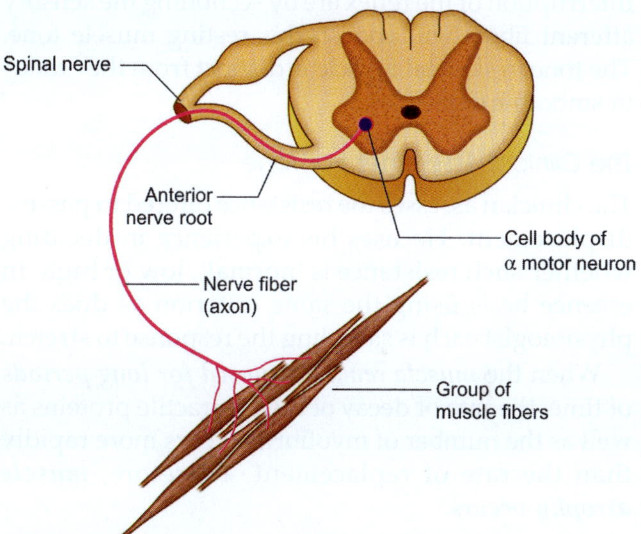

Fig. 3.15: A motor unit. Consists of a motor neuron and a group of muscle fibers that it innervates

Factors Responsible for Grading of Muscular Activity

There is little spontaneous activity in skeletal muscles of normal individuals at rest. With minimal voluntary activity a few motor units act, with *increasing voluntary effort more* and **more motor units** are brought into action. This process is called ***recruitment of motor units***.

In addition, **increase in frequency** of discharge of impulse in a nerve fiber results in stronger contractions of muscle fibers it supplies (tension developed during tetanic contraction being stronger).

SKELETAL MUSCLE TONE

The skeletal system supports the body mass efficiently when the tone is normal. Muscles relaxed in the body are firm, this tone is due to low level of contractile activity in some motor units and it is a reflex activity arising from some receptors in the muscle.

Motor units when discharging impulses asynchronously produce smooth contractions and do not fatigue; it is so during maintenance of muscle tone. The amount of energy used for muscle contraction that is required to maintain a standing posture is small.

Muscles with less than the normal degree of tone are said to be *flaccid*. When muscle tone is greater than normal, the muscles are *spastic*.

Isolated (i.e. denervated) unstimulated muscles are in a relaxed state and are said to be flaccid. However, relaxed muscles in the body are comparatively firm. This firmness, or tone, is caused by low levels of contractile activity in some of the motor units and is driven by reflex arcs from the muscle spindles. Interruption of the reflex are by sectioning the sensory afferent fibers will abolish this resting muscle tone. The tone in skeletal muscle is distinct from the "tone" in smooth muscle.

The Clinical Assessment of Tone

The clinician assesses the resistance offered to passive displacement. He uses his experience in deciding whether such resistance is 'normal', low or high. In essence he is using the same criterion as does the physiologist each is sampling the response to stretch.

When the ***muscle remains unused for long periods*** of time, the rate of decay of the contractile proteins as well as the number of myofibrils occurs more rapidly than the rate of replacement. Therefore, ***muscle atrophy occurs***.

Fatigue

The causes for it are not clearly understood. Fatigue may occur in any of the process from the brain to the muscles and in the process of muscle contraction, as well as in systems involved in maintaining ***energy and oxygen*** supplies including cardiovascular and respiratory functions.

Experimentally when muscles are ***stimulated by tetanic stimuli*** after some time the strength of contraction gradually decreases, as *there is depletion of glycogen and creatine phosphate and accumulation of lactic acid*; these factors are responsible for fatigue that starts occuring.

Most persons tire and cease exercise long before there is any motor unit fatigue. ***General physical fatigue*** is a state of ***disturbed homeostasis*** produced by work. The basis for discomfort or pain *probably involves many factors, like lowering of plasma glucose levels and accumulation of metabolites*.

Highly motivated and trained athletes are able to bear the discomfort and will exercise to the point where some motor units fatigue occurs.

Growth and Development

When the total mass of a muscle enlarges this is called muscle hypertrophy. When it decreases the process is called muscular atrophy.

All muscle hypertrophy results from hypertrophy of the individual muscle fibers, which is called **fiber hypertrophy**. This usually occurs in response to *contractions of muscle at almost maximal force*. Only a few strong contractions each day are required to cause almost maximal hypertrophy in 6 to 10 weeks.

It is seen that rate of synthesis of muscle contractile proteins is far greater during developing hypertrophy than their rate of decay, leading to progressively greater number of both actin and myosin filaments in the myofibrils. In turn the myofibrils themselves split within each muscle fiber to form new myofibrils.

It is mainly this **great increase in member of additional myofibrils** that cause muscle fibers to hypertrophy. *The enzyme systems that provide energy also increase, especially enzymes of glycolytic system, providing energy for short-term forceful muscle contractions.*

Transmission of Impulse from Nerve to Skeletal Muscle (Neuromuscular Junction)

When the impulse reaches the nerve ending it releases a chemical transmitter, acetylcholine. The voltage change at presynaptic membrane with arrival of action potential causes opening up of voltage gated Ca^{2+} channels resulting in influx of Ca^{2+} that causes fusion of synaptic vesicles with presynaptic membrane which breaks down to release acetylcholine. The **acetylcholine** then passes across the small gap between the nerve and the muscle membrane (gap is called ***synaptic cleft***) and it binds with the receptors, ***nicotinic acetylcholine receptors*** present on the postsynaptic muscle membrane which at this junction is specialized to form **motor end plate** (Fig. 3.16).

The binding of acetylcholine to its receptors on the motor end plate results in change in permeability of the muscle membrane to ions; opening of Na^+ and K^+ channels. Influx of Na^+ results in depolarization of postsynaptic membrane called endplate potential (EPP) that with local current flow between EPP and adjacent sarcolemma results in action potential (or impulse) which travels along the muscle membrane (sarcolemma) of the fiber and produces contraction. The acetylcholine is then removed from its receptors

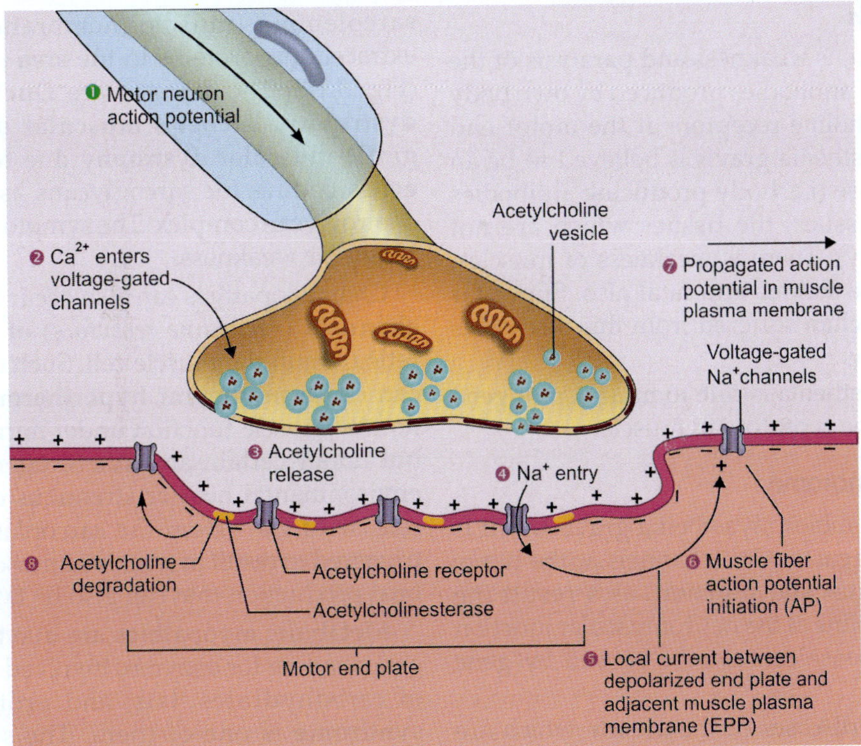

Fig. 3.16: Electron microscopic appearance showing the ultrastructure of the junction between an axon terminal and the muscle fiber membrane. The invagination of the sarcolemma forms the synaptic trough into which the axon terminal protrudes. The space between the plasma membrane of the axon and the invaginate sarcolemma is the synaptic cleft. The invaginate sarcolemma (postjunctional/postsynaptic membrane) has many folds which increase its surface area. Acetylcholine is stored in the synaptic vesicles in the axon terminal. Acetylcholine receptor protein and acetylcholinesterase are both associated with the postjunctional membrane.

by the action of an enzyme, **acetylcholinesterase** present around the motor end plate.

Table 3.2 summarizes the events leading to contraction of skeletal muscle.

Clinical Application

Skeletal Muscles in the Intact Organism

Destruction of nerve supply to the skeletal muscle causes **muscle atrophy**. It also leads to abnormal excitability of the muscle and increases sensitivity to the circulating acetylcholine. Fine irregular contractions of individual fibers, fibrillations appear. Atrophy is progressive in humans with degeneration of cells after 3–4 months. Most of the muscles fibers are replaced by fat and connective tissue after 1–2 years.

These changes are all reversed if re-innervation occurs within a few months, if motor nerve regenerates. The fibrillations disappear. Re-innervation is normally achieved by growth of the peripheral stump of the motor nerve axon along the old nerve sheath.

If the nerve regenerates muscle fiber function is restored. Nerve supply to a muscle fiber may be restored if:

- Regeneration of the nerve to the muscle takes place.
- There is the growth of a terminal from another axon that is supplying the adjacent muscle fiber.

Table 3.2: Sequence of events in contraction and relaxation of skeletal muscle

Steps in contraction

1. Impulse from motor neuron.
2. Release of transmitter (acetylcholine) from axon terminal at motor end plate.
3. Binding of acetylcholine to nicotinic acetylcholine receptors at motor end plate.
4. Increased Na^+ K^+ conductance in motor end plate membrane.
5. Generation of end plate potential (EPP).
6. Generation of action potential in muscle fibers.
7. Inward spread of depolarization along T tubules.
8. Release of Ca^{2+} from terminal cisterns of sarcoplasmic reticulum and diffusion to thin filaments.
9. Binding of Ca^{2+} to troponin C, uncovering myosin-binding sites on actin.
10. Formation of cross-linkages between actin and myosin, sliding of thin on thick filaments, producing shortening.

Steps in relaxation

1. Ca^{2+} pumped back into sarcoplasmic reticulum.
2. Release of Ca^{2+} from troponin.

Cessation of interaction between actin and myosin

Myasthenia Gravis

In this disease there is weakness and paralysis of the muscles because of antibodies produced by own body against its acetylcholine receptors at the motor end plate. Hence, myasthenia gravis is believed to be an autoimmune disease (i.e. body producing antibodies against its own tissues, the tissues which are not foreign to the body). There is weakness of muscles. This disease can be serious and fatal also. Superstar **Mr Amitabh Bachchan** suffered from this disease; is fully recovered now.

Congenital myasthenia is due to mutation of gene for the acetylcholine receptors in muscle.

Lambert-Eaton Syndrome

This condition resembles myasthenia gravis but it is due to antibodies against Ca^{2+} channels at the nerve ending at neuromuscular junction, as a result the release of acetylcholine at the neuromuscular junction decreases. The disease can also be caused by gene mutation.

There are other diseases of the muscle which are due to mutation in the genes coding for various components of dystrophin-glycoprotein complex which is present in the skeletal muscle and forms connection for contractile protein, for actin to the sarcolemma (muscle membrane) and also with extracellular proteins in the area around the muscle (Fig. 3.17). The diseases are **Duchenne's muscular dystrophy, Becher's muscular dystrophy. Limb-girdle muscular dystrophy due to mutation of the** genes coding for sarcoglycans associated with the dystroglycan complex. The symptoms are progressive muscular weakness.

Channelopathies can also occur in the **Ca^{2+} release channels** (*ryanodine receptors*) of the sarcoplasmic reticulum in the muscle cell. Such channel mutations can cause **malignant hyperthermia** where there is normal muscle function under normal circumstances but under certain anaesthetic agents or under high environmental heat or strenuous exercise abnormal release of Ca^{2+} from the sarcoplasmic reticulum is triggered to result in sustained muscle contraction and heat production that can also be fatal.

Metabolic myopathies are due to mutation in the genes coding for enzymes involved in the metabolism of carbohydrates, fats, and proteins. **McArdle's syndrome** is one of them. The symptoms of this diseases differ according to the enzyme defective but the common features are exercise intolerance and possibly of muscle breakdown due to accumulation of toxic metabolites.

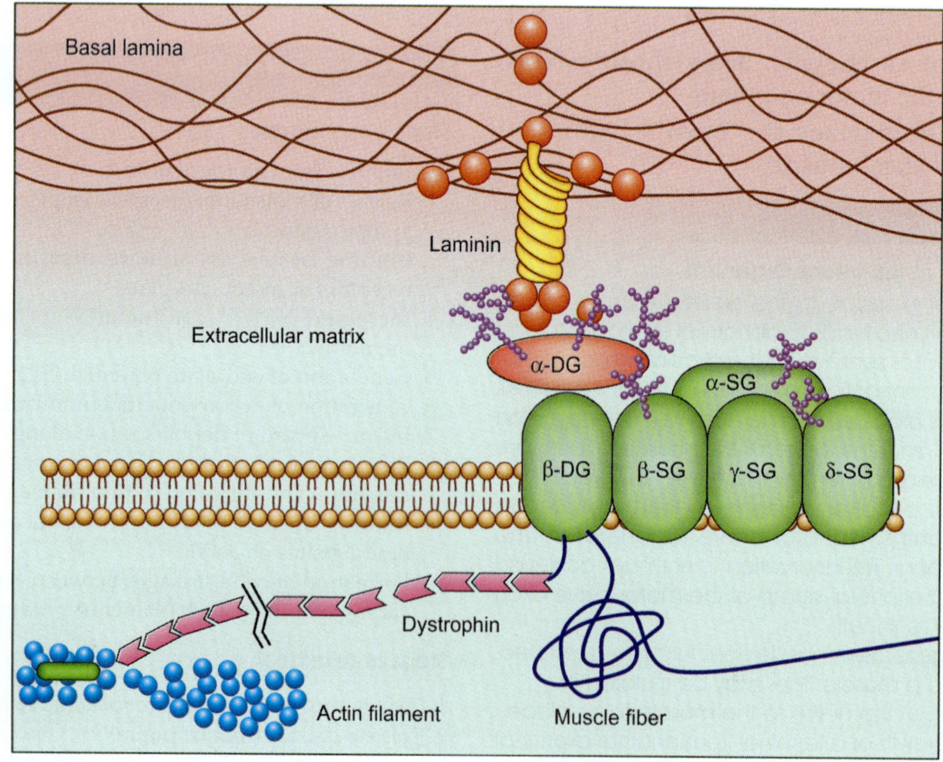

Fig. 3.17: Dystroglycan complex

Myotonia, in various forms; the muscle relaxation is prolonged after voluntary contraction. Diseases are also due to mutation of genes.

Muscle Injury

Muscle fiber may be damaged accidentally or be cut during surgery. Healing depends upon the extent of damage. Damaged tissue is removed by phagocytosis and replaced by granulation tissue.

- If the injury is slight the small gap in the muscle fiber is bridged by outgrowth from the surviving ends of the fiber and recovery occurs.
- In more extensive injury the muscle fiber outgrowths may not be able to bridge the gap by extending into granulation tissue, and so the remaining granulation tissue becomes fibrosed and scar tissue forms. In time this contracts and may restrict the joint movement.
- In cases of crush injury there may be systemic serious effects. Ischemia of muscle results in massive muscle necrosis. Myoglobin and other necrotic products are released from damaged muscle and enter blood. This material is highly toxic to the kidneys and acute renal failure may develop. Complication is infection especially with anaerobic microbes causing gas gangrene. Healing of such extensive injury is by fibrosis.

CARDIAC MUSCLE

It is ***striated*** but functionally it is ***involuntary*** and the nerve supply is by ***autonomic nerves***. It regularly originates its own beat for contraction from the ***pacemaker region***. *This* property is called ***auto-rhythmicity***.

Myocardium: The myocardium is formed of muscle fibers which like the skeletal muscle fibers are *cross striated on microscopic* examination but muscle is *not* under voluntary control. The muscle *fibers branch* but each fiber is surrounded by *complete cell membrane;* where end of one muscle fiber comes in contact with another, the membrane of both fibers are bound together to form dense structures, ***intercalated disks*** (Fig. 3.18), *which provide a strong union between fibers,* maintaining a cell-to-cell cohesion so that pull of one contractile unit can be transmitted along its axis to the next.

There are ***functional connections*** between individual muscle fibers and the impulse can spread from one fiber to another fiber, i.e. cardiac muscle is a ***functional syncytium*** (there are no anatomical connections between muscle fibers yet due to presence of ***gap junctions between adjoining fibers***, there is *transmission of impulse to the adjoining fibers*).

Action potential in the cardiac muscle fiber has ***long duration*** that lasts almost the period of contraction and during this time muscle is refractory to another stimulus (Fig. 3.19). Hence, tetanus by repeated stimuli of the type in skeletal muscle cannot be produced in cardiac muscle. This fact is of advantage to cardiac muscle.

Contractile Responses

The contractile response begins just after the start of depolarization. The role of Ca^{2+} in excitation and contraction coupling is similar to skeletal muscle, but here influx of Ca^{2+} from the extracellular fluid through 'T' system triggers release of Ca^{2+} from sarcoplasmic reticulum. This involves the role of Ca^{2+} ATPase and Na^+/Ca^{2+} exchanger in expelling the extra Ca^{2+} entry into ECF after the contraction is over.

Cardiac muscle ***resembles slow skeletal muscle*** as it has myosin isoenzymes with low ATPase activities.

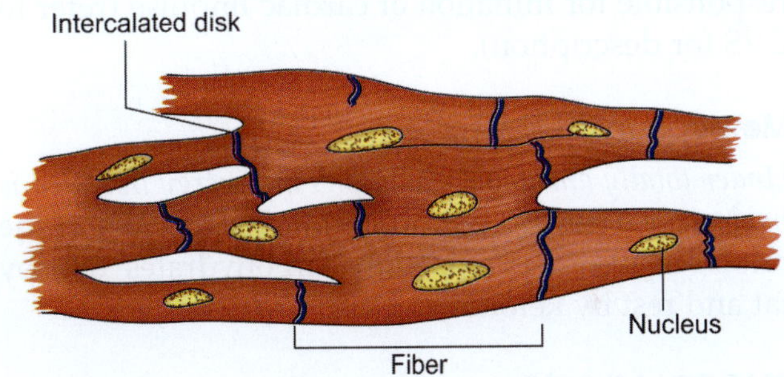

Fig. 3.18: Cardiac muscle under light microscope

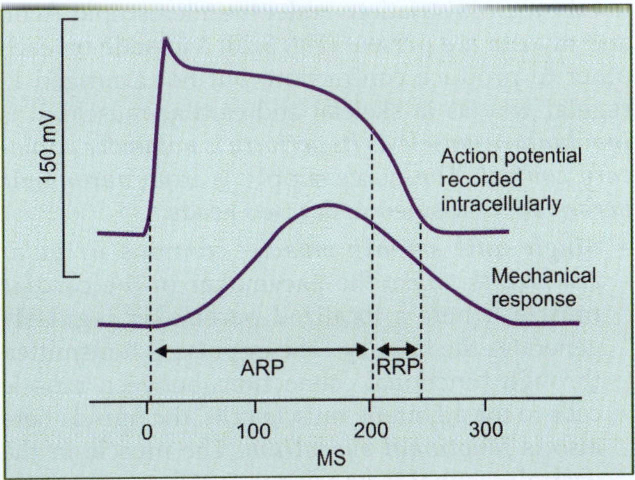

Fig. 3.19: Action potential and contractile response of mammalian cardiac muscle fiber plotted on the same time axis. ARP, absolute refractory period; RRP, relative refractory period

Since it is continuously active muscle ***it is almost entirely oxidative and is highly sensitive to interruption to its blood supply. Muscle fibers have high myoglobin content and numerous mitochondria.***

Correlation between Muscle Fiber Length and Tension

The developed tension increases as the diastolic volume increases until it reaches a maximum and then tends to decrease. ***Starling's law of the heart states that force of contraction is proportional to the initial length of muscle fibers*** within physiological limits.

The force of contraction of cardiac muscle can also increases with catecholamines and this occurs without a change in muscle length. This is positive inotropic effect of catecholamines mediated by β adrenergic receptors.

The nerve supply is by the *autonomic nerves*. The *nerves only modify the rate of heart beat* which is *initiated* by the *pacemaker* in the heart. *Activity of the vagal nerves* (parasympathetic nerves) *slows the heart rate whereas the activity of the sympathetic nerves increases the heart rate*. The pacemaker potential has the features responsible for initiation of cardiac impulse (refer to CVS for description).

Metabolism

Under totally anaerobic conditions the energy liberated is inadequate to sustain ventricular contractions 35% of the caloric heads are provided by carbohydrates 60% by fat and rest by ketones and amino acids.

SMOOTH MUSCLE

Smooth muscle is found in hollow organs and it does not show cross-striations under the microscopic. Actin and myosin are present (Fig. 3.20) and slide on each other to produce contraction, but not arranged in regular way as in skeletal and cardiac muscle. It is ***involuntary muscle as its activity is not under voluntary control***. The nerve supply is from ***autonomic nerves.*** It is classified under two heads.

- ***Single unit smooth muscle***; contains *irregular pacemakers unlike* the pacemaker in the cardiac muscle, where a localized pacemaker regularly generates the impulse. The impulse is transmitted through functional connections between muscle cells to the adjoining muscle cells, the muscle here also is ***functional syncytium***. The muscle in the **gastrointestinal tract** belongs to this group.
- ***Multiunit smooth muscle.*** In this group of smooth muscles the activity *in one fiber does not* spread to another fiber. *Contractions are discrete and in response to nerve impulses* of the *autonomic nervous system (involuntary nervous system)*. There is *no spontaneous activity* as no pacemakers are present. These muscles are involved in *fine, discrete, graded contractions. This type is* present in the **iris** and **ciliary muscles** of the eye.

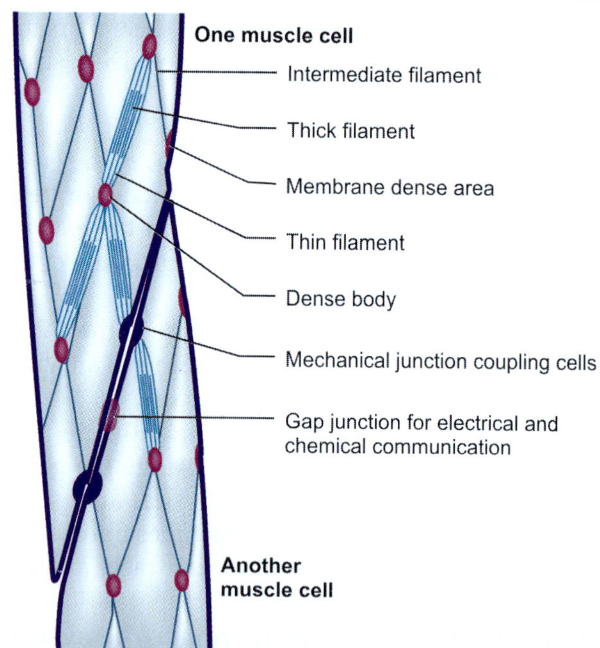

Fig. 3.20: The cytoskeleton and myofilaments in smooth muscles. Small contractile elements equivalent to a sarcomere underlie the similarities in between smooth and skeletal muscles. But regular striation are absent. Linkages functionally couple the contractile apparatus of adjacent cells

Single unit smooth muscle is present in gastrointestinal tract, where the function is to mix and propel the contents. Coordination of contraction of the muscle fibers occurs because of a nerve plexus present between the longitudinally and circularly arranged muscle fibers. The plexus is linked to autonomic nerves.

The muscle cells show *fluctuating membrane potential* (Fig. 3.21) unlike the steady resting membrane potential of skeletal muscle cells. The ***membrane potential decreases*** (*excitability of muscle increases*) with acetylcholine, parasympathetic stimulation **cold** and **stretch** of the muscle; whereas *sympathetic stimulation and epinephrine increase the membrane potential making the muscle less excitable.*

The mechanism of contraction is slightly different in smooth muscle; instead of calcium combining with troponin to lead to contraction it combines with ***calmodulin*** a protein present in the muscle cell and the events for contraction follow. The relaxation may not follow for some time when the calcium ions have

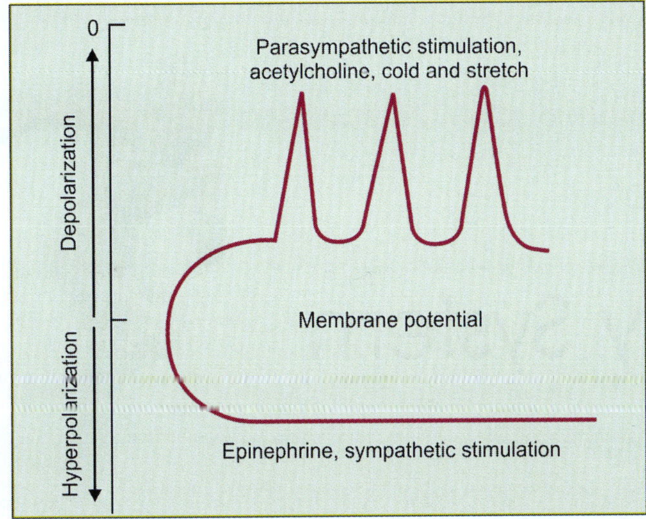

Fig. 3.21: Effects of various agents and membrane potential of intestinal smooth muscle

Table 3.3: Sequence of events in contraction and relaxation of visceral smooth muscle

1. Binding of acetylcholine to muscarinic receptors in the cell membrane
2. Influx of Ca^{2+} into the cell (influx from extracellular fluid). In skeletal muscle, instead Ca^{2+} released from terminal cisterna no unflux from ECF.
3. Activation of calmodulin-dependent myosin light chain kinase, when Ca^{2+} binds to calmodulin.
4. Phosphorylation of myosin
5. Increased myosin ATPase activity and binding of myosin to actin
6. Results in contraction
7. Dephosphorylation of myosin by myosin light chain phosphatase
8. Results in relaxation, or sustained contraction due to the latch bridge and other mechanisms.

been withdrawn from the cell cytoplasm because of mechanism described as latch bridge mechanism (Table 3.3).

Smooth muscles in the wall of circular structures, such as urinary bladder or rectum passively allow the organ to increase in size with accumulation of urine or feces in each case. The cells are so arranged that they reduce the internal volume to zero during urination or defecation in each case.

Growth of Smooth Muscle

Proliferation of smooth muscle cells occurs in hypertension. Growth factors involved are catecholamines and angiotensin II which stimulate growth.

Dihydropyridine Receptors (DHPR)

The action potential causing depolarization of 'T' tubule triggers release of Ca^{2+} from terminal cisterns of sarcoplasmic reticulum next to T system. DHPR are voltage-gated Ca^{2+} channels in the T tubule membrane. In cardiac muscle influx of Ca^{2+} via these channels triggers release of Ca^{2+} stored in sarcoplasmic reticulum by activating there the ryanodine receptors (RyR). RyR is a ligands gated Ca^{2+} channel. In skeletal muscle Ca^{2+} entery from ECF by this route is not required for Ca^{2+} release in sarcoplasm. Instead DHPR serves as a voltage sensor to unlock the nearby RyR in terminal cisterna of sarcoplasmic reticulum to release Ca^{2+}.

IMPLICATIONS AND APPLICATIONS

- Feel the normal tone of the muscles. Feel the loss of tone in paralysed muscle.
- Perform the actions of important muscles of neck, e.g. sternocleidomastoid, trapezius; muscles of upper limb, e.g. biceps brachii, triceps brachii, deltoid; of lower limb, e.g. quadriceps femoris, hamstrings, gluteus maximus, gluteus medius, tibialis anterior and tendocalcaneus.
- Contract muscle against resistance and feel the strength of the muscle. Feel the peristaltic movements of intestine.
- Feel important bony land marks especially those assisting in giving intramuscular injections.

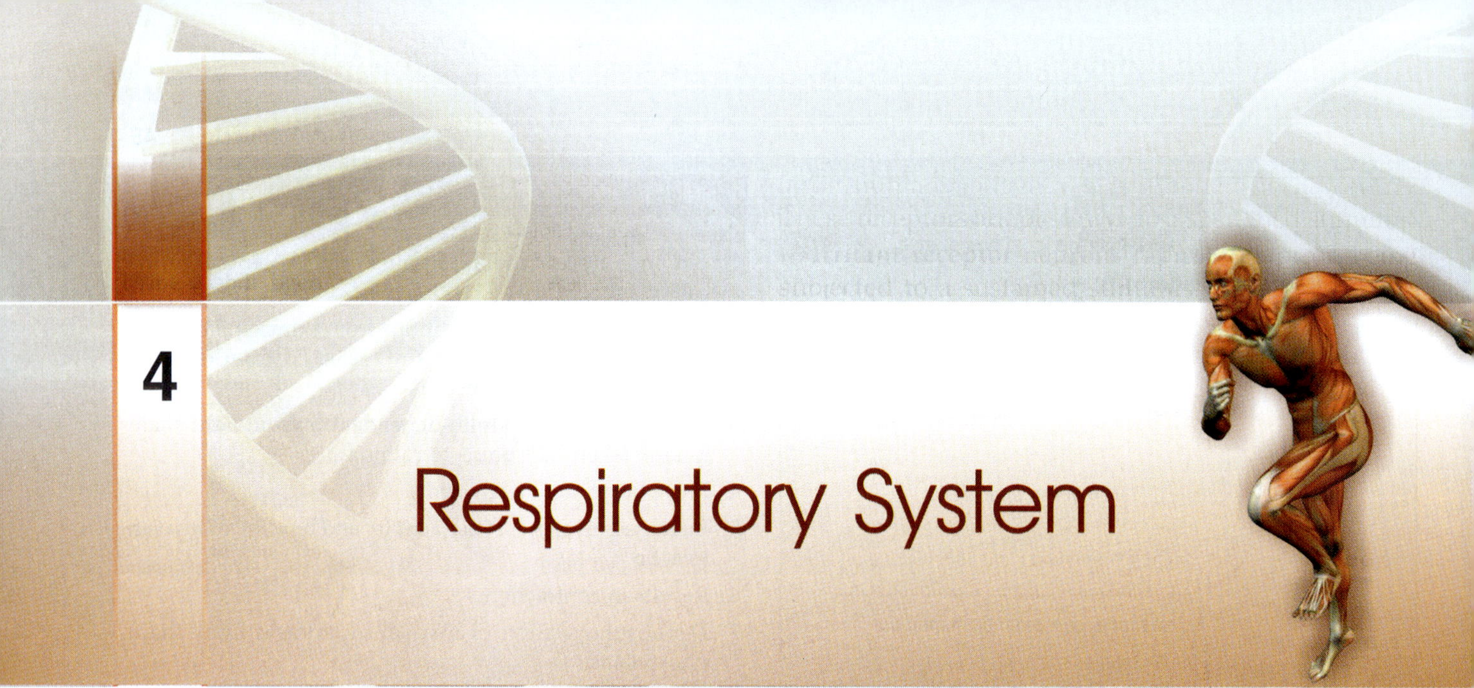

4 Respiratory System

Breathing is **automatic, rhythmic** process *regulated by* **neurons in the brainstem,** in the central nervous system. The activity of the neurons produce contractions and relaxations of the ***skeletal muscles of diaphragm, rib cage and abdomen*** which cause air to move in and out of terminal respiratory units, where exchange of gases takes place across the blood capillaries of the lung.

Respiration includes two processes:

- ***External respiration,*** the absorption of O_2 and removal of CO_2 from the body.
- ***Internal respiration,*** the utilization of O_2 and production of CO_2 by cells and the exchange with tissue fluid.

EXTERNAL RESPIRATION

The respiratory system is made-up of gas exchange organs, the lungs with their coverings, the pleura; and the respiratory muscles, which increase and decrease the size of thoracic cavity. The areas in the brainstem (Pons and Medulla) control the muscles and are responsible for successive inspirations and expirations. In quiet breathing the inspiration is an active process produced by the contractions of the muscles of inspiration, expiration is a passive process produced when the inspiratory muscles relax. *During inspiration the size of the thoracic cavity is increased by descent of the diaphragm due to its contraction, and by outward movement of the ribs due to contraction of external intercostals muscles.* The diaphragm is supplied by motor neurons of C3, 4 and 5; and intercostals muscles by motor neurons of T1 to T12. Both these sets of neurons are stimulated by impulses from inspiratory center of the ***respiratory center*** complex *in the brainstem*. The *elastic lungs* follow this thoracic expansion passively and room air enters into the depths of the lungs. *At the end of inspiration the external intercostals muscles and diaphragm relax; the recoil of the thoracic wall and lungs cause passive expiration.*

During inspiration, air enters by nose and mouth and passes through the glottis to the trachea and then by two main bronchi and their branches to bronchioles the terminal and then to the respiratory bronchioles, which give rise to alveolar ducts (Fig. 4.1) which lead to the pulmonary alveoli. The pulmonary alveoli consist of single layer of large flat thin epithelial cells against which lie numerous pulmonary capillaries (Fig. 4.2).

At rest, an adult person **breathes 12–15 times a minute**, about **500 ml air** is inspired and expired per breath (this volume is known as ***tidal volume***) amounting to 6 to 8 L of air breathed in or out in a minute. The air breathed in mixes with air that is present in the alveoli; the capillary blood is around the alveoli, exchange of O_2 by diffusion from alveoli into capillary blood and CO_2 from capillary blood into alveoli takes place.

During expiration, the air is breathed out but the alveoli do not empty completely; with next breath the inspired air mixes with alveolar air already present.

Under ordinary resting conditions, **250 ml of O_2 enters** the body **per minute** and **200 ml of CO_2 is expelled per minute** with these respiratory movements.

For successful respiration to occur, oxygen and nutrients must be brought to the vicinity of the tissue

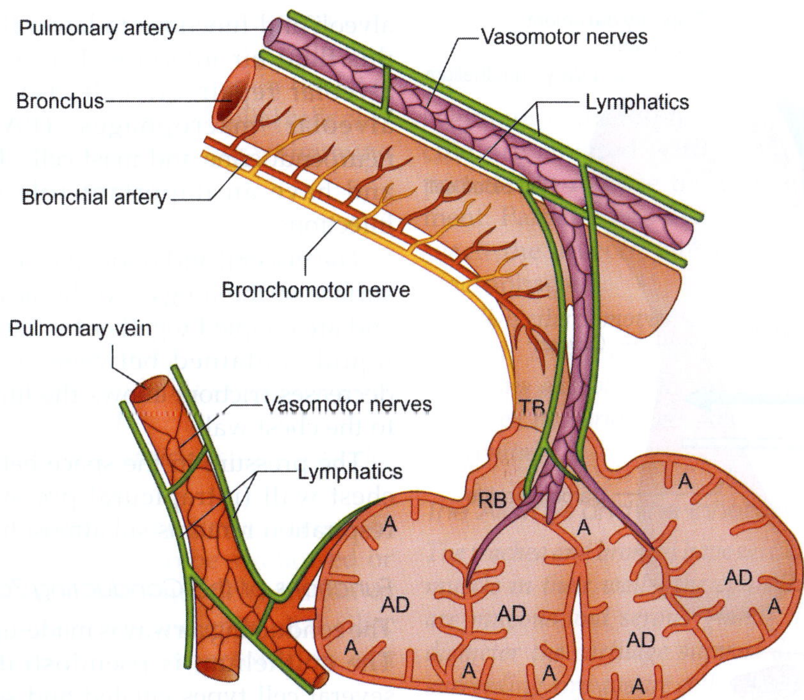

Fig. 4.1: Structure of the lung. A alveolus: AD. alveolar duct: RB, respiratory bronchiole; TB, terminal bronchiole. The air filling respiratory passages up to TB does not take part in gas exchange (anatomical dead space). Further down from respiratory bronchioles it takes place

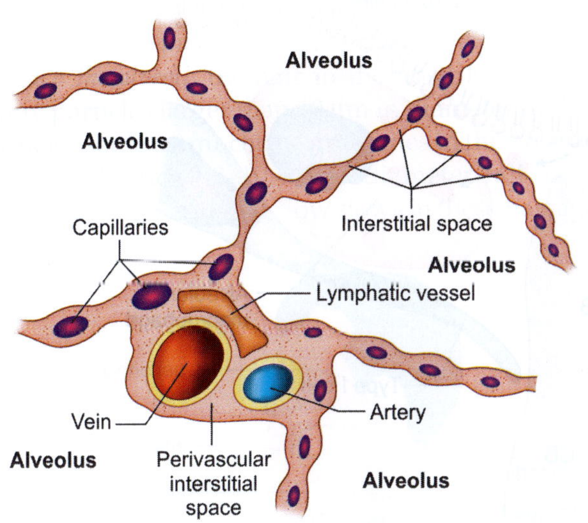

Fig. 4.2: Alveoli surrounded by capillaries

cells, whereas CO_2 and other waste products must be taken away from these cells; the *circulatory system* carries whatever is needed *to* and *from* the tissue cells and to and from the lungs.

When the air is expired from the lungs, the alveoli do not empty completely; this permits exchange of gases to continue in the alveoli and capillary blood throughout the respiratory cycle.

The partial pressure of for oxygen is 100 mmHg and that of carbon dioxide is 40 mmHg in the alveolar air.

Gases diffuse from areas of higher pressure to the lower pressure; the rate of diffusion depends upon concentration gradient and nature of barrier. Venous blood from pulmonary artery reaches the lungs, and under ordinary conditions has partial pressure of oxygen at 40 mmHg and partial pressure of carbon dioxide at 46 mmHg. The gases diffuse from higher pressure to lower pressure; the barrier between the air in the alveoli and blood in the capillaries around it is thin (Fig. 4.3) permits the exchange of gases to take place.

The ***conducting zone*** of the airways transports gas through trachea, bronchi, bronchioles and terminal bronchioles. The ***gas exchange occurs*** in respiratory bronchioles, alveolar ducts and alveoli. The total cross section area is greatly increased from trachea to the alveoli, hence velocity of air flow declines to low values in the terminal airways.

The alveoli are lined by two types of epithelial cells. Type I cells are flat cells with large cytoplasmic extensions and are primary lining cells. Type II cells, the granular cells (Fig. 4.4) are thicker and contain numerous inclusion bodies. These cells secrete **surfactant,** which is present in the fluid lining the

Anatomical Dead Space

With inspiration the air which remains in the ***conducting parts of airways***, i.e. nose, mouth, pharynx, larynx, trachea, bronchi and terminal bronchioles (Fig. 4.7) no exchange of gases takes place and is called **anatomical dead space.** The same amount of air fills the passages during expiration. With a tidal volume of 500 ml, approximately 150 ml is anatomical dead space and 350 ml enters the respiratory exchange area in one breath and this is *alveolar ventilation per breath*; this volume increases with increase in tidal volume since the anatomical dead space would remain the same. When there is rapid shallow breathing there is much less alveolar ventilation than per breath when there is deep breathing.

Physiological Dead Space (Wasted Ventilation)

In a perfect lung all the alveoli receive ventilation ($\dot{V}$) and blood flow ($\dot{Q}$) in the same proportion. This is referred to as *uniform ventilation/perfusion* ratio ($\dot{V}/(\dot{Q})$ ratio). Though the ideal condition may not exist in healthy individuals but it can be markedly abnormal in diseased lungs.

Ventilation of anatomical dead space is necessary, but it is wasted as no exchange takes place. But in addition if terminal lung units do not receive any pulmonary blood flow, though are ventilated, that part of ventilation is wasted; this forms ***alveolar dead space*** (present in diseased conditions). Hence under these conditions the total dead space becomes more than anatomical dead space. Physiological dead space (which means total dead space) is the ***sum*** of *anatomical dead space* and any *alveolar dead space. In health the anatomical and physiological dead space are identical (the same value), as there is no alveolar dead space.*

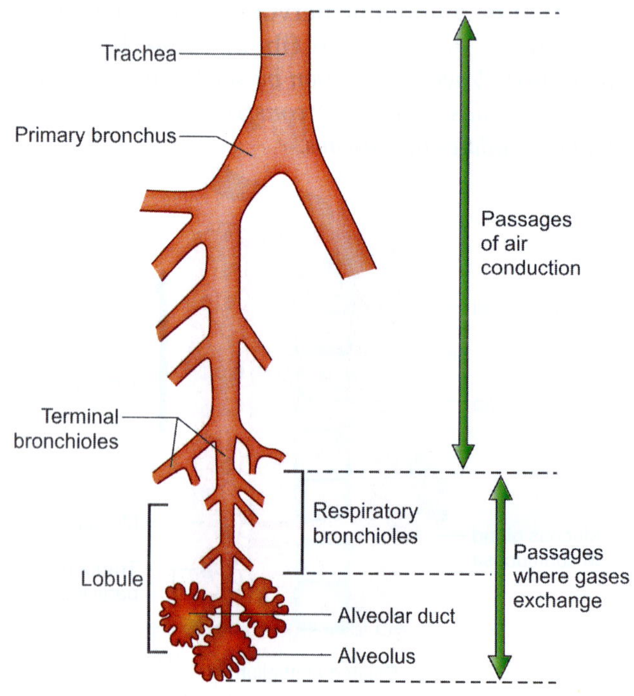

Fig. 4.7: Lower respiratory tract

Pulmonary Ventilation Per Minute

Alveolar Ventilation Per Minute

Pulmonary ventilation per minute (respiratory minute volume) at any time is the air breathed in one breath multiplied by the rate of respiration. When an adult is in resting condition (with a tidal volume of 500 ml and respiratory rate of 12 per min) it is about = 12 × 500 ml = 6L/min.With this tidal volume the air that *ventilates the alveoli*, would be 350 ml × 12 = 4200 ml = 4.2L/per minute. This is called **alveolar ventilation per minute.**

MECHANICS OF RESPIRATION

The Chest Wall

The breathing is affected by the movements of chest wall, which includes rib cage, diaphragm and anterior abdominal wall. The lungs are passive during breathing and it is the muscles of the chest wall and diaphragm which expand the thoracic cavity and cause inspiration. The thoracic cavity enlarges during inspiration. The rib cage rotates upwards and outwards (pump-handle movement), increasing anterior posterior diameter and to some extent transverse diameter also; and the diaphragm descends into abdomen, increasing vertical diameter of the chest cavity (Fig. 4.8).

Intrapleural Pressure

The pressure in the space between the lungs and chest wall (intrapleural pressure) remains subatmospheric in normal quiet respiration.

The lungs at the end of quiet expiration have a tendency to recoil from the chest wall, and the recoil pressure of the lungs (inward recoil) is balanced by the recoil pressure of the chest wall to recoil in the opposite direction (outwards).

Hence, if the chest is opened, the lungs collapse; and also in the conditions in which the lungs lose their elasticity the chest expands and becomes barrel-shaped as in emphysema.

Respiratory Muscles

Inspiratory Muscles. Movements of ***diaphragm*** are important for the changes in intrathoracic volume

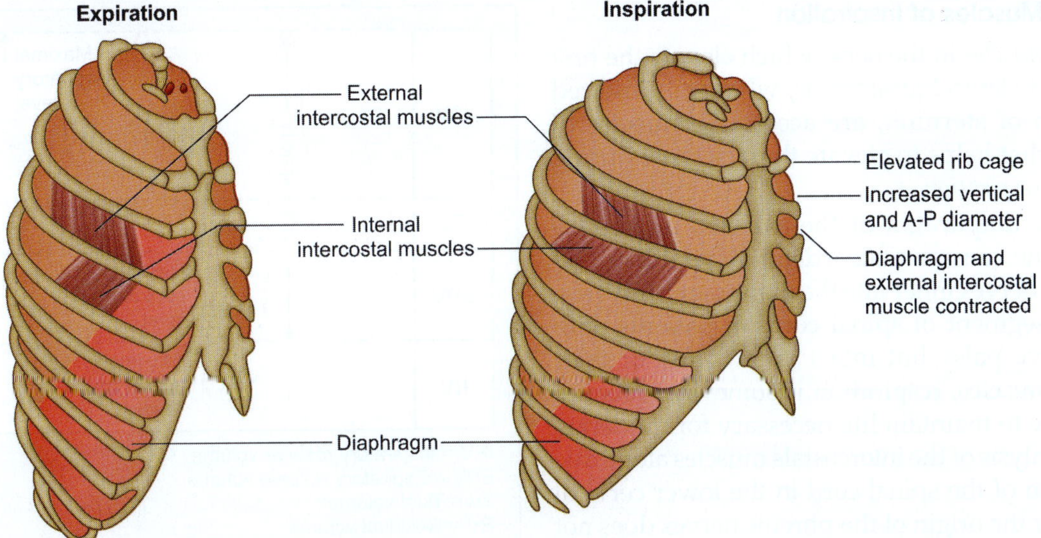

Fig. 4.8: Representation of the position of the thoracic cage and diaphragm in expiration (left) and inspiration (right)

during quiet inspiration. The distance it moves ranges from 1.5 cm to as much as 7 cm with deep inspiration.

The other important inspiratory muscles are ***external intercostal muscles*** which run downwards and forward from rib above to the rib below. Their contractions elevate the lower rib. This pushes the sternum outward and increases the anteroposterior diameter of the chest. The transverse diameter also increases but to a lesser degree.

The intrapleural pressure at the base of the lungs is normally about –2.5 mmHg (relative to atmospheric) at the start of inspiration, decreases as the chest expands with inspiration to about –6 mmHg (Fig. 4.9). With the negative pressure the lungs are pulled to expanded position. The pressure in the airways becomes slightly negative and air flows into the lungs. At the end of inspiration, with the relaxation of inspiratory muscles the lungs recoil due to elasticity and pull the chest wall back into expiratory position.

The pressure in the airways with lung recoil becomes slightly positive and air flows out of the lungs.

During strong inspiratory efforts intrapleural pressure is reduced to values as low as – 30 mmHg which produces greater lung inflation.

Expiration during *quiet breathing* is ***passive*** as no muscles contract to decrease the intrathoracic volume. When pulmonary ventilation is increased (as during exercise and in forced respiratory maneuvers), the extent of lung deflation is also increased by active contractions of **expiratory muscles**, that decrease the intrathoracic volume and forced expiration results. The muscles producing active expiration are the *internal intercostals* because they pass obliquely downwards and posteriorly from rib to rib and therefore pull the rib cage downwards when they contract; the contractions *of the muscles of anterior abdominal wall* aid expiration by pulling the rib cage downwards and also increasing the intra-abdominal pressure which pushes the diaphragm upward.

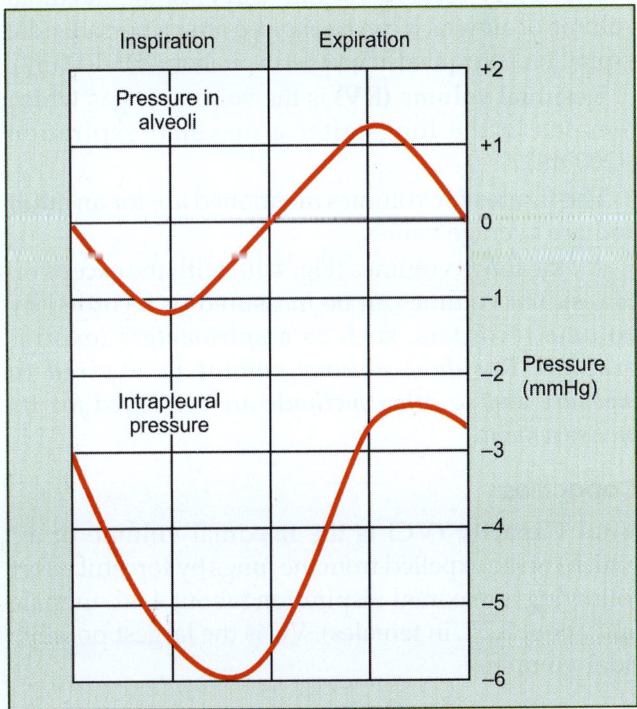

Fig. 4.9: Changes in intrapleural and intrapulmonary pressure relative to atmospheric pressure during inspiration and expiration

Accessory Muscles of Inspiration

The *scalene muscles* in the neck, which elevate the first two ribs and *sternocleidomastoids*, which are inserted into the top of sternum, are accessory muscles of inspiration that helps to elevate thoracic cage during *deep labored respiration*.

Either the diaphragm or the external intercostal muscles alone can maintain adequate ventilation *at rest*. Phrenic nerves innervate the diaphragm and arise from C3–5 segment of spinal cord. In patients with phrenic nerve palsy but intact innervation of their intercostal muscles, respiration is somewhat labored but adequate to maintain life necessary for moderate activity. Paralysis of the intercostals muscles alone due to transection of the spinal cord in the lower cervical region below the origin of the phrenic nerves does not seriously affect breathing as diaphragm is very effective.

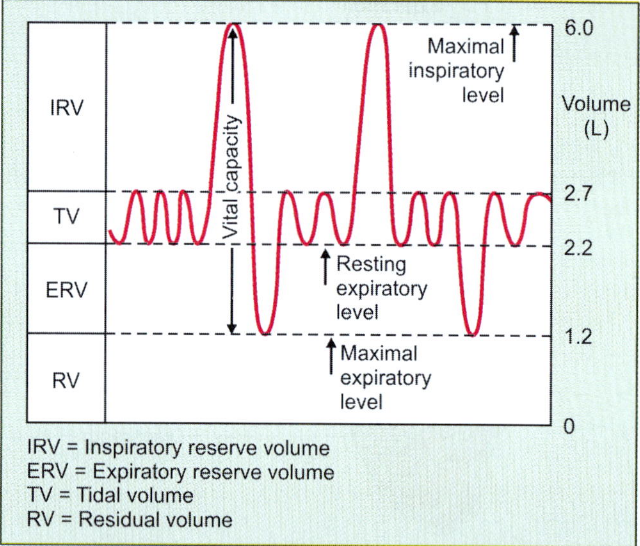

Fig. 4.10: Recording of lung volumes by spirometer

LUNG VOLUMES AND CAPACITIES

Volumes

Tidal volume (TV) is the volume of air breathed in or out during quiet respiration (about 500 ml).

Inspiratory reserve volume (IRV) is the maximal volume of air which can be inspired after completing a normal tidal inspiration, i.e. inspired over and above a normal tidal inspiration (2000–3000 ml).

Expiratory reserve volume (ERV) is the maximal volume of air which can be expired after a normal tidal expiration, i.e. expired after quiet expiration (750–1000 ml).

Residual volume (RV) is the volume of gas which remains in the lungs after a maximal expiration (1200 ml).

The figures for volumes mentioned are for an adult and are average values.

All the lungs volumes (Fig. 4.10) with the exception of residual volume can be measured or recorded by volume recorders, such as a *spirometers* (expirographs). ***Residual volume cannot be expired to measure and so other methods are employed for its measurement.***

Capacities

Vital Capacity (VC) is the maximal volume of air which can be expelled from the lungs by forceful effort following a maximal inspiration (about 4.8 L in male and about 3.2 L in females). VC is the largest possible tidal volume.

Factors Affecting Vital Capacity

Vital capacity is correlated with (1) age, (2) sex, (3) body build of an individual. It is 2.6 L/sq m surface area in male and 2.1 L/sq m in female. In old age it decreases. Vital capacity is altered by (4) posture and is less in supine position due to increase in pulmonary blood volume.

Timed Vital Capacity

FEV_1

The fraction of vital capacity expired during first second of forced expiration is called FEV_1 (or timed vital capacity). Normal value for FEV_1 is 80% of the vital capacity. In obstructive lung diseases, e.g. asthma and COPD, FEV_1 is reduced, even if the forced vital capacity is not decreased, due to increased airway resistance; it is a better index of severity of the obstructive disease than is provided by vital capacity. In restrictive lung diseases this fraction FEV_1 of FVC is not decreased.

Timed vital capacity is measured with a recording spirometer. For measurement the person inspires maximally to the total lung capacity, then exhales into spirometer with maximum expiratory effort as rapidly and as completely as possible. The down slope of the record against time (Fig. 4.11) represents forced vital capacity (FVC). In a record for airway obstruction, there is decrease in the amount of air expired in first second (FEV_1).

Inspiratory capacity is the maximal volume of air that can be inspired after a quiet expiration.

Functional residual capacity (FRC) is the volume of air left in the lungs after a quiet expiration. It is sum of residual volume and expiratory reserve volume.

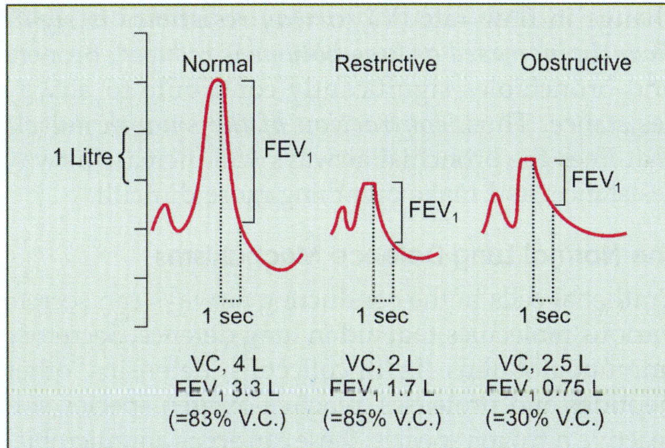

Fig. 4.11: Records of spirometer tracings. After a deep inspiration the subjects breathed out as forcefully and as rapidly as they could. Restrictive record shows here that although the vital capacity is gravely reduced the proportion of the vital capacity expired in the first seconds is normal unlike that in the 'obstructive' patient

Conditions Affecting FRC

FRC is increased in conditions of hyperinflation of lungs that may result from asthma or emphysema; in asthma due to increased expiratory airway resistance and in emphysema due to destruction of lung elastic tissue. Under these conditions the muscles of inspiration work at a disadvantage for to generate lower pleural pressures to cause lung expansion.

Total lung capacity is the volume of gas contained in the lungs after a maximal inspiration. It is equal to vital capacity plus the residual volume and is about 6000 ml in an adult male. Table 4.1 shows normal values in adults.

Diseases of the lungs or chest wall affect lung volumes and capacities in various ways. The most frequent change is in the vital capacity (VC) that is reduced. The reduction may be caused by limited expansion (restrictive disease) or due to an abnormally large residual volume (obstructive airway disease).

Table 4.1: Lung volumes and some measurements related to the mechanics of breathing

		Volume (L)		
		Men	*Women*	
Vital capacity	IRV	3.3	1.9	Inspiratory capacity
	TV	0.5	0.5	
	ERV	1.0	0.7	Functional residual capacity
	RV	1.2	1.1	

Respiratory minute volume (rest): 6 L/min
Alveolar ventilation (rest): 4.2 L/min
Maximal voluntary ventilation (BTPS): 125–170 L/min
Timed vital capacity: 83% of total VC in 1 S; 97% in 3 S

In strenuous exercise tidal volume may have to increase to one half of the vital capacity to ensure adequate alveolar ventilation. Hence, an early sign of lung disease that limits VC is limitation of exercise capacity.

Maximal Voluntary Ventilation (MVV)

Maximal voluntary ventilation formerly called the maximum breathing capacity (MBC) is the largest volume of air that can be moved into (or out of lungs) in one minute by voluntary effort. The normal MVV is 125–170 L/min. It depends upon muscular forces of the subject, and on the compliance of the thoracic walls and of lungs, and on the airway resistances. It is profoundly reduced in patients of emphysema or in the patients with airway obstruction.

Compliance of the Lungs and Chest Wall

Compliance is the index of expandability of elastic organs and defined as the change in the volume per unit change in pressure ($\Delta V/\Delta P$); compliance measures the stretchability (or distensibility) of the lung and chest wall (it can also be measured for lung or chest separately). The normal value is 0.2 L/cm H_2O. But the compliance of an individual with only one lung is half as approximately half the ΔV for a given ΔP.

The compliance is affected by *tissue elasticity* and the *surface tension of the film of fluid lining the alveoli.*

High compliance means that lung and chest wall expand easily. Low compliance means that they resist expansion.

Variation of Compliance

Compliance is decreased by pulmonary congestion and interstitial pulmonary fibrosis. Pulmonary fibrosis is a progressive disease in which there is stiffening and scarring of the lung.

Compliance is increased in emphysema due to destruction of elastic tissue.

Alveolar Surface Tension

An important factor affecting the compliance of the lungs is the surface tension of the film of fluid lining the alveoli. In experiments it is found that the surface tension of the fluid lining the alveoli is much lower than the expected surface tension at water-air interface of the same dimensions. The **low surface tension** is due to the presence in the fluid lining the alveoli of a lipid surface tension lowering agent, called **surfactant** which increases the lung compliance.

Surfactant

1. It is a phospholipid protein material (contains dipalmitoylphosphatidylcholine, DPPC);

2. It is produced by type 2 alveolar epithelial cells (Fig. 4.4) and secreted into alveolar surface. If the surface tension is not kept low the alveoli collapse when they become smaller during expiration.
3. Lung surfactant is continually replaced as some old molecules leave the surface film and some new ones enter it.
4. Continuous metabolism of the type 2 alveolar epithelial cells produces and recycles the surfactant (Fig. 4.4).

In the third trimester of fetal life the pulmonary surface active material is produced as the lungs mature to become ready for air breathing. Immediately after birth liquid filled lungs fill with air. The first cry of the newborn indicates that the lungs have been successfully inflated with air. Although surfactant has no role to make the initial air inflation easier, it does keep the alveoli inflated at end expiration. This inflation makes subsequent breathing easier to achieve.

The role of the lung surfactant is:

- It reduces the muscular effort to expand the lungs
- It lowers the elastic recoil at low lung volume (FRC) preventing the alveoli from collapsing at the end of each expiration.
- Surfactant also helps to prevent pulmonary edema.

When the alveoli become smaller during expiration the molecules of surfactant move closer together reducing the surface tension still more and preventing collapse of alveoli.

Surfactant Deficiency

Surfactant deficiency is the basic defect in ***infant respiratory distress syndrome*** (IRDS; hyaline membrane disease); that occurs in lungs of underdeveloped newborns.

Maturation of surfactant in the lungs is accelerated by glucocorticoid hormones. There is an increase in the fetal and maternal glucocorticoids near term and the lungs are rich in glucocorticoid receptors.

Patchy atelectasis develops with ***surfactant deficiency*** (1) with occlusion of one pulmonary artery or (2) long-term inhalation of 100% O_2 (3) there is decrease in surfactant in cigarette smokers.

Airway Resistance

Airway resistance is defined as the change of pressure (ΔP) from the alveoli to the mouth divided by the change in flow rate (V) ***Airway resistance is significantly increased as lung volume is reduced.*** Bronchi and bronchioles significantly contribute to airway resistance. Thus, ***contraction of the smooth muscle*** that lines the bronchial airways will increase airway resistance, and make breathing more difficult.

The Normal Lung Defence Mechanisms

Epithelial cells in the conducting airways can secrete various molecules that aid in lung defence. Secretory immunoglobulins (IgA), collectins, defensins, other peptides and proteases, reactive oxygen species and reactive nitrogen species; these can act as antimicrobial directly. The lungs also contain (1) alveolar macrophages (PAMs), (2) lymphocytes, (3) plasma cells, (4) APUD cells the neuroendocrine cells and (5) mast cells. **PAMs** (Fig. 4.4) are important for pulmonary ***defence mechanisms***. They are phagocytes and ingest bacteria and small particles. PAMs help to process inhaled antigen for immunologic attack; secrete substances to stimulate granulocyte and monocyte formation in bone marrow; and attract granulocytes to lungs. *When the macrophages ingest large amounts of substances in cigarette smoke, they may release lysosomal enzymes in the extracellular space; which produces inflammation.*

The **mast cells** contain histamine, heparin, and various other substances (lipids and proteases) that ***participate in allergic reactions.***

Bronchial Tone

The bronchi dilate during inspiration and constrict during expiration. There is **circadian rhythm** in bronchial tone, with *maximal constriction at about 6 am and maximal dilation at about 6 pm.*

1. Sympathetic discharge produces dilatation
2. Parasympathetic discharge produces constriction.
3. Cool air causes bronchoconstriction.
4. Exercise induced asthma is common in people who have hyperirritable airways.
5. Inhalation of smoke, dust and irritant substances, e.g. sulfur dioxide reflexly constrict the airways via the vagal nerves.
6. Some substances directly constrict airways, e.g. histamine, acetylcholine.
7. Many cytokines and inflammatory products produce constriction, e.g. leukotrienes.
8. Airway smooth muscle has ***adrenergic receptors*** so that local diffusion of the sympathetic postganglionic neurotransmitter, norepinephrine, ***inhibits airway constriction.***

Pulmonary Circulation

All the *impure blood* from the body passes through pulmonary artery (this artery carries impure blood) to the pulmonary capillary bed, where it is oxygenated and returned to the left atrium via pulmonary veins (these veins carry pure blood).

The conducting airways receive their blood supply from branches from the systemic arterial system. There are anastomoses between bronchial circulation and pulmonary capillaries and veins. Some of the bronchial impure blood enters the bronchial veins but some also enters the pulmonary capillaries and veins, causing minor dilution in its oxygenation, as this is venous blood. The bronchial circulation nourishes upper respiratory tract and does not reach terminal or respiratory bronchiole or alveolus but also nourishes pleura.

Pulmonary artery walls are about 30% as thick as the walls of aorta and the walls of small arteries have very little muscle in their walls; as a result the ***entire pulmonary vascular system is distensible low pressure system.***

Systolic pressure in the pulmonary artery is about 25 mmHg (Fig. 4.12).

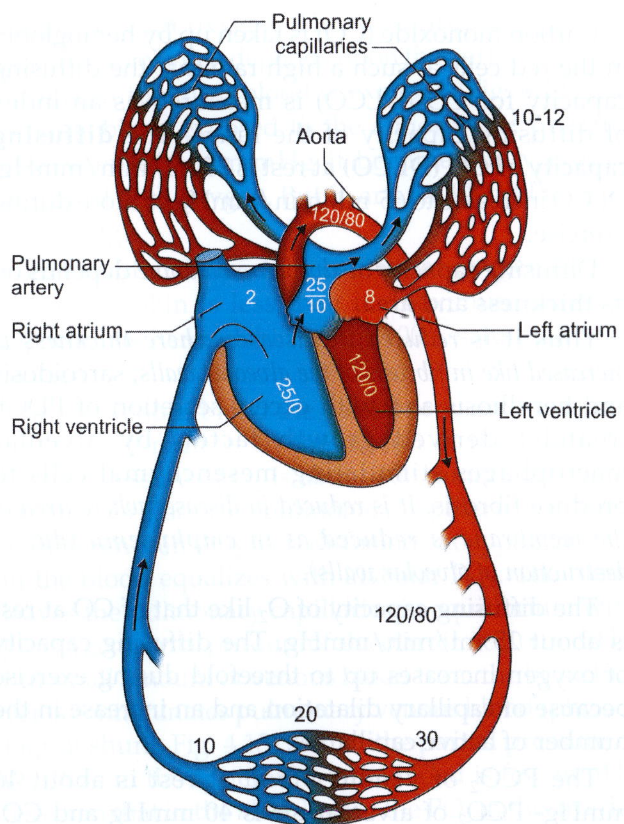

Fig. 4.12: Blood pressures (mmHg) in the pulmonary and systemic circulation

Diastolic pressure is about 10 mmHg;

Mean pressure is about 15 mmHg.

The pressure in the left atrium during diastole is about 8 mmHg so the pressure gradient for the flow of blood towards it is about 7 mmHg as compared to a much higher pressure gradient in the systemic circulation for flow into right atrium.

Pulmonary Capillary Pressure

Pulmonary capillary hydrostatic pressure is about 10 mmHg but the colloidal osmotic pressure of plasma proteins (oncotic pressure) is 25 mmHg so there is inward directed pressure gradient of about 15 mmHg which keeps the alveoli free of fluid.

If the pulmonary capillary hydrostatic pressure becomes more than 25 mmHg as may happen when there is left ventricular failure and due to the "backward failure", there is rise in the left atrial pressure, the lungs become congested; resulting in edema of the lungs.

Effect of gravity on pulmonary circulation from the top to the bottom of the lung the hydrostatic pressure in the pulmonary circulation varies approximately 1 cm H_2O per cm height in the direction of gravity (increase from top to bottom).

There is steady fall in blood flow per unit of alveolar volume from the bottom to the apex of the lung when the subject is sitting or standing; the apical flow is almost zero. Exercise increases blood flow in all regions and flow becomes equal in all regions.

Posture also modifies this distribution. When supine the apical blood flow increases, basal flow remains the same and two become almost equal. When supine the posterior regions receive more blood flow than do the anterior.

Ventilation Perfusion Ratios

The ratio of ventilation to pulmonary blood flow for the whole lung is about 0.8 (4.2 L/per min. alveolar ventilation 5.5 L per min pulmonary blood flow). There are differences in this ratio in different parts of the lung as a result of gravity.

Ventilation as well as perfusion in the upright position declines in a linear fashion from the bases to the apices of the lungs. But the ventilation perfusion ratios are high in the upper portions of the lungs.

Local changes in this ratio are common in disease; when if are widespread the non-uniform ventilation and perfusion in the lungs can cause CO_2 retention and decline in systemic arterial PO_2.

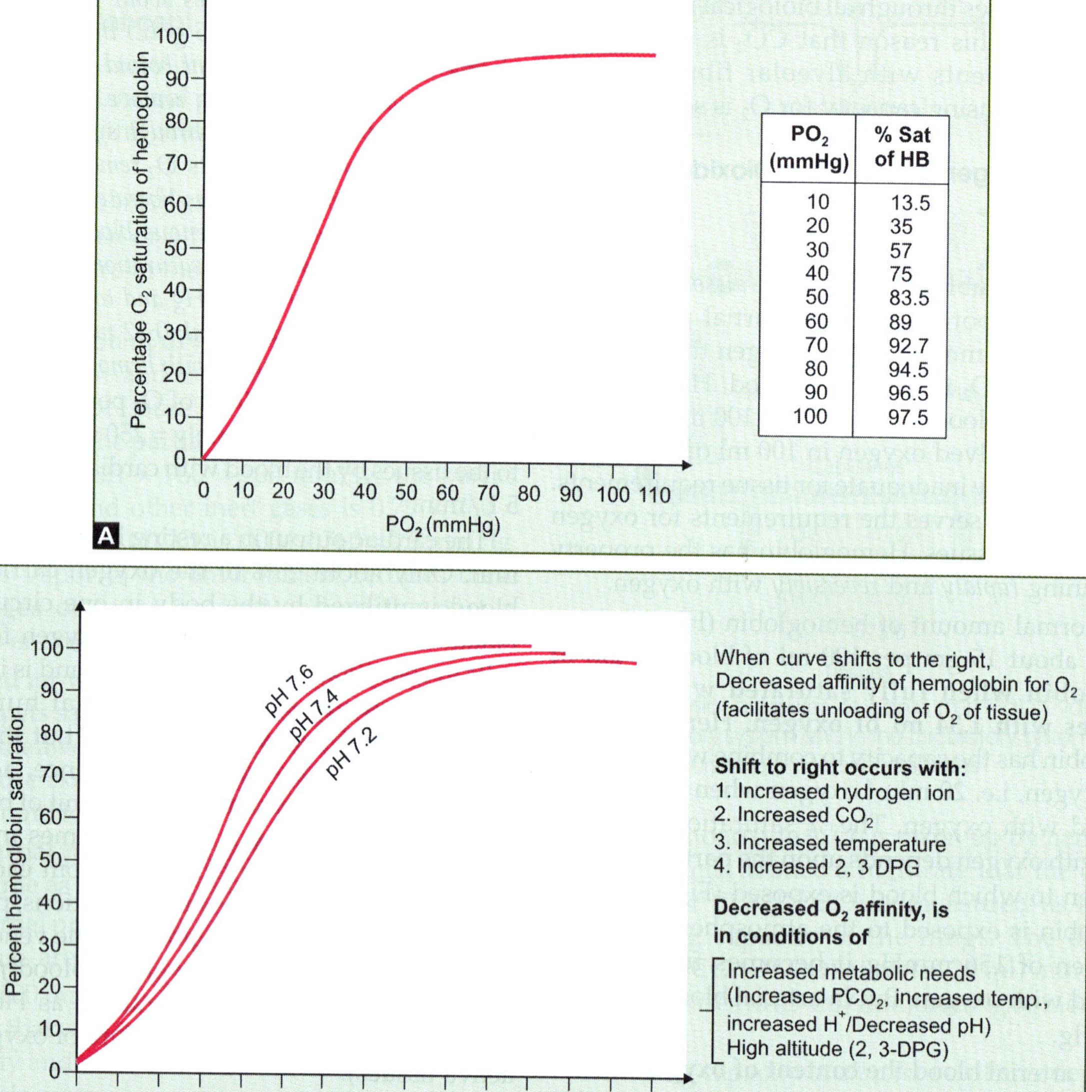

Figs 4.14A and B: (A) Oxygen-hemoglobin dissociation curve at pH 7.40 and temperature 38°C and (B) Effect of pH on the oxygen hemoglobin dissociation curve

Table 4.2: Gas content of blood

	mL/dL of blood containing 15 g of Hemoglobin			
	Arterial Blood *PO_2 95 mmHg; PCO_2 40 mmHg; Hb 97% saturated)*		*Venous Blood* *(PO_2 40 mmHg; PCO_2 46 mmHg; Hb 75% saturated)*	
Gas	*Dissolved*	*Combined*	*Dissolved*	*Combined*
N_2	0.98	0	0.98	0
O_2	0.29	19.5	0.12	15.1
CO_2	2.62	46.4 (HCO_3^- and carbamino compounds)	2.98	49.7 (HCO_3^- and carbamino compounds)

Pulmonary Circulation

All the *impure blood* from the body passes through pulmonary artery (this artery carries impure blood) to the pulmonary capillary bed, where it is oxygenated and returned to the left atrium via pulmonary veins (these veins carry pure blood).

The conducting airways receive their blood supply from branches from the systemic arterial system. There are anastomoses between bronchial circulation and pulmonary capillaries and veins. Some of the bronchial impure blood enters the bronchial veins but some also enters the pulmonary capillaries and veins, causing minor dilution in its oxygenation, as this is venous blood. The bronchial circulation nourishes upper respiratory tract and does not reach terminal or respiratory bronchiole or alveolus but also nourishes pleura.

Pulmonary artery walls are about 30% as thick as the walls of aorta and the walls of small arteries have very little muscle in their walls; as a result the ***entire pulmonary vascular system is distensible low pressure system.***

Systolic pressure in the pulmonary artery is about 25 mmHg (Fig. 4.12).

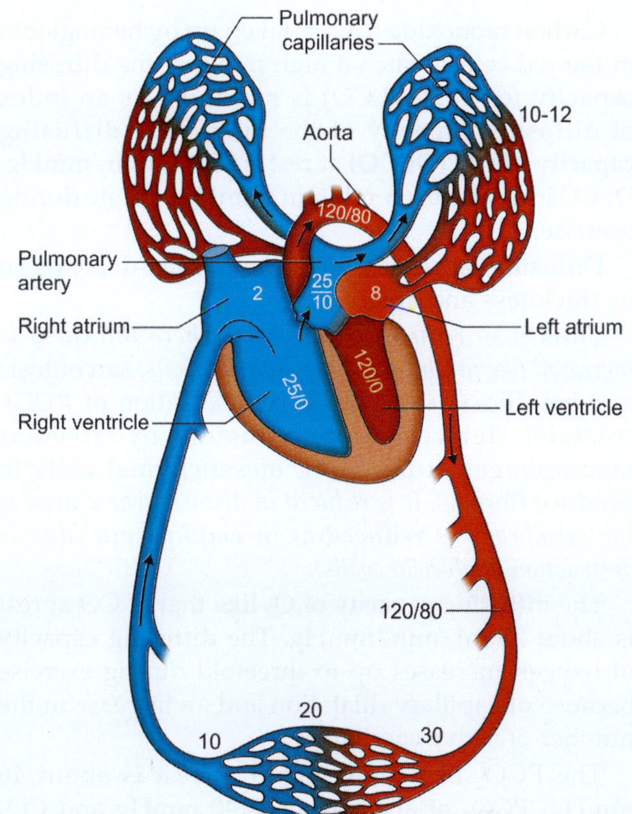

Fig. 4.12: Blood pressures (mmHg) in the pulmonary and systemic circulation

Diastolic pressure is about 10 mmHg;

Mean pressure is about 15 mmHg.

The pressure in the left atrium during diastole is about 8 mmHg so the pressure gradient for the flow of blood towards it is about 7 mmHg as compared to a much higher pressure gradient in the systemic circulation for flow into right atrium.

Pulmonary Capillary Pressure

Pulmonary capillary hydrostatic pressure is about 10 mmHg but the colloidal osmotic pressure of plasma proteins (oncotic pressure) is 25 mmHg so there is inward directed pressure gradient of about 15 mmHg which keeps the alveoli free of fluid.

If the pulmonary capillary hydrostatic pressure becomes more than 25 mmHg as may happen when there is left ventricular failure and due to the "backward failure", there is rise in the left atrial pressure, the lungs become congested; resulting in edema of the lungs.

Effect of gravity on pulmonary circulation from the top to the bottom of the lung the hydrostatic pressure in the pulmonary circulation varies approximately 1 cm H_2O per cm height in the direction of gravity (increase from top to bottom).

There is steady fall in blood flow per unit of alveolar volume from the bottom to the apex of the lung when the subject is sitting or standing; the apical flow is almost zero. Exercise increases blood flow in all regions and flow becomes equal in all regions.

Posture also modifies this distribution. When supine the apical blood flow increases, basal flow remains the same and two become almost equal. When supine the posterior regions receive more blood flow than do the anterior.

Ventilation Perfusion Ratios

The ratio of ventilation to pulmonary blood flow for the whole lung is about 0.8 (4.2 L/per min. alveolar ventilation 5.5 L per min pulmonary blood flow). There are differences in this ratio in different parts of the lung as a result of gravity.

Ventilation as well as perfusion in the upright position declines in a linear fashion from the bases to the apices of the lungs. But the ventilation perfusion ratios are high in the upper portions of the lungs.

Local changes in this ratio are common in disease; when if are widespread the non-uniform ventilation and perfusion in the lungs can cause CO_2 retention and decline in systemic arterial PO_2.

BLOOD GAS TRANSPORT

Partial Pressure Concept

In any volume the *total gas pressure* of all the gases is the sum of the individual pressures of each gas that it would exert even if it was present alone in the same volume.

The *partial pressure of gas dissolved in water or blood plasma* or *interstitial* or *intracellular liquids* is equal to the partial pressure in the gas phase with which it is in equilibrium.

The **composition of dry atmospheric air** is O_2 21%, CO_2 0.04%, N_2 78% and the rest are other inert gases. The barometric pressure at sea level is 760 mmHg (1 atmosphere). The partial pressure of O_2 at sea level is therefore as, $0.21 \times 760 = 160$ mmHg; the partial pressure of N_2 and other inert gases is $0.79 \times 760 = 600$ mmHg and that of CO_2 is $.0004 \times 760 = 0.3$ mmHg. The water vapor in the environment reduces these percentages of gases present and so the partial pressures are reduced to a slight extent.

Inspired air while passing through the respiratory passages gets saturated with water vapor by the time it reaches the alveoli; and at 37°C, (the body temperature) the pressure exerted by water vapor in the alveoli is about 47 mmHg.

The partial pressures of gases in the inspired air are the same as that in the atmospheric air (Fig. 4.13).

The partial pressures of gases in the air of the alveoli of the lungs are;

PO_2 is 100 mmHg, CO_2 is 40 mmHg (Fig. 4.13); due to the fact that with expiration the alveoli do not empty completely and air remains in the alveoli, with which inspired air mixes.

The expired air is a mixture of dead space air and expired alveolar air and its composition is dependent on that.

Oxygenated blood leaving the lungs via pulmonary veins is pumped by the left ventricle through the systemic arteries to the capillaries associated with the cells of the body. Also the principal waste product of metabolism, CO_2 is transported away from the cells via systemic veins to the lungs for elimination (Fig. 4.13). The transport of O_2 and CO_2 is important part of respiration.

Diffusing Capacity of the Lungs

The diffusing capacity of the lungs for a gas is defined as the amount of that gas which diffuses across the lungs into the blood per minute when there is pressure difference of 1 mmHg.

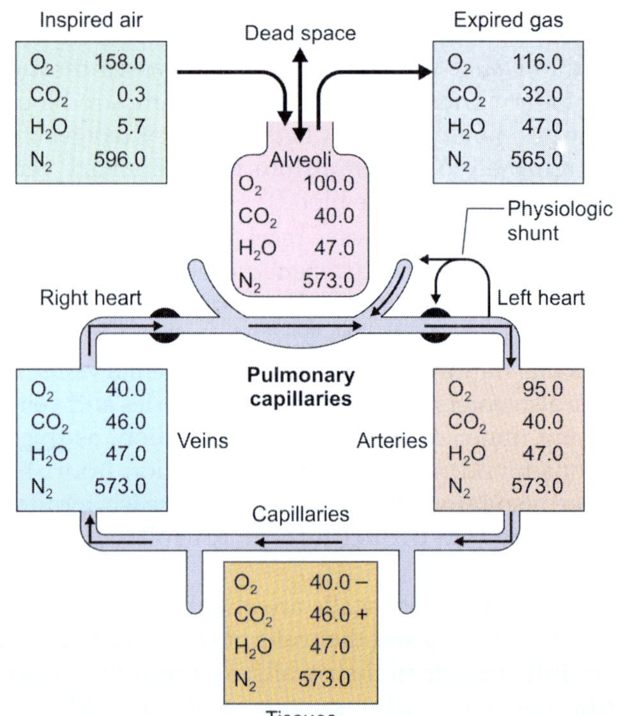

Fig. 4.13: Partial pressures of gases (mmHg) in various parts of the respiratory system and in the circulatory system. Diffusion of gases occurs in pulmonary capillaries

Carbon monoxide (CO) is taken up by hemoglobin in the red cells at such a high rate that the diffusing capacity for CO (DLCO) is measured as an index of diffusing capacity of the lungs. The **diffusing capacity of CO (DLCO)** at rest is 25 ml/min/mmHg. DLCO increases to 65 ml/min/mmHg or more during exercise.

Diffusing capacity of *alveolar membrane* depends on its **thickness** and **area**.

Thus it is *reduced in diseases where thickness is increased like in fibrosis of the alveolar walls;* sarcoidosis and berylliosis and with excess secretion of PDGF (platelet derived growth factor) by alveolar macrophages stimulating mesenchymal cells to produce fibrosis. *It is reduced in diseases where* ***area*** *of the membrane is* ***reduced*** *as in* ***emphysema*** *(due to destruction of alveolar walls).*

The diffusing capacity of O_2 like that of CO at rest is about 25 ml/min/mmHg. The diffusing capacity of oxygen increases up to threefold during exercise because of capillary dilatation and an increase in the number of active capillaries.

The PCO_2 of venous blood at rest is about 46 mmHg- PCO_2 of alveolar air is 40 mmHg and CO_2 diffuses along this gradient into the alveoli of lungs from the blood.

Hence, PCO_2 of blood leaving the lungs is 40 mmHg. CO_2 passes through all biological membranes easily. It is for this reason that CO_2 is not a great problem in patients with alveolar fibrosis when reduction in diffusing capacity for O_2 is severe.

Carriage of Oxygen and Carbon Dioxide by the Blood

O_2 Transport

O_2 is not very soluble in plasma. The *dissolved* oxygen *in plasma* is proportional to the partial pressure of oxygen, for each mmHg PO_2 of oxygen there is 0.003 ml of dissolved O_2 in 100 ml of blood. Hence, at the normal arterial blood with a PO_2 of 100 mmHg there is 0.3 ml of dissolved oxygen in 100 ml of blood; this quantity is grossly inadequate for tissue requirements. The hemoglobin serves the requirements for oxygen carriage to the tissues. Hemoglobin has the property of combining *rapidly* and *reversibly* with oxygen.

The normal amount of hemoglobin (Hb) in circulation is about 15 gm per 100 ml of blood; **1 gm of hemoglobin when fully saturated with oxygen combines with 1.34 ml of oxygen.** Hence, 15 g of hemoglobin has the capacity to combine with 15 × 1.34 ml of oxygen, i.e. 20 ml of oxygen when Hb is 100% saturated with oxygen. The % saturation of hemoglobin with oxygen depends upon the partial pressure of oxygen to which blood is exposed (Fig. 4.14A). If hemoglobin is exposed to the atmospheric pressure of oxygen of 156 mmHg it becomes fully (100%) saturated with oxygen. But in arterial blood PO_2 is 97 mm of Hg.

In the arterial blood the **content of oxygen** carried by hemoglobin is less than its maximum carrying capacity; as hemoglobin is not 100% saturated with oxygen.

In the venous blood the partial pressure of oxygen is about 40 mmHg. In the alveoli of the lungs the partial pressure of O_2 is about 100 mmHg **diffusion of O_2** takes place into pulmonary capillary blood due to **difference in PO_2** with diffusion of oxygen the PO_2 in the blood equalizes with alveolar PO_2. The blood leaves the pulmonary capillaries in equilibrium with the oxygen partial pressure of alveolar air, i.e. 100 mmHg. But small amount of venous blood from the bronchial veins contaminates pulmonary venous blood (physiological shunt, Fig. 4.13) so that the partial pressure of O_2 (PO_2) in the systemic arterial blood is few mmHg less than that in the alveolar air; the PO_2 in the **arterial blood is about 97 mmHg**; at this partial pressure hemoglobin is only **97% saturated with oxygen.**

Hence, 100 ml of arterial blood at normal partial pressure of oxygen of 97 mmHg carries about 19.8 ml of oxygen; (when Hb concentration is 15 g/dL) that dissolved in the plasma is 0.3 ml, and 19.5 ml bound to hemoglobin. At resting conditions the tissues remove 4.6 ml of O_2 from each 100 ml of blood passing through systemic circulation; of which 0.17 ml of represents O_2 removed from solution and the remainder O_2 that was liberated from hemoglobin (Table 4.2). Hence, in the venous blood in resting state hemoglobin remains at 75% saturation with oxygen at a partial pressure of 40 mm of Hg and total oxygen content in the blood at 15.2 per 100 ml; 0.12 ml in dissolved form and 15.1 ml in combination with hemoglobin.

In this way about 250 ml of O_2 per minute (4.6/100 × 5 L = 230 ml, approximately = 250 ml) is transported to the tissues by the blood with cardiac output of about 5 L/min.

The cardiac output in a resting human adult is 5 L/min. Only about 25% of the oxygen carried in the blood is utilized by the body in one circulation of blood. This provides a reserve of oxygen for use by cells in conditions when oxygen demand is increased. In heavy steady exercise by normal humans the cardiac output increases by 3 times but the oxygen usage may increase six fold and hence, **additional** oxygen must be released from each unit of blood. The oxygen released is by is (1) three times increase in blood flow; (2) oxygen extraction from each unit of blood is increased from resting conditions; producing greater reduction of hemoglobin in the venous blood (% saturation of Hb in the venous blood ***falls*** from the resting level of 75% saturation; as Hb is more reduced with lower partial pressure of oxygen in the active tissues).

Hence, the transport of oxygen from the environment to the cells of the body is affected by two processes, (1) the ventilation and (2) blood flow in the pulmonary capillaries and to the tissue cells. The normal process of diffusion at both sites is necessary for the oxygen transport and supply.

Reaction of Hemoglobin with Oxygen

The reaction with oxygen is rapid (time is in milliseconds). The deoxygenation is also very rapid. If blood is equilibrated with 100% O_2 (PO_2 = 760 mmHg) outside the body the normal hemoglobin becomes 100% saturated.

The **oxygen carrying capacity of hemoglobin** is the maximum amount of O_2 that can be bound to hemoglobin; but in the arterial blood hemoglobin is less than 100% saturated with oxygen. *In vivo* the hemoglobin in the blood at the end of the pulmonary

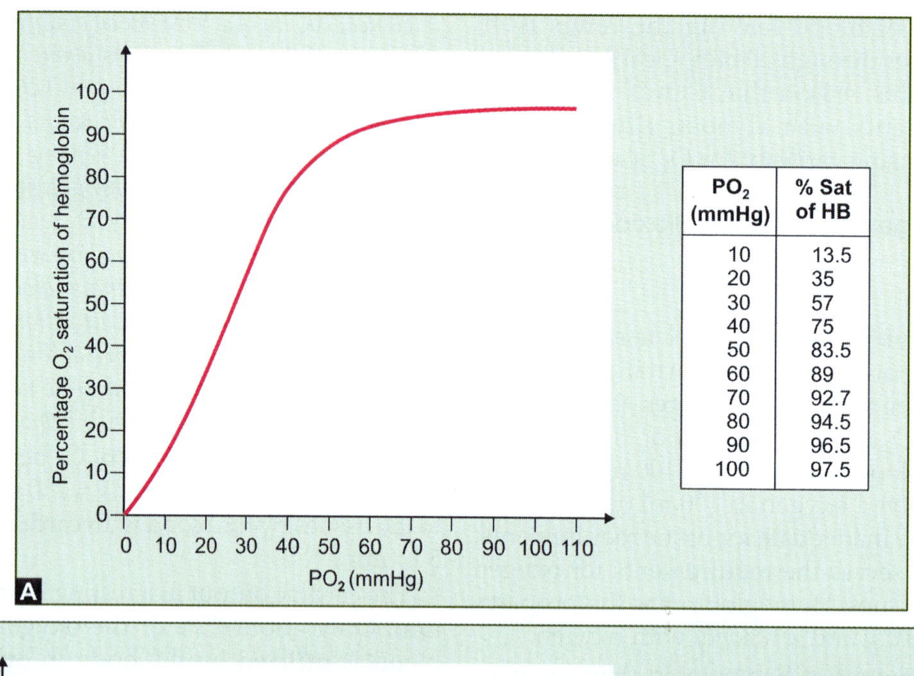

PO_2 (mmHg)	% Sat of HB
10	13.5
20	35
30	57
40	75
50	83.5
60	89
70	92.7
80	94.5
90	96.5
100	97.5

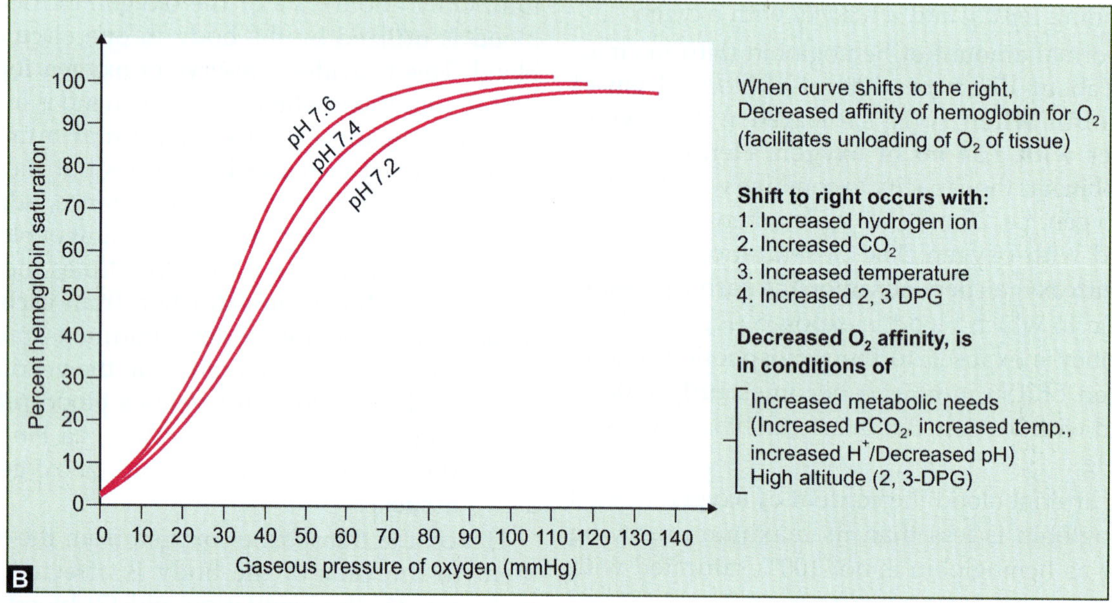

When curve shifts to the right, Decreased affinity of hemoglobin for O_2 (facilitates unloading of O_2 of tissue)

Shift to right occurs with:
1. Increased hydrogen ion
2. Increased CO_2
3. Increased temperature
4. Increased 2, 3 DPG

Decreased O_2 affinity, is in conditions of

- Increased metabolic needs (Increased PCO_2, increased temp., increased H^+/Decreased pH)
- High altitude (2, 3-DPG)

Figs 4.14A and B: (A) Oxygen-hemoglobin dissociation curve at pH 7.40 and temperature 38°C and (B) Effect of pH on the oxygen hemoglobin dissociation curve

Table 4.2: Gas content of blood

	mL/dL of blood containing 15 g of Hemoglobin			
	Arterial Blood (PO_2 95 mmHg; PCO_2 40 mmHg; Hb 97% saturated)		*Venous Blood (PO_2 40 mmHg; PCO_2 46 mmHg; Hb 75% saturated)*	
Gas	*Dissolved*	*Combined*	*Dissolved*	*Combined*
N_2	0.98	0	0.98	0
O_2	0.29	19.5	0.12	15.1
CO_2	2.62	46.4 (HCO_3^- and carbamino compounds)	2.98	49.7 (HCO_3^- and carbamino compounds)

capillaries and with slight admixture with bronchial venous and cardiac venous blood is only 97% saturated with oxygen as described above.

Oxygen Dissociation Curve of Hemoglobin is Sigmoid-shaped Curve

The oxygen dissociation curve has been plotted in experimental conditions to show percentage saturation of hemoglobin at different partial pressures of oxygen in blood (Figs 6.14A and B). It is not a linear curve but a sigmoid curve (S-shaped); the amount of oxygen combined with hemoglobin increases rapidly up to a PO_2 of 50 mmHg here curve is steep but the curve becomes flatter at a higher PO_2.

The **flat upper portion** of the curve has the advantage that oxygen taken up by hemoglobin is little affected if PO_2 in the arterial blood falls below the normal of 97 mmHg to up to 60 mmHg that could happen wtih fall in the oxygenation of the blood in the lungs; **the steep portion of the curve** has the advantage that the release of oxygen is facilitated when there is fall in oxygen tension in the tissues below the resting value of 40 mmHg (40 mmHg to 25 mmHg or less) when there is increased activity of tissues.

Three conditions further affect the ability of hemoglobin to combine with oxygen at these partial pressures of oxygen (Fig. 4.14B). These conditions are:

1. pH of the blood
2. temperature of the blood
3. the concentration of 2,3-diphosphoglycerate (2,3-DPG) in the red cells.

Hence, the curve in the venous blood, i.e. oxygen-hemoglobin dissociation curve is affected by pH, the temperature of the tissues and the concentration of 2,3–DPG in the red cells.

A rise in temperature or a fall of pH shift the curve to the right resulting in oxyhemoglobin releasing more oxygen at the same partial pressures of oxygen (Fig. 4.14B). ***Most of the desaturation*** of hemoglobin that occurs in tissues ***is due to fall in PO_2***, *but some extra desaturation is due to rise in tissue partial pressure of CO_2 (PCO_2), amounting to about 1–2% effect in desaturation. Fall in pH with rise in partial pressure of PCO_2 shifts the dissociation curve to the right (called the Bohr effect).*

Role of 2,3-DPG

2,3-DPG is very plentiful in red cells. An increase in the concentration of 2,3-DPG in the red cells shifts the reaction to the right, causing more oxygen to be liberated. 2,3-DPG concentration in the red cells increases when there is rise in pH (more alkaline) as happens at high attitudes. There is sustained rise in 2,3-DPG concentration in red cells due to rise in pH. But it falls to normal levels upon return to sea level.

2,3-DPG concentration in the red cells is increased in anemia and in a number of diseases in which there is chronic hypoxia. This facilitates the delivery of oxygen to the tissues.

Exercise also produces an increase in 2,3-DPG within an hour; the rise does not occur in trained athletes.

During exercise more O_2 is removed from each unit of blood flowing through tissues because the tissue PO_2 declines producing greater diffusion gradient; also at lower level of PO_2 the oxygen-hemoglobin dissociation curve is steep releasing more oxygen (against a similar fall in the partial pressure of oxygen at higher partial pressures). There is also rise in active tissues temperature and CO_2 and metabolites accumulate, lowering the pH further assisting in release of oxygen.

There is greater affinity of **fetal hemoglobin** than that of adult hemoglobin (hemoglobin A) for O_2; this facilitates the movement of O_2 from the maternal circulation. The cause of the greater affinity is the poor binding of 2,3-DPG by the gamma polypeptide chains in fetal hemoglobin that replace β chains. The oxygen binding sites in hemoglobin also bind nitric oxide (NO) the affinity is increased by O_2, so hemoglobin binds NO in the lungs and releases in the tissues; there it promotes vasodilation.

Hemoglobin has four functions:

1. facilitates oxygen transport
2. it facilitates CO_2 transport
3. important role as buffer
4. transports NO (nitric oxide)

If reduced or oxygenated hemoglobin is treated with an oxidizing agent Fe^{2+} is oxidized to ferric iron (Fe^{3+}). The compound is called methemoglobin, it cannot unite reversibly with gaseous oxygen, O of the OH cannot be given off. Reduced hemoglobin is commonly represented as Hb, oxyhemoglobin as HbO_2 methemoglobin as HbOH.

Carbon monoxide (CO) has more than 250 times the affinity than that of oxygen for Hb; and its combination blocks the union for oxygen.

Because carbon monoxide combines readily with Hb; HbCO does not dissociate unless partial pressure of carbon monoxide is very low; hence, the danger of carbon monoxide poisoning even when its concentration is low in the atmosphere. The affinity of CO for Hb is so great relative to that of O_2 that even with a very low concentration of CO in alveolar air, large quantity of HbCO will be formed in the blood.

Carbon Dioxide Transport

In the ***arterial blood partial pressure of CO_2 (PCO_2) is 40 mm*** *and the* ***content of CO_2 is 49 ml per 100 ml at 37°C.*** At this partial pressure of CO_2 the amount of ***CO_2 dissolved in plasma in 2.6 ml per 100 ml*** (CO_2 is much more soluble than oxygen in plasma). *Dissolved form is a small fraction* of the total amount of CO_2 in blood *most of the CO_2 is carried in the combined form. It is carried in the form* ***of bicarbonate,*** *mostly in* ***plasma*** *but also in the* ***red cells;*** *and carried in the form of* ***carbamino compounds,*** *i.e. carbon dioxide combined with amino groups of hemoglobin and other proteins* (Table 4.3).

Hence, of 49 ml of CO_2 in each 100 ml of arterial blood is as:

1. 2.6 ml is in dissolved form
2. 43.8 ml is in HCO_3^-
3. 2.6 ml is in carbamino compounds

In the ***tissues*** *the* ***partial pressure of CO_2*** *is higher* ***(more than 46 mmHg)*** and so the CO_2 diffuses into the blood in the capillaries and enters the plasma and red cells; *it is hydrated to form* ***carbonic acid,*** the reaction being ***rapid in the red cells*** due to the presence of enzyme **carbonic anhydrase**; the carbonic acid dissociates to form H^+ ions (which are buffered by Hb) and HCO_3^- ions; ***70% of the HCO_3^-*** ions formed in the red cells enter plasma in ***exchange with chloride ions that enter the red cells*** (Fig 4.15).

Table 4.3: Fate of CO_2 in blood

In plasma	*In red blood cells*
1. Dissolved	1. Dissolved
2. Hydration formation of H_2CO_3, H^+ buffered, HCO_3^- in plasma	2. Hydration, H^+ buffered, 70% of HCO_3^- enters the plasma in exchange for Cl^-
3. Formation of carbamino compounds with plasma proteins	3. Formation of carbamino-Hb

CO_2 diffusing into the blood also enters into *combination with hemoglobin and plasma proteins to form* ***carbamino compounds.***

As a result of these changes with ***PCO_2 in the venous blood*** *of about* ***46 mmHg*** the ***content of CO_2 increases by 3.7 ml per 100 ml of blood; increase of 0.4 ml in solution, 0.8 ml in carbamino compounds and 2.5 ml in HCO_3^-.***

The pH of the venous blood drops from 7.4 to pH 7.36. The CO_2 added to the red cell increases either HCO_3^- or chloride in the red cell, these are osmotically active particles; the red cells take up water and increase in size; hence, the hematocrit of venous blood is 3% higher than that in the arterial blood.

In the lungs the ***changes are reversed*** and 3.7 ml of CO_2 is given off in the alveoli.

In this way 200 ml of CO_2 3.7/100 × 5L (cardiac output) = 185 ml, approximately = 200 ml per minute. at rest and much larger amounts in exercise are transported from the tissues to the lungs and removed.

Deoxygenated hemoglobin binds more H^+ than oxygenated hemoglobin and forms carbamino compounds more readily, facilitating carbon dioxide removal from tissues; binding of O_2 to hemoglobin reduces its affinity for CO_2 facilitating CO_2 release in the lungs (Haldane effect).

REGULATION OF RESPIRATION

Rhythmic discharge of neurons in the **medulla** and **pons** produce **automatic respiration**. The neurons discharge impulses to the motor neurons controlling the respiratory muscles. **Voluntary control** over the respiration is located in the **cerebral cortex** but it is only limited control and respiration cannot be held voluntarily except for a brief period.

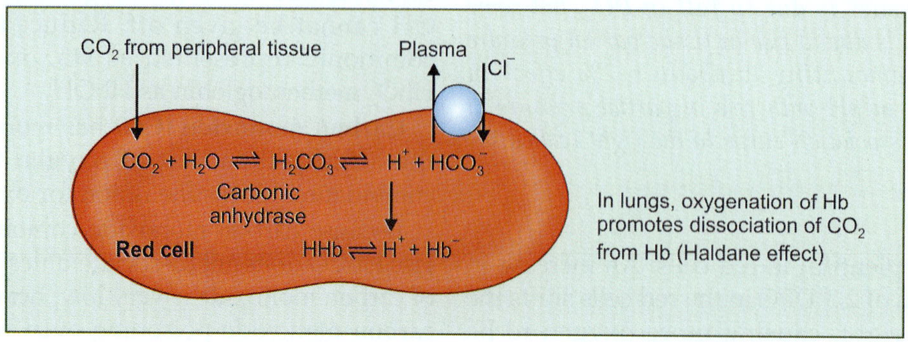

Fig. 4.15: CO_2 transport in red cells from tissues to lungs

The automatic control is present in medulla and pons. The efferent connections from this system control the respiratory neurons in the spinal cord, which innervate the respiratory muscles. The nerve fibers mediating inspiration converge on the motor neurons of phrenic nerve located in the spinal cord in ventral horns from C3 to C5, and to the neurons of the external intercostal nerves in the ventral horns throughout the thoracic spinal cord. The fibers concerned with expiration converge mainly on the motor neurons for internal intercostals muscles in the thoracic spinal cord. The main control of automatic respiration is exerted by the neurons located in the medulla. ***These are small groups of neurons called pre-Botzinger complex located on both sides of medulla.***

There are in addition dorsal and ventral groups of respiratory neurons in the medulla and probably they effect respiration by the projections on pre-Botzinger pacemaker neurons.

Pontine and Vagal Influences

The spontaneous discharge of neurons in the medulla for respiration is modified by neurons in the pons; and also by afferents in the vagal nerves from receptors in the airways and lungs. An area known as *apneustic center* located in the lower pons contains neurons active during inspiration; *pneumotaxic center* situated in the upper pons contains neurons active during expiration. The normal function of pneumotaxic centre is unknown, but it may play a role in switching between inspiration and expiration.

When the pneumotaxic centre area is damaged respiration becomes slower and tidal volume greater; if vagal nerves are **also cut** in anesthetized animals there is prolonged inspiratory spasms (called apneusis), resembling breath holding (Fig. 4.16).

During respiration the stretch of the lungs during inspiration initiates impulses in afferent pulmonary vagal fibers. These impulses are normally inhibitory to inspiratory discharge. Hence, after vagotomy (i.e. vagal nerves are cut) the depth of inspiration is increased.

When the activity of the inspiratory neurons is increased in intact animals, the rate and depth of breathing is increased.

CHEMICAL CONTROL OF RESPIRATION

There are three chemical factors which regulate pulmonary ventilation: arterial PO_2 fall; arterial PCO_2 change; arterial pH change. The receptors which sense these changes are located at two sites: (1) peripheral chemoreceptors in the carotid and aortic bodies (Fig. 4.17) which are stimulated by decline in arterial blood PO_2, or a rise in PCO_2 or H^+ concentration of arterial blood; (2) central chemoreceptor zone, the site affected by the increase of arterial PCO_2 or decline in pH.

Decline of arterial PO_2 stimulates the respiratory centre because of impulses from the peripheral chemoreceptors (carotid and aortic bodies) that are stimulatory to the respiratory centre. Though, oxygen lack at respiratory centre is a direct depresant of respiration. A fall in **PO_2 stimulates respiration** but when the fall in it is small stimulant effect is low.

On the other hand changes in arterial PCO_2 both at the level of **medullary chemoreceptors**, (situated in the medulla in the vicinity of respiratory centre) and

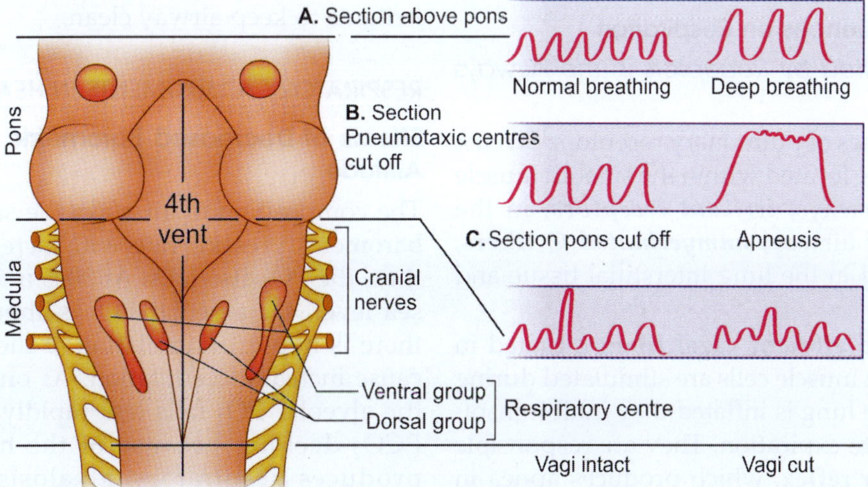

Fig. 4.16: Respiratory neurons in the brainstem. Dorsal view of brainstem; The effects of various lesions with brainstem transections in animals are shown. The spirometer tracings at the right indicate the depth and rate of breathing

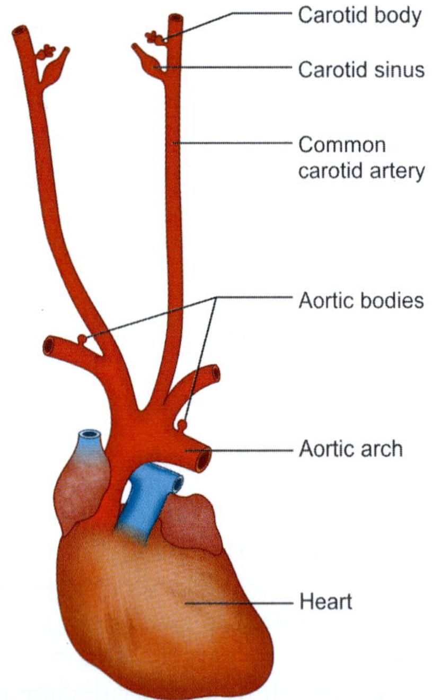

Fig. 4.17: Location of carotid and aortic bodies

peripheral chemoreceptors in the carotid and aortic bodies stimulate respiration but affect more at the central chemoreceptors; only 30–35% of the response is due to stimulation at the peripheral chemoreceptors.

A rise in **PCO_2 is a powerful stimulant** of respiration, a fall in PCO_2 is inhibitory to respiration. Increase in arterial **blood H^+ concentration** is stimulatory to respiration affecting through peripheral chemoreceptors, although larger changes exert some effect at central level in brainstem.

Asphyxia which is oxygen lack and carbon dioxide excess is a **powerful stimulant** of respiration; obstruction of trachea produces it.

Nonchemical Influences on Respiration

Responses Mediated by Receptors in the Airways and Lungs

There are three types of pulmonary receptors: ***Stretch receptors*** which are located within the smooth muscle of pulmonary airways; ***irritant receptors***, in the epithelial cells of airway; ***unmyelinated* C fibers**, which are situated in the lung interstitial tissue and alveolar walls.

The myelinated afferent vagal fibers situated in the airway smooth muscle cells are stimulated during inspiration. As the lung is inflated they inhibit inspiration and promote expiration. They are responsible for **Hering-Breuer reflex**, which produces apnea in response to large lung inflations and reinforces expiratory muscle contraction. This reflex is weak in adult humans, but may be prominent in newborns. These receptors adapt slowly to a sustained stimulus.

Irritant receptor neurons rapidly adapt on being subjected to a sustained stimulus. Irritant receptors are stimulated by noxious agents, such as sulfur dioxide, ammonia, or inhaled antigens (pollens). Irritant receptor excitation constricts the airways, promotes rapid, shallow breathing.

The chemical mediators released in the lungs during allergic reactions (histamine, leukotrienes or bradykinin) also stimulate irritant receptors. The increase in the breathing frequency produced by irritant receptor excitation may enhance ventilation during asthmatic attacks and the work of breathing is increased.

The **unmyelinated C fibers** are close to pulmonary vessels and have been called J (juxtacapillary) receptors; excited by changes in the lungs interstitial tissue, such as edema and by some chemicals, including histamine. Stimulation of C fibers causes laryngeal closure and apnea, followed by rapid, shallow breathing, bradycardia and hypotension. Stimulation of C fibers, together with irritant receptors may be responsible for tachypnea (rapid breathing) seen in patients with multiple pulmonary emboli, lung edema or pneumonia.

Coughing and Sneezing

Coughing begins with deep inspiration followed by forced expiration against a closed glottis. This increases intrapleural pressure to about 100 mm of Hg or more. The glottis is then suddenly opened producing an explosive outflow of air at very high velocities. Sneezing is similar expiratory effort with a continuously open glottis. These reflexes help to expel irritants to keep airway clean.

RESPIRATORY ADJUSTMENTS IN HEALTH AND DISEASE

Effects of Decreased Barometric Pressure at High Altitude

The composition of air stays the same, but the total barometric pressure falls with increasing altitude and thus, the PO_2 also falls. At 3000 m (~10,000 ft) above sea level, the alveolar PO_2 is about 60 mmHg and there is hypoxic stimulation of the chemoceptors to cause increased ventilation. As one ascends higher, the alveolar PO_2 falls less rapidly and the alveolar PCO_2 declines because of the hyperventilation, produces respiratory alkalosis. A number of compensatory mechanisms operate over time to increase altitude tolerance **(acclimatization)**. In unacclimatized persons, mental symptoms, such as irritability appear at about 3700 m. At 5500 m the hypoxic symptoms are severe; and at above altitudes of 6100 m (20,000 ft), consciousness is usually lost.

Effect of Exercise

Oxygen needs are increased and cardiovascular and respiratory systems operate in an integrated fashion to meet the tissue needs and extra CO_2 and heat must be removed from the body. There is increase in the extraction of oxygen from the blood flowing to the active tissues hence, the blood is more reduced; cardiac output is increased; and ventilation increases to make more oxygen available for the increased requirement of the flow in pulmonary capillaries; the flow increases with increase of cardiac output; the increased ventilation gets rid of extra CO_2 and some of the heat produced.

Ventilation is increased to:

- Supply increased demand of O_2
- To get rid of increased production of CO_2
- To get rid of some heat

The amount of O_2 entering the blood increases due to:

- Amount of oxygen added to each unit of blood is increased. The blood flowing into pulmonary capillaries has lower partial pressure of oxygen from the resting level of 40 mmHg to 25 mmHg or less, hence alveolar-capillary PO_2 gradient is increased and more O_2 enters the blood per unit of blood.
- Pulmonary blood flow per minute is increased.

Blood flow per minute is, increased from 5.5 L/min to may be as much as 20–35 L/min. The total amount of O_2 entering the blood hence, increases from 250 ml/min at rest to a value as high as 4000 ml/min. The amount of CO_2 removed from each unit of blood is increased and CO_2 excretion increases from 200 ml/min to as much as 8000 ml/min.

The increase in O_2 uptake is proportionate to work load up to a maximum. Above the maximum, the O_2 consumption does not increase and blood lactate level starts to rise. The lactate comes from the muscle in which the oxygen available cannot supply all the energy requirements and oxygen debt is incurred.

After exercise is over the respiratory rate does not reach basal levels until oxygen debt is repaid; that may take up to 90 minutes. The stimulus to ventilation after exercise is not the arterial PCO_2 which is normal or low or arterial PO_2 which is normal or high but the elevated arterial H^+ concentration due to lactic acidemia. The magnitude of oxygen debt is the amount by which O_2 consumption exceeds basal consumption from the end of exertion until the O_2 consumption has returned to the pre-exercise basal levels.

Hypoxia

Hypoxia (sometimes called Anoxia) is **O_2 deficiency** at the tissue level. Hypoxia has been divided into 4 types:

1. **Hypoxic Hypoxia (Hypoxemia):** Partial pressure of O_2 is reduced. PO_2 of arterial blood is reduced (it occurs in physiological condition as at high altitudes where barometric pressure is reduced that results in the reduction of partial pressure of O_2) in alveoli and hence in arterial blood. *In diseased conditions it could be (1) with gas exchange deficit, e.g. in pulmonary fibrosis, pneumonia or ventilation perfusion imbalance; (2) congenital heart disease in which large amounts of blood are shunted from venous to arterial side; and (3) in conditions in which respiratory pump fails (morphine or other drugs) or (4) due to mechanical defects, such as pneumothorax or bronchial obstruction that limit ventilation.*
2. **Anemic Hypoxia.** It is less serious in its effect than hypoxic hypoxia because the partial pressure of oxygen is normal in the blood; but the content of oxygen is reduced because the amount of hemoglobin is reduced. As the oxygen partial pressure is normal rate of tissue oxidation is maintained at its normal level.

   If the 19 ml of oxygen per 100 ml of blood is present in the arterial blood, only 5 ml are used in resting conditions. If a person has 50% hemoglobin it would carry 9.5 ml oxygen per 100 ml of blood, the resting requirements are readily satisfied but the capacity to do work is greatly diminished, because the reserve to draw upon is decreased.

   In severe anemia the venous blood is very much reduced. During exercise the chief method available to increase the oxygen supplies to the tissues is by increase in cardiac output. Alteration in pulse rate occurs with slight exertion.

   Carbon monoxide poisoning

   Small amounts of carbon monoxide are formed in the body. In larger amounts it is poisonous. It is formed by incomplete combustion of carbon in the atmosphere.

   CO is toxic because it reacts with hemoglobin to form carbonmonoxyhemoglobin (carboxyhemoglobin COHb) and COHb cannot take up O_2 at it combines on the site for oxygen binding.

Since there is deficiency of hemoglobin to carry oxygen it is classified as anemic hypoxia. COHb has cherry red color which is visible in the skin, nail beds and mucous membrane. Death occurs if 70–80% of circulating Hb is converted into HbCO.

Treatment of CO poisoning consists of immediate termination of exposure and adequate ventilation with oxygen, artificial respiration preferable (hyperbaric oxygen if available).

3. **Stagnant Hypoxia.** When the circulation is slow and tissues suffer from oxygen lack it is called stagnant hypoxia. This can occur in heart failure.
4. **Histotoxic Hypoxia.** The tissue enzyme system is paralyzed and tissues are unable to use oxygen, though the oxygen supply is adequate, e.g. cyanide poisoning.

Venous to Arterial Shunts

When there is congenital cardiovascular abnormality, such as interatrial septal defect there is mixing of unoxygenated venous blood with the oxygenated blood (right to left shunt), and causes hypoxic hypoxia and cyanosis; in this type of hypoxic hypoxia oxygen therapy is of limited value as it **only** increases the dissolved amount of oxygen in the blood.

Cyanosis

Cyanosis is bluish coloration of skin and/or of mucus membranes. It is caused by presence in the blood of reduced hemoglobin more than 5 gm per 100 ml of blood. Two causes of cyanosis are: hypoxic hypoxia and stagnant hypoxia. Individuals who suffer from methemoglobinemia show similar coloration like cyanosis. Sufferers from carbon monoxide poisoning do not show cyanosis, because of the cherry red color of the compound with hemoglobin.

Collapse of the Lung

When a bronchus or bronchiole is obstructed, the gas in the alveoli beyond the obstruction is absorbed and lung collapses. Collapse of alveoli is called **atelectasis.** Some blood is diverted from the collapsed area to better ventilated portions of the lung.

Another cause of atelectasis is absence or inactivation of surfactant.

Collapse of the lung may also be due to presence in the pleural space of air (pneumothorax) or tissue fluid (hydrothorax) or blood (hemothorax).

Respiratory disorders are usually classified as:

1. Obstructive disorders (increased air flow resistance), i.e. asthma; chronic obstructive bronchitis; emphysema.
2. Restrictive disorders (small lung volumes), i.e. restrictive lung disorders of the lung parenchyma; restrictive disorders in the chest wall (rib fractures, kyphoscoliosis, pneumothorax, pleural effusions)

Asthma

It is an acute obstructive lung disease, due to bronchoconstriction, hypersecretion and edema of the bronchial wall.

There is episodic or chronic wheezing, cough and a feeling of tightness in the chest as a result of bronchoconstriction. The cause is still unknown. Three abnormalities are present: *airway obstruction* which is usually partially reversible; *airway inflammation; airway hyper-responsiveness* to a variety of stimuli.

The usual cause is hypersensitivity of the airways to substances in the air. In younger persons under the age of 30 years the usual cause is allergic hypersensitivity especially to plant pollens. In older persons the cause is hypersensitivity to non-allergic irritants like pollutants in the air.

When there is a link to allergy the plasma IgE levels are frequently elevated. In asthma these antibodies mainly attach to mast cells in the lungs. When the person breathes the pollen to which the person is sensitive (has developed antibodies to it), the pollen reacts with the antibodies attached to mast cells, these cells release several different substances, among them are histamine, slow reacting substance of anaphylaxis (which is mixture of leukotrienes), eosinophil chemotactic factor and bradykinin. Products released from eosinophils, in the inflammatory reaction may damage the airway epithelium and contribute to hyper-responsiveness. Leukotrienes released from cosinophils, mast cells enhance bronchoconstriction. Some other substances that may affect the bronchial smooth muscle or produce inflammation may also be involved.

Numerous other amines, neuropeptides, chemokines, an interleukins have effects on bronchial smooth muscle or produce inflammation and they may be involved in asthma.

The bronchiolar diameter becomes more reduced during expiration than during inspiration, therefore the person inspires quite adequately but expires with difficulty, hence measurements of maximum expiratory rate and FEV1 (Fig. 4.11) are greatly reduced.

The FRC and RV are greatly increased during asthmatic attacks because of difficulty in expiration.

Asthma attacks are more severe in the late night and early morning hours; at this time there is maximal constriction of bronchial smooth muscle with **circadian rhythm** of bronchial tone. **Cool air** and

exercise which normally cause bronchoconstriction also trigger asthmatic attacks, some are triggered by **aspirin (5% cases)**. Other substances have also been found to trigger asthmatic attacks.

Physiological basis of the treatment. Beta2 adrenergic agonists have been used for treatment. **Beta2 adrenergic receptors mediate bronchodilation.** Inhaled and systemic **steroids** are also used.

Emphysema

It is degenerative disease, the lungs lose their elasticity as a result of disruption of elastic tissue and the walls between the alveoli breakdown so that alveoli are replaced by large air spaces. It is a **chronic obstructive lung disease** with degenerative loss of radial traction on bronchial walls. There is also destruction of pulmonary capillaries. There are destructive and obstructive changes in the lungs. There is marked loss of lung parenchyma, hence greatly **decreased diffusing capacity** of the lungs, decreasing the capacity to oxygenate the blood and remove carbon dioxide. Physiological dead space is greatly increased as some parts have high $\dot{V}/(\dot{Q})$ ratio. Some portions of the lungs are well ventilated others are poorly ventilated, hence there is **abnormal ventilation perfusion ratio ($\dot{V}/(\dot{Q})$**, is very low in some parts; as a result **severe hypoxia develops**. Expiration during natural breathing at rest is achieved by the passive recoil of the lungs, which maintains the pressure in the airways above that in the intrapleural space and drives the air up to the mouth. In emphysema this elastic recoil is mostly lost, and the flow resistance is considerably increased; expirations are labored and work of breathing is greatly increased. The chest becomes enlarged and barrel-shaped because the chest wall expands as the opposing elastic recoil of the lung declines.

FRC is greatly increased, compliance is increased; FEV1 is greatly reduced (obstructive lung disease), expiration time is prolonged.

The hypoxia leads to **polycythemia**.

Destruction of alveolar walls includes the capillary bed with increased vascular resistance causing **pulmonary hypertension**. Pulmonary hypertension develops and the right side of the heart enlarges and then fails.

The **most common** cause of emphysema is very *heavy cigarette smoking*.

Pneumonia

It is inflammatory condition of the lungs in which the alveoli are filled with fluid and blood cells. The disease begins with infection of the alveoli; pulmonary membrane becomes inflamed and highly porous so that blood cells pass out of it into the alveoli; there is reduction in the surface area of the respiratory membrane, alveolar ventilation gets reduced due to accumulation of fluid in the alveoli; resulting in reduction of the total surface area of the respiratory membrane and reduced $\dot{V}/\dot{Q}$ ratio; both reduce diffusing capacity, which produces hypoxia and hypercapnia.

Tuberculosis

The tubercle bacilli cause reaction in the lungs which includes invasion by macrophages and walling off the lesion with fibrous tissue to form tubercle. Walling off the lesion prevents transmission in the lungs and is a protective effect. If the walling off process fails the bacilli spread throughout the lungs with destruction of tissue and formation of large abscess cavities. Thus, it may cause large areas of fibrosis reducing functioning lung tissue. The effects result in increased work of breathing and reduced vital capacity and reduced respiratory surface area with increased thickness of the membrane resulting in reduced diffusing capacity and abnormal $\dot{V}/\dot{Q}$ ratio that further reduces diffusing capacity.

There is predilection of tuberculosis for apical region of the lung; the reason perhaps is that relatively higher $\dot{V}/\dot{Q}$ ratio in the apical portion of the lungs in upright position may provide favorable environment for growth of the bacteria.

Oxygen Therapy in different types of Hypoxia

It is of great value in some types of hypoxia and of no value in others.

In ***high altitude*** it is of great value. In *hypoventilation hypoxia* it is again beneficial as it increases amount of oxygen in the alveoli of the lungs but is of no value as cure for hypercapnia caused by hypoventilation, it is again of *value in impaired diffusion.*

In hypoxia caused by anemia, circulatory deficiency or physiological shunt it is of much less value because plenty of oxygen is already available in the alveoli for oxygenation of hemoglobin. The small amount of extra oxygen transported as dissolved amount may become important in some cases.

In histotoxic hypoxia it possibly is of no use.

Oxygen Toxicity

O_2 is also toxic. Some infants treated with O_2 for respiratory distress syndrome develop chronic condition in the lungs or retinopathy of prematurity, producing opaque vascular tissue in the eyes, which can lead to serious vascular defects.

When 80–100% oxygen is given for periods of 8 hours or more, respiratory passages become irritated, and produce substernal distress, nasal congestion, irritation of throat and coughing.

Toxicity is believed to be due to production of superoxide anion, (which is free radical), and H_2O_2.

Treatments which deliver less than 100% O_2 are of value; both acute and chronic administration of O_2 24 hours per day for 2 years in this manner has been shown to reduce the suffering of diseases and the mortality of chronic obstructive pulmonary diseases.

But in those hypercapnic patients in severe pulmonary failure, the CO_2 level may be so high that it depresses rather than stimulates respiration. Some of these patients keep breathing only because of carotid and aortic chemoreceptors drive to the respiratory centre. If the hypoxic drive is withdrawn by administration O_2 breathing may stop. During resultant apnea, arterial PO_2 drops but breathing may not start again because increased PCO_2 further depresses the respiratory centre. Therefore O_2 therapy must be started with care in **severely hypercapnic** patients.

Administration of **hyperbaric oxygen** accelerates the onset of toxicity but administration of 100% O_2 at 2–3 atmospheres can increase dissolved O_2 in arterial blood to the point that arterial O_2 tension is greater then 200 if exposure is limited to 5 hours or less at these pressures O_2 toxicity is not a problem.

Therefore hyperbaric O_2 therapy is used in carbon monoxide poisoning, radiation induced tissue injury, gas gangrene, very severe blood loss, anemia, diabetic leg ulcers and for their wounds slow to heal. It is also primary treatment for decompression sickness and air embolism.

Hypercapnia

Retention of CO_2 in the body (hypercapnia) initially stimulates respiration. Retention of larger amounts produces symptoms of depression of central nervous system. Hypercapnia is rarely a symptom of pulmonary fibrosis. It occurs in **ventilation perfusion inequality** and in various forms of **pump failure** and in **circulatory deficiency** in association with hypoxia. The effect is increased in fevers as 13% increases in CO_2 production with each 1°C rise in temperature occurs. In other types of hypoxia, i.e. anemic hypoxia, histotoxic hypoxia hypercapnia would not exist along with it.

Hypocapnia

It is a result of hyperventilation. The chronic effects are seen in neurotic patients who chronically hyperventilate. Cerebral blood flow may be reduced by 30% or more because of direct constrictor effect of hypocapnia on his cerebral vessels.

Other consequences of hypocapnia are due to the associated respiratory alkalosis, the blood pH being increased to 7.5 or 7.6. The plasma HCO^- level is low. The plasma total calcium level does not change but the plasma Ca^{2+} level falls and hypocapnic individuals develop carpopedal spasm, a positive Chvostek's sign and other signs of tetany.

Asphyxia

Occlusion of airway produces asphyxia, i.e. acute hypercapnia and hypoxia together. There is pronounced stimulation of respiration with violent respiratory efforts, BP and heart rate rise and catecholamine secretion is increased and blood pH drops.

Finally the respiratory efforts cease, the BP falls and heart slows. If artificial respiration is not started cardiac arrest occurs in 4–5 minutes.

Drowning

1. Drowning is asphyxia caused by immersion in water. In some cases it would be that on losing struggle not to breathe, the first gasp of water triggers laryngospasm and death results from asphyxia with no water in the lungs.
2. In other cases the glottic muscles then relax and fluid enters the lungs.

Fresh water is rapidly absorbed, diluting plasma and causing intravascular hemolysis.

Ocean water is markedly hypertonic and draws fluid from the vascular system into the lungs, decreasing plasma volume.

The immediate goal is resuscitation, but long-term treatment also takes into account the circulating effects of water in the lungs.

Sleep Apnea

Episodes of apnea during sleep can be central in origin due to the failure of discharge in the nerves producing respiration or they can be due to airway obstruction (obstructive sleep apnea). **Central apnea** is characterized by cessation of all breathing efforts; **obstruction apnea** despite persisting breathing effective airflow ceases because of total obstruction of the upper airways. This can occur at any age and is produced when the pharyngeal muscles relax during sleep. In some cases during inspiration genioglossus muscles fail to contract during inspiration and tongue falls back and obstructs the airway contributing to blockage. After several increasing strong respiratory efforts, the patient wakes up takes a few normal breaths and falls back to sleep.

Patients with chronic bronchitis and emphysema may complain of sleep apnea.

Symptoms of loud snoring, headache, fatigue and day time sleepiness may occur. When it is severe and prolonged may causes hypertension.

Periodic Breathing

It occurs in a number of different diseases. The person breathes deeply for a short period of time and then breathes slightly or not at all for an additional interval with cycles repeating over and over again; a common type is **Cheyne-Stokes breathing** in which there is instability of respiratory control. Tidal volume waxes and wanes cyclically with repeated periods of apnea (Fig. 4.18). The blood concentration of oxygen and carbon dioxide fluctuates markedly. It may occur during hypoxia, or sleep or immediately after voluntary hyperventilation. In cardiac failure the respiratory controller may react inappropriately and produce Cheyne-Stokes breathing; it may also occur in uremia, and in patients with brain disease.

Sudden Infant Death Syndrome (SIDS)

Cause is not completely understood. There is evidence that incidence of SIDS is increased in infants of mothers who smoke. It is increased by putting the infant to sleep in the prone position. Some of the cases could be due to cardiac causes of long QT interval causing arrythmias.

Work of Breathing

The work of taking a breath is done on the lung by the inspiratory muscles. Work is low under normal conditions so that there is large reserve capacity. In certain diseases the fatigue of chest wall muscles, especially diaphragm may occur.

The work of breathing rises during exercise but energy cost of breathing in normal individuals represents less than 3% of the total energy expenditure during exercise.

In many diseases FRC is increased, e.g. in asthma with marked expiratory airway resistance and emphysema due to destruction of lung elastic tissue. Under these conditions the muscles of inspiration work at a disadvantage. Their ability to generate lower pleural pressures that cause lung expansion is reduced. The work of breathing is greatly increased in these conditions; and so also in congestive heart failure with dyspnea and orthopnea. The respiratory muscles are so severely stretched that they contract with less strength; they can become fatigued and with the pump failure it leads to inadequate ventilation.

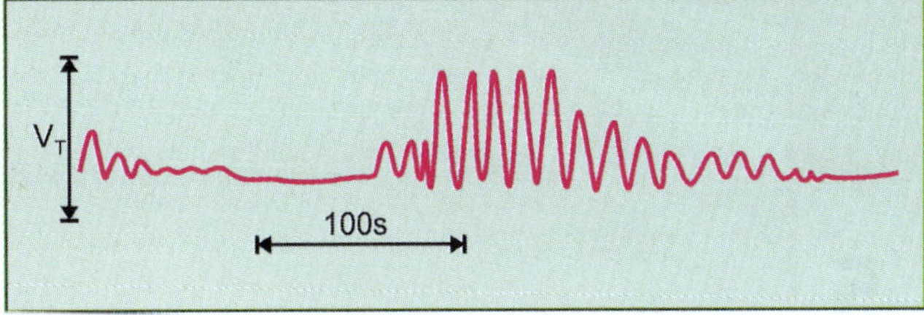

Fig. 4.18: Cheyne-Stokes breathing during sleep. Two periods of apnea are separated by an increase and then a smooth decrease in tidal volume

Normal Differences in Ventilation and Perfusion of the Lung in Upright Position

At apex the intrapleural pressure is more negative, greater transmural pressure, larger alveoli, lower intravascular pressure, less blood flow, so less ventilation and perfusion. Ventilation per unit lung volume is greater at the base than at the apex. The reason is that at the start of inspiration, intrapleural pressure less negative at the base than at the apex, and the intrapulmonary intrapleural pressure difference is less than at the apex, the lung is less expanded. At the apex, the lung is more expanded; that is, the percentage of maximum lung volume is greater. The stiffness of the lung, the increase in lung volume per unit increase in pressure is smaller when the lung is initially more expanded, and ventilation is consequently greater at the base. Blood flow is also greater at the base than the apex. The relative change in blood flow from the apex to the base is greater than the relative change in ventilation, so ventilation/perfusion ratio is low at the base and high at the apex.

The ventilation and perfusion difference tend to disappar in the supine position.

IMPLICATIONS AND APPLICATIONS

- Count the respiratory rate/minute in normal children, adults and senior citizens.
- Count the respiratory rate in various diseased conditions.
- Know about tracheostomy.
- Know about insertion of endotracheal tube. See the normal X-ray of chest and identify lobes of lungs, bronchi, etc.

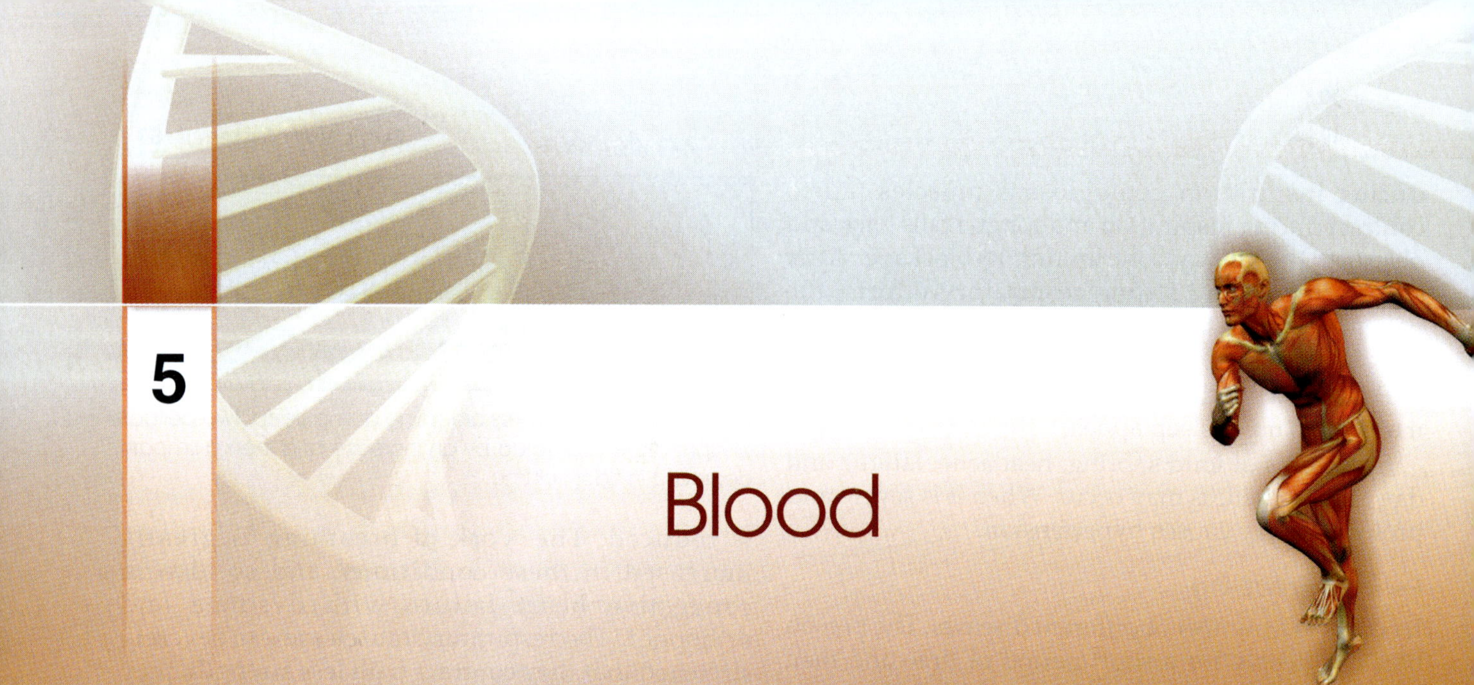

5 Blood

COMPOSITION AND FUNCTIONS OF BLOOD

Blood is a means of transport to and from all parts of the body for the requirements of all the cells. Its composition is **plasma** and cells. The cells are **red cells**, **white cells**, and **platelets**. The white blood cells are further classified as granulocytes (neutrophils, eosinophils, and basophils), and agranulocytes (lymphocytes and monocytes).

The functions of blood can be grouped as:

- Transport of oxygen from lungs to tissues; CO_2 from tissues to lungs. Hemoglobin present in red cells has very important role in these functions. The red color of blood is due to hemoglobin present in the red blood cells.
- Transport of nutrients absorbed from gastro-intestinal tract.
- Transport of metabolic waste to kidneys, lungs, and skin for removal from the body.
- Transport of hormones from glands to different sites for action
- Provides buffers for maintenance of acid base balance in the body. **The normal pH 7.4 of blood** is maintained.
- Distributes heat for the maintenance of body temperature.
- Provides defence against infections. White blood cells and antibodies in plasma proteins are important for the function.
- The clotting properties of plasma factors and platelets prevent the loss of blood during an injury of a blood vessel.
- Plasma proteins exert osmotic pressure which influences exchange of fluid across the capillaries between blood and tissue fluid.
- Transfusion of blood, if it is required, is possible by finding a compatible blood group donor or by planned autotransfusion.

Blood Volume and Plasma Volume

The blood volume is about 8% of the body weight. Plasma forms about 55% of the blood and the rest 45% is cell volume (Fig. 5.1).

With an average weight of 70 kg in an adult the blood volume is about 5.6 L.

Plasma

Plasma can be separated from the blood, to which an anticoagulant has been added (to inhibit coagulation),

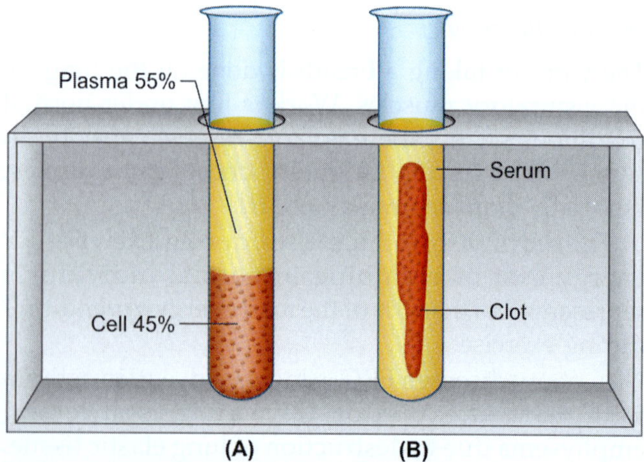

Figs 5.1A and B: (A) The proportions of blood cells and plasma in whole blood to which anticoagulant has been added, (B) Clot in blood sample as no anticoagulant added

by centrifugation, the cells settle down due to higher density leaving clear yellow liquid plasma on the top.

Blood kept without adding anticoagulant clots; after coagulation, the cell-depleted fluid phase of blood, is called the *Serum* (Fig. 5.1b). Plasma also clots on standing, remains fluid only if an anticoagulant is added. Serum has the same composition as plasma except its fibrinogen and some clotting factors (II, V, and VIII) have been consumed; and serotonin has added because of breakdown of platelets during clotting.

Plasma volume is about 5% of the body weight and is roughly 3.5 L in an adult with body weight about 70 kg.

The Constituents of Plasma

- Water (90–92%)
- Rest is dissolved substances, which are:

Proteins: There are three main fractions of proteins: Albumin; globulin (including antibodies); fibrinogen. The globulin is further subclassified into groups and includes the clotting factors.

Electrolytes: Sodium; potassium; chloride; bicarbonate; calcium; phosphorus; iron; copper; magnesium.

Nutrients: Glucose; amino acids; fatty acids; cholesterol; phospholipids; glycerol; triglycerides; vitamins.

Waste products: Urea; uric acid; creatinine.

Hormones

Gases: oxygen, carbon dioxide, nitrogen

The chief inorganic cation of plasma is sodium present normally at an average concentration of 142 meq/L, range 135–145 meq/L.

Plasma contains potassium in smaller amounts than sodium; calcium in the ionic and combined form; magnesium and some other microelements like iron and copper (Table 5.1). The principle anion of plasma is chloride; other anions are bicarbonate; plasma proteins; and in smaller amounts phosphates, sulfate and organic acids.

Plasma Proteins

Plasma proteins have a concentration of 6–8 gm/dL (100 ml = 1 dL).

Plasma proteins consist of **albumin, globulin** and **fibrinogen** fractions; the average concentrations are; albumin, 4.8 gm/dL; globulin, 2.3 gm/dL; fibrinogen, 0.3 gm/dL. The globulin fraction is subdivided usually into alpha 1; alpha 2; beta 1; beta 2; gamma globulins; fibrinogen. Prothrombin is also a globulin.

Table 5.1: Constituents of plasma in adult

Ionic constituents of plasma	
Cations	
Sodium (mEq/L)	135–145
Potassium (mEq/L)	3.5–5.0
Calcium in ionic form (mEq/L)	2.2–2.5
(Total plasma calcium is 8.5–10.5 mg/dL)	
Magnesium (mEq/L)	1.5–2.0
Hydrogen (pH)	7.35–7.45
Anions	
Chloride (mEq/L)	95–107
Bicarbonate (mEq/L)	22–26
Lactate (mEq/L)	1.0–1.8
Sulfate (mEq/L)	1.0
Phosphate (mEq/L)	2.0
(Total inorganic phosphorus is 2.5–4.5 mg/dL)	
Some constituents of serum	
Proteins (gm/dL)	**6.0–8.0**
Albumin (g/dL)	3.4–5.0
Total globulin (g/dL)	2.2–4.0
Transferrin (mg/dL)	250
Ceruloplasmin (mg/dL)	25–45
Ferritin (µg/L)	15–300
Nonproteins	
Cholesterol (mg/dL)	120–200
Glucose (mg/dL)	70–110
*Urea nitrogen (mg/dL)	6–23
Uric acid (mg/dL)	4.1–8.5
Creatinine (mg/dL)	0.7–1.4
Iron (µg/dL)	50–100

*The urea in plasma is measured as the portion of nitrogen in the urea molecule or blood urea nitrogen (BUN)

Molecular Weight and shape of Plasma Proteins. The approximate size and shape of plasma proteins relative to each other; and in relation to a molecule of glucose are shown in the Fig. 5.2. The molecular weight of plasma albumin is the smallest and is about 69,000; that of fibrinogen is high and is about 340,000.

Functions of Plasma Proteins

The protein molecules cannot pass through capillaries into tissue fluid as the molecular weights are high (and because of shape of the molecules as that of fibrinogen). Largely plasma proteins are retained within the blood in the capillaries being too large to pass through capillary pores into the tissues spaces; (though small amounts of albumin having smallest molecular weight, and even the other proteins in small

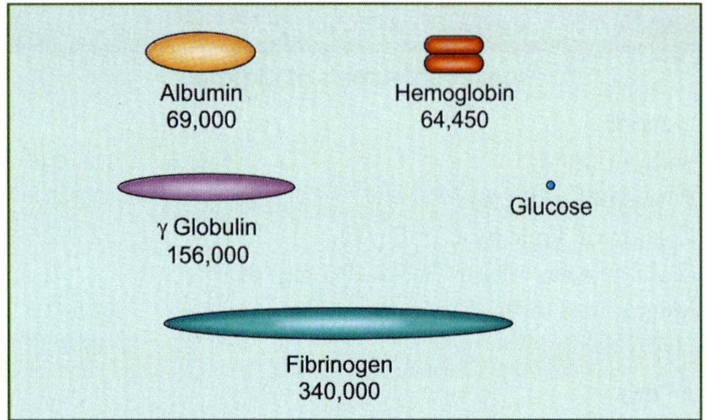

Fig. 5.2: Relative dimensions and molecular masses of some of the proteins and relative to a molecule of glucose

amounts pass through to the tissue fluid and from there are reabsorbed in lymph, and through it re-enter the circulation). As the proteins are retained in the blood in the capillaries they are responsible for **colloid osmotic pressure** (also called oncotic pressure); of about 25 mmHg that pulls water into blood at the capillaries. *Albumin fraction of the plasma proteins contributes to about 80% of this pressure*, as its concentration is highest and its molecules smallest and osmotic pressure dependents on the number of molecules in solution.

If plasma protein levels fall, especially if it involves albumin fraction, plasma oncotic pressure is reduced and fluid moves into the tissue spaces (edema) and body cavities (ascities in peritoneal cavity or as effusions in pleural or pericardial cavities).

Plasma proteins also act as ***carriers*** *for some substances in the blood, e.g. certain steroid hormones; bilirubin; plasma lipids, the triglycerides, cholesterol, and phospholipids.*

The plasma proteins act as **buffers** as contain both carboxyl and amino group in the maintenance of blood pH and are responsible for 15% of the buffering capacity of blood.

Plasma proteins, such as **antibodies** (*immunoglobulins*) are required for defence against infection.

Many plasma proteins function in **blood clotting** and have specific functions.

Origin of Plasma Proteins

Immunoglobulins are synthesized in lymphoid organs by the plasma cells. Plasma cells are transformed from B lymphocytes, when the lymphocytes are exposed to antigen.

Antigens are substances which are foreign to the body and evoke formation of specific antibodies. The antigens which form antibodies are proteins or polypeptides in structure.

Albumin and most of the other plasma proteins are formed in the liver. In diseases of liver the concentration of albumin may fall in the plasma. Albumin synthesis is carefully regulated to maintain plasma concentration. It is decreased during fasting and increased in conditions of nephrosis (kidney disease) when large amounts of albumin are lost in the urine.

Vitamin K is required for the synthesis of prothrombin, factors VII, IX and X in the liver, the proteins required for blood clotting.

Hypoproteinemia

- In **prolonged starvation** and in **malabsorption syndrome** (due to intestinal diseases) plasma protein levels are low (hypoproteinemia). They are also low in **liver diseases**, because hepatic protein synthesis is depressed and in **nephrosis (a kidney disease)** when large amounts of protein are lost in the urine and liver is unable to form at the rate at which they are lost.

  Because of decrease in the plasma oncotic pressure, edema tends to develop in hypoproteinemia.
- There can be congenital absence of one or another plasma protein fraction, e.g. **afibrinogenemia,** resulting in defective blood clotting. Congenital deficiency of any other clotting factor, also results in defective blood clotting.

CELLULAR CONTENTS OF BLOOD

There are three types of blood cells (Fig. 5.3).

1. Erythrocytes or red cells
2. Leukocytes or white cells (5 different types):
   Classified in two groups as:
   a. Granulocytes – neutrophils,
      – eosinophils,
      – basophils.
   b. Agranulocytes – lymphocytes,
      – monocytes.
3. Thrombocytes or platelets.

Bone Marrow

At and after birth **blood cells** (red blood cells, most white blood cells, and platelets) are formed only in the bone marrow, though most lymphocytes are formed in the lymphoid tissues.

All blood cells originate from *pluripotential stem cells, which are uncommitted* stem cells and go through several stages of development. These, the pluripotential stem cells differentiate into different *committed* stem cells called the *progenitor cells*, each type of which gives rise to only one type of blood cells.

Therefore, there are progenitor cells in the bone marrow for megakaryocytes which form platelets;

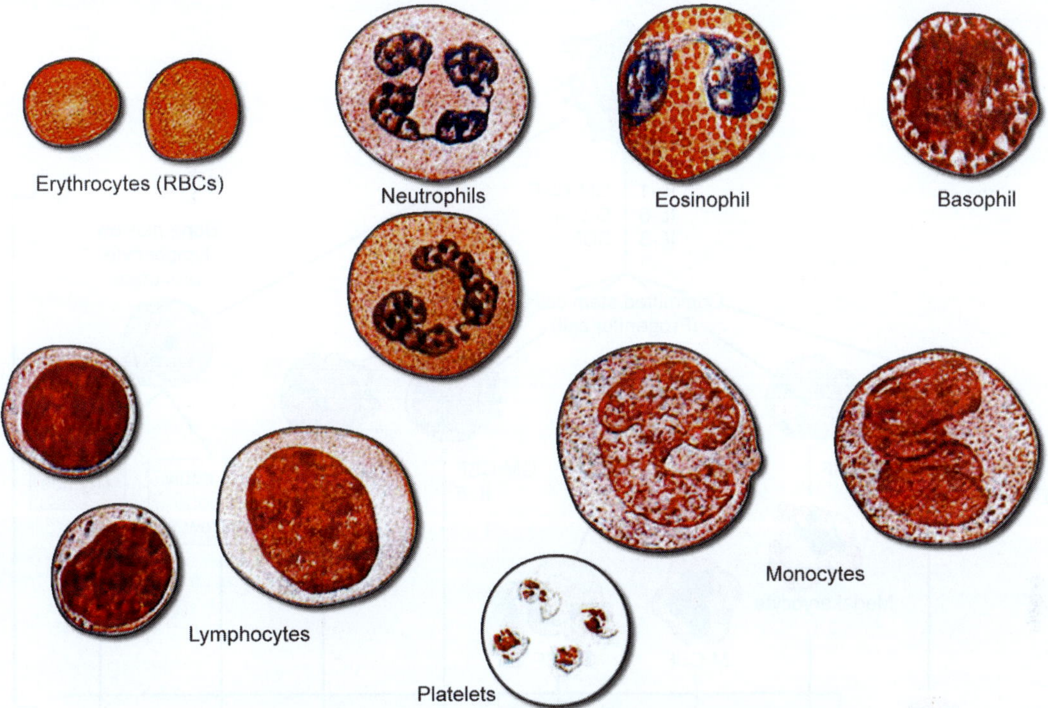

Fig. 5.3: Different blood cells in stained blood smear

progenitor cells that form red cells; progenitor cells that form eosinophils; progenitor cells that form basophils; whereas common progenitor cells form neutrophils and monocytes (Fig. 5.4).

The bone marrow where blood cells are formed is the active cellular marrow and is called *red marrow*, inactive marrow infiltrated with fat is called *yellow marrow* because of its fat content.

At birth marrow in all bones is red, actively producing blood cells. During growing age gradually some marrow becomes fatty, this occurs in an organized manner as the child develops, the process setting in first in the distal bones of the limbs (tarsus and carpus), then in the intermediate bones (tibia, fibula, radius and ulna), and finally in the proximal bones (femur and humerus). By the age of 20 the marrow in cavities of all *long bones* with *exception of* the upper ends of humerus and femur becomes inactive. **Hence, in adults red marrow is present in the axial skeleton; skull, pelvis, ribs, sternum, vertebrae; and proximal ends of femur and humerus.** Normally 75% of the cells in the active marrow belong to white blood cells (myeloid series) and only 25% are maturing red cells (erythroid series); although there are over 500 times as many red cells in the blood circulation as there are white cells. This difference is due to the fact that average life span of white cells is shorter.

The pluripotential cells are few in number but are capable of replacing the bone marrow when injected into a host whose own bone marrow has been completely destroyed. The bone marrow stem cells are also source of osteoclasts, Kupffer cells, mast cells dendritic cells and Langerhans cells. The best source for these hematopoietic stem cells, is umbilical cord blood. The pluripotential cells are in turn derived from uncommitted *totipotent* stem cells that possibly can be stimulated to form any cell of the body. These are a few in adults but can be obtained from blastocysts of embryos.

Hematopoiesis

This term means process of generating all types of blood cells.

Originally all blood cells including lymphocytes are derived from the **pluripotential stem cell.** All white blood cells; the white blood cells (except lymphocytes), after fetal life are formed only within the bone marrow and therefore referred to as myeloid cells. *Lymphocytes* though originating from marrow precursors cells, mature and proliferate outside the marrow in the *thymus* and *peripheral lymphoid tissues*.

In the fetal life blood cells arise from totipotent stem cells from blood islands in the embryonic yolk sac, the cells then colonize in the liver, spleen and marrow.

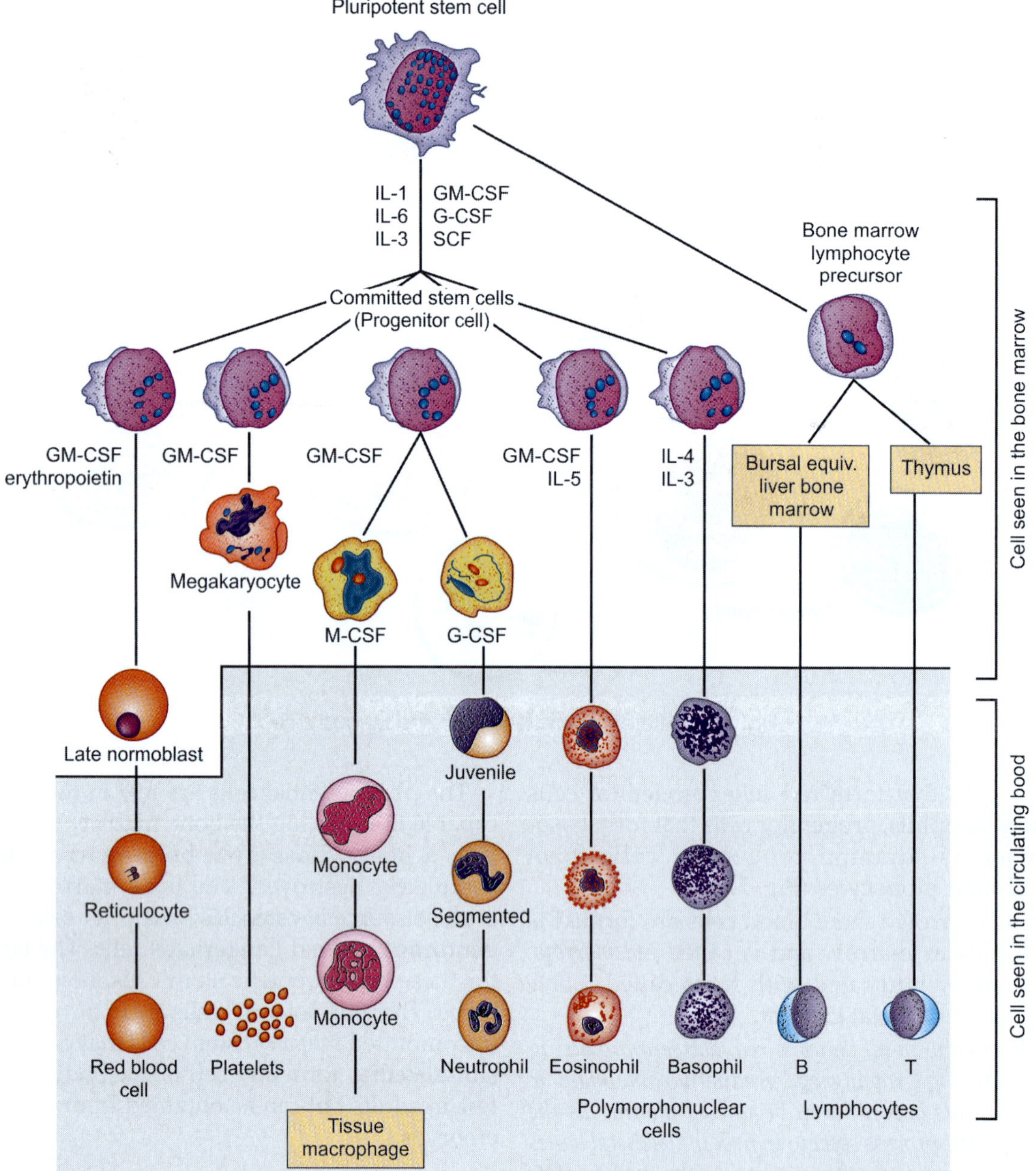

Fig. 5.4: Development of various formed elements of the blood from bone marrow cells. Cells below the horizontal line are found in normal peripheral blood. The principal sites of action of erythropoietin and the various colony-stimulating factors (CSF) that stimulate the differentiation to the components are indicated. G, granulocyte; M. Macrophage; IL interleukin.

Note: Differentiation and maturation of cells are stimulated by agents called colony-stimulating factors (CSF) and interleukins. These agents are small polypeptides, hormone like substances

In the 2nd trimester of fetal life, the cells are formed in the liver and spleen. (In an adult bone formation **may** start in liver or spleen in diseases in which bone marrow becomes diseased or fibrosed). Blood cell formation gradually shifts to marrow, and by the time of birth the development only takes place in the marrow tissues. In the fetus lymphocytes too are derived first in the liver and spleen and later in the bone marrow.

The totipotent stem cells differentiate into stem cells that are precursors of either lymphocytes or pluripotential stem cells that develop into committed stem cells for either erythrocytes or the different types of WBC or platelets (Fig. 5.4).

As these cells mature in marrow there are some common features during the development of all types of cells; the earliest cells of all the types consist of **blast cells** that are large in diameter have *large nuclei* with nucleoli and with *scanty cytoplasm;* further division (mitosis) and development results in *decrease in cell size, shrinkage of nucleus, loss of nucleoli,* and expansion of cytoplasm and appearance of granules of maturity and in the case of red cells loss of nucleus.

The differentiation and maturation of these cells are stimulated by agents called, colony-stimulating factors (CSF) and interleukins (Fig. 5.4). These agents are small polypeptides and hormone like substances.

The normal differentiation and maturation of marrow cells depends upon adequate supply of **vitamin B_{12}** and **folic acid**. These agents are required for formation of DNA, i.e. essential for cell division.

Vitamin B_{12} (cyanocobalamin) is a cobalt- containing compound. The vitamin cannot be synthesized by man but is furnished in the diet by foods of animal origin. In stomach vitamin B_{12} is bound to "**intrinsic factor**" that is secreted by the parietal cells of the stomach.

In the mucosal cells in the lower portion of the ileum, vitamin B_{12} is split from the complex and vitamin B_{12} is absorbed.

Folic acid is also furnished by diet particularly vegetables and diary products.

RED BLOOD CELLS

The red blood cells carry hemoglobin in the circulation. The cells are *circular, biconcave, non-nucleated* disks (Fig. 5.5). The cells lose their nuclei before entering the circulation. The shape of the red cell is flexible and can accommodate extra fluid without rupturing. They have **life span of about 120 days**. They are solely dependent on glucose for metabolism.

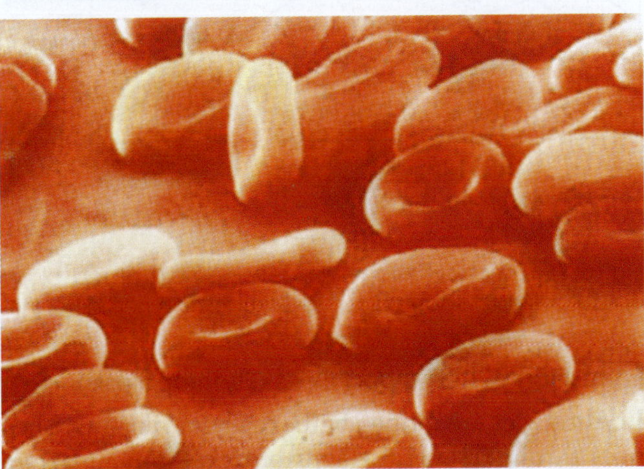

Fig. 5.5: Red blood cells

The average red cells count in the blood is 5.4 million/cu mm in men and 4.8 million/cu mm in women (Table 5.2). A red blood cell is about 7.5 μm in diameter (range 6.5–8.8); 2 μm thick at the edges and 1 μm at the center; mean corpuscular volume 87 cu vm; and contains approximately 29 pg of hemoglobin.

The viability of red cell depends upon the integrity of its membrane. The membrane is freely permeable to water. The ATP pump mechanism keeps the concentration of sodium ions low and potassium ion concentration high inside the cell. When red cell metabolism ceases as in cold-stored blood the ions move according to their concentration gradients.

The red cell membrane can be broken down by some stimuli which are used to test if the membrane is abnormally fragile.

Red Cell Fragility

Mechanical Fragility. The red cells when shaken with glass beads for one hour, 2–5% of the cells hemolyse (i.e. the cell membrane breaks down and hemoglobin is liberated). The test is undertaken to detect if the fragility of cells is increased. It is increased in some hemolytic anemia.

Osmotic Fragility. Red blood cells like other cells, shrink in solutions that have osmotic pressure greater than that of normal plasma (normal plasma is isotonic

Table 5.2: Characteristics of human red cells

		Male	Female
Hematocrit (Hct)(%)		47	42
Red blood cells (RBC) (10^6/μl)		5.4	4.8
Hemoglobin (Hb) (g/dL)		15	14
Mean corpuscular volume (MCV) (fL) 1 fL = 10^{-15} L	$\frac{Hct \times 10}{RBC (10^6/\mu l)}$	87	87
Mean corpuscular hemoglobin (MCH) (pg)	$\frac{Hb \times 10}{RBC (10^6/\mu l)}$	29	29
Mean corpuscular hemoglobin concentration (MCHC) (g/dL)	$\frac{Hb \times 100}{Hct}$	34	34
Mean cell diameter (MCD) (μm)		7.5	7.5

Cells with MCVs >95 fL are called macrocytes; cells with MCVs < 80 fL are called microcytes; cells with MCHCs <25 g/dL are called hypochromic.

with **0.9% NaCl**), as they lose water due to greater osmotic pressure in the surrounding fluid. In solutions with a lower osmotic pressure they swell, becoming spherical rather than disk-shaped, as water enters the cells; in more dilute solutions the cell wall breaks with loss of hemoglobin (hemolysis).

Normal red cells begin to hemolyse (i.e. some cells hemolyse) when suspended in 0.5% saline and hemolysis is complete, i.e. all cells hemolyse in 0.35% saline.

In disease state of **hereditary spherocytosis** the cells are spherocytic in normal plasma and hemolyse more readily than normal cells in hypotonic solutions of sodium chloride, i.e. the cells hemolyse in higher concentrations of saline than the normal cells.

Packed Cell Volume (PCV/hematocrit)

The percentage of the volume of blood made-up of erythrocytes is defined as hematocrit. The cell volume in a sample of blood to which an anticoagulant is added is measured in a Wintrobes tube; which is a narrow tube filled with blood up to 100 mark and in it the blood is *centrifuged* so that the cells being heavier settle down leaving clear plasma on the top. The volume of cells (settled, packed) is measured and it is **normally about 45% of the blood volume.** Below 40% is taken as low, indicates anemia.

Erythrocyte Sedimentation Rate (ESR)

When blood to which an anticoagulant has been added is allowed to *stand vertically* in a narrow tube (usually Westergrens tube), the red cells gradually settle down to the bottom part of the tube, leaving clear plasma on the top. The reading of plasma formed on the top after one hour is taken and if desired after the second hour also. The reading of column of clear plasma on the top gives the sedimentation rate after one hour; and after two hours if required. The cells settle down because of greater density; more the rouleaux formation (pilling of cells on top of each other) the greater the rate of settling of cells and larger the column of plasma on the top, i.e. higher the sedimentation rate.

The sedimentation rate is measured for ***evaluating the progress of chronic diseases;*** it is high in diseases where there is tissue destruction and serial checks that show rise in the rate indicate that there is worsening of the disease. It also **rises in cancer** when there is tissue destruction, the released products increase the rouleaux formation and so the ESR.

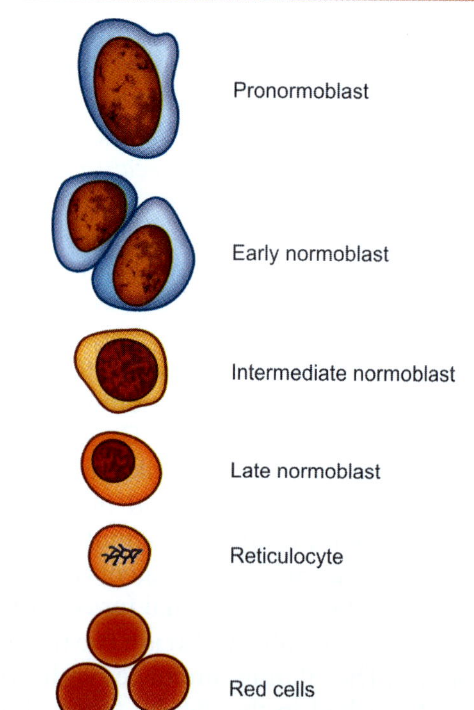

Fig. 5.6: Stages in erythropoiesis

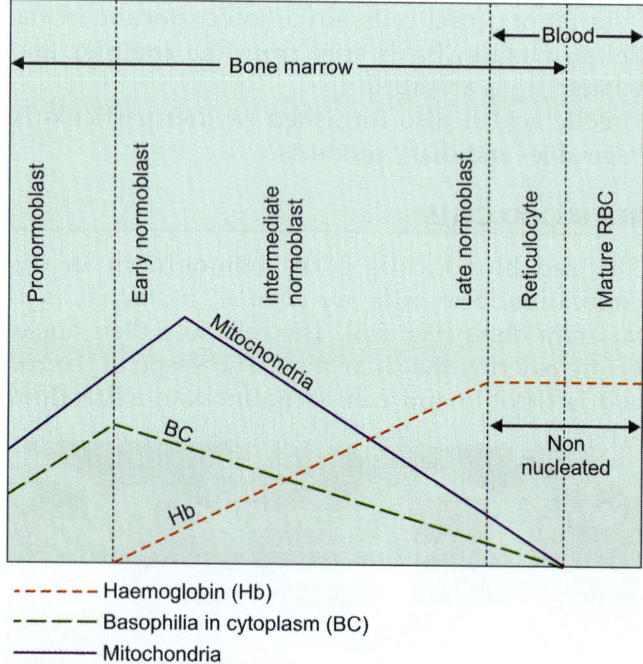

Fig. 5.7: Summary—Stages in development of red blood corpuscles and appearance and increase in hemoglobin

Formation of Red Blood Cells (Erythropoiesis)

Erythrocytes are formed in the red bone marrow. They pass through several stages of development before entering blood.

The development of red blood cells from pluripotential stem cells takes place about 7 days and is called **erythropoiesis**. It is characterized by two main features:

- Maturation of the cell
- Formation of hemoglobin inside the cell
- Loss of nucleus

Earliest *committed erythroid precursor* cells differentiate into nucleated erythroblasts *(pronormoblasts)*, large cell size, with prominent nucleoli and relatively scanty cytoplasm (Fig. 5.6).

Further cell division and differentiation brings about the formation of the more mature cells; the nucleoli disappear; and begins the synthesis of hemoglobin the cell is called normoblast, with the stages named as *early normoblast; intermediate normoblast; late normoblast;* (Fig. 5.7) in these successive stages the cells size decreases, the nuclear chromatin is condensed, cytoplasm becomes less basophilic due to decrease of ribonucleic acid, and appearance of hemoglobin, the late normoblasts lose their nuclei (Figs 5.4 and 5.6) and are released as erythrocyte (red blood cell) through the capillaries of the marrow into the bloodstream. A young erythrocyte in which remnants of ribonucleic acid (not the remnants of nucleus) are still present in the cytoplasm is called a **reticulocyte**.

In a newborn 2–6% of red cells in the circulation are **reticulocytes**, the number falls during the first week to less than 1%. It remains at **1% level** throughout life; the number increases whenever the red cells formation is increased in the bone marrow.

Normal blood has about 15 gm/dL of hemoglobin in adult men and about **13.5 g/dL in adult women.**

The cytoplasm also **contains enzymes** to provide energy to preserve the integrity of the cell membrane, to maintain the intracellular concentration of potassium above that in the surrounding plasma, to convert carbon dioxide to bicarbonate ion (i.e. carbonic anhydrase); and to prevent the oxidative transformation of hemoglobin to a nonfunctional protein methemoglobin.

Hemoglobin

It is a protein with a molecular weight of 68,000 and is synthesized in the marrow by the nucleated cells that develop into erythrocytes. The synthesis of hemoglobin requires: **protein**; vitamins (vitamin **B_{12} and folic acid**); minerals especially **iron**. At birth hemoglobin concentration is high about 23 gm/dL in the blood, and falls to 10 gm/dL at the end of third month. The concentration then rises to reach 12 gm/dL at one year. **Hemoglobin concentration is an indication of oxygen carrying capacity of blood.** One gram of hemoglobin when fully saturated combines with 1.34 ml of oxygen.

Functions of Hemoglobin

It has very important role in **oxygen carriage** in the blood. It also **carries carbon dioxide** in the blood. It is an important **buffer** in the blood for maintenance of pH. It has a role in transport of NO from lungs to tissues where it causes vasodilation.

Composition of Hemoglobin

Hemoglobin is composed of **heme** and protein **globin**. There are **four heme units** in a molecule of hemoglobin, and **four polypeptide chains in globin portion**; each heme unit is attached to one polypeptide chain in the molecule (Fig. 5.8A). **Each heme unit is a tetrapyrole in structure** and it contains one **atom of iron**. The iron is in the **ferrous state** and it combines with one molecule of **oxygen in a loose and reversible combination** (Fig. 5.8B). Hence, each molecule of hemoglobin when fully saturated with oxygen carries four molecules of oxygen.

Compounds of Hemoglobin

In carbon monoxide poisoning the place on ferrous atom is occupied by carbon monoxide blocking the attachment of oxygen.

Carbon monoxide reacts with hemoglobin to form carbonmonoxy-hemoglobin **(carboxyhemoglobin)**. The affinity of hemoglobin for carbon monoxide is much higher, about 250 times than that for oxygen, hence, it displaces O_2 from hemoglobin, reducing O_2 carrying capacity of blood. Therefore, the danger of carbon monoxide poisoning when it is present in the environment.

If the iron in the hemoglobin is **oxidized to ferric** iron it cannot combine reversibly with gaseous oxygen nor can it give up its oxygen from the OH bond. The compound is called **methemoglobin**, which is dark colored and when it is present in large quantities in the circulation, it causes dusky discoloration of the skin resembling cyanosis. Some oxidation of hemoglobin to methemoglobin occurs normally but the enzyme systems in the red blood cells convert methemoglobin back to hemoglobin. Congenital absence of this system is one of the causes of methemoglobinemia.

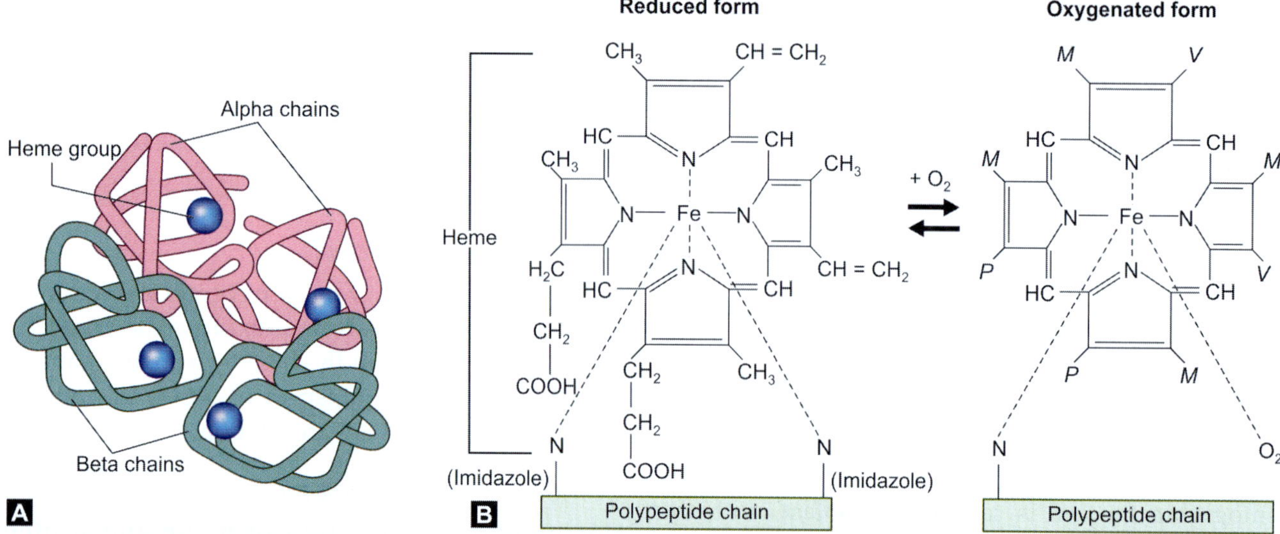

Figs 5.8A and B: (A) Structure of hemoglobin, each heme unit is attached to one polypeptide chain. One molecule of hemoglobin has 4 heme units and 4 polypeptide chains (B) Reduced hemoglobin, and reaction of heme with O_2. The abbreviations M, V, and P stand for the groups shown on the molecule on the left

Composition of Globin Part of Hemoglobin

The globin part of hemoglobin is composed of four polypeptide chains, of which two are of one type and the other two of another type, i.e. two alpha chains and two nonalpha chains in one molecule of hemoglobin (Fig. 5.8A).

Varieties of Hemoglobin

In humans several varieties of hemoglobin appear; in all the heme unit is the same, the differences are **due to variation in the composition of the polypeptide chain** of the globin portion.

Physiological Varieties of Hemoglobin

Adult Hemoglobin is of two types:

Hemoglobin A is the main type. In adult hemoglobin called HbA there are two alpha chains and two are β chains, in a molecule of hemoglobin.

Hemoglobin A_2: A small proportion, up to 3% of hemoglobin in an adult is made-up of two alpha (α) and two delta (δ) chains.

Hemoglobin F: In the fetus the fetal hemoglobin (HbF) is present and in it instead of β chains there are two gamma chains. *Hence, fetal hemoglobin is composed of two alpha and two gamma chains.* In a newborn most of the hemoglobin is composed of hemoglobin F, the proportion starts declining soon after birth; by about 2 months HbF has almost disappeared; it may fails to disappear in abnormal conditions. The fetal hemoglobin has greater affinity for oxygen it binds 2,3-DPG less avidly; hence it picks up more oxygen at lower pressures of oxygen that is useful in picking up oxygen from placental blood.

ABNORMALITIES OF HEMOGLOBIN

There are two major types of inherited disorders of hemoglobin in humans.

Hemoglobinopathies in which abnormal polypeptide chains are formed due to substitution of an unusual amino acid in polypeptide chain of hemoglobin. Many of the abnormal hemoglobins are harmless. Others cause anemia, e.g. *hemoglobin S* (sickle cell anemia); it occurs due to substitution of amino acid valine for glutamic acid in beta chain of HbA. It occurs in 10–20% of Negroes.

Thalassemias are disorders in which chains are normal in structure but synthesis of the chain is suppressed. There are α and β thalassemias due to decreased or absent α and β polypeptides chains respectively.

The Breakdown of Red Blood Cells

The **life span** of red blood cell is about 120 days.

As the red cell age the senile red cells are engulfed by *macrophages* mainly in the *liver* and *spleen*. In the macrophages hemoglobin is released from the cells and split into globin and heme. The globin is broken down by cellular enzymes into amino acids, which are reused for protein synthesis (Fig. 5.9).

The heme which is tetrapyrrole in structure is split off enzymatically, and its iron is released, the remainder molecule forms biliverdin. The released iron is stored in the body; reused mostly in erythropoiesis to form heme. The biliverdin is reduced to bilirubin which is released into plasma;

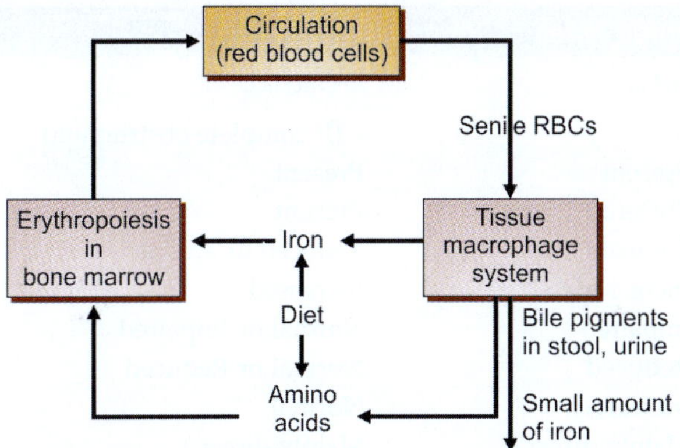

Fig. 5.9: Red cell formation and products of destruction

it being water insoluble is bound to albumin for transportation; hence being bound cannot be excreted in urine; reaches the liver cells; in liver it is conjugated to glucuronic acid to form water soluble glucuronides of bilirubin; conjugated bilirubin is excreted into the bile and through it into the intestine. Most of it undergoes reduction by bacterial enzymes in the gut to form urobilinogen (stercobilinogen); part of which is reabsorbed from the gut to enter portal circulation and re-excreted by the liver in bile, in small amounts excreted in the urine; the rest of urobilinogen in the intestines is colorless is excreted in the stool as urobilin (stercobilin) (Fig. 5.10) that is brown in color.

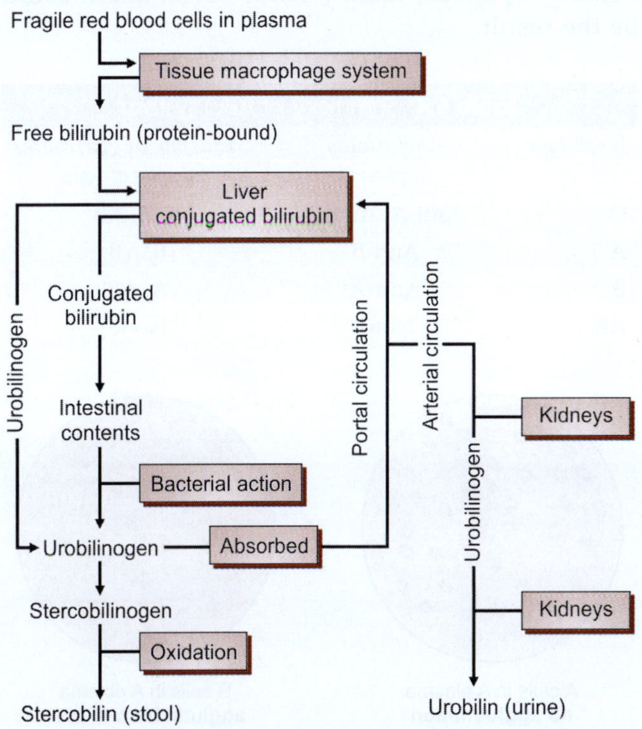

Fig. 5.10: Fate of bilirubin on destruction of RBCs

JAUNDICE

It is yellow color of the skin, conjunctiva and other tissues caused by presence of **excess of bilirubin** in the plasma and tissue fluids. (The normal range of plasma bilirubin is 0.3 to 1 mg/dL)

Jaundice can result from:

- Excess breakdown of red blood cells (hemolytic jaundice)
- Infective or toxic damage to liver cells (hepatic jaundice)
- Obstruction of the bile ducts (posthepatic jaundice)

Different types of jaundice can be distinguished by features that are presented in the table (Table 5.3). In the hemolytic type it is water insoluble bilirubin which is in excess in the blood, it is not excreted in the urine but urobilinogen is increased in urine as red cell destruction is increased. In obstructive type it is water soluble bilirubin which accumulates in the blood. Water soluble is excreted by the kidneys and *present in the urine*. In hepatic jaundice both types of bilirubin may be increased in blood as liver function is decreased and swelling of liver cells produces obstruction to the excretion in bile.

Jaundice of the Newborn

Bilirubin formed during fetal life can cross the placenta and excreted through maternal circulation; but immediately after birth the only means of excretion falls on the liver; in infants the **liver, for the first week functions poorly** and bilirubin concentration rises to an average of 5 mg/dl in first three days after birth then gradually falls back to normal.

Phototherapy (exposure to light) has value in treating infants with jaundice. Exposure of the skin to white light converts bilirubin to lumirubin which has shorter half life than of bilirubin.

Rh Incompatibility

The other cause of rather serious neonatal jaundice is the Rh incompatibility due to Rh positive fetus in Rh negative mother; the mother may form antibodies to Rh positive cells of the fetus resulting in excessive destruction of fetal red cells.

Control of Erythropoiesis

The red cells count in the blood is maintained constant; hence, bone marrow produces erythrocytes at the rate at which they are destroyed. This is due to homeostatic negative feedback mechanism.

The primary stimulus to increase erythropoiesis is hypoxia, i.e. deficient oxygen supply to body cells. Hypoxia increases the production of hormone **erythropoietin** that is produced **mainly by the kidney.** The hormone **stimulates the production of erythrocytes** in the bone marrow. The increased formation of

Table 5.3: Different features in three types of Jaundice

	Prehepatic	*Hepatic*	*Posthepatic*
Urine urobilinogen	+ +	+	– (If complete obstruction)
Urine–bile salts	Absent	Present	Present
Urine bilirubin	Absent	Present	Present
Fecal urobilinogen	Increased	Reduced	Reduced or absent
Fecal fat	Absent	Increased	Increased
Liver function tests	Normal	Impaired	Normal or Impaired
Plasma albumin	Normal	Reduced	Normal or Reduced
Plasma γ-globulin	Normal	Increased	Normal
Vandenberg	Indirect +	Mainly direct +	Mainly direct +

red cells increases the oxygen carrying capacity of the blood and reverses tissue hypoxia (negative feedback effect).

The formation of red cells requires adequate amounts of materials; like **iron** in the body, and vitamins, in particular the **vitamin B_{12}** and **folic acid**. Deficiency of any of these can result in anemia. *Proteins* supply the amino acids for formation of globin.

Deficiency of **intrinsic factor** formed by stomach mucosa and required for absorption of vit B_{12} also causes anemia.

BLOOD GROUPS

The membranes of the red blood cells contain a variety of blood group antigens, which are also called agglutinogens. The most important are A and B antigens but there are many others. Of the others Rh system antigens are of great clinical importance.

Blood group of an individual depends upon the antigens, (agglutinogens) present on the red cells and this characteristic is inherited.

ABO Blood Groups

Individuals are divided into four blood groups. **Group A, Group B, Group AB, and Group O,** depending upon the presence or absence of aggutinogens called A and B on the red cell membrane. A Group has A antigen on the red cells; B group has B antigen on red cells; AB has both A and B antigens on red cells; group O has absence of both on the red cell.

Antibodies (agglutinins) are present in the plasma to the antigen that is absent on the red cells in that individual and not to the one that is present in that individual. Individuals who are blood group A, have agglutinogen A on their red cells, and anti-B agglutinins in their plasma; those with blood group B have B agglutinogen on the red cells and anti-A agglutinins in the plasma; those belonging to AB group have both A and B agglutinogens on the red cells and no agglutinins in the plasma; those belonging to O blood group have no agglutinogen on their red cells but both anti-A and anti-B agglutinins in the plasma (Table 5.4).

Blood group of an individual can be determined by blood typing, i.e. mixing the individuals red cells with antisera containing the various agglutinins; on a slide and observing for agglutination (Fig. 5.11).

For blood transfusion individual is transfused with blood of his own blood group. If transfused with mismatched blood, transfusion reaction with main signs of clumping of red cells followed by hemolysis, shock, kidney failure even death could be the result.

Table 5.4: Summary of ABO system

Blood type	*Agglutinins in plasma*	*Plasma agglutinates red cells of type*
O	Anti-A, Anti-B	A, B, AB
A	Anti-B	B, AB
B	Anti-A	A, AB
AB	None	None

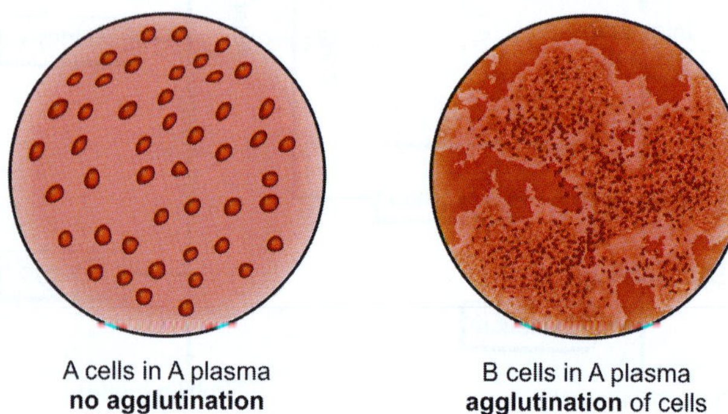

Fig. 5.11: Red cell agglutination in incompatible plasma

Person with AB blood group are called *"universal recipients"* because they have no circulating agglutinins and can receive blood of any group without developing transfusion reaction due to ABO incompatibility, though it is preferred to give them their own blood group blood. Type O individuals are called*"universal donors"* because they lack A and B antigens, and type O blood can be given to anyone without producing a transfusion reaction due to ABO incompatibility, though again own blood group transfusion is preferred. But this term of universal donor is avoided, since it does not take into account the Rh incompatibility.

Antigens of **Rh system** are also of great clinical significance. Most individuals are Rh positive. The Rh negative individuals do not have antibody against Rh factor in their plasma but can develop it under certain circumstances: (1) if Rh negative mother gets pregnant with Rh positive fetus and if some fetal cells cross placenta to reach maternal circulation to form antibodies which travel back to fetal circulation can cause destruction of fetal cells; (2) or if Rh positive blood is given to Rh negative individual it would form antibodies. The antibodies to Rh+ cells are usually anti-D bodies. The formation of such anti-D can cause severe reaction if another Rh+ transfusion is given to the individual or if it is a female and gets pregnant with Rh+ fetus. Hence, to avoid incompatibility due to ABO grouping and Rh grouping, both groups are tested in an individual and compatibility determined by crosschecking of the blood of the donor with that of recipient. Blood is not transfused without being crossmatched except in most extreme emergencies.

In **crossmatching** donor red cells are mixed with recipient plasma (major crossmatch) on a slide and checked for agglutination. Action of donor plasma on recipient cells (minor crossmatch) is in addition often checked, though this is rarely a source of trouble as plasma in the transfusion is usually so much diluted in the recipient that it rarely causes agglutination in the recipient even when the titer of agglutinins is high.

A procedure of **autologous transfusion** has become popular as it prevents infections that could be transmitted through contaminated blood.

Rh blood group factor has significance during pregnancy. Women who are Rh negative may develop antibodies against Rh factor if they carry Rh positive fetus who has inherited the Rh factor from the father. Some fetal cells may cross into maternal circulation and this can happens especially during labor, and form antibodies in the mother. The maternal antibodies can cross the placenta to the fetus and destruction of fetal erythrocytes by maternal antibodies can take place (hemolytic disease of the newborn, or erythroblastosis fetalis). If the hemolysis in the fetus is severe infant may die in the uterus; or develop anemia, severe jaundice and edema the condition is called hydrops fetalis. Another affect can be **kernicterus** when unconjugated bilirubin is deposited in the basal ganglia, as blood brain barrier is more permeable in infants and high concentration of the pigment may result in its deposition.

Usually the first pregnancy is normal but subsequent pregnancies can be affected if the fetus is again Rh positive. Since sensitization of Rh negative mothers by carrying an Rh+ fetus generally occurs during labor, the first child is usually normal; hemolytic disease occurs in about 17% of the Rh positive fetuses born to Rh negative mothers who have been pregnant one or more times with Rh positive fetuses.

With transfusion of Rh positive blood to Rh negative individuals about 50% of the Rh negative individuals are sensitized (develope anti Rh titre), and in the case of women in reproductive period this can affect an Rh positive fetus in case of such pregnancy later in life.

ANEMIAS

Anemia is decrease in the number of red cells or hemoglobin. It may result from:

- Decreased formation of red cells or hemoglobin
- Premature destruction of RBCs' (hemolytic anemias)
- Loss of blood through hemorrhage

Decreased formation results:

- Due to deficiency of iron required for formation of heme
- Due to deficiency of vitamin B_{12} or folic acid required for maturation of red cells
- Due to decreased activity of bone marrow
- Suppression of erythropoiesis due to kidney disease
- Disorders of stem cells. Aplastic anemia

Iron Deficiency Anemia

It is the most common type of anemia. It occurs either due to *blood loss* or when dietary intake of iron is not enough for **increased demands** during *pregnancy, growth* or even *menstruation.*

The red cells in iron deficiency anemia are smaller than normal (microcytic) and pale from deficiency of hemoglobin (hypochromic).

Deficiency of Vitamin B_{12} and Folic Acid

Erythrocytes are larger in size than normal (macrocytic). In bone marrow erythroblasts are abnormally large (megaloblasts) and they are less mature in appearance than normal. The types of megaloblastic anemia are:

1. Pernicious anemia in which gastric mucosal atrophy results in deficient secretion of intrinsic factor essential for absorption of vitamin B_{12} from terminal ileum.
2. Folate deficiency may occur from inadequate dietary intake, such as occurs in alcoholics, or when there is increased demand. B_{12} and folic acid are required for DNA synthesis each in a different way.

Aplastic Anemia

Hemopoietic stem cells must continually supply progenitor cells for the production of new cells; failure of the function results in **aplastic anemia**; in which mature forms of *all blood cells* formed in the bone marrow are markedly decreased (pancytopenia). Damage to the stem cell pool by ***environment toxins or radiation; suppression*** of stem cell proliferation and self renewal by immune mechanisms, could result in this effect. The individual becomes highly susceptible to bacterial infections because of granulocytopenia (decreased granulocyte count) and to serious bleeding due to thrombocytopenia (decreased platelet count).

Hemolytic Anemias

They are caused either by the abnormality of the red cell structure or by the presence of a hemolytic agent in the circulating blood.

Of the first type is the **sickle cell** anemia and of the latter type is the **hemolytic disease of the newborn.** Acquired hemolytic anemias have several causes like **some drugs**; chemicals in the work environments, e.g. lead or arsenic compounds; toxins produced by bacteria. Still other causes of hemolytic anemias include parasitic diseases like **malaria; ionising radiation** due to X-rays or radioisotopes; physical damage to red cells as in **crush injuries** or in kidney dialysis machines.

Sickle Cell Anemia

There is defect in the globin portion of hemoglobin; cause is genetic; abnormal hemoglobin is designated as hemoglobin S. The red cells have shorter life span and hence, this is hemolytic anemia.

Thalassemias are inherited disorders characterized by deficient synthesis of α or β chains. They are inherited as ***autosomal recessive*** traits.

The Therapy of Anemia

It depends on its pathogenesis. Iron is needed in iron deficiency anemia, or **vitamin B_{12}** by injections to treat pernicious anemia. In severe cases red cells transfusion may be required. Administration of **erythropoietin** is helpful in certain refractory anemias and in chronic kidney disease.

POLYCYTHEMIA

Polycythemia means RBC count is above normal limits. Physiological stimulation occurs at high attitudes due to hypoxia due to low barometric pressure, stimulating erythropoiesis and hence polycythemia occurs.

Pathological causes include impaired oxygen saturation of hemoglobin: due to diseases of lungs; or when there is congenital heart disease with shunting of blood from the right side to the left side of the heart without passing through the lungs; these conditions may increase red cell count in the blood. Great increase in the red cell count increases the viscosity of the blood, which increases the peripheral resistance and there is slowing of the blood flow velocity, that result in other pathological effects.

Polycythemia vera is a proliferative disorder of the stem cells in which erythroid (red cell) precursors arising from abnormal clones that do not respond appropriately to normal regulatory mechanisms in the bone marrow; there is great increase in the red cell count.

Table 5.5 Lists some important disorders that affect red blood cells.

WHITE BLOOD CELLS

Development Blood cells arise through a succession of steps from stem cells as described above.

All committed cells for white cells differentiate through similar steps (described in hemopoiesis) from blast cells to mature cells (Fig. 5.4). The characteristics (Fig. 5.12) of neutrophils, eosinophils, basophils or monocytes develop in mature cells.

Lymphocytes are generated from primitive hematopoietic stem cells in the marrow from where they enter the bloodstream and colonize in the lymphoid organs principally the thymus, spleen, lymph nodes, tonsillar tissue and Peyer's patches in the intestine.

In the peripheral lymph organs, the lymphocytes can reproduce and further differentiate and return to the circulation.

T lymphocytes (or T cells) are thought to be derived from lymphocytes that have migrated from the

Table 5.5: Causes of anemias

Disorder	*Sole or Major Cause*
Iron deficiency anemia	Inadequate intake or excessive loss of iron
Methemoglobinemia	Intake of excess oxidants (various chemicals and drugs)
Sickle cell anemia	Sickle cell gene, resulting in substitution of valine for glutamic acid in β-globin chain
α-Thalassemias	Mutations in the α-globin genes
β-Thalassemia	A very wide variety of mutations in the β-globin gene
Megaloblastic anemias deficiency of vitamin B_{12}	Decreased absorption of B_{12}, often due to a deficiency of intrinsic factor, normally secreted by gastric parietal cells
Deficiency of folic acid	Decreased intake, defective absorption, or increased demand (e.g. in pregnancy) for folate
Hereditary spherocytosis[1]	Deficiencies in the amount or in the structure of RBC membrane (of a or b spectrin, ankyrin, band 3 or band 4.1)
Glucose-6 phosphate dehydrogenase (G6PD) deficiency	A variety of mutations in the gene (X-linked) for G6PD

The last three disorders cause hemolytic anemias, as do a number of the other disorders listed.

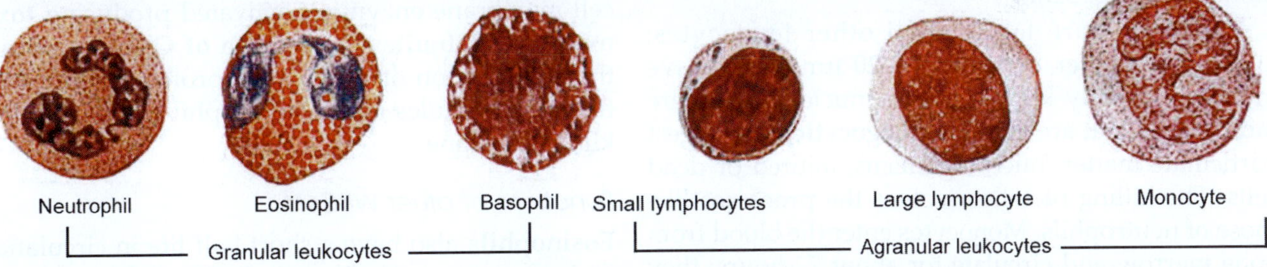

Fig. 5.12: The different white blood cells as in stained blood film

marrow to the cortex of thymus gland. They proliferate and migrate to the medulla of the thymus where they mature and then migrate to other lymphoid tissues.

B-cells probably mature in **bone marrow** and then migrate to the various **lymphoid tissues** where they reproduce themselves. Synthesis of immunoglobulins takes place in those lymphocytes that have migrated to lymphoid organs, where they are transformed on antigenic stimulation to antibody producing plasma cells.

In the lymphoid organs **T-cells and B-cells** segregate in separate zones. **Both types of cells freely re-circulate between lymphoid organs and peripheral blood.**

Characteristics of WBCs (Leucocytes)

There are 4000–11000 per microliter white blood cells in the blood. Normal % of different types of white blood cells is: granulocytes 70% (neutrophils 50–70%, eosinophils 1–4%, basophils 0–1%); agranulocytes are the lymphocytes 20–40%, and monocytes 2–8% (Table 5.6).

Table 5.6: Normal values for the WBCs in blood

Cell	*Cells/μl (average)*	*Approximate normal range*	*Percentage of total WBC*
Total WBC	9000	4000–11,000	...
Granulocytes			
Neutrophils	5400	3000–6000	50–70
Eosinophils	275	150–300	1–4
Basophils	35	0–100	0.4
Agranulocytes			
Lymphocytes	2750	1500–4000	20–40
Monocytes	540	300–600	2–8
Platelets	3,00,000	2,00,000–5,00,000	—

The Granulocytes

The cells have granules in the cytoplasm that contain active substances involved in **inflammatory** and **allergic** reactions. The diameter of the cells is about 12 to 15 μm, they have small multilobed nuclei and there is abundant cytoplasm. The three types of cells are distinguished by the nature of granules in their cytoplasm (Fig. 5.12).

Neutrophils contain neutrophilic granules and the young neutrophil has a horseshoe-shaped nucleus that becomes mutilobed as the cell grows older as a result usually cells have 2 to 5 lobes in the nuclei. The average half life of a neutrophil in the circulation is 6 hours. Many of the neutrophils enter the tissues. They pass through the walls of the capillaries between endothelial cells by a process called **diapedesis** especially if triggered by infection or by inflammatory cytokines. Many of those that leave circulation enter gastrointestinal tract and are lost from the body.

Eosinophils show coarse red granules on staining with acidic dyes. Eosinophil has 2 or 3 lobes in the nucleus.

Basophils have purple black basophilic granules and nucleus is covered by granules.

The Agranulocytes

These are of two types: The lymphocytes and monocytes (Fig. 5.3).

Monocytes are larger than other leucocytes; average diameter of about 15–20 μm. They have indented, usually kidney shaped nucleus. They are **motile cells** that are **actively phagocytic**; they ingest particulate matter, microorganisms, injured or dead cells. The killing of cells involves the processes like those of neutrophils. Monocytes enter the blood from bone marrow and circulate for about 72 hours; they then enter tissues and become **macrophages**. Some of them end up as the multinucleated giant cells seen in chronic infections, such as tuberculosis.

The tissue macrophages include the **Kupffer cells** of the liver, **pulmonary alveolar macrophages** and **microglia** in the brain; in the past they have been called reticuloendothelial system.

The macrophages become **activated by lymphokines** from T lymphocytes. The activated cells respond to chemotactic stimuli and engulf and kill bacteria like neutrophils. Macrophages also **secrete many substances** that affect lymphocytes, other cells, and clot promoting factors; **macrophages have important role in immunity.**

Lymphocytes have large round nuclei and scanty cytoplasm; the amount of cytoplasm depends on their size; the size varies from 6 to 20 μm.

All leukocytes act together to provide the body powerful defenses against: tumors; infections by viral, bacterial and parasitic microorganisms.

The Inflammatory Response on Invasion by Bacteria

The bone marrow is stimulated, produces and releases large number of neutrophils; blood count of WBCs is increased (**leucocytosis**).

Chemotaxis: The bacterial products interact with plasma factors and cells to produce substances chemokines which attract neutrophils to the infected area, this effect is called chemotaxis.

Opsonization: Bacteria when acted upon by some plasma factors become tasty to phagocytosis and this is called opsonization. Products that coat the bacteria are immunoglobulins (of IgG class) and **complement proteins** (described below in immunity).

Phagocytosis: The coated bacteria then bind to receptors on the membrane of neutrophils, and stimulate increased motor activity of the cell that leads to ingestion of bacteria by endocytosis; this is phagocytosis (Fig. 5.13).

Degranulation. Then there is degranulation; the neutrophils discharge their content of phagocytic vacuoles containing bacteria, by exocytosis into the interstitial space. The granules contain various **proteases** plus **antimicrobial proteins.** In addition the cell membrane enzyme is activated producing **toxic oxygen metabolites (generation of O^- free radical);** the combination of which with proteolytic enzymes from the granules makes neutrophil a very effective killing machine.

Functions of other WBCs

Eosinophils also have a short half life in circulation and enter tissues by diapedesis. The cells are motile like neutrophils and phagocytic and destroy organisms through oxidative mechanisms similar to but not identical to neutrophils. *Like neutrophils they release proteins, cytokines and chemokines* that produce inflammation and are capable of killing invading organisms. They are especially abundant in the *mucosa*

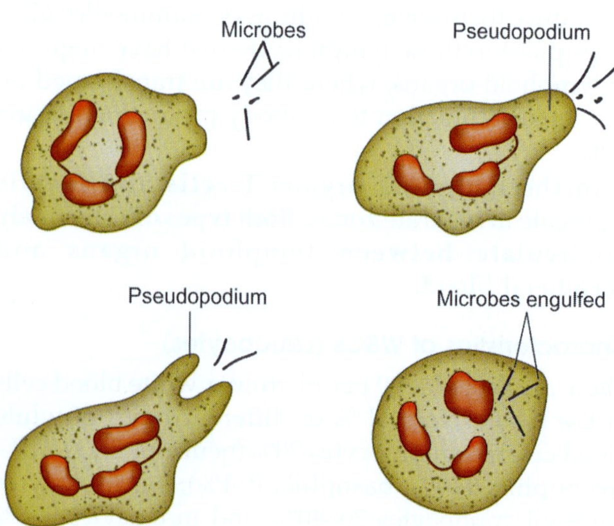

Fig. 5.13: Phagocytosis by neutrophils

of the gastrointestinal tract, where they defend against parasites; and in the *mucosa of respiratory and urinary tracts.* Circulating eosinophils are increased in allergic conditions or hypersensitive states, such as asthma, or in parasitic infestations.

Basophils also enter tissues and release proteins and cytokines. They resemble but are not identical to mast cells; like mast cells they contain **histamine**. They *release histamine and other inflammatory mediators when activated by a histamine releasing factor secreted by T lymphocytes* and are responsible for immediate type **hypersensitive reactions**; from mild urticaria and rhinitis to severe anaphylactic shock.

Mast cells are not present in the blood but are wandering cells, heavily granulated that are found in *areas rich in connective tissue* and they are abundant beneath epithelial surfaces. *Their granules contain histamine heparin and many proteases. They have IgE receptors on their cell membranes and like basophils, they degranulate when IgE coated antigens bind to their surface.* They are involved in inflammatory responses initiated by immunoglobulins IgE and IgG. *The inflammation fights parasites; is involved in acquired immunity; participates in the nonspecific natural immunity that fights infections.*

Marked mast cell degranulation produces clinical manifestations of allergy including anaphylaxis.

Lymphocytes are important in the production of immunity. After birth some lymphocytes are formed in the bone marrow but most are formed in the **lymph nodes, thymus and spleen.** Lymphocytes enter the bloodstream mostly via lymphatic vessels.

Lymphocytes are of three types: B lymphocytes; T lymphocytes (again of 3 types, cytotoxic, helper and memory cells); natural killer cells (NK cells).

In acquired immunity T and B lymphocytes are activated by specific antigens. Acquired immunity has two components; humoral immunity and cellular immunity.

Humoral immunity is major defense against bacterial infections, is mediated by B lymphocytes. The activated B lymphocytes proliferate and transform into plasma cells. *Plasma cells form antibodies which attack foreign proteins.* But for **full activation and antibody production B lymphocytes must contact helper T cells (CD4 T cells).** After invasion is over, a small number persist as **memory B cells** so that a second invasion by the same antigen provokes a prompt and magnified immune attack.

Cellular immunity is mediated by T lymphocytes. Cellular immunity is the major defense *against infections that are due to viruses, fungi and some bacteria, such as tubercle bacilli. It also defends against tumors. It is responsible for delayed allergic reactions and rejection of transplant.*

Cytotoxic T cells (mostly CD8 cells) destroy the cells that have antigen that activated them.

Natural killer (NK), cells are lymphocytes but are *not T cells; they are cytotoxic cells* capable of destroying certain tumor cells, virus infected cells, or tissue cells that have been coated with antibody; these cells are called natural killer (NK) cells. *NK cells differ from cytotoxic T cells in that they produce lysis of sensitive cells on first contact without a prior requirement for antigen sensitization.*

IMMUNITY

Immunity is of two types:

1. **Innate Immunity** (Natural Immunity): It is defense which is *immediate* and *general* against vide variety of invading organisms. *Also present at birth.*
2. **Acquired Immunity:** Immunity develops on contact with a *particular invading organism.* It takes *time to develop* and involves *activation of specific lymphocytes,* which *combat the specific infection.*

Some terms used in immunity are:

The chemotaxic agents are a part of family of chemokines and include a component of complement system (C_{5a}); leukotrienes and polypeptides from lymphocytes mast cells and basophils.

Cytokines: These are hormone like substances that regulate immune responses. Mostly have paracrine effects. *They are secreted by lymphocytes, macrophages and many other cells in the body;* if the chemical composition of anyone of the cytokines is understood its name is changed to interleukin. Hence, there are number of cytokines and interleukins which are known to participate in immune responses. Some of them have systemic and local effects. IL-1; IL-6; tumor necrosis factor alpha cause fever.

Chemokines. These are cytokines that attract **neutrophils and other white cells** to the *site of inflammation or immune responses.* They also have a role in regulation of **cell growth and angiogenesis** (growth of blood vessels to the tissue).

Complement system: The *innate* and *acquired* immunity are mediated in part by a system of *plasma enzymes* called complement system because they **complement the effects of antibodies:**

The proteins that are produced **have three functions.**

- They help kill the invading organisms by opsonization, chemotaxis and later lysis of cells

- They serve also as an bridge from innate to acquired immunity by activating B cells and aiding immune memory
- They help dispose off waste products after apoptosis (cell death). There are more than 30 proteins in this system.

Interferons are proteins made and released by host cells in response to the presence of pathogens, such as viruses, bacteria, parasites or tumor cells.

Antigen: It is a substance that is foreign to the normal body and is immunogenic, i.e. an antigen can induce the formation of antibody (immunoglobulins) that can combine in a specific way with antigen.

Innate Immunity

The natural immunity is present in the body against infections; it is *not specific for any specific type of infection.* There are receptors present in the body that bind sequences of sugars, fats or amino acids in common bacteria and activate various defense mechanisms. The activated defenses include phagocytosis, production of antibacterial peptides, and activation of complement system. Innate Immunity provides the first line of defense against infections and stimulates more specific acquired Immunity (Fig. 5.14). On activation the immune cells communicate by means of cytokines and chemokines. They kill viruses, bacteria and other foreign cells by secreting other cytokines and activating complement system.

Cells that mediate it are neutrophils, macrophages and natural killer (NK) cells.

Acquired Immunity

It has two components: Humoral immunity and cellular immunity (Fig. 5.15). The T and B lymphocytes are activated by *specific antigens* that attack the body.

Humoral immunity *It is mediated by circulating immunoglobulin antibodies.* Immunoglobulins are produced by B lymphocytes. The activated B lymphocytes form clones that produce more antibodies, which attack and neutralize antigens and activate complement system. After the invasion is repelled small numbers of B lymphocytes persist as memory cells so that second exposure to the same antigen provides a quicker and exaggerated immune attack. The lymphocytes produce antibodies that are specific for the infection that occurs.

Cellular Immunity

It is mediated by T lymphocytes (Fig. 5.15). T cells are of three types; **Cytotoxic T cells; helper T cells** and **memory T cells.**

Cytotoxic T cells destroy the cells that have antigen which activated them; kill by inserting perforins and by initiating apoptosis (cell death). *Cellular immunity*

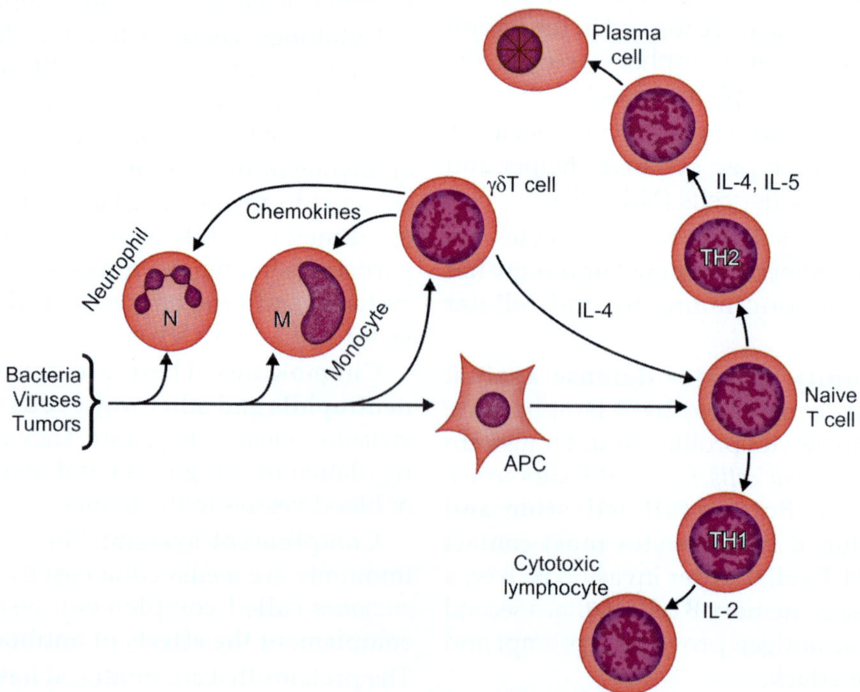

Fig. 5.14: Bacteria, viruses, and tumors trigger innate immunity and initiate the acquired immune response. APC, antigen-presenting cell; TH1 and TH2, helper T cell type 1 and type 2, respectively

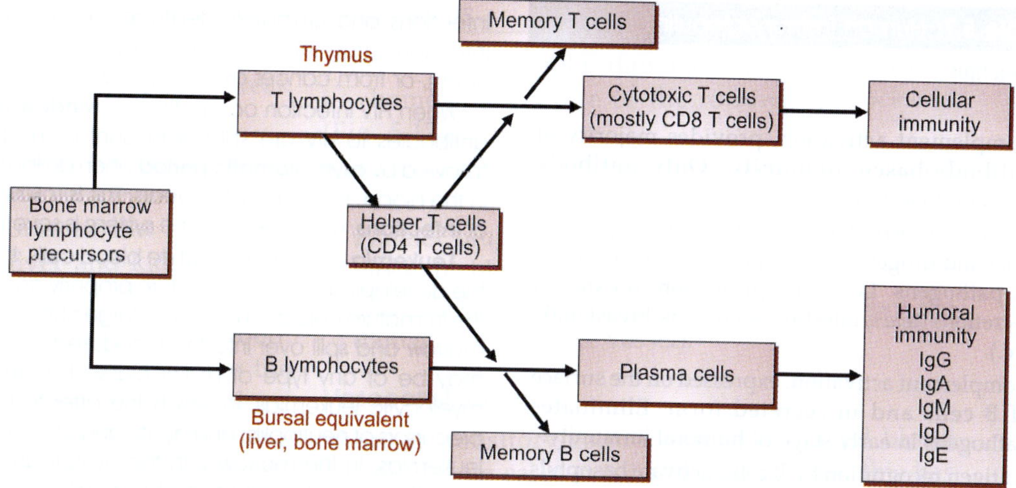

Fig. 5.15: Development of the system mediating acquired immunity

is major defense against infections due to viruses, fungi and tubercle bacteria and tumors. It is also responsible for rejection of transplanted tissue.

Helper T cells also are of two types, the T cells which stimulate the B cells for the formation of antibody, the B cells get transformed to plasma cells in the lymphoid tissues which form antibodies; and the other type of helper T cells are those that stimulate cytotoxic T cells (Fig. 5.14).

Memory T cells act for producing a prompt and exaggerated response on another invasion by the same antigen and lie in the lymphoid tissues.

The Antibodies

The antibodies circulate in the globulin fraction of plasma proteins and are called immunoglobulins. They protect the host by:

- binding and neutralizing some protein toxins,
- blocking the attachment of some viruses and bacteria to cells,
- opsonizing bacteria, and
- activating complement.

Five different types of antibodies are produced by plasma cells (Fig. 5.15). The basic component of each is the symmetrical unit containing four polypeptide chains. Two long chains are heavy chains, the other two chains are light chains; chains are linked by interchain disulfide bonds (Fig. 5.16).

The immunoglobulins are divided on the basis of difference in the heavy chains, into five major classes: IgM, IgG, IgA, IgD, IgE.

The function of the different antibodies are enumerated in table (Table 5.7).

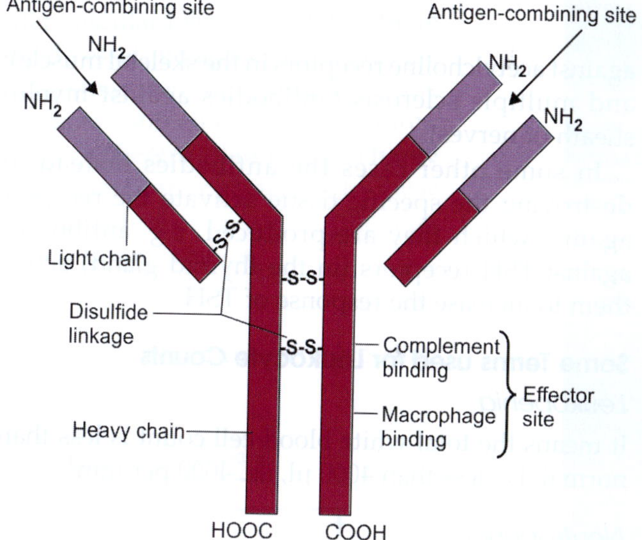

Fig. 5.16: Typical immunoglobulin shows portion of the molecule that is concerned with antigen binding and site of effector portion of the molecule

Recognition of Self

The T and B cells do not form antibodies against cells and organs of the individual. The mechanism though not very clearly understood, is believed to be, that *during development there is tolerance developed to individuals own antigens.*

Autoimmunity

Sometimes the process that eliminates own antigens fails, and antibodies are produced against ones own tissues, producing autoimmune diseases. These can be T cell mediated or B cell mediated. The diseases include: type 1 diabetes mellitus (antibodies against pancreatic islets B cells); myasthenia gravis (antibodies

FIBRINOLYTIC SYSTEM

Blood also has the capacity to re-dissolve clots that might form within blood vessels. This is mainly due to the formation of, in the plasma of proteolytic enzyme, **plasmin**; plasmin (**fibrinolysin**) is generated from its inactive precursor, **plasminogen**, present in the blood (Fig. 5.20). In the process of blood clotting plasmin is formed from plasminogen by the action of thrombin and tissue type plasminogen activator (tPA). The enzyme **plasmin** *lyses fibrin and fibrinogen* with production of fibrinogen degradation products (FDP) that *inhibit thrombin.*

The endothelium of blood vessels except in the cerebral vessels produces **thrombomodulin**, a thrombin binding protein, when thrombin binds it **becomes anticoagulant** and this prevents extension of clots into blood vessels.

Plasminogen receptors are present in many cells including endothelial cells, when *plasminogen binds to these receptors* it gets activated, so that *intact blood vessels* have a mechanism of *inhibiting coagulation.*

Integrity of blood vessel is important in hemostasis. The supporting structures are defective in scurvy **(vitamin C deficiency)** and *hemorrhagic tendency result.*

Formation of *intravascular clots is promoted by stasis of flow* (slow blood flow); inhibited by rapid blood flow.

In vivo, when plasma Ca^{2+} level is low enough to interfere with blood clotting that level is incompatible with life; hence, *in vivo* calcium deficiency does not produce defects in blood coagulation. **But clotting can be prevented *in vitro* if Ca^{2+} is removed** from the blood by addition of substances, such as oxalates, which form insoluble salts with Ca^{2+} or by **chelating agents** which bind ionic calcium, *as calcium in the ionic form is necessary for blood coagulation.*

Dicumarol and **warfarin** drugs are effective anti-coagulants, **they inhibit the actions** of **vitamin K,** which is necessary for the formation of prothrombin (factorII), VII, IX, X in the *liver.*

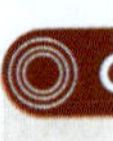

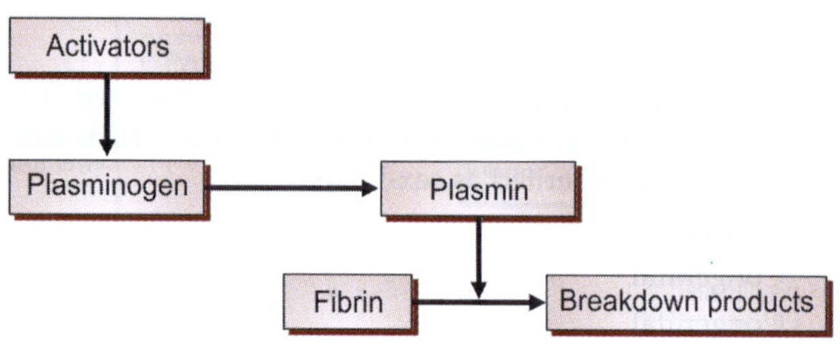

Fig. 5.20: Anticlotting mechanism

Abnormalities of Hemostasis

Clotting abnormalities are due to *platelets disorders*, and hemorrhagic diseases **(hemophilia)** that are produced by selective *deficiencies of the clotting factors* (Table 5.9). Uncontrolled bleeding even from a minor wound may occur, or ordinary activities can cause spontaneous internal bleeding into a joint, causing swelling and lead to deformities. **Hemophilia A** is caused by deficiency of factor VIII, called classical hemophilia it is most common hereditary disorder in the intrinsic pathway; in this disease the titer of antihemophilic factor (factor VIII) is decreased: classical hemophilia is X chromosome linked disorder. It affects only males; abnormal gene is carried by daughters (Fig. 5.21) but since there is another X chromosome the disease only affects them if the other X chromosome also carries abnormal gene; hence, daughters are usually carriers. In turn half their sons are hemophilic and half the daughters are carriers, who are asymptomatic.

von Willebrand factor forms a complex with factor VIII and regulates its plasma levels. Congenital deficiency of von Willebrand factor causes a bleeding disorder. **von Willebrands disease** is hereditary disorder may occur in either sex and is inherited as an autosomal dominant, in which affected individuals have symptoms suggestive of mild hemophilia.

The absorption of vitamin K *along with other fat-soluble vitamins is depressed in obstructive jaundice because of the lack of bile in the intestines and depression of fat absorption.* The resulting deficiency of clotting factors which depend on the vitamin K can cause the bleeding tendency.

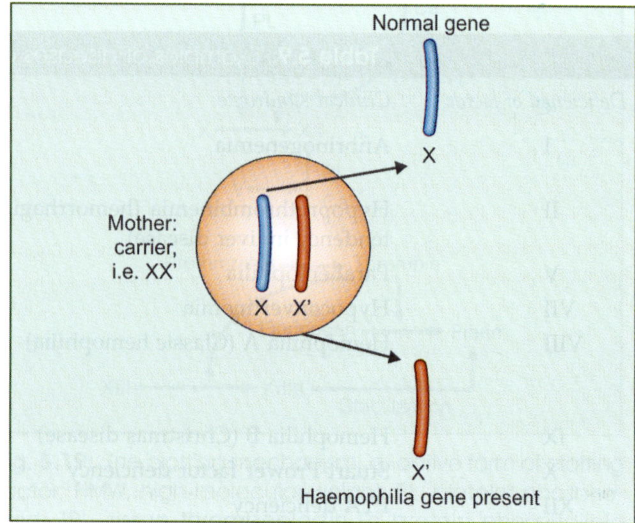

Fig. 5.21: The sex-linked haemophilia gene

Thrombosis

Formation of clot inside blood vessels is called thrombosis. It is particularly prone to occur where blood flow is sluggish, e.g. in the veins of the legs after operation and delivery, because the slow flow permits activated clotting factors to accumulate instead of being washed away.

It also occurs in vessels over areas of damage, such as in coronary and cerebral arteries at sites where the endothelium of blood vessel (inner lining) is damaged by atherosclerotic plaques.

Bits of thrombi sometimes break off and travel in the bloodstream (**emboli**) to distant sites, damaging other organs.

THROMBOCYTOPENIA

The platelet count is low. In this condition the clot retraction is poor and there is poor constriction of ruptured vessel.

Normal platelet count is about 300,000/μL (Table 5.6). Clotting abnormalities can be produced by platelet disorders, if the blood platelets count falls below 150,000/μL, but spontaneous capillary bleeding does not usually occur unless the count falls below 30,000/μL.

Anticoagulants for Clinical Use

In some thromboembolic conditions it is desirable to delay the coagulation process. Therefore anti-coagulants have been developed for treatment of these conditions. The most useful clinically are heparin and coumarins.

Heparin is used as intravenous anticoagulant in the treatment of the patient. Too much heparin can cause serious bleeding.

Coumarins as Anticoagulants

When coumarin, such as warfarin is given to a patient, the plasma levels of prothrombin and Factors VII, IX and X formed by the liver begin to decrease, *Warfarin blocks the action of vitamin K for formation of prothrombin and other clotting factors mentioned.*

Prevention of Blood Coagulation Outside the Body

Blood removed from the body and put in glass test tubes normally *clots in about* **six minutes,** blood collected in *siliconized continers does not clot for as long as an hour or so, as the containers prevent contact activation of platelets and Factor XII.*

Heparin can be used for preventing coagulation outside the body as well as in the body. Heparin is especially used in Surgical procedures in which blood is passed through a heart lung machine or artificial kidney and then back into the body.

Various substances that decrease the concentration of calcium ions in the blood can be used for preventing blood *coagulation outside the body*, e.g. small quantities of soluble oxalate compounds mixed with blood sample cause precipitation of calcium oxalate from the plasma, decrease the ionic calcium levels so much that blood coagulation is blocked.

Another calcium deionizing agent used is *sodium citrate,* the citrate ion combines with calcium in the blood to cause an unionized calcium compound and lack of ionic calcium prevents coagulation.

Oxalate anticoagulant is toxic to the body whereas **moderate** quantities of citrates are not so.

Blood Coagulation Tests

Bleeding Time

If a sharp knife is used to pierce the tip of the finger or lobe of the ear, *bleeding ordinarily lasts 1 to 6 minutes.* The time also depends on the depth of the wound and the degree of hyperemia.

Lack of several clotting factors can prolong the bleeding time, but this is *especially prolonged by lack of platelets.*

Clotting Time

Many methods have been deviced for determining clotting time. The one most widely used is to collect blood in a chemically clean glass test tube and *tube is moved back to forth until blood is clotted. By this method the clotting time is about* ***6 to 10 minutes****.*

Clotting time is dependent on the *condition of the glass itself and even the size of the tube;* which makes standardization important.

A typical condition that causes *prolonged clotting time is hemophilia A,* but deficiency of *any clotting factor* in the intrinsic pathway for clotting can cause it.

Prothrombin Time

It gives an indication of the total quantity of prothrombin in the blood. Blood is removed in the patient and is immediately oxalated so that none of the prothrombin can be change to thrombin. Later excess quantities of calcium ions and tissue thromboplastins are mixed for extrinsic pathway for coagulation and time required for coagulation to take place is noted; normally it is about 12 seconds.

Thromboplastin Generation Test

This test is used to detect the deficiency of anyone of the clotting factors. When all the other factors (except the one being tested) is added to the oxalated blood and coagulation time noted. It the factor is deficient coagulation will be prolonged.

Table 5.10 gives a summary of functions and other characteristics of blood cells.

Table 5.10: Summary of formed elements in blood

Name and appearance	*Number*	*Characteristics**	*Functions*
Red blood cells (RBCs) or erythrocytes	4.8 million/µl in females; 5.4 million/µl in males.	7–8 µm diameter, biconcave discs, without a nucleus; live for about 120 days.	Hemoglobin within RBCs transports most of the oxygen and part of the carbon dioxide in the blood.
White blood cells (WBCs) or leucocytes	4000–11,000/µl	Most live a few hours to a few days.+	Combat pathogens and other foreign substances that enter the body.
Granular leucocytes			
Neutrophils	50–70% of all WBCs	12–15 µm diameter; nucleus has 2–5 lobes connected by thin strands of chromatin; cytoplasm has very fine, pale lilac granules.	Phagocytosis. Destruction of bacteria with lysozyme, defensins, and strong oxidants, such as superoxide anion, hydrogen peroxide, and hypochlorite anion.
Eosinophils	1–4% of all WBCs	12–15 µm diameter; nucleus has 2 or 3 lobes; large, red-orange granules fill the cytoplasm	Combat the effect of histamine in allergic-antibody complexes, and destroy certain parasitic worms.
Basophils	0.5–1% of all WBCs	12–15 µm diameter; nucleus has 2 lobes; large cytoplasmic granules appear deep blue-purple.	Liberate heparin, histamine, and serotonin in allergic reactions that intensify the overall inflammatory response.
Agranular leucocytes			
Lymphocytes (T cells, B cells, and natural killer cells)	20–45% of all WBCs	Small lymphocytes are 6–9 µm in diameter; large lymphocytes are 10–20 µm in diameter; nucleus is round or slightly indented; cytoplasm forms a rim around the nucleus that looks sky blue; in larger cell, the more cytoplasm is visible.	Mediate immune responses, including antigen-antibody reactions. B cells develop into cells, which secrete anti-bodies. T cells attack invading viruses, cancer cells, and transplanted tissue cells. Natural killer cells attack a wide variety of infectious microbes and tumor cells Phagocytosis of bacteria,
Monocytes	2–8% of all WBCs	15–20 µm diameter; nucleus is kidney shaped or horseshoe shaped; cytoplasm is blue-gray and has foamy appearance	dead cells, kill bacteria, involved in immune responses (transform into macrophages).
Platelets (thrombocytes)	150,000–350,000/µl	2–4 µm diameter that live for 5–9 days; contain many vesicles but no nucleus	Form platelet plug in hemostasis; release substances to promote vascular spasm and blood clotting.

+ Some lymphocytes, called T and B memory cells, can live for many years.

IMPLICATIONS AND APPLICATIONS

- Understand the causes of anemia.
- The role of WBC's in infections.
- Precautions when blood transfusion is ordered.
- Role of platelets in blood clotting.
- Hemophilia A-inheritance.
- Plasminogen activators in thrombolysis.

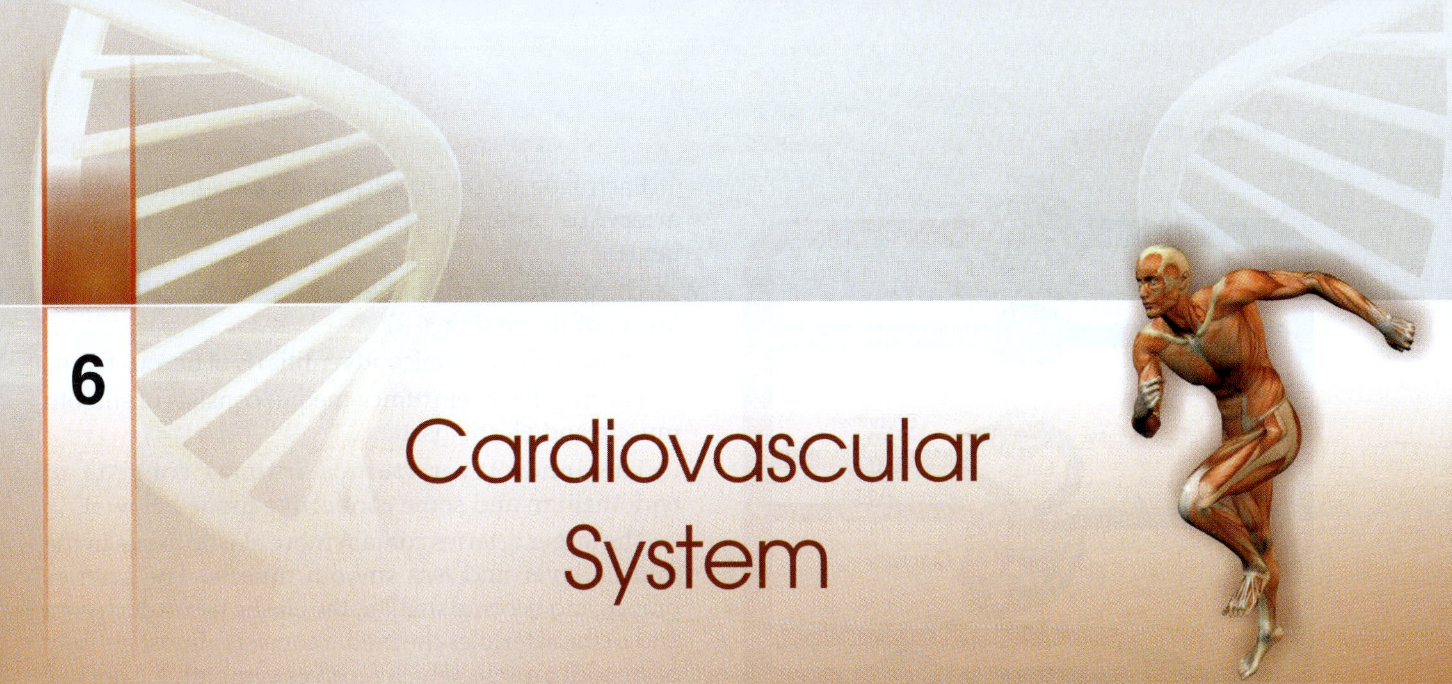

6 Cardiovascular System

The system includes:

- **The heart,** which acts as pump.
- The **blood vessels** through which the blood circulates.
- The **lymphatic system** consisting of lymph nodes and lymph vessels through which lymph flows and is associated with the system.

Functions of the System Overview

- Transport of oxygen and essential substances for the tissues needs
- Removal of waste products of metabolism of the cells
- Transport of hormones
- Regulation of body temperature
- Regulation of blood flow during varying needs of body, e.g. regulation during exercise, digestion, etc.
- Endothelial cells secrete certain substances, e.g. growth factors and vasoactive substances
- Lymph nodes have role in immunity; lymph vessels remove excess fluid from tissue spaces.

To meet these requirements the parts of circulatory system function as:

- Heart pumps blood into a large artery (aorta and pulmonary artery) so that the pressure is provided to the blood for its circulation.
- A series of distributing tubes (arteries, and their smaller branches and finally the arterioles), carry blood from the heart to the capillaries.
- Single layered endothelial vessels, the capillaries, permit exchange between the blood and tissue fluid, which surrounds the cells.
- Collecting tubes, the venules and veins which carry away the blood from the capillaries to the heart.
- The control mechanisms regulate the distribution of blood to the different tissues as per their requirements, e.g. the flow of blood to the skeletal muscle is increased during exercise; during digestion the blood flow to the gastrointestinal tract is increased.

The heart pumps blood through two circulations.

- The **pulmonary circulation**
- The **systemic circulation**

The heart consists of two pumps in series (Fig. 6.1). The right ventricle of the heart pumps deoxygenated blood into pulmonary artery which divides into smaller branches in the lungs, which form pulmonary capillaries, gas exchange occurs, oxygen enters the blood and carbon dioxide diffuses into alveoli of the lungs, purifying the blood which reaches via pulmonary veins to the left atria of the heart. This forms the pulmonary circulation. ***Pulmonary artery is an artery which carries deoxygenated blood.*** Details of this part of circulation are in the chapter on respiration.

The left ventricle of the heart pumps blood into the aorta, which gives branches to supply all parts of the body; that divide into smaller arteries and then into arterioles which open into capillaries where exchange of gases, nutrients and waste products takes place, hence pure blood is supplied to all parts of the body from where the waste products are removed into circulation and via veins which join to form larger veins the impure blood reaches the right atrium. This is **systemic circulation.**

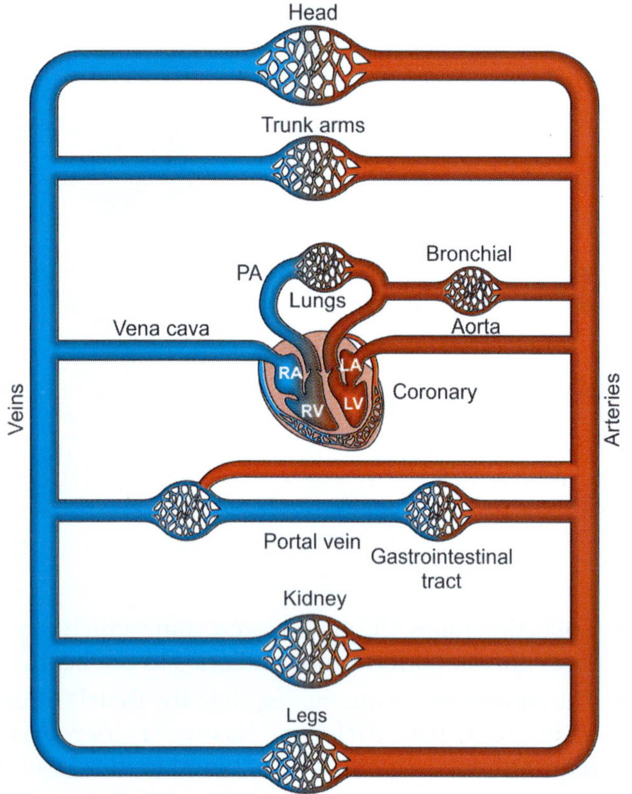

Fig. 6.1: The pulmonary and systemic circulations. The pulmonary circulation is connected in series to the systemic circulation. In systemic circulation the organ systems operate in parallel circuits. PA, pulmonary artery; RA, right atrium; RV, right ventricle; LA, left atrium; LV, left ventricle

If the supply of oxygen were to become inadequate to any part of the body, tissue damage would result.

Each side of the heart pumps blood into a large artery, i.e. arteries transport blood away from the heart.

The **arterial walls** of blood vessels consist of three layers of tissue (Fig. 6.2).

The outer layer (tunica adventitia) is of fibrous tissue.

The middle layer (tunica media) consists of smooth muscle and elastic tissue.

The inner layer (tunica intima) consists of endothelium and some connective tissue below it.

The larger arteries contain more elastic tissue in the middle layer and less smooth muscle. The arteries branch and become smaller, the elastic tissue decreases and in the arterioles the media consists almost entirely of smooth muscle, which receives sympathetic nerves; hence, these nerves regulate the diameter of small arteries and of arterioles. Increased activity of the sympathetic nerves causes contraction of smooth muscle decreasing the diameter of the vessels. Small changes in the diameter of arterioles result in large changes in the blood flow to the organ supplied by them.

Arterioles offer most of the peripheral resistance to the blood flow and are called **resistance vessels.** Widespread constriction of arterioles in the body increases the total peripheral resistance and so the level of blood pressure and this is the physiological response in large hemorrhage, to maintain the blood pressure.

Local chemical factors produced **as a result of the activity** of the tissue also act on the smooth muscle of the vessels.

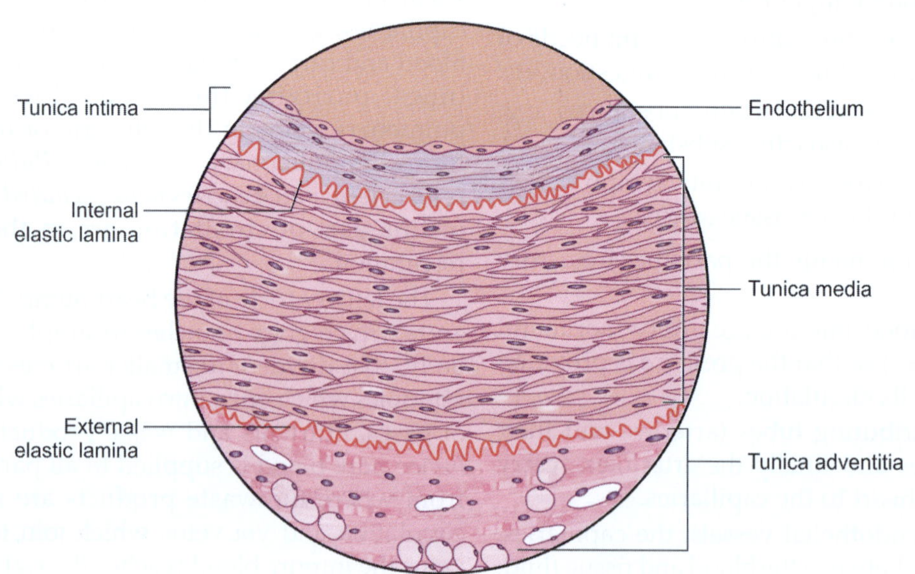

Fig. 6.2: Structure of a normal artery

The larger arteries *are elastic vessels with little smooth muscle tissue and hence diameter does not change much with sympathetic nerve activity.* But *aorta and large arteries are stretched when blood is ejected into them during systole of ventricles.* The contraction (systole) of the left ventricle pumps blood into aorta providing pressure for circulation of blood in the body (average pressure in a young adult is about 120 mmHg, the systolic pressure); aorta distends due to elastic fibers in its wall; when the ventricle muscle relaxes (diastole), the blood flow into aorta stops, pressure falls to about 80 mmHg as there is forward flow of blood to tissues; the *elastic recoil of the walls of aorta contribute to maintain the pressure head for forward flow of blood to enable continuous flow towards periphery throughout diastole.* ***This effect is called Windkessel effect and vessels are called Windkessel vessels.*** *In old age this effect decreases due to some loss of elastic tissue resulting in wide pulse pressure (systolic pressure minus diastolic pressure).*

Arteries have thicker walls than veins and they are able to withstand the high pressure of arterial blood. The pressure of blood is low in veins and their walls are thinner, they have the same three layers of tissue, but there is much less smooth muscle and elastic tissue in the media. Smooth muscle in veins is also innervated by sympathetic nerves. Marked constriction occurs on injury to stop bleeding from a vein. Noradrenergic impulses of the sympathetic nervous system and circulating vasoconstrictors cause constriction to decrease the capacity of veins, when ever required.

When an artery is cut blood spurts at high pressure; while if vein is cut slow, steady flow of blood takes place till vein collapses.

The veins of the limbs especially the **lower limbs** possess **valves** which prevent backflow of blood. This is important when an individual is standing as the blood travels against gravity and the valves prevent back flow. Valves are not present in the arteries and in very small veins, or in veins in the brain or viscera. Valves are a fold of intima strengthened by connective tissue. The cusps of the valves are semilunar in shape with a concavity towards the heart.

The arterioles lead to a network of *capillaries*. ***The wall of the capillaries consists of only a single layer of endothelial cells, exchange of substances across them takes place.*** *Blood cells and plasma proteins do not pass through the capillary walls.* Capillaries do not have smooth muscle fibers in the walls and there is no nerve supply.

The capillary bed is the site of exchange of substances between the blood and tissue fluid, which bathes the body cells. Fluid is **filtered** and added to the tissue fluid *at the arterial end of the capillary,* and almost same amount of it is absorbed back into circulation at the venous end of the capillary carrying the waste substances. But any extra amount not entered into circulation is carried back by lymphatic system and via it again enters the circulation. This prevents accumulation of fluid in tissue spaces.

In certain organs, i.e. in **bone marrow, spleen** and **liver,** vessels somewhat different from capillaries called **sinusoids** are present; these are wider than capillaries and have extremely thin walls separating blood from neighboring cells. In some places they even have distinct spaces between the endothelial cells. Present among the endothelial cells, there may be some phagocytic cells (macrophages), e.g. Kuffers cells in the liver.

Sympathetic nerves supply the media of the blood vessels. There is **no parasympathetic supply to most blood vessels** and so the diameter of the vessel is determined by degree of sympathetic stimulation.

There is a constant sympathetic nerve activity to the smooth muscle in the arterial wall and this input of nerve impulses is altered; decreased or increased by regulatory mechanisms in the body to affect the blood supply to an organ. Decrease in the number of impulses leads to increase in the diameter of the vessel (**vasodilation**), which increases the blood flow to the organ supplied by the vessel. An increase in the number of impulses to the smooth muscle causes contraction of the smooth muscle decreasing the diameter of the vessel (vasoconstriction), which results in decrease in blood supply to the organ.

The smooth muscle of arterioles is also affected by local accumulation of ***metabolites*** *in their surroundings. The metabolites like CO_2, lactic acid, lack of oxygen, dilate the arterioles in active tissues to increase the blood supply, to meet the demands of tissue.*

Veins also receive sympathetic impulses to the thin smooth muscle in their walls and when the impulses increase there is venoconstriction which *decreases the capacity of veins and more blood is released into the circulation. In hemorrhage this occurs.*

Blood flow in the aorta and large arteries is rapid; but as the arteries branch into smaller arteries the velocity of blood flow decreases.

The resistance to blood flow is small in larger arteries and so the drop in blood pressure during flow through them is small; fall in pressure is moderate in small arteries but is maximum in the arterioles, due to smaller diameter and hence there is maximum fall in blood pressure in the arterioles (Figs 6.3 and 6.4). Due to the marked fall of blood pressure across the arterioles the pressure is low in capillaries.

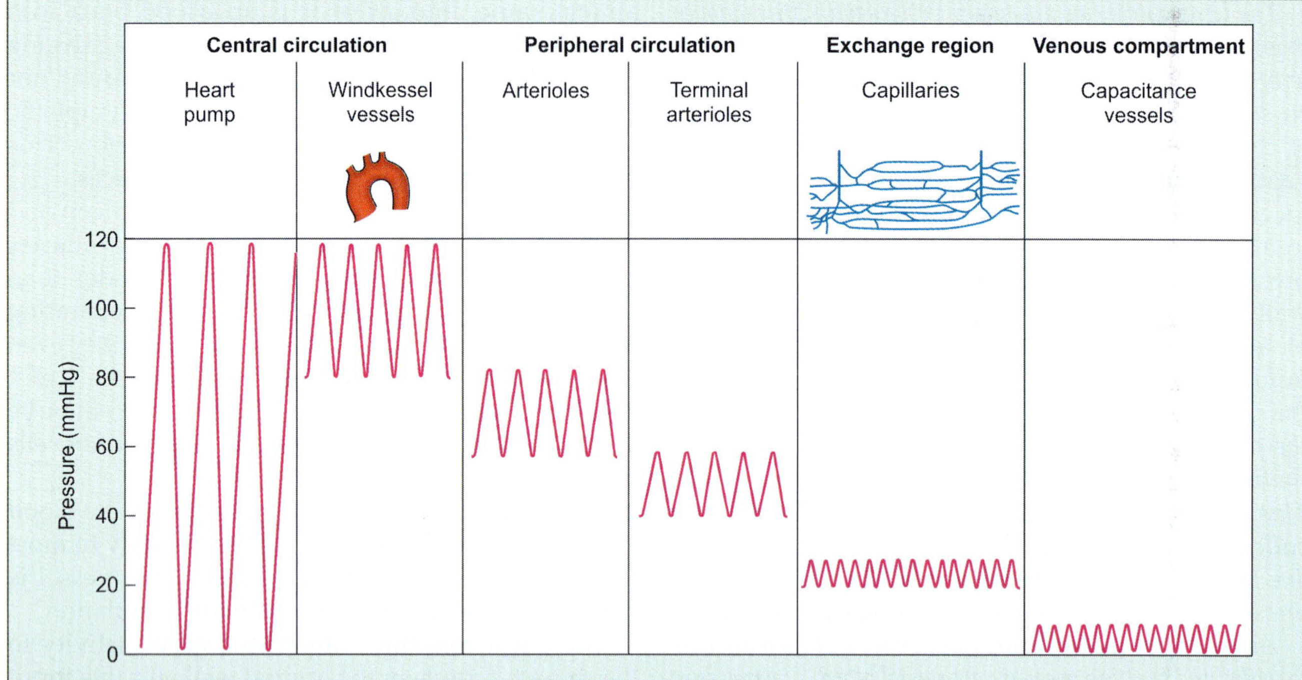

Fig. 6.3: Blood pressures in different regions of the systemic circulation. The greatest pressure drop and reduction of pulse pressure in arterioles

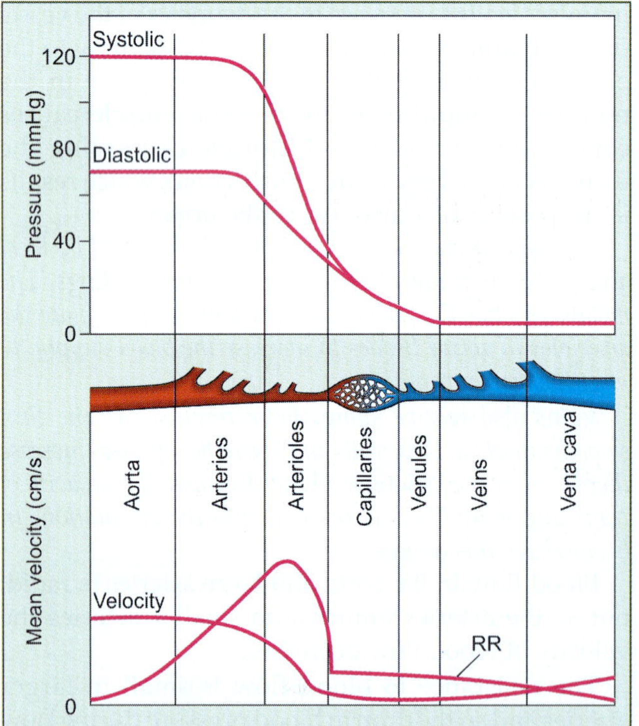

Fig. 6.4: Diagram of the changes in pressure and velocity as blood flows through the systemic circulation. RR, relative resistance, which is highest in the arterioles

Many capillaries arise from each arteriole and **though** the lumen of each capillary is smaller but as a **number** of capillaries form from an arteriole there is an increase in the total surface area of the capillary bed, that **slows blood flow velocity** (Fig. 6.4) providing an ideal condition for exchange across capillary walls.

The capillary blood passes into venules and then through veins of increasing size till it reaches right atrium.

The venous side contains most of the blood in circulation (about 50% of the blood volume is contained in systemic veins) and hence ***veins*** are called **capacitance vessels.** When there is venoconstriction (due to sympathetic activity) the capacity of veins decreases and more blood enters into the circulatory system.

Blood entering the right atrium from the systemic veins enters the right ventricle and is pumped into the pulmonary arterial system at a systolic pressure of about 25 mmHg which is much lower than that in the systemic arteries. During diastole the pressure falls to about 10 mmHg in the pulmonary arterial system.

The blood passes into pulmonary capillaries and returns to the left atrium from there flows to the left ventricle to be ejected on ventricular systole (Fig. 6.5) in the aorta. In the pulmonary circulation unlike the systemic circulation, blood is equally distributed among the arterial, capillary and venous vessels.

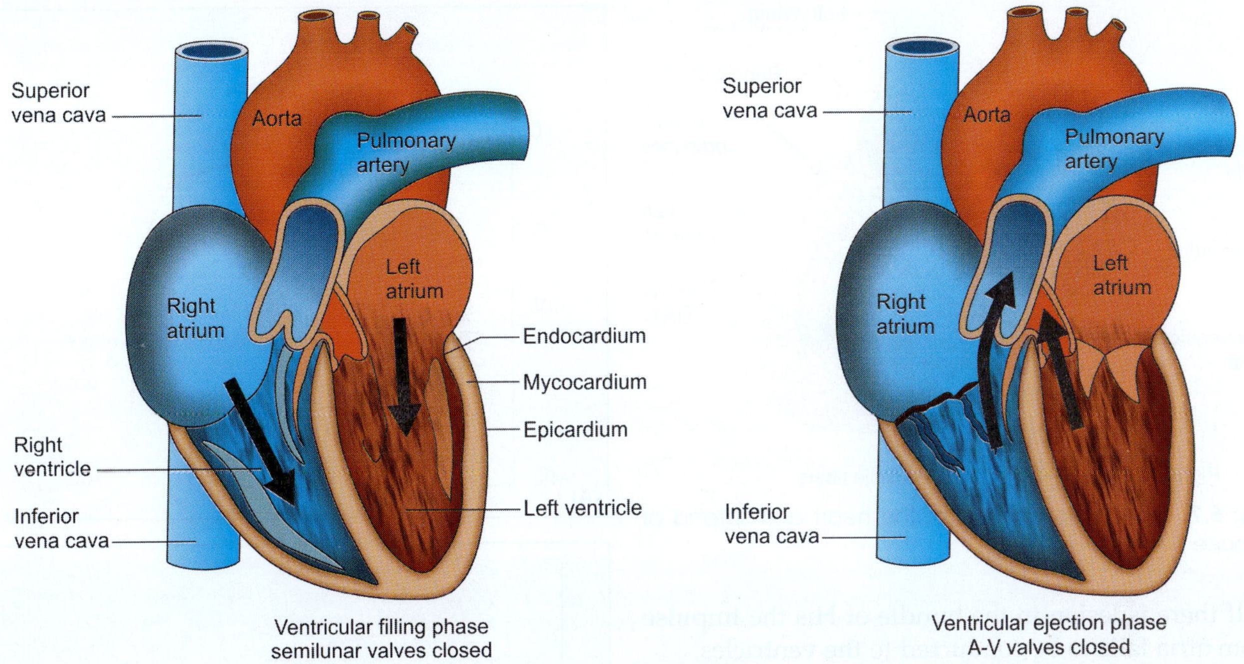

Fig. 6.5: Ventricular filling phase and ventricular ejection phase

Functional Anatomy of the Heart

The heart is composed of three layers of tissue (Fig. 6.5): pericardium, myocardium and endocardium.

Pericardium: The two layers cover the heart. **Endocardium:** It forms the **lining** of the chambers of the heart and forms the **heart valves.** It consists of flattened cells.

Myocardium is the middle layer formed of muscle fibers (Fig. 6.6).

Important feature of the cardiac muscle is the presence of ***gap junctions between adjacent fibers; the gap junctions provide a low resistance pathway for conduction of an impulse between muscle cells.*** This arrangement enables the spread of impulse to all the atrial muscle fibers to contract as a unit. Similarly when the impulse reaches ventricle muscle fibers it can be conduct to all ventricle muscle fibers due to such junctions; but in the ***ventricle a fast conducting system, Purkinje fibers normally conducts at a faster*** **rate than muscle to muscle conduction** (Table 6.1) and so ventricular muscle fibers contract in a coordinate manner necessary for efficient functioning. When there is lesion in the conductive system in one ventricle the impulse can reach from the other ventricle via cell to cell conduction; though time taken is longer for the impulse to reach that ventricle. Hence, the ***cardiac muscle is said to be a functional syncytium.*** Syncytium, because impulse spreads from muscle fiber to muscle fibers; functional because the impulse is conducted despite all fibers being completely surrounded by cell membrane with no protoplasmic continuity between them; spread is through gap junctions.

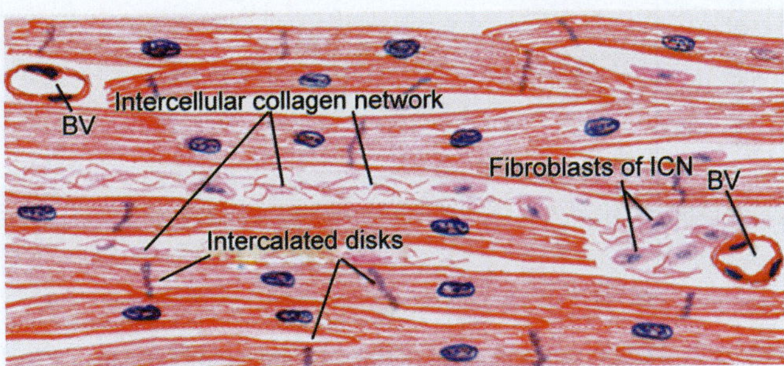

Fig. 6.6: Cardiac muscle under microscope

Atrial muscle fibers provide one functional syncytium and ventricular muscle fibers provide another. Atrial muscle fibers do not connect with ventricular muscle fibers. *However, between the atria and ventricles there is fibrous tissue ring and hence a pathway is necessary for the conduction of impulse from atria to ventricles and this is provided by* **bundle of His** (Fig. 6.7), *a conducting pathway for the impulse.*

Table 6.1: Conduction speeds in cardiac tissue

Tissue	*Conduction rate (m/s)*
SA node	0.05
Atrial pathways	1
AV node	0.05
Bundle of His	1
Purkinje system	4
Ventricular muscle	1

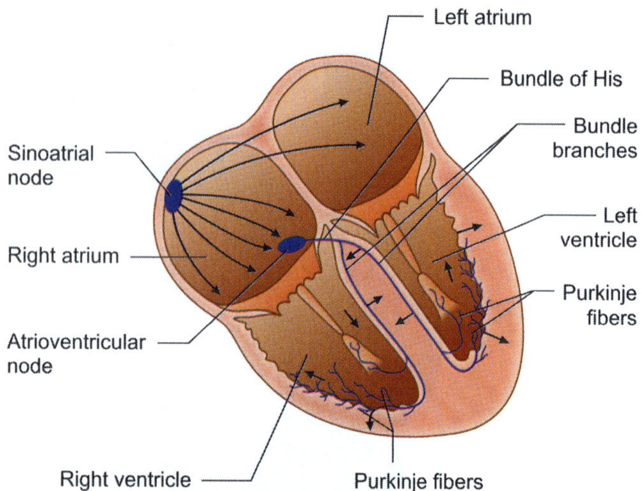

Fig. 6.7: Conduction system of the heart and spread of impulse

If there is lesion in the bundle of His the impulse from atria fails to be conducted to the ventricles.

Another property of cardiac muscle is that *the muscle cannot be tetanized (the contractions cannot be summed up). This is due to the fact that cardiac muscle has a long duration action potential* (Fig. 6.8A) *which almost lasts the duration of muscle contraction* (Fig. 6.8B), *and the next action potential that could result in another contraction is produced when the previous contraction is almost over. This property that tetanus cannot occur is beneficial for cardiac muscle.* Fig. 6.9 *shows the comparison with action potential in skeletal muscle where contractions can add on.*

The cardiac muscle has long duration of action potential because after the initial increase in membrane permeability to sodium ions that produces Na^+ *influx and depolarization it is followed by increase in calcium permeability of the membrane that prolongs the action potential due to* Ca^{2+} *influx; this phase in not present in the skeletal muscle. There is then repolarization due to decreases in calcium permeability and increase in K permeability* (Fig. 6.10).

Cardiac Muscle Action Potential and its Ionic Basis

Resting membrane potential of cardiac muscle is 90 mV (Fig. 6.10). An impulse to the muscle opens up Na^+ channels in the membrane which results in inward movement of Na^+ into the muscle producing depolarization of membrane (phase 0), the membrane potential reaches to +20 mV, but as the Na^+ channels open momentarly closure produces phase 1 in action potential, this is followed by plateau phase of action potential (phase 2) which is due to opening of Ca^{2+} channels (known as slow Ca^{2+} channels) and influx of Ca^{2+}in the cell. As the Ca^{2+} channels close the efflux

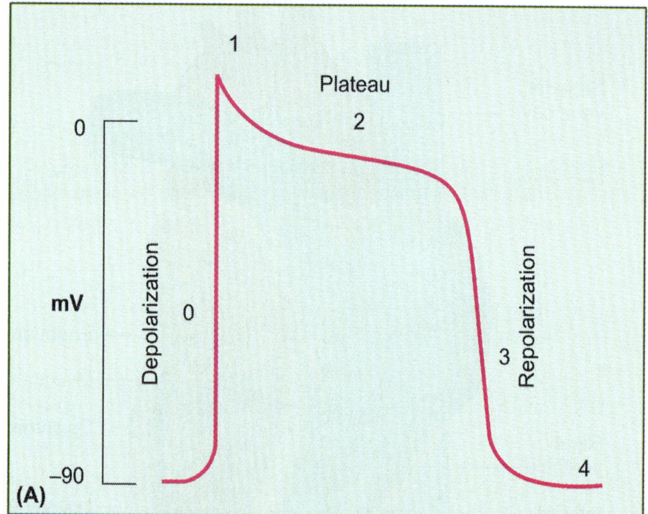

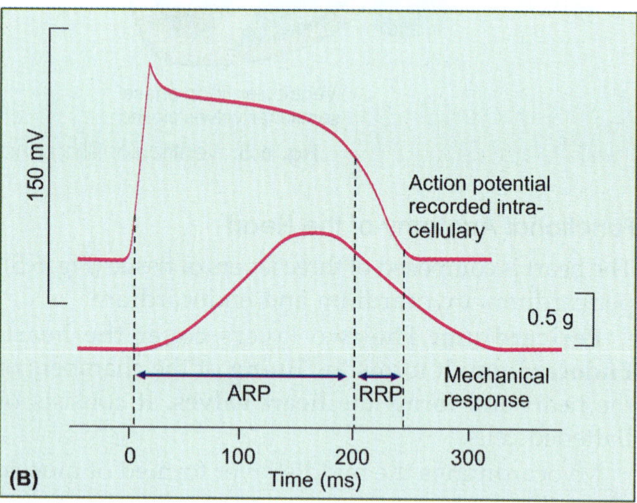

Figs 6.8A and B: (A) Cardiac muscle action potential-intracellular recording, (B) Cardiac muscle action potential and mechanical response of muscle

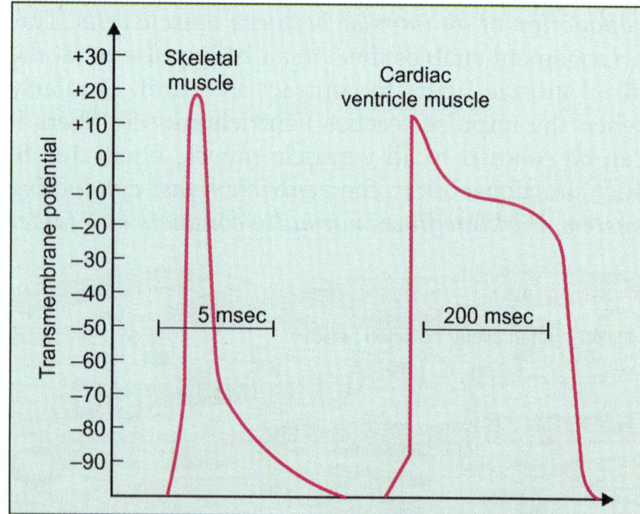

Fig. 6.9: Action potentials of different time periods as recorded from skeletal muscle cell and cardiac ventricle muscle cell

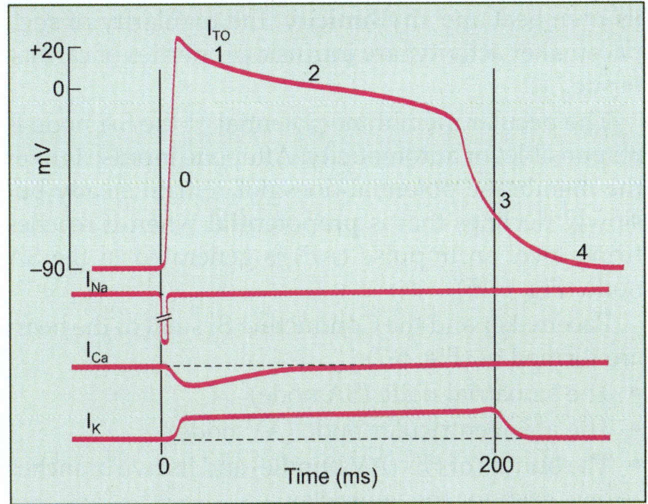

Fig. 6.10: Ionic changes producing action potential in cardiac muscle. Influx is shown downward and efflux as upward. Phase 0: due to inward movement of Na^+ Phase 2: due to inward movement of Ca^{2+} (This phase is not present in skeletal muscle) Phase 3: due to outward movement of K^+, Phase 4: resting membrane potential

of K^+ causes repolarization of membrane potential (phase 3). The resting membrane potential is phase 4 (–90 mV). This is the electrical activity of ventricular muscle which results in contraction of the muscle (Fig. 6.10). Plateau phase is not present in action potential of skeletal muscle and hence, there the duration of action potential is short (Fig. 6.9).

BLOOD SUPPLY TO THE HEART

Arterial Supply

The heart is supplied by right and left coronary arteries (Fig. 6.11), which originate from aorta closely after the aortic valves. They supply the entire blood supply to the myocardium. The right coronary artery supplies mainly the right ventricle and atrium; the left coronary artery, which divides near its origin into anterior descending and the circumflex branches, supplies mainly the left ventricle and atrium, but there is some overlap. In 50% humans the right artery is dominant. Coronary arteries branch and form network of capillaries. There are a few anastomoses between coronary arterioles and extracardiac arterioles especially around the mouth of great veins, it is believed that these may enlarge and increase in number in coronary artery disease.

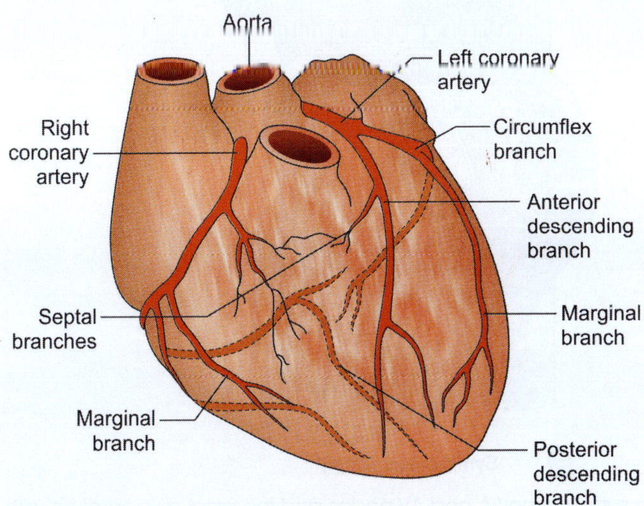

Fig. 6.11: Coronary arteries and their principal branches

Venous Drainage

Most of the blood is collected into several small veins that join to form coronary sinus, which opens into the right atrium. The remainder drains directly into heart chambers through different types of small channels (Fig. 6.12).

Nerve Supply

The nerves of the heart are autonomic nerves which originate in the cardiovascular centers (vasomotor center and cardioinhibitory center) in the medulla and reach the heart through autonomic nerves. The nerves belonging to parasympathetic system are the two vagal nerves (Xth cranial nerves, the right vagus and the left vagus).

There is sympathetic nerve supply the heart.

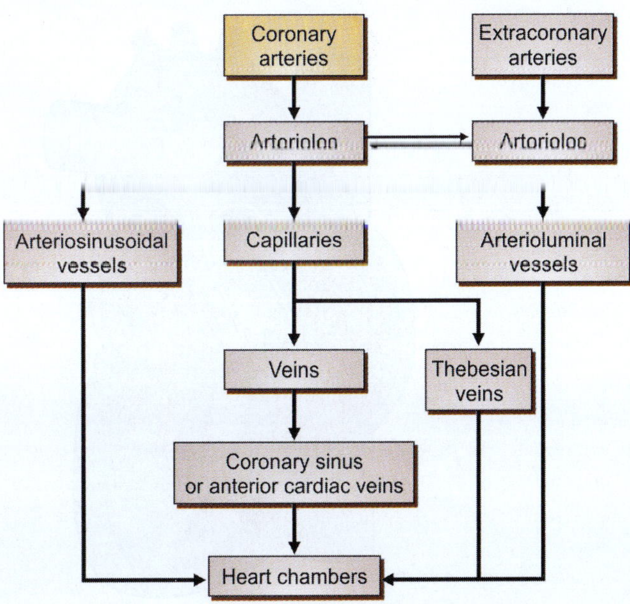

Fig. 6.12: The coronary circulation, venous blood drains mainly by coronary sinus into right atrium but also by other routes into the heart

Influence of autonomic nerves: The vagal nerves supply the SA node, AV node and atrial muscle, but the fibers to the ventricular muscle are few (Fig. 6.13A). **Parasympathetic stimulation decreases the heart rate** by influencing the activity of SA node, **decreases the conduction velocity** of impulse through the AV node and decreases the force of contraction of atrial muscle fibers, effect on ventricular contractility is small.

The sympathetic nerves supply the SA node, AV node, atrial and ventricular muscle (Fig. 6.13B).

Sympathetic stimulation increases the heart rate by influencing the activity of SA node; increases the **excitability** of heart muscle; increases the **speed of impulse** conduction through the conducting system; increases the **force of contraction** of ventricular muscle and hence the output of ventricles. The most prominent effects being **increase in heart rate and force of contraction** of ventricles.

Any effect on the heart rate is referred as **chronotropic** effect; since the sympathetic nerves increase the heart rate, the effect of sympathetic nerves on heart rate is *positive* **chronotropic** effect. Any effect on force of contraction is called **inotropic** effect hence sympathetic nerves have *positive* **inotropic** effect.

Initiation and Conduction of Cardiac Impulse

The cardiac muscle initiates its own beat, and this function does not require intact nervous pathways. The property of **automaticity** (the ability to initiate its own beat and **rhythmicity** (the regularity of such pacemaker activity) are intrinsic properties of cardiac tissue.

The pecular membrane potential of the SA node is responsible for automaticity. After one inpulse is over the membrane potential does not remain steady but slowly declines that is **prepotential** when it reaches firing level an impulse (AP) is generated in the SA node (Fig. 6.15).

Pacemaker and the Conducting System of the heart are formed of (Fig. 6.7):

- The sinoatrial node (SA node)
- The atrioventricular node (AV node)
- The bundle of His (AV bundle) and its two branches one, each for the ventricles
- The Purkinje system.

Sinoatrial Node (SA Node)

It is a small mass of cells in the wall of right atrium near the opening of the superior vena cava. It is the pacemaker of the heart; the impulse for the heart beat originates in this tissue and is conducted to atrial muscle (Fig. 6.7) which as a result contracts (atrial contraction).

Atrioventricular Node (AV Node)

It is also a small mass of cells situated in the right atrium in the posterior portion of interatrial septum. The impulse which originated in the SA node spreads in both atria reaches AV node, it is conducted through

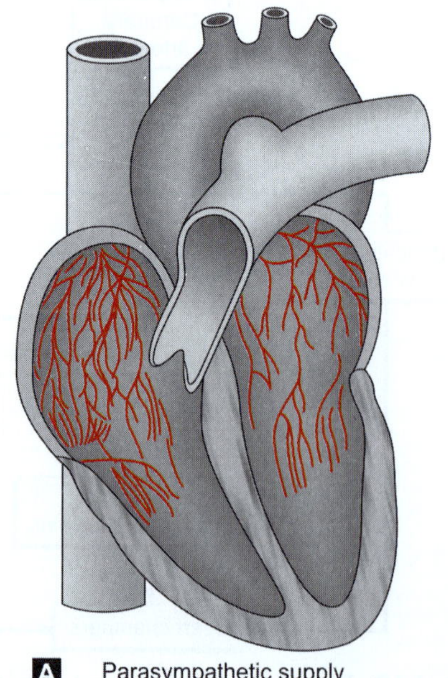

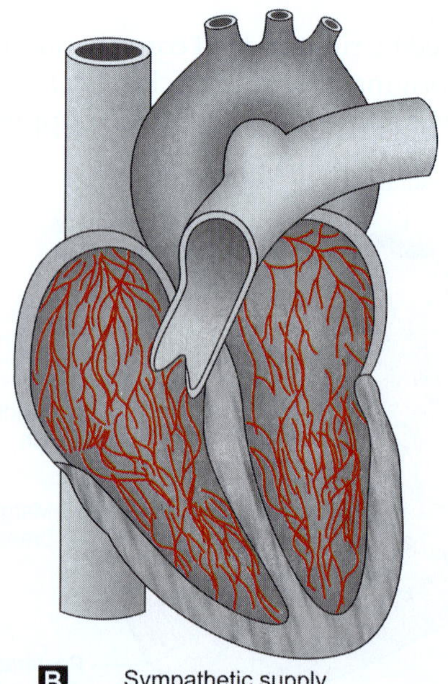

Figs 6.13A and B: (A) The parasympathetic system predominantly supplies the SA and AV nodes and the atrial myocardium with only a few branches to the ventricles; (B) Sympathetic innervation is to the SA node, AV node and to atrial and ventricular myocardium

it to the bundle of His, but after a short delay at AV node, due to slow conduction through it. This helps the atrial contraction to be over before ventricular contraction.

Bundle of His (AV Bundle)

It originates from AV node, crosses the fibrous ring that separates atria from ventricles and passes down the right side of interventricular septum for 1 cm and then divides into **right and left bundle branches** for the right and left ventricles respectively. Within the ventricles the branches break up into fine fibers, called **Purkinje fibers**. The impulse passing through the bundle of His spreads to its two branches and then through Purkinje fibers to all parts of myocardium. It reaches the apical region first and then spreads to the bases of the heart (Fig. 6.14). The conducting system of bundle of His, its branches and the Purkinje fibers conduct the impulse at a fast rate (Table 6.1), which results in almost simultaneous contraction of all of the myocardial fibers, with the spread of the impulse. Thus, the contractions are very effective for the output of the ventricles and the contraction are coordinated at both sides.

The **Pacemaker which is the SA node** regularly **initiates an impulse** for the heart beat. It does not require nervous pathways for its function and initiates the impulse even in the absence of nerves (e.g. cardiac transplant patient can function well and adapt to stressful situation).

Membrane Potential of SA node: The SA node acts as a pacemaker because of characteristic resting membrane potential; that does not remain steady but slowly declines (called prepotential) and when it reaches the firing level (threshold level), an action potential (impulse) is originated (Fig. 6.15). The rate at which action potential is originated depends on the slope of prepotential, which is influenced by the activity of autonomic nerves and other factors and it determines the rate of the heart beat.

Ionic movements producing pacemaker potential. The slow depolarization producing prepotential is because of decline in K^+ permeability and action potential is produced due to opening of Ca^{2+} channels.

The nerves *influence* the Pacemakers activity. The rate of impulse generation is modified by autonomic nerves (Fig. 6.15B), due to influence on the slope of prepotential.

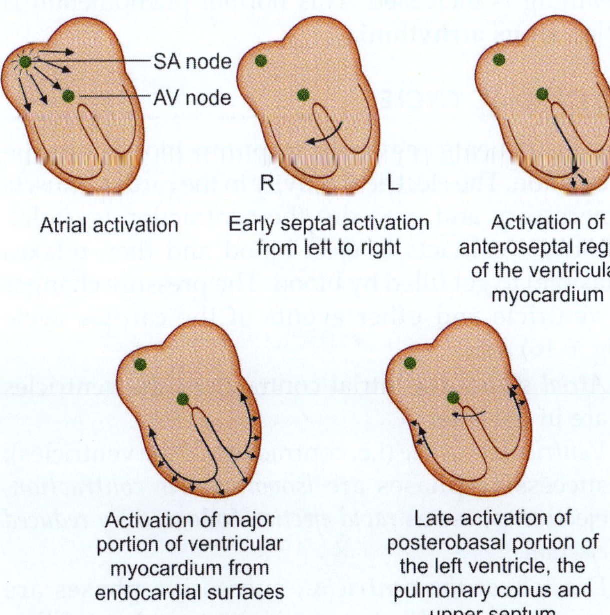

Fig. 6.14: Normal spread of electrical activity in the heart

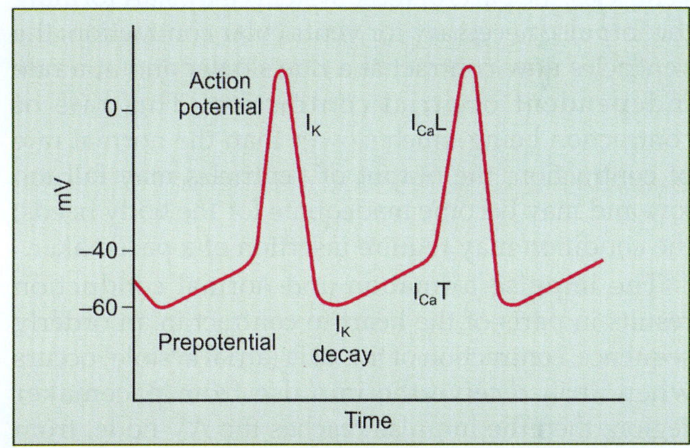

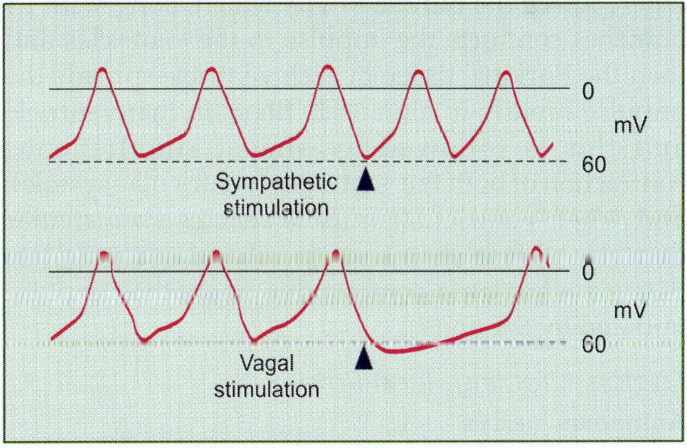

Figs 6.15A and B: (A) Diagram of the membrane potential of pacemaker tissue. The current responsible for each part of the potential is shown under or beside the component. L, long-lasting; T, transient. The resting membrane potential of pacemaker tissue is somewhat lower than that of atrial and ventricular muscle and slowly declines to reach firing level; (B) Effect of sympathetic (noradrenergic) and vagal (cholinergic) stimulation on the membrane potential of the SA node. Reduced slope of the prepotential after vagal stimulation and the increased spontaneous discharge after sympathetic stimulation

SA node is normal cardiac pacemaker, its rate of discharge determines the rate at which heart beats (normal sinus rhythm, NSR).

The **Atrioventricular node** (AV node) is another region which has the ability to initiate the heart beat but it initiates at a slower rate, so normally the SA node overrides its activity and acts as the pacemaker. AV node only initiates the beat if the SA node is depressed or fails to generate an impulse; in that case the AV node takes over the function and starts forming the impulse but it forms at a slower rate and the heart beats at slower but regular rate.

The bundle of His, its branches, and the Purkinje system also have a property of automaticity, i.e. they are capable of impulse generation. In complete heart block, the impulse from atria fails to reach the ventricles, the parts of these systems may start forming the impulse necessary for ventricular contraction; the ventricles now contract at a rate slower and at a rate independent of atrial contraction. This rate of contraction being much slower than the normal rate of contraction, the output of ventricles may fall too low and may become inadequate for the body needs; the condition may require insertion of a pacemaker.

The impulse formation and normal conduction results in parts of the heart to contract in an orderly sequence, contraction of the atria (atrial systole) occurs when atria receive the impulse from pacemaker region; then the impulse reaches the AV node, from where arises the bundle of His which along with its branches conducts the impulse to the ventricles and then the Purkinje tissue in each ventricle spreads the impulse rapidly to all muscle fibers in that ventricle and this is followed by almost simultaneous contraction of both the ventricles (ventricular systole), and when ventricular muscle relaxes (ventricular diastole) all four chambers are relaxed except in late diastole when atria contract due to another impulse initiated by SA node.

Factors Affecting Heart Rate

Autonomic nerves

- Increase in sympathetic nerve activity increases the heart rate.
- Increase in parasympathetic nerve activity (increase in ***vagal tone***) decreases the heart rate.

The heart rate is determined by the balance of the activities of the sympathetic and parasympathetic nerves, as both types of nerves innervate the pacemaker. The vagal activity is referred to as vagal tone.

The actions of the parasympathetic and sympathetic nerves are opposite to each other. Under resting conditions, the parasympathetic and sympathetic systems interact; and normal resting conditions parasympathetic activity predominates; the heart beats at a rate of about 72 beats per minute. If the activity of vagal nerves is blocked in an individual the heart rate increases to about 180. If even sympathetic activity is blocked the rate falls to 100.

Circulating Hormones

Epinephrine (adrenaline) and norepinephrine (noradrenaline) secreted by adrenal medulla have the same effect as sympathetic stimulation. *Thyroid hormones* increase the heart rate. In hyperthyroidism the heart rate is fast and in hypothyroidism it is slow.

Exercise: Increases the heart rate

Emotional States: During *excitement*, *fear* or *anxiety* the heart rate increases, during depression it is decreased.

Age: In children, the heart rate is faster than in adults.

Body Temperature: Heart rate increases with rise of body temperature and decreases if the body temperature falls.

The average heart rate is 72 beats per minute in an adult under resting conditions. Normally varies from 60 to 80 beats per minute. Increase in heart rate above normal is called in **tachycardia** and decrease below normal is called **bradycardia**.

In healthy normal individuals breathing at a normal rate, the heart rate varies with the phases of respiration; it accelerates during inspiration and decelerates during expiration, especially if depth of breathing is increased. This normal phenomenon is called **sinus arrhythmia.**

THE CARDIAC CYCLE

The heart beats regularly to pump blood into the circulation. The electrical activity in the cardiac muscle is necessary and precedes the contraction (systole). The heart contacts to eject blood and then relaxes (diastole) to get filled by blood. The pressure changes in ventricle and other events of the cardiac cycle (Fig. 6.16) are:

- *Atrial systole* (i.e. atrial contraction) the ventricles are in diastole.
- *Ventricular systole* (i.e. contraction of the ventricles); successive phases are *isovolumetric contraction*, ejection phase as *rapid ejection* followed by *reduced ejection*.
- *Diastole of the ventricles;* successive phases are *isovolumetric relaxation, rapid filling, reduced filling*, then atrial contraction.

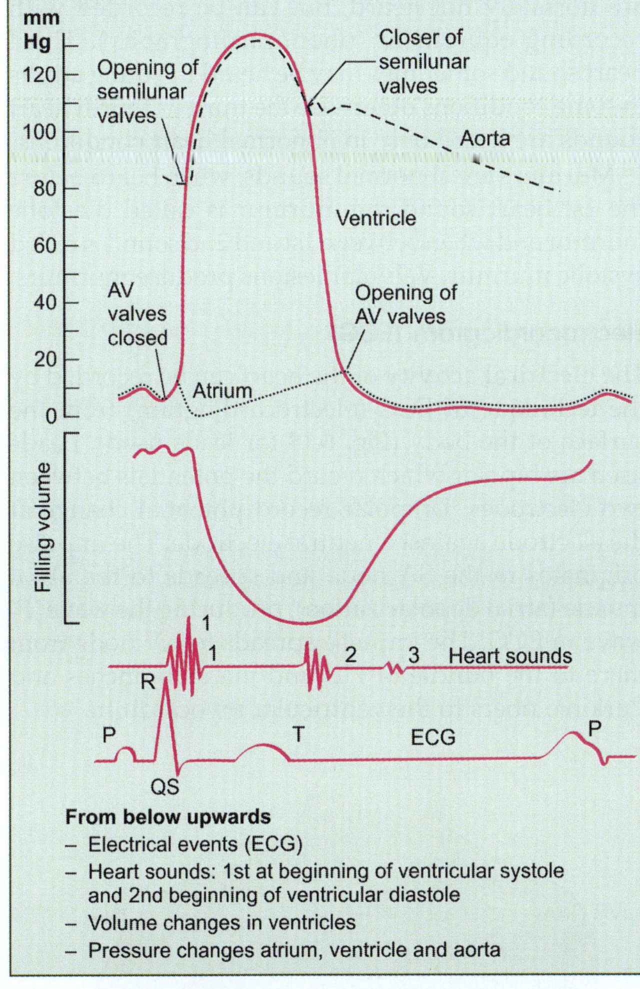

Fig. 6.16: Events in the cardiac cycle

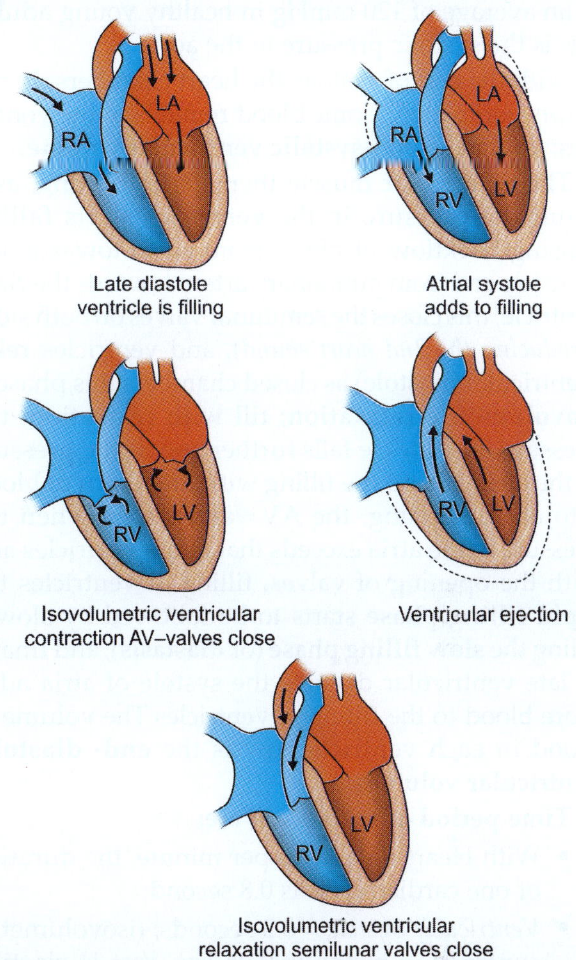

Fig. 6.17: Blood flow in the heart during the cardiac cycle. RA and LA, right and left atria; RV and LV, right and left ventricles

Ventricular diastole: The superior vena cava and the inferior vena cava bring deoxygenated blood to the right atrium and at the same time the pulmonary veins bring oxygenated blood from the lungs to the left atrium.

The blood from each of the atria flows into the respective ventricles AV valves being open and blood fills the ventricles (Fig. 6.17). The impulse arises in the SA node, spreads to all the atrial muscle fibers and produces contraction of the atria (atrial systole), which further adds blood to the filling of each ventricle, both ventricle are in diastole still.

The filling of the ventricles is over, that impulse spread to the AV node which conducts the impulse to the bundle of His, there is little delay in the conduction at the AV node which ensures that the atrial contraction is over before the ventricles contract on being excited by the impulse.

With ventricular systole, i.e. contraction of the ventricles, pressure in the ventricles rises. With onset of the rise of the pressure the AV valves close on each side of the heart (*producing 1st heart sound*) and prevent back flow of blood from ventricles into atria. The ventricles contract as closed chambers, both AV and semilunar valves are closed and as the pressure rises further in the each ventricle and exceeds the pressure in aorta on the left side and pulmonary artery on the right side; the semilunar valves open up (Fig. 6.17); **ending** the **isovolumetric contraction phase.** As semilunar valves open on each side of the heart, blood is ejected into the pulmonary artery on the right side and on the left side is ejected into the aorta, this is the ejection phase.

On the right side the maximum pressure built-up in the ventricle is lower than the pressure built-up in the left ventricle so the work of the right heart is lower. The ejection of blood is rapid at first and then reduced; these phases are called **rapid ejection phase** and **reduced ejection phase of systole.** The ejection of blood into the aorta results in aortic pressure to rise to an average of 120 mmHg in healthy young adults; this is the systolic pressure in the aorta.

With the end of systole, the heart chambers do not empty completely, some blood remains in the ventricles; volume is **end-systolic ventricular volume.**

The ventricular muscle then starts relaxing; as a result the pressure in the ventricles starts falling causing backflow of blood from aorta towards left ventricle and from pulmonary artery towards the right ventricle; this closes the semilunar valves on both sides (*producing the 2nd heart sound*), and ventricles relax (ventricular diastole) as closed chambers this phase is **isovolumetric relaxation**; till with relaxation, the pressure in ventricle falls further and as the pressure in the atria, due to the filling with the return of blood into atria, is rising, the AV valves open when the pressure in the atria exceeds that in the ventricles and with the opening of valves, filling of ventricles the **rapid filling phase** starts to be followed by slower filling the **slow filling phase** (or **diastasis**), and finally in late ventricular diastole the systole of atria adds more blood to the filling of ventricles.The volume of blood in each ventricle now is the **end- diastolic ventricular volume.**

Time period of each event are:

- With Heart Rate of 75 per minute, the duration of one cardiac cycle is 0.8 second.
- *Ventricular Systole* = 0.3 seconds; (isovolumetric contraction phase is 0.05 sec, rest is ejection phase).
- *Ventricular Diastole* = 0.5 seconds (0.08 sec isovolumetric relaxation phase, 0.12 sec rapid filling phase, 0.2 sec diastasis, 0.1 sec atrial systole).

When the heart rate increases both systole and diastole shorten but diastole shortens more and at very fast rates due to shortening of diastole the filling of ventricles may decrease to low levels.

Heart Sounds

The character of the first heart sound is different from that of the second heart sound.

The **first heart sound** is like word "**Lubb**", low pitched, prolonged as compared to the **second heart sound** which is high pitched, shorter in duration (brief) and sharp ending and like the word "**dup**". The first heart is produced at the beginning of systole of the heart and second heart sound at the beginning of diastole of the heart.

These are the two heart sounds which are normally heard. There are also the 3rd, 4th heart sounds which are normally not heard, but can be recorded with recording equipment (phonocardiography). Third heart sound sometimes may be heard in young adults in some conditions otherwise the third or fourth heart sounds are heard only in abnormal heart conditions.

Murmurs are abnormal sounds; when heard before the 1st heart sound the murmur is called diastolic murmur and when between 1st and 2nd sound is called systolic murmur. Valvular lesions produce murmurs.

Electrocardiogram (ECG)

The **electrical activity** of the heart can be recorded by the technique of ECG (electrocardiogram) from the surface of the body (Fig. 6.18 for leads used). Leads used are bipolar which record the potentials between two electrodes. Unipolar record potential change at the electrode against a neutral electrode. The impulse originates in the SA node and spreads to the atrial muscle (atrial depolarization), producing the wave 'P' wave in ECG. The impulse spreads to AV node from there to the bundle of His and via its branches and Purkinje fibers to the ventricular myocardium.

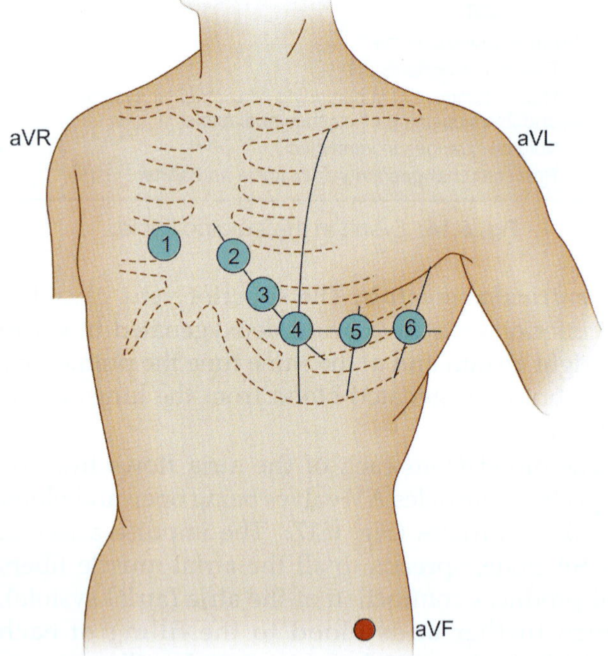

Fig. 6.18: Electrocardiographic leads, Unipolar limb leads are aVR, aVL and aVF and chest leads V_1, fourth intercostal space to right of sternum, V_2, fourth intercostal space to the left of sternum, V_4, fifth intercostal space in midclavicular line, V_3, midway between V_2, and V_4. V_5, anterior axillary line V_6, mid axillary line both fifth intercostal space. Other electrodes positions are bipolar leads; Lead I between Right arm and Left arm; Lead II between Right arm and Left leg; Lead III between Left arm and Left leg

The spread of the impulse in the ventricular myocardium (ventricular depolarization) produces the 'QRS' complex in ECG (Fig. 6.19). The up wave is 'R' wave down wave is 'S' wave, 'Q' wave a small down wave may or may not be present. The time taken for the impulse to spread from the atria to the ventricles is 'PR' interval (if Q wave is absent) or 'PQ' interval (if Q wave is also present) ; this interval also includes the time taken in the bundle of His. It gives information about the conduction time through AV node. If there is delay in the spread of the impulse at the AV node or in the bundle of His the PR interval is prolonged. If it is more than the upper limit of normal of 0.2 seconds, this is called first degree of heart block. Following the QRS complex the record returns to the base line and records another wave 'T' wave which is due to repolarization of the ventricle muscle fibers. The ST segment is isoelectric. The duration and amplitude of the waves (Fig. 6.19) is measured in the recordings. The standardization of the recording apparatus before a record is taken enables the interpretation of the amplitude and duration of waves (Table 6.2).

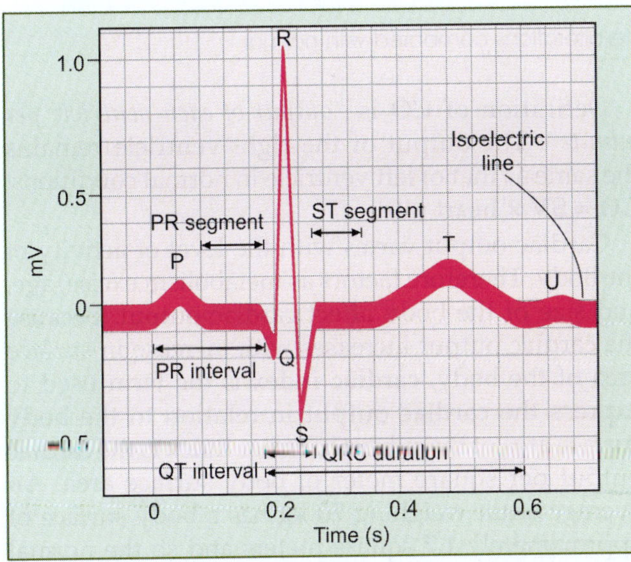

Fig. 6.19: Waves and intervals in the ECG

When there is *inadequate* blood supply to the ventricular muscle the ST segment may be deviated from normal isoelectric line to be depressed or elevated. The 'T' wave in the leads where it is upright if it gets inverted is also abnormal finding. ECG is used for diagnosis of **ischemia** of cardiac muscle or **myocardial infarction** (infarction is irreversible changes or death of myocardial fibers), or for some other abnormalities in heart function.

Heart Block

If the AV node function is not normal and some impulses pass through AV node to the ventricles while some do not it is called second degree heart block and is incomplete heart block. Fist degree of heart block has been described above.

When **all the impulse** from atria **fail** to reach the ventricles, due to disease of the AV node it is called complete heart block. When there is **complete** block of impulses fail to reach from atria to ventricles, the ventricles beat at their own rate (**idioventicular rhythm**) the rate is 30 to 45 beats per minute. The block may be in the AV node (AV nodal block) or in the conducting system (Bundle of His, below the node, infranodal block). Differential diagnosis can be made with special technique of His bundle electrogram (HBE).

Bundle branch block. Sometime there is bundle branch block, one branch of the bundle is blocked, the excitation passes normally down the normal side but muscle to muscle conduction activates the blocked side; since this conduction is slower the QRS complex is prolonged with its duration more than normal.

Abnormalities in ECG are also recorded in certain **systemic diseases** and when there are changes in **ionic composition of blood/ECF**; hyperkalemia (increase in potassium ion concentration or hypokalemia decrease in K ion concentration) result in characteristic abnormalities in ECG (Fig. 6.20).

Table 6.2: ECG intervals

Intervals	*Normal duration (sec.)*		*Events in the heart during Interval*
	Average	*Range*	
PR interval[1]	0.18^{+}	0.12–0.20	Atrial depolarization and conduction through AV node
QRS duration	0.08	to 0.10	Ventricular depolarization and atrial repolarization
QT interval	0.40	to 0.43	Ventricular depolarization plus ventricular repolarization

[1]Measured from the beginning of the P wave to the beginning of the QRS complex

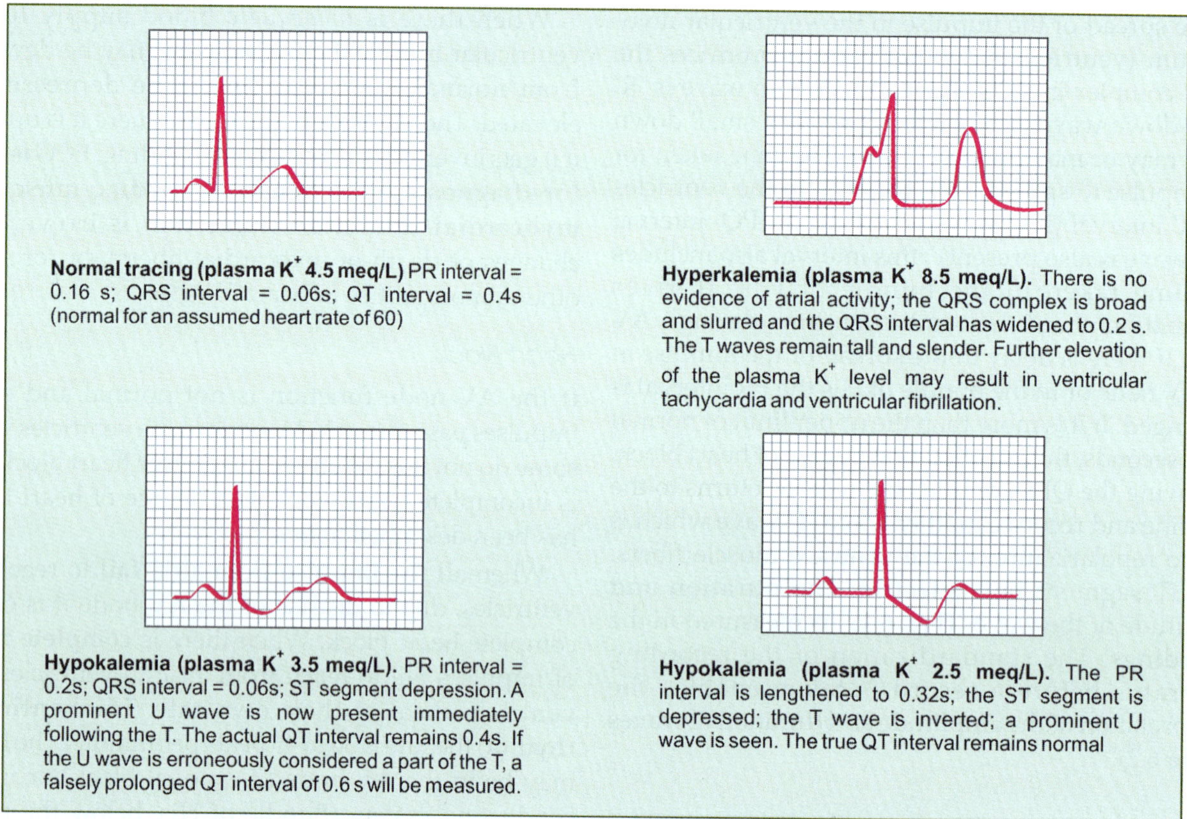

Fig. 6.20: Changes in ECG with electrolyte alterations compared with normal

LONG QT INTERVAL

In people in whom the QT interval is prolonged, there is irregular cardiac repolarization and increased incidence of ventricular arrhythmias with dangers of sudden death.

Increase is produced by a number of drugs, by electrolyte abnormalities, by myocardial ischemia or it can be congenital.

CARDIAC OUTPUT (CO)

The blood pumped out by *each ventricle* in *each systole* (into aorta on the left side or pulmonary artery on the right side) is called **Stroke volume** (**SV**). The stroke volume is about 70 ml on the left side and the same on the right side.

The stroke volume multiplied by the heart rate per minute amounts to output of each ventricle per minute, i.e. if the heart rate is 72 per min the output of the left ventricle would be 72 × 70 ml = 5040 ml per minute or 5L per min; the same would be output on the right side.

CO in adult individual in resting state is about 5L/per min, while activity causes increase in the cardiac output to supply the increased demands of the tissues.

Definition of **CO** is *"output of each ventricle per minute"*. The output of the right ventricle remains the same as that of left ventricle in normal conditions. **CO = SV × heart rate.**

Cardiac output varies with the level of activity of the body. Therefore factors as metabolism excise, age, and size of the body affect cardiac output. Because the cardiac output increases with increase in surface area of the body, **cardiac index** is the term used to express the cardiac output in relation to the body surface area of the subject. Cardiac index is the cardiac output per square meter of body surface area. An average adult weighing 70 kg has a body surface of approximately 1.7 square meters and so the normal average cardiac index for adult in resting condition is 3L/min/sqm. Expressing in terms of cardiac index helps in assessing the cardiac output in individuals with different surface areas.

Cardiac Output in various conditions (Table 6.3):

- There is great *increase* in CO during exercise. In exercise CO may reach 24 to 30 L/min.
- CO *increases* during digestive activity.
- Anxiety and excitement cause *increase* in cardiac output.
- High environmental temperature *increases* CO

Table 6.3: Effect of various conditions on cardiac output

Sleep	*No change*
Increase	
Anxiety and excitement	50–100%
Eating	30%
Exercise	Up to 700%
High environmental temperature	
Pregnancy	
Decrease	
Sitting or standing from lying position	20–30%
Heart disease	

Approx. percent changes mentioned.

- Sitting or standing from lying down position *decreases* the cardiac output
- Cardiac output increases during pregnancy.

Control of Cardiac Output

As mentioned, cardiac output = **SV × heart rate**. Either factor if it increases would increase the CO provided any change in other factor does not balance the effect.

During exercise there is increase in venous return to the heart; it results in greater stretch of the ventricular muscle fibers; which results in greater force of contraction of the fibers; and increase in the cardiac output. This effect of greater stretch of muscle fibers resulting in increase in the force of contraction is called **'Starlings' law of the heart.** Law states: **"Force of contraction is proportional to the initial length of the muscle fibers within physiological limits".** The physiological limit is specified because if the muscle is overstretched (beyond a limit) the effect may be counter productive (Fig. 6.21).

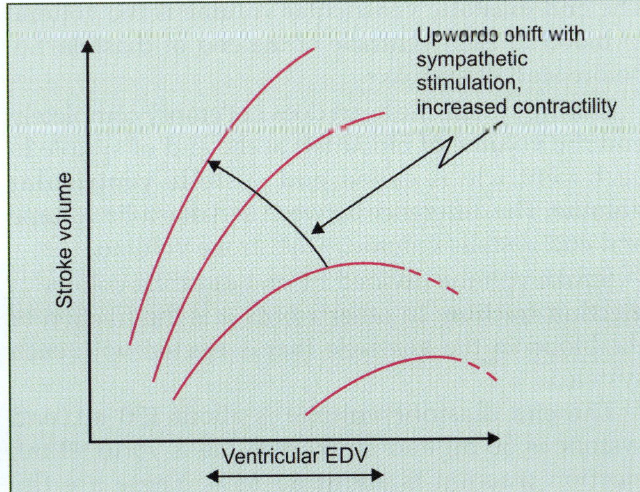

Fig. 6.21: Starling curves. Sympathetic stimulation shifts the whole curve because of increased contractility at the same length

The second factor which affects cardiac output is the **contractility of the ventricular muscle** which depends upon the degree of stimulation by the *sympathetic impulses* to the ventricular muscle. The sympathetic nerve activity increases the force of contraction at any length of the muscle fibers of the heart (Fig. 6.21). With increased activity of sympathetic nerves there is increase in the force of contraction at the same length of muscle fibers (or the same filling of the heart). Increased activity of the sympathetic system increases the force of contraction of the ventricular muscle by altering its contractility. Since there is increase in contractility with sympathetic nerve stimulation, the effect of sympathetic stimulation on contractility is *positive* inotropic effect. The regulation of cardiac output by effect on contractility is called **homometric regulation** of the cardiac output (regulation independent of the length) in contrast to **heterometric regulation** which is due to increase in the filling of ventricles causing increase in muscle length, leading to increase in force of contraction (Starling's law).

Some factors that influence contractility are as in Fig. 6.22.

Venous Return

Venous return is the quantity of blood flowing from veins into right atrium each minute.

The return of the blood to the heart (venous return) determines the filling of the chambers of the heart and the filling determines the output (cardiac output); more the filling more the output as explained with CO. The venous returns to the heart increases under following conditions.

- Pumping action of contractions of muscles on blood vessels; as during exercise (muscular pump).
- An increase in the pulmonary ventilation; which builds more negative pressure in the thoracic cavity,

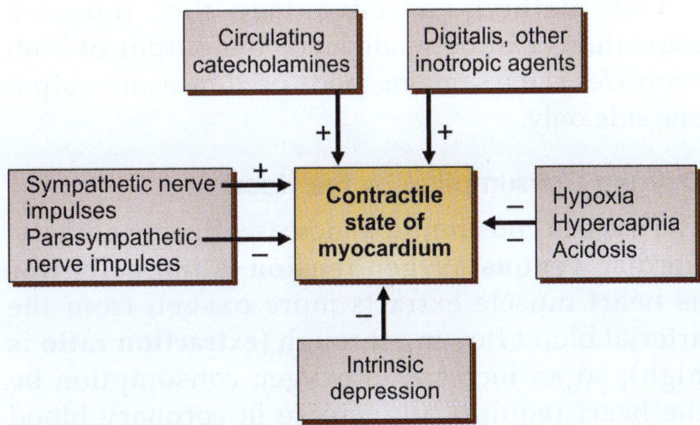

Fig. 6.22: Factors affecting contractility of myocardium

aids in the return of the blood towards to the heart (the thoracic pump).

- Increase in heart rate results in drawing the blood towards the heart (cardiac pump).
- Constriction of veins decreases the reservoir capacity of veins and more blood enters the circulation.

Methods of Measurement of CO

In humans Doppler combined with echocardiography and direct Fick method and indicator dilution method are used.

Fick principle states that the amount of substance taken up by an organ (or by whole body) per unit of time is equal to arteriovenous difference times the blood flow.

The principle used to measure CO is measuring maount of O_2 consumed by the body in a given period divided by A-V difference across the lungs.

$$= \frac{O_2 \text{ consumption (ml/min)}}{[AO_2]-[VO_2]}$$

$$\text{e.g. } \frac{25 \text{ ml/min}}{190 \text{ ml/L} - 140 \text{ ml/L}} = \frac{250}{50}$$

$$= 5 \text{ L/min}$$

Indicator Dilution Technique

A known amount of substance, dye or radioactive isotope is injected and average concentration of indicator in arterial blood after single circulation through heart is measured.

A popular indicator dilution technique is use of cold saline, which is injected into right atrium through a double lumen catheter and temperature change is recorded in the pulmonary artery. The temerature change is inversely proportional to the amount of blood flowing through pulmonary artery.

This method has advantage that repeated estimations can be made since the output of both ventricles is the same methods used measure output one side only.

Oxygen Consumption by the Heart

The oxygen consumption increases during activity. Cardiac **venous oxygen tension** is normally **low** as heart muscle extracts more oxygen from the arterial blood flowing through (**extraction ratio is high**); so an increase in oxygen consumption by the heart requires an increase in coronary blood flow.

Oxygen consumption depends: on the *heart rate; contractile state* of the myocardium (increase in contractility consumes more oxygen); the *intramyocardial tension* (which depends on the systolic pressure which the heart builds up and on the radius of the ventricles); dilated heart requires more oxygen to built-up same pressure.

The oxygen consumption per beat is related to the work of the heart per beat. The work is product of stroke volume and mean arterial pressure. Though increase in either of these factors should affect the work in the same way but pressure work produces greater increase of oxygen consumption (reasons not understood). It means that it is more dangerous for coronary artery disease person to be *angry* raising his blood pressure than to be involved in some *exercise* in which the stroke volume increases producing similar increase of stroke work.

Oxygen Requirements of Exercise

The venous return is greatly increased during exercise because of the factors mentioned above; as a result there is an increase in the cardiac output. There is activation of sympathetic system during exercise to increase the cardiac output.

An increase in cardiac output results in increased in the blood flow to the active muscles. The arterioles in the active muscles dilate due to accumulation of products of increased metabolism this further increase the blood flow as it diverts more blood flow to the active muscles at the cost of that to the digestive system and splanchnic circulation.

Ejection Fraction

The **end-diastolic ventricular volume** is the volume of blood in each ventricle at the end of diastole, i.e. before start of systole.

During systole the heart does not empty completely and the volume of blood left at the end of systole in each ventricle is called **end systolic ventricular volume**. The difference between end diastolic volume and end systolic volume is the stroke volume.

Stroke volume divided by end diastolic volume is **ejection fraction**. In other words it is the fraction of the blood in the ventricle that is ejected with each systole.

The end diastolic volume is about 130 ml; end systolic is 50 ml and stroke volume is 70 to 90 ml; ejection fraction is about **60–65%**. These are the average figures in an adult. Ejection fraction is measured to assess the ventricular function. The value falls low in heart failure.

Arterial Pulse

As the blood is pumped into the aorta, with each ventricular systole, the aorta which is already full, its wall expand and this sets up a pressure wave long the vessel wall, which travels to the peripheral arteries and can be felt (as pulse) at a place where the artery is superficial, e.g. the radial artery which is superficial and over the bone.

The pulse wave travels at a rate faster than the velocity of blood flow and it is independent of it. The pulse wave gives the following indications.

- Rate of pulse beat per minute indicates the heart rate per minute.
- Regularity of the pulse beat indicates that the heart beat is regular
- The amplitude of the pulse indicates the magnitude of pulse pressure (systolic BP—diastolic BP)
- The strength of the pulse, i.e. the pulse is weak in shock and strong during exercise.

Clinical Application

When the aortic valve is incompetent (aortic insufficiency) the pulse is large in volume and water hammer in type (collapsing, Fig. 6.23). In some diseased conditions of the heart the pulse rate may be lower than the heart rate, i.e. if in some extra beats (extrasystoles) the heart is not able to pump enough blood into the aorta to set up a pressure wave.

DYNAMICS OF BLOOD FLOW

The blood flowing into arteries is brought back by the venous system into the heart. Some tissue fluid formed from the blood in the capillaries which is not reabsorbed back into the capillaries enters the lymphatic and passes via these vessels to the vascular system.

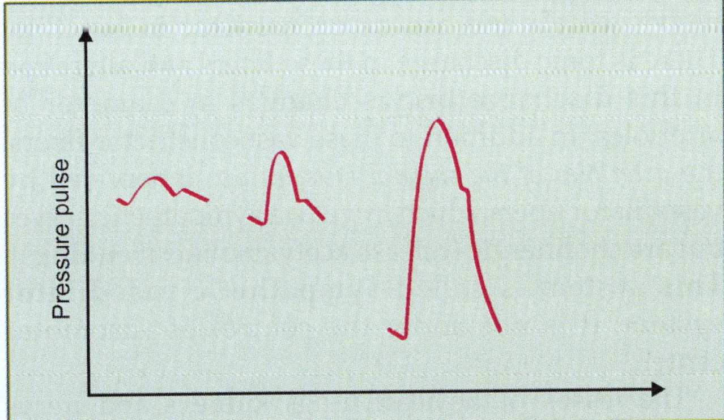

Fig. 6.23: Factors affecting the arterial pulse pressure and the arterial wave form. Beat 1 is normal. Beat 2 shows the effects of an increased stroke volume. Beat 3 indicates the consequences of aortic valve regurgitation

Blood flows through the vessels mainly because of the forward motion imparted to it by the **pumping action of the heart**, and is assisted (in the systemic circulation only) by the recoil of the walls during diastole; because in the large arteries with their elastic tissue which is stretched during filling of blood in systole, the wall recoils during diastole and the potential energy is released which helps in propulsion of blood in the arteries.

Compression of veins by the skeletal muscles also helps in the propulsion of blood, and the negative pressure in the thorax also helps to move the blood forward.

The resistance to flow depends mainly on the diameter of the vessels, majority of the ***peripheral resistance*** resides in the arterioles. The blood flow to each tissue is regulated by **local chemical factors** and **general neural** and *humoral* mechanisms, which dilate or constrict the arterioles of the tissue (Table 6.4).

In the pulmonary circuit all the output of the right ventricle flows through the lungs but in the systemic circulation there are different circuits in parallel, an

Table 6.4: Factors affecting the caliber of the arterioles

Constriction	*Dilation*
Local factors	
Low temperature	Increased CO_2 and decreased O_2.
	Increased K^+, adenosine, lactate, etc. (Products of metabolism)
	Decreased local pH
	High temperature
Endothelial products	
Endothelin–1	NO (nitric oxide)
Locally released platelet-serotonin	Kinins
	Prostacyclin
Thromboxane A_2	
Circulating hormones	
Epinephrine (except in skeletal muscle and liver)	Epinephrine in skeletal muscle and liver
	Atrial natriuretic peptide
Norepinephrine	CGRP
Angiotensin II	Histamine
Arginine vasopressin	Substance P
Neuropeptide Y	Vasoactive intestinal
polypeptide	
Neural factors	
Increased discharge of noradrenergic sympathetic nerves	Decreased discharge of nor-adrenergic sympathetic nerves
	Activation of sympathetic cholinergic dilator fibres to skeletal vasculature muscle

arrangement that permits wide variations in regional blood flow without changing total blood flow, e.g. in exercise proportions of cardiac output distributed to the active muscles is much increased; in hemorrhagic shock the output to the vital organs is better maintained with cut down of the flow to nonvital regions.

The walls of the arterioles contain less elastic tissue but much more smooth muscle (Fig. 6.2). The muscle is innervated by sympathetic noradrenergic nerve fibers, which are constrictor in function.

In an active tissue the locally produced metabolites, cause vasodilatation so that the blood flow is increased for the increased requirements. The metabolites that produce vasodilatation are decreased in the O_2 tension, fall in pH, increased in CO_2 tension, rise of temperature and some products of metabolism.

The veins act as blood reservoir. Normally they are partially collapsed and oval in section. A large amount of blood can be added to the venous system before they fill to a point where further addition would raise pressure. The veins are therefore called **capacitance vessels**. The venous system is also affected by circulating vasoactive factors as by sympathetic stimulation; venoconstriction takes place during blood loss in hemorrhage. The blood from the capacitance vessels which hold it in great proportion is released into the circulation to tide over the effects of blood loss.

The small arteries and arterioles are referred to as **resistance vessels,** as most of the resistance to the blood flow is in these vessels, as has been already mentioned.

Flow, Pressure and Resistance

Blood flows from areas of high pressure to that of low pressure. The relationship between mean flow, mean pressure and resistance in the blood vessel is as:

$$\text{Flow (F)} = \frac{\text{Pressure (P)}}{\text{Resistance (R)}}$$

Flow in any portion of the vascular system is equal to the effective perfusion pressure in that portion divided by the resistance. The effective perfusion pressure is the mean intraluminal pressure at the arterial end minus pressure at the venous end.

Resistance to blood flow is determined by radius of the blood vessels and viscosity of blood. *In vivo* the viscosity has little role except in polycythemia, when it increases workload on heart.

Localized vasoconstriction occurs in injured arteries and arterioles due to liberation of serotonin from platelets. A drop in tissue temperature causes vasoconstriction and thus local response to cold plays a part in temperature regulation.

Endothelial Cells

They secrete growth factors and many vasoactive substances. The vasoactive substances are *prostaglandins, thromboxanes,* ***nitric oxide*** and *endothelins.* Prostaglandin H_2 (PGH_2) is the precursor for various other prostaglandins, for thromboxanes and prostacyclin.

Whereas **prostacyclin** secreted by endothelial cells inhibits platelet aggregation and promotes vasodilation, thromboxane A_2 secreted by platelets promotes platelet aggregation and vasoconstriction; the balance between the two determines localized platelet aggregation and clot formation, and prevents excessive extension of the clot and maintains blood flow around it in conditions when clots form.

The thrombaxane A_2, prostacyclin balance can be shifted towards prostacyclin by administration of low doses of aspirin, which reduces production of both, but endothelial calls can regain the function in matter of hours, but not the platelets, being nonnucleated (no nuclei) the level rises only when new platelets enter circulation (half-life of platelets is 4 days). Therefore administration of small amounts of aspirin daily reduces clot formation and is of value in preventing myocardial infarction, unstable angina, transient ischemic attacks and stroke.

Nitric oxide (NO) produced by endothelial cells is a vasodilator. **Endothelin-1** produced by endothelial cells is one of the most potent vasoconstrictors; whether it has any role in hypertension there is no evidence as yet.

Innervation of Blood Vessels

Sympathetic noradrenergic fibers are present on all blood vessels and are vasoconstrictor in function. There is tonic discharge in these fibers and alteration in this discharge brings changes in diameter of arterioles. In addition to these vasoconstrictor fibers, the *arterioles of the skeletal muscles* are innervated by vasodilator fibers which travel via sympathetic nerves but are cholinergic (release acetylcholine at endings). This system is called **sympathetic vasodilator system**; it is not under the control of vasomotor center.

The **vessels** of the heart, lungs, kidneys, and uterus also receive parasympathetic impulses but there is no tonic discharge in these fibers.

The various factors that influence the tone of arterioles are summed up in Table 6.4.

ARTERIAL BLOOD PRESSURE

The arterial pressure in the aorta and in the brachial and other large arteries rises to *a peak value* during ventricular systole of each cardiac cycle this is the **systolic blood pressure;** and the pressure falls to *a minimum value* during ventricular diastole of the cardiac cycle, the *lowest pressure* recorded in the large vessels is the **diastolic pressure**.

In a young adult it rises to an average value of 120 mmHg systolic and falls to about 70 to 80 mmHg diastolic. The arterial pressure is expressed as systolic over the diastolic pressure, e.g. 120/70 mmHg or 120/80 mmHg.

The **pulse pressure** is the difference between systolic and diastolic pressures and is normally about 50 mmHg. The **mean pressure** is average pressure throughout the cardiac cycle. As systole is shorter than diastole, the mean pressure is not midway between systolic and diastolic but roughly equal to diastolic pressure plus 1/3rd of the pulse pressure.

Definitions: Systolic blood pressure is the maximum pressure during systole of the ventricle measured in large arteries. Diastolic pressure is the lowest pressure during the diastole of the ventricles measured in large arteries. The pulse pressure is the difference between the systolic and diastolic pressures. Mean pressure is the average pressure during cardiac cycle and is calculated by adding to diastolic pressure one thirds of pulse pressure.

Methods of Measuring Blood Pressure

Clinically the arterial BP is measured by:

- Auscultatory method
- Palpatory method
- Automated machines employing the auscultatory or other methods are used for continuous monitoring of blood pressure in hospital practice and in the home.

Auscultatory Method

The arterial blood pressure is clinically measured in humans by this method. An inflatable covered rubber cuff (Riva-Rocci cuff) is attached to a mercury manometer (sphygmomanometer). It is wrapped around the upper arm and a stethoscope is placed over the brachial artery at the elbow (Fig. 6.24).

The cuff is rapidly inflated to raise the pressure to above the expected level of systolic pressure in the artery or else to 180–200 mmHg. The artery gets occluded and no sound is heard with the stethoscope. The pressure is then lowered slowly (at the rate of 2–3 mm per sec).

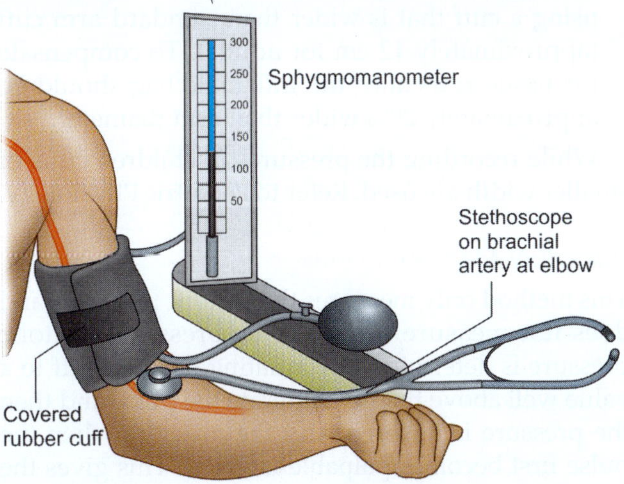

Fig. 6.24: Determination of blood pressure by the auscultatory method

The point where a sound is first heard the pressure is noted. This is a systolic pressure; at this time the systolic pressure in the artery just exceeds the cuff pressure and a part of blood passes through with each heart beat during systole and a tapping sound is heard due to turbulent blood flow; as the cuff pressure is lowered further the sound become louder, then dull and muffled, and finally disappears as the blood flow becomes continuous; the first disappearance gives the diastolic blood pressure. Sometimes especially in children and in adults after exercise the disappearance of sounds may not be made out and in that case diastolic pressure is recorded when the sound becomes muffled or appears to be disappearing. This is also true in diseases, such as hyperthyroidism and aortic insufficiency.

The sounds heard during the recordings are called **Korotkoff's sounds** after the scientist who first described them.

The auscultatory method is accurate but some precautions need to be taken, as:

1. The cuff on the artery must be at the heart level.
2. Patients should be resting for at least 5 minutes and should not have smoked during the last 30 minutes before the measurement.
3. When BP is measured in the thigh with the stethoscope over the popliteal artery, (with subject in prone position so that cuff is at heart level), where there is more tissue between the cuff and artery, some cuff pressure is dissipated due to this, so that pressures recorded are high and this is also true in obese arms (where there is more fat) when pressure is measured over brachial artery. In both these conditions accurate measurements are obtained by

using a cuff that is wider than standard arm cuff (approximately 12 cm for adults). To compensate for tissue resistance the inflatable bag should be approximately 20% wider than arm diameter.

While recording the pressures in children cuffs of smaller width are used. Refer to Pediatric Physiology.

Palpatory Method

This method only measures the systolic pressure, and does not measure the diastolic pressure. Systolic pressure is determined by inflating the arm cuff to a value well above that to obliterate the pulse and then the pressure is lowered, and the pressure when the pulse first becomes palpable is noted. This gives the systolic pressure, which may be 2 to 5 mm lower than that recorded by auscultatory method.

When using auscultatory method it is helpful to palpate the radial pulse while inflating the pressure and to note the systolic pressure in addition to making measurements with auscultatory method.

Normal Arterial Blood Pressure

In a young adult under resting condition, sitting or lying; measured in the brachial artery the pressures are approximately 120/70 mmHg or 120/80 mmHg. The systolic pressure may be range up to 140 mmHg; and the normal range for diastolic pressure is 60 to 90 mmHg. The blood pressure rises with advancing age. There is steady rise in systolic and the diastolic pressures until the age of 50–60 years but later the diastolic pressure falls. Hence, there is marked increase in pulse pressure in elderly individuals. The increase in systolic and pulse pressures is due to increased stiffness of the arteries.

Determinants of Blood Pressure

The arterial pressure is **product of cardiac output and peripheral resistance**; it is affected when they change. Emotions of anxiety increase cardiac output and peripheral resistance and hence the blood pressure.

Conditions Affecting Blood Pressure

Blood pressure falls by about 20 mm during sleep. The fall is reduced or absent in hypertensive patients.

The blood pressures are lower in women as compared to men until the age of menopause, but in postmenopausal women pressure readings are similar to men of the same age. The lower readings in earlier life of women may be one of the factors contributing to their longevity in relation to men.

The blood pressure readings taken during different times of the day may vary.

Blood pressure recorded in different postures may vary.

The Blood Pressures in Smaller Vessels

The pressures fall very slightly in large and medium sized arteries because the resistance to the flow is small; but fall rapidly in small arteries and arterioles which are the main sites of peripheral resistance.

The mean pressure at the *end of the arterioles* is 30–38 mmHg. Pulse pressure also declines to about 5 mm at the end of arterioles. The magnitude of the pressure drop along arterioles varies considerably depending on whether they are constricted or dilated.

Capillary Circulation

At anyone time only 5% of the circulating blood is in the capillaries but this 5% is very important part of blood volume because it is across the systemic capillary walls that O_2 and nutrients enter the interstitial fluid and CO_2 and waste products enter the bloodstream. Muscle fibers are not present in capillary wall (Fig. 6.25).

Capillary pressures vary considerably in different parts of the body; in human nail bed the pressure is

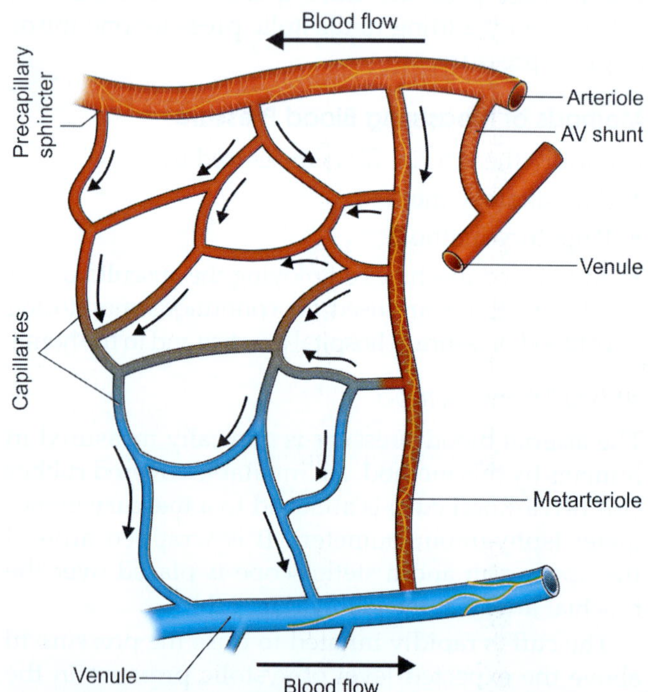

Fig. 6.25: Microcirculation. The color on the arteriole and venule represent smooth muscle fibers; branching solid lines represent sympathetic nerve fibers. The arrows indicate the direction of blood flow

32 mmHg at the arteriolar end and 15 mmHg at the venous end of capillary.

Exchange across Capillaries and Tissue fluid formation.

Capillary wall is thin membrane made-up of endothelial cells. Substances pass through its wall by *diffusion, filtration* and *vascular transport*. O_2 and glucose diffuse from the blood into the interstitial fluid (tissue fluid) and CO_2 diffuses in the opposite direction.

The rate of filtration and formation of tissue fluid at any point in the capillary wall depends upon the hydrostatic pressure and osmotic pressure. The net hydrostatic pressure is the capillary hydrostatic pressure minus the hydrostatic pressure of the tissue fluid. The net osmotic pressure is osmotic pressure of the blood minus the osmotic pressure of the tissue fluid. At the arterial end of the capillary **hydrostatic pressure** is about 35 mmHg. This tends to push the fluid out the capillary wall into the interstitial fluid. The colloidal osmotic pressure due to plasma proteins in the capillaries is about 25 mmHg, (it is due to the large molecules of proteins which are unable to pass through the capillary wall), and the tissues fluid has very low concentration of proteins hence this colloidal osmotic pressure in capillaries tends to retain fluid in the capillaries.

The difference between the net hydrostatic pressure and colloidal osmotic pressures at the arterial end of the capillaries is positive, i.e. hydrostatic pressure is more and fluid, along with small molecular weight substances like glucose is filtered out of capillary. At the venous end of the capillary the colloidal osmotic pressure is more than the hydrostatic pressure which has fallen due to fluid loss; fluid is absorbed into the capillary circulation (Fig. 6.26). Not all the filtered water is reabsorbed in the blood capillaries. The excess is drained by lymphatic channels, which originate as blind capillaries, more permeable than blood capillaries and water and some waste substances are returned via lymphatic circulation to the blood circulation. Any protein that left by vascular transport is reabsorbed via lymphatic vessels which are more permeable than capillaries.

Active and Inactive Capillaries

In *resting tissues* most of the capillaries are collapsed, blood for most part flows through the thoroughfare vessels from the arterioles to the venules (Fig. 6.25). In *active tissues*, the metarterioles and precapillary sphincter dilate and blood flows through most capillaries. Relaxation of the smooth muscle of metarterioles and precapillary sphincter is due to the action of vasodilator metabolites formed in active tissue.

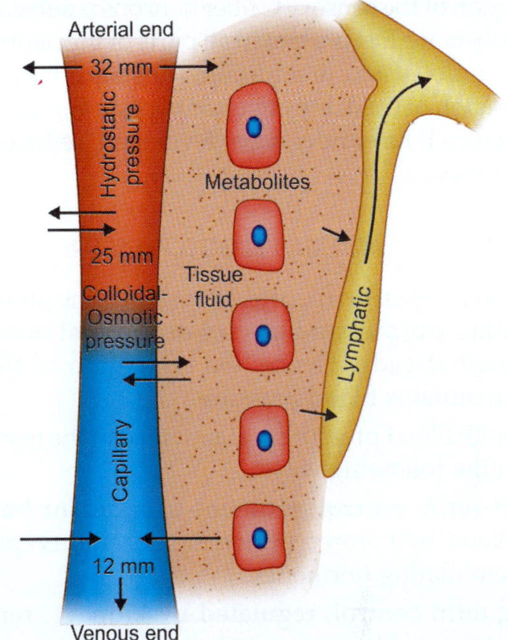

Fig. 6.26: Fluid interchanges between capillary, tissue spaces, and lymphatics

After noxious stimulation, substance P released by the axon reflex increases capillary permeability. Bradykinin and histamine also increase capillary permeability.

White reaction: When a pointed object is drawn lightly over the skin, the stroke lines become pale (white reaction). The mechanical stimulus apparently initiates contraction of the precapillary sphincters, and blood drains out of the capillaries and small veins.

Triple response: When the skin is stroked more firmly with a pointed instrument, instead of the white reaction there is reddening (red reaction) at the site that appears in about few seconds. This is followed by local swelling and diffuse reddening around the injury in few minutes. The initial redness is due to capillary dilation, a direct response of the capillaries. The swelling (wheal) is local edema due to increased permeability of the capillaries and postcapillary venules. The redness spreading out from the injury (flare) is due to arteriolar dilation. This three-part response—is called the **triple response** and is part of the normal reaction to injury. It is due to an **axon reflex,** a response in which impulses initiated in sensory nerves by the injury are relayed antidromically down other branches of the sensory nerve fibers. The transmitter released at the central termination of the sensory C fiber neurons is substance P and substance P is present in all parts of the neurons. Dilate arterioles and in addition, substance P causes extravasation of fluid. Effective nonpeptide antagonists to substance P have now been developed, reduce the extravasation.

REGULATION OF ARTERIAL BLOOD PRESSURE

The blood pressure in the arterial system is the product of cardiac output and peripheral resistance as mentioned already. Hence, the regulation of these factors maintains blood pressure.

In health blood pressure is maintained at the normal level by the following ways:

- Short-term control, moment-to-moment basis, regulated by baroreceptor reflex, chemoreceptors and circulating hormones.
- Long-term control, regulated by kidneys, renin-angiotensin aldosterone system.

Baroreceptor Reflex

There are group of neurons in the *medulla oblongata* called the cardiovascular centers (or the vasomotor center and cardioinhibitory center) which regulate and maintain blood pressure. Regulation is by the impulses via autonomic nerves to the heart and blood vessels; the sympathetic impulses to the heart regulate the heart rate (chronotropic effect) and force of contraction (inotropic effect), and the impulses to the arterioles regulate the peripheral resistance; the parasympathetic impulses via vagal nerves decrease the heart rate. Cardiovascular centers receive input from baroreceptors that sense the level of blood pressure. The baroreceptors are pressure receptor formed by nerve endings situated in the carotid sinus, and aortic arch (Fig. 6.27). The receptors are also located in the right and left atria, entrance of superior and inferior vena cava and in pulmonary circulation. In the carotid sinus they are endings of IXth cranial nerve (glossopharyngeal nerves) and in the aorta they are nerve endings of Xth cranial nerve (vagal nerves); the impulses carried by these nerves (also called buffer nerves) inhibit the vasomotor center. When there is fall in blood pressure less number of impulses are carried by these nerves (as receptors are sensing the pressure) to the vasomotor centre, as a result the activity of the center is increased; center regulates efferent autonomic discharge to the heart and blood vessels to raise the pressure back to the normal. The sympathetic discharge to the heart and blood vessels is increased in this situation. The increased activity of

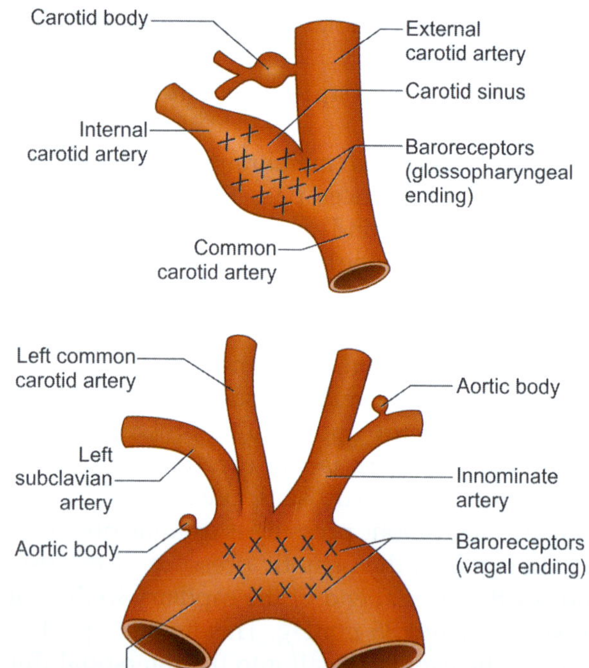

Fig. 6.27: Baroreceptor areas in the carotid sinus and aortic arch (Marked as XX)

sympathetic nerves to the heart increase the heart rate and the force of contraction of ventricles; this results in increase in the cardiac output; increased sympathetic nerve impulses to the arterioles cause arteriolar constriction which increase the peripheral resistance to the blood flow; both factors raise the pressure back to the normal. This is the homeostasis of blood pressure.

On the contrary if high pressure is sensed by these baroreceptors, the vasomotor center is inhibited by increased impulses from baroreceptors; that decreases the sympathetic discharge to the heart and arterioles; that decrease cardiac output and peripheral resistance; and lower the pressure to normal (Normally there is always some sympathetic discharge to the heart and blood vessels). Baroreceptor impulses also stimulate cardioinhibitory center, the vagal nerves are stimulated and vagal tone to the heart increases which also decreases the heart rate affecting the cardiac output (Figs 6.28A and B).

Other Factors that Affect the Vasomotor Center

Chemoreceptors

These are the nerve endings situated in the carotid bodies and aortic bodies (Fig. 6.27), the endings of glossopharyngeal nerves and vagal nerves respectively; their main influence is on respiration. But

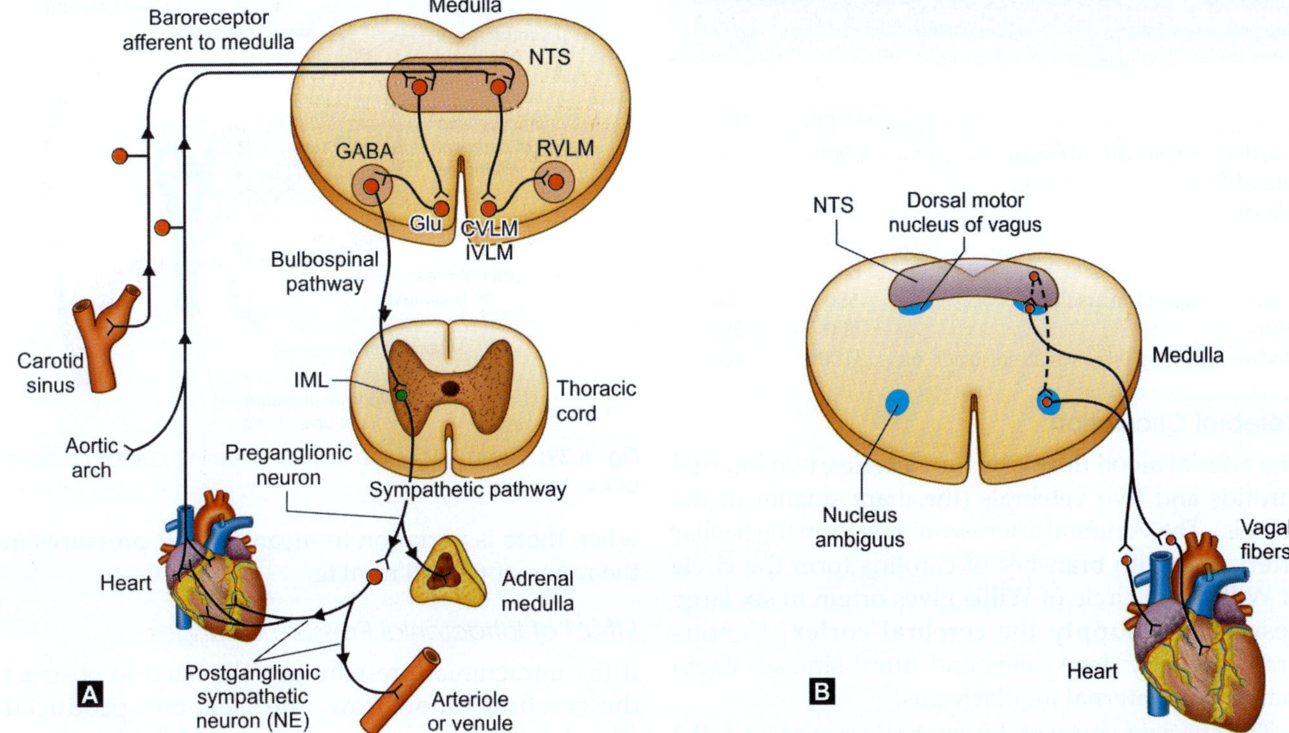

Figs 6.28A and B: (A) Basic pathways involved in the medullary control of blood pressure, (B) The vagal efferent pathways that slow the heart rate

the influence on BP becomes important in large hemorrhage; when there is blood loss that results in chemical changes in the blood, like oxygen lack and CO_2 excess or fall in pH; the chemoreceptor nerve endings get stimulated and impulses reach the vasomotor centre to stimulate it to raise the blood pressure.

Higher Brain Centers

Input from the cerebral cortex into the cardiovascular center due to emotional states; of fear, anxiety, pain and anger raise the blood pressure.

Table 6.5 sums up the factors affecting vasomotor center.

Table 6.5: Factors affecting the activity of the vasomotor area in the medulla

Direct stimulants
CO_2
Hypoxia
Excitatory inputs
From cortex via hypothalamus (Emotions)
From carotid and aortic chemoreceptors
From pain pathways
Somatic afferents
Inhibitory inputs
From cortex via hypothalamus (Emotions)
From carotid, aortic, and cardiopulmonary baroreceptors
From lungs (inflation afferents)

Long-Term Regulation of Blood Pressure

When there is low pressure in the renal arteries it causes release of renin from the kidneys, renin is an enzyme that acts on a plasma protein called

angiotensinogen to produce angiotensin 1, which is inactive, another enzyme called converting enzyme in the lungs and other tissues changes angiotensin 1 to an active form called **angiotensin 11**, which is a potent **vasoconstrictor** and also stimulates the **secretion of aldosterone** from adrenal cortex that causes sodium retention in the body leading to water retention and hence increase in extracellular fluid volume. This is the mechanism of long-term regulation of blood pressure involving **renin angiotensin system.**

CIRCULATION THROUGH SPECIAL REGIONS

The cardiac output is distributed in accordance to the specific functions being performed by the different regions (Table 6.6). The general features of circulation apply to all the regions but different regions have some *specific features.*

Table 6.6: Cardiac output and regional blood flow in a sedentary man quiet standing and exercise

	Quiet Standing	*Exercise*
Cardiac output (in ml/min)	5,900	24,000
Blood flow (in ml/min) to:		
Heart	250	1000
Brain	750	750
Active skeletal muscle	650	20,850
Inactive skeletal muscle	650	300
Skin	500	500
Kidney, liver, gastrointestinal tract, etc.	3100	600

Cerebral Circulation

The arterial blood flow is by four arteries; two internal carotids and two vetebrals (these are smaller of the vessels). The vertebral arteries unite to form the basilar artery and with branches of carotids form the circle of Willis. The circle of Willis gives origin to six large vessels that supply the cerebral cortex. Venous drainage is by deep veins and dural sinuses, drain mainly into internal jugular veins.

The special feature of the cerebral circulation is the **blood brain barrier**. The choroid plexuses contain gaps between the endothelial cells in the capillary wall, but the choroid epithelial cells covering them separate them from CSF and are connected to one another by tight junctions.

The other capillaries in the brain are *non-fenestrated* capillaries and there are tight junctions between the endothelial cells that limit the passage of substances through these junctions and these capillaries are surrounded by endfeet of astrocytes. The end feet induce tight junctions between the endothelial cells.

These features contribute to the **blood brain barrier** that prevents proteins from entering the brain in adults and slows the passage of smaller molecules. The blood brain barrier maintains the constant composition of the environment of the neurons in the CNS, and protects from the endogenous and exogenous toxins in the blood; and prevents escape of neurotransmitters from the brain.

Blood flow in various parts of the brain. Technique **positron emission tomography** (PET) has been used for measuring **regional blood flow** in different parts of the brain in conscious humans.

The main factors that affect **total cerebral blood flow** are outlined in Fig. 6.29.

Autoregulation is prominent feature in cerebral circulation. By this process blood flow to the brain is maintained relatively constant despite variation in the perfusion pressure; brain blood flow remains constant when there is variation in mean arterial pressures in the range of 65–140 mmHg.

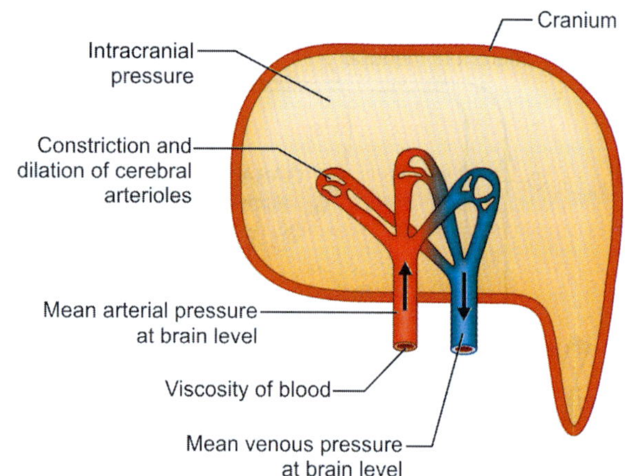

Fig. 6.29: Summary of the factors affecting overall cerebral blood flow

Effect of Intracranial Pressure Changes

If the intracranial pressure gets elevated to obstruct the cerebral blood flow, the ischemia produced stimulates the vasomotor center and blood pressure rises (**Cushing reflex**), this helps to maintain cerebral blood flow; but bradycardia via baroreceptor reflex occurs. The respiration is slowed.

Further details of cerebral circulation are described in the nervous system.

Coronary Circulation

The Special Features Only

The coronary arteries are compressed when the heart beats, especially in the left ventricle (Fig. 6.30) where higher pressure is built; as a result the blood flow in the **left ventricle in the subendocardial regions**, where compression effect is most; **only occurs during diastole.** As diastole is shorter when the heart rate is high, left ventricular flow is reduced during tachycardia hence this region is prone to ischemic damage. On the right side pressure difference between the aorta and right ventricle is higher during systole than diastole, hence flow is high, in right coronary vessels during systole.

Another special feature of coronary circulation is that at rest the **heart extracts 70–80% of oxygen from the arterial blood flow** in coronary arteries hence very *little reserve* to draw upon when the requirement increases with activity. The blood flow per min must increase to supply the requirements of oxygen.

At rest the coronary **blood flow is 250 ml/min**.

The **local chemical factors** regulate the coronary blood flow according to **metabolic requirements,** O_2 lack, increased concentrations of CO_2, H^+ ions, K^+ ions,

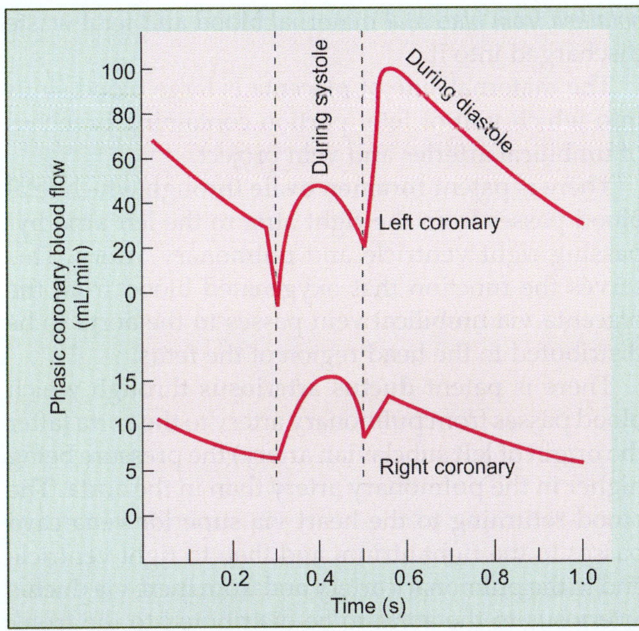

Fig. 6.30: Blood flow in the left and right coronary arteries during phases of the cardiac cycle

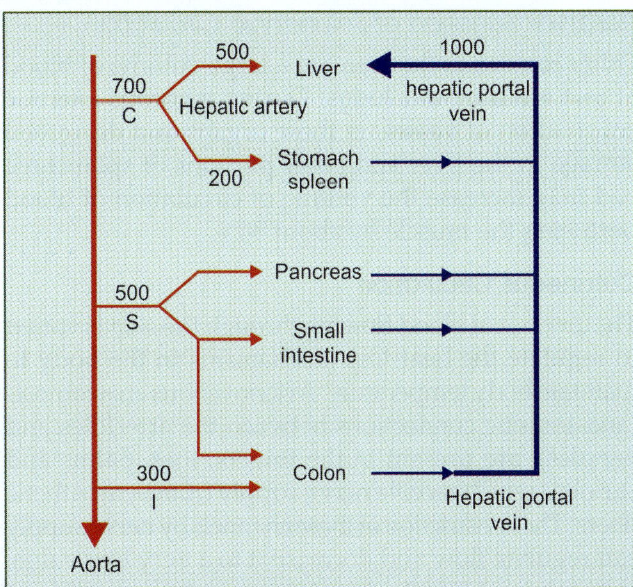

Fig. 6.31: Splanchnic circulation. The liver receives blood from the hepatic artery and the portal vein. The figures are average blood flows (mL/min). C, celiac artery; S, superior mesenteric artery; I, inferior mesenteric artery

lactate, and adenosine cause dilation of **arterioles. Nerves do not affect the flow very much** except that when sympathetic nerves get stimulated the increased metabolism of the myocardium, due to production of local metabolites, results is increase in the blood flow.

Splanchnic Circulation

The blood from the intestine, pancreas, stomach and spleen drains via the hepatic portal vein to the liver and from the liver via the hepatic veins to the inferior vena cava (Fig. 6.31).

Intestinal Circulation

Superior and inferior mesenteric arteries supply the intestine. Blockage of a large intestinal artery produces infarction of intestine.

Hepatic Circulation

The liver receives about 1000 ml/min of blood from portal vein and 500 ml/min from the hepatic artery (Fig. 6.31). The functional unit of liver is an acinus. Each acinus contains terminal branches of portal vein, hepatic artery and bile ducts. Blood flows from the center of this functional unit to the terminal branches of the hepatic veins at the periphery, with the result that central part is well oxygenated and peripheral zone is least well oxygenated and is most susceptible to hypoxic damage. The sinusoids in the liver show large gaps and are highly permeable.

Portal venous pressure is about 10 mmHg and hepatic venous pressure is about 5 mmHg.

The intrahepatic portal vein has smooth muscle in the wall that receives sympathetic fibers. The hepatic artery also is innervated by sympathetic fibers as are other arteries. At rest the circulation in the peripheral portions of the liver is sluggish and only a portion of the organ is actively perfused.

When systemic venous pressure rises, the portal vein parts are dilated passively and the amount of blood in the liver increases, thus in congestive heart failure the hepatic congestion may be extreme. Large quantities of plasma water may transduce from the liver into the peritoneal cavity; such a fluid accumulation in the abdomen is known as **ascites.** Fibrosis of the liver, in the various types of **hepatic cirrhosis,** leads to pronounced increase in hepatic vascular resistance and raises pressure in portal venous system. As a result increase in capillary hydrostatic pressure through the splanchnic circulation leads to extensive fluid into the abdominal cavity. The pressure may rise substantially in other veins that anastomose with the portal vien. The esophageal veins may enlarge considerably to form **esophageal varices.** These may rupture and may lead to severe internal bleeding. In the opposite situation when the blood pressure falls and diffuse sympathetic discharge is produced intrahepatic portal vessel parts constrict, portal pressure rises and blood flow through the liver is brisk and bypasses most of the organ; and most of the blood in the liver enters the systemic circulation. Constriction of the hepatic arterioles diverts blood from the liver; constriction of the mesenteric arterioles reduces portal blood flow. In severe shock the hepatic blood flow may be reduced so much that it may result in patchy necrosis in the liver.

Reservoir Function of Splanchnic Circulation

Other reservoirs that contain a large volume of blood at rest are skin and lungs. During vigorous exercise constriction of vessels in these organs and decreased storage in the liver and other portions of splanchnic bed may increase the volume of circulation of blood perfusing the muscle by about 30%.

Cutaneous Circulation

The amount of blood flowing through the skin is varied to regulate the heat loss mechanisms in the body to maintain body temperature. Arteriovenous anastomosis (anastomotic connections between the arterioles and venules), are present in the fingers, toes. palms and earlobes which receive nerve supply from sympathetic fibers. The constriction of these channels by nerve supply can regulate flow and decrease it to a very low value.

Subdermal capillary and venous plexus are blood reservoir of significance.

Fetal Circulation

The peculiar features of fetal circulation are:

The placenta serves the function of oxygenation of fetal blood (not lungs as in postnatal life); nutrients are also obtained from placental maternal blood and fetal waste discharged into it.

The maternal side of placenta is large blood sinus into which villi of fetal portion containing branches of umbilical arteries and vein project.

There is patent **foramen ovale** through which fetal blood passes from the right atria to the left atria bypassing right ventricle and pulmonary artery. This serves the function that oxygenated blood from the placenta via umbilical vein passes to the aorta to be distributed to the head region of the fetus.

There is patent **ductus arteriosus** through which blood passes from pulmonary artery to the aorta (after the origin of left subclavian artery) the pressure being higher in the pulmonary artery than in the aorta. The blood returning to the heart via superior vena cava passes to the right atrium and then to right ventricle and to the pulmonary artery and from there via ductus arteriosus to the aorta to be distributed to the trunk and lower part of fetal body; from iliac veins arise the umbilical arteries that pass through umbilical cord to the placenta for purification of blood (Fig. 6.32).

The blood returning from placenta via umbilical vein passes into inferior vena cava via ductus venosus

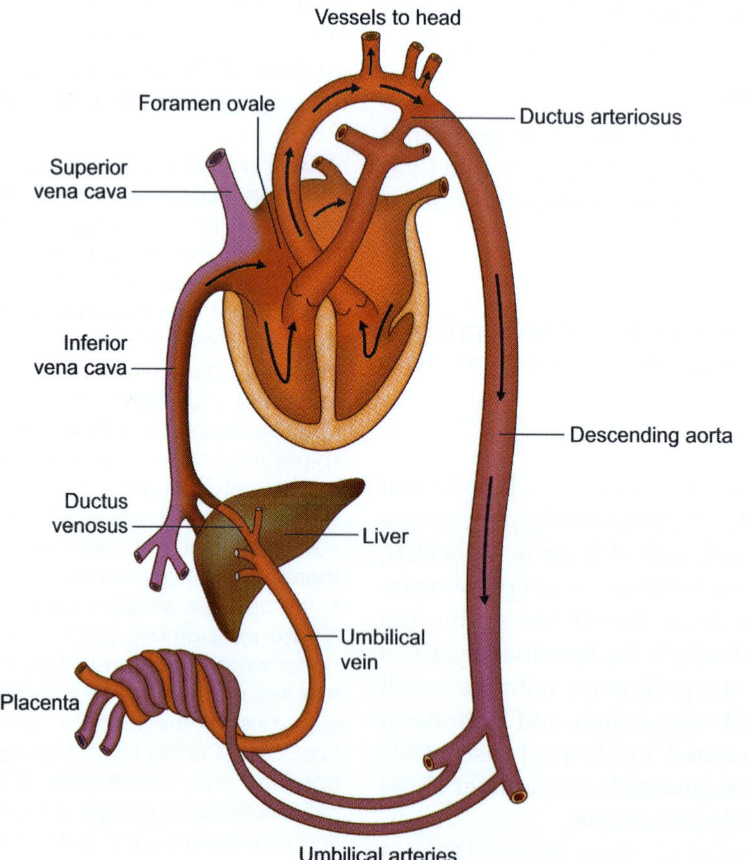

Fig. 6.32: The normal fetal circulation

and another part into portal circulation from thereto inferior vena cava. This is the oxygenated blood that passes to head region of the fetus. Most of the blood from superior vena cava via right atrium and then right ventricle is expelled into pulmonary artery.

Though the arterial oxygen saturation in placental blood is low but due to the presence of fetal hemoglobin blood is able to pick-up enough oxygen; the fetal hemoglobin has higher affinity for oxygen as compared to adult hemoglobin.

After birth *the blood that returns to the left atrium from lungs raises the pressure in the left atrium, closing foramen ovale by pushing a valve that guards it. The ductus arteriosus constricts within a few hours producing a functional closure and permanent closure follows in following 24–48 hours. In many premature infants ductus fails to close spontaneously; treatment with drugs may be required.*

LYMPHATIC SYSTEM

An another system of vessels, the lymphatic system starts as lymph capillaries and transports lymph fluid, which is tissue fluid containing large protein molecules, fragments of damaged tissue cells and microbes from the tissues. The vessels pour this into the venous system, as the larger lymph vessels enter the right and left subclavian veins at their junction with the respective internal jugular veins. In the lymphatic capillaries, the junctions between the cells are open there are no tight intercellular junctions. The proteins which have large molecules enter the lymphatic vessels possibly at these junctions between the endothelial cells and proteins are thus returned to the bloodstream via lymph vessels. The extra fluid in the tissue spaces, which is not drained by blood capillaries, is drained away by this lymphatic system and this prevents the tissue fluid pressure from rising. Normally the fluid which leaves the capillaries at the arterial end is more than the fluid that enters into the capillaries at the venous end, the remaining fluid enters the lymphatic vessels to enter the circulation again. This produces about 2 to 4 L, 24 hours lymph flow.

The lymph vessels are divided into two types; initial lymphatics and collecting lymphatics. Initial lymphatics lack valves and smooth muscle in their walls; the fluid is massaged mainly by muscle contractions and they drain into collecting lymphatics, which have valves and smooth muscle in their walls and contract in peristaltic manner propelling the lymph, the flow is aided by movements of skeletal muscle, the negative intrathoracic pressure and suction effect of the venous circulation into which they drain.

The agents which increase the lymph flow are called lymphagogues.

In the intestine absorption of long chain fatty acids and cholesterol as chylomicrons is into lymphatic vessels (refer to digestive system).

Along the lymph vessels lymph glands are situated. The glands have the function of filtering, microbes and other noxious substances and waste materials from the lymph circulation. The lymph glands also form lymphocytes, the white blood cells involved in immunity.

Among the other causes of edema, one cause is lymphatic obstruction, it is known as lymphedema, and edema fluid has high protein content. If it persists it causes a chronic inflammatory reaction that can produce fibrosis in the interstitial tissue. In cases of radical mastectomy for cancer breast where lymph glands are removed on one side complication of lymphedema occurs in some patients.

Another cause of lymphedema is filariasis in which parasitic worms migrate into lymphatics and produce obstruction, usually causing swelling of the legs and scrotum that is called elephantiasis.

CARDIOVASCULAR HOMEOSTASIS IN HEALTH AND DISEASE

Effect of Gravity

In standing position, as a result of the effect of gravity on the blood the mean arterial pressure in the feet of a normal adult is 180–200 mmHg and venous pressure is 85–90 mmHg. The arterial pressure at head level is 60–75 mmHg and the venous pressure is zero. If the individual **stands still (does not move)**, 300–500 ml of blood would pools in venous vessels of the lower limbs, fluid would accumulate in the tissue spaces due to increased hydrostatic pressure in the capillaries and the stroke volume would decrease. **If the compensatory mechanisms did not come into action unconsciousness would result.** However the compensatory mechanisms protect. The baroreceptors sense the fall in blood pressure and the heart rate increases to maintain cardiac output. Circulating levels of renin and aldosterone increase, that result in constriction of arterioles by angiotensin II, that maintains the blood pressure.

Exercise

In anticipation of exercise the vagal nerve impulses to the heart are inhibited and the sympathetic system is activated. This results in increased heart rate and myocardial contractile force.

With exercise vascular resistance in skin, kidney, splanchnic regions increases; resulting in decrease of blood flow to these regions so that blood is diverted to active muscles. The cardiac output increases (Fig. 6.33) mainly caused by increase in heart rate, and

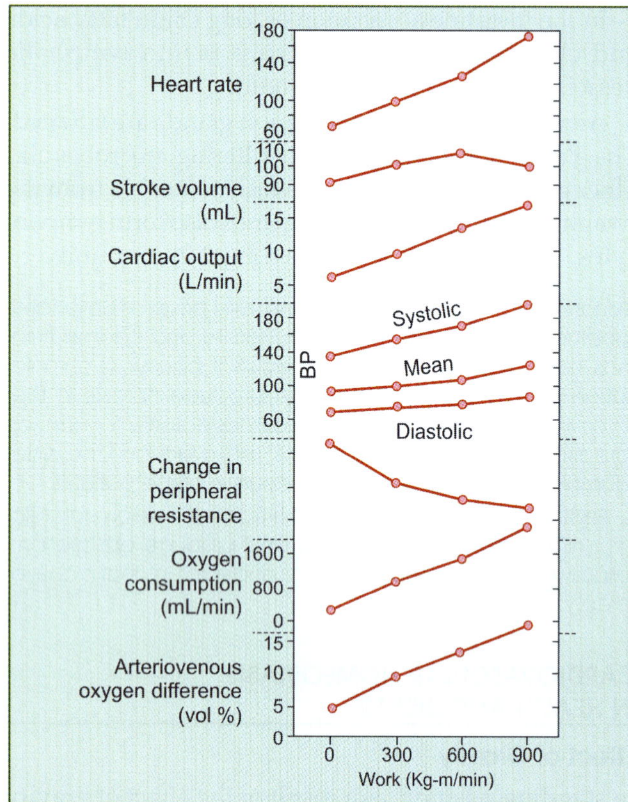

Fig. 6.33: Effects of different grades of isotonic exercise

some increase in stroke volume; this also results in increased blood flow to the active tissue. Total peripheral resistance decreases, due to vasodilation in active regions. Systolic and mean blood pressure increase slightly. Oxygen consumption and blood oxygen extraction increase. If the body temperature increases during exercise the skin blood vessels dilate. The limiting factor in exercise performance is the delivery of blood to the active muscle.

Refer to Chapter on Physiology of Muscular Exercise for details.

SHOCK

The cardiac output is inadequate to maintain tissue perfusion. It occurs when metabolic requirements of tissues are not met with the blood flow. Cardiac output may be inadequate due to reduction in circulating blood volume, or due to increase in the size of vascular system due to vasodilation (even though the blood volume is normal). Shock can also be cardiogenic shock due to inadequate output with inadequate pumping action of the heart. Hence causes of Shock can be:

- Cardiogenic shock. When the cardiac output falls as may be in myocardial infarction, congestive heart failure or arrhythmias.
- Septic shock, due to infection that causes hypovolemia due to increased capillary permeability with loss of fluid into tissues.
- Neurogenic shock as in fainting
- Anaphylactic shock due to sudden fall of BP.
- Obstuctive shock due to tension pneumothorax, pulmonary embolism, cardiac tumor.

Hypovolemic Shock

It occurs when blood volume is reduced. The venous return is decreased, and so the cardiac output. It may occur due to:

- Severe hemorrhage. Whole blood is lost.
- Trauma or extensive superficial burns (Serum is lost and blood cells at the site are burnt).
- Dehydrating condition: severe vomiting and diarrhea due to water and electrolyte loss, or heat stress
- Perforation of an organ

Hypovolemic shock is also called 'cold shock'. Hemorrhagic shock is characterized by hypotension; rapid thready pulse; and a cold pale skin which may have grayish tinge because of stasis of blood in the capillaries with some amount of cyanosis; intense thirst; rapid respiration; restlessness or stupor.

Immediate Changes

Physiological attempt is to restore an adequate blood circulation. There is generalized vasoconstriction sparing only the brain and heart, it is most marked in the skin, kidneys and viscera. There is venoconstriction. GFR is decreased and if hypotension is prolonged there may be severe renal tubular damage. Chemoreceptor activity is the main cause of stimulation of respiration and it also stimulates vasomotor center augmenting its activity.

If the shock persists, long-term changes may be irreversible.

Hormonal Changes

As blood pressure falls hormone secretions increase to restore homeostasis.

- Increased secretion of adrenal medulla
- Sympathetic system stimulation
- Water retention by the kidney by stimulation of antidiuretic hormone.
- Stimulation of renin-angiotensin-aldosterone system

In shock of moderate intensity the circulation to the heart and brain is maintained at the expense of circulation to nonvital regions.

Refractory Shock

In hemorrhagic shock depending upon the blood lost some patients may die after hemorrhage and others recover as the compensatory mechanisms, aided by proper treatment, gradually restore the circulation to normal.

In intermediate group of patients, shock persists for hours and gradually progress to a state in which there is no longer any response to vasopressor drugs and in which even if the blood volume is restored to normal, cardiac output remains depressed. This is known as refractory shock.

Various positive feedback mechanisms contribute to the production of refractory shock. Severe cerebral ischemia leads to depression of the vasomotor center and cardiac center causing vasodilation and bradycardia; these make the BP to fall further decreasing blood flow to the brain. Another cause is myocardial failure due to decrease in coronary blood flow because of hypotension and tachycardia, even though coronary vessels are dilated. Acidosis due to accumulation of lactic acid because of inadequate availability of oxygen to the body this contributes to myocardial depression.

Cardiogenic Shock

In acute myocardial damage (myocardial infarction) heart muscle is enable to maintain adequate cardiac output and BP falls.

Septic Shock

This is caused by severe infections usually due to gram-negative bacteria that release endotoxins. There is vasodilation and increased permeability with loss of plasma into tissues and hence decrease in cardiac output. Due to release of cytokines and coagulant reactions it can lead to multiple organ failure.

Neurogenic Shock

Sudden acute pain, severe emotional experience, spinal anesthesia, and spinal cord damage, there is sudden autonomic activity producing vasodilation in these conditions. Parasympathetic nerve impulses reduce heart rate and result in decrease in cardiac output.

The venous return may also be reduced by the pooling of blood in dilated veins. The blood supply to the brain is reduced causing fainting.

Postural syncope is fainting due to pooling of blood in dependent parts of the body on standing, e.g. Standing up quickly from a sitting or lying position. It may be seen in patients receiving sympatholytic drugs, as in treatment of hypertension or when there is damage to the sympathetic nervous system as in diabetes or syphilis.

The sympathetic system fails to bring about the compensatory effects on the pooling of blood in lower parts of the body (the gravity effect) that occurs in a normal individual, the regulation via baroreceptors through vasomotor centre and increased activity of sympathetic system to restrict the pooling of blood in lower parts of the body.

Fainting

It is neurogenic shock also called distributive shock, as the capacity of the circulation is increased due to which, with a normal cardiac output there is shock. It is also warm shock. There is sudden autonomic activity producing vasodilation, pooling of blood in extremities and fainting. This is called vasovagal attack and is short lived and benign.

Pressure on the carotid sinus, as by tight collars can produce bradycardia and vasodilation producing fainting this is called **carotid sinus syncope**.

Anaphylactic Shock

The reaction of antigen with antibody may be severe enough to cause release of large quantities of histamine to cause increased capillary permeability and widespread arterial vasodilation resulting in sudden fall of blood pressure. There may be contraction of smooth muscle of bronchi (bronchospasm).

The vasodilation increases the capacity of circulation and this condition is also called warm shock and the skin is not cold and clammy.

Disorders of Blood Pressure

Hypertension

Hypertension is sustained elevation of the systemic arterial pressure.

In over 90% of patients with elevated blood pressure the cause of hypertension is unknown and this hypertension is called ***essential hypertension***.

Essential hypertension is treatable but not curable. Effective lowering of the blood pressure can be produced by drugs. Some hypertensives appear to be salt-sensitive, i.e. increased intake of salt reflects in hypertension; others have only slight increase in blood pressure when fed high salt diet.

Secondary hypertension in a few cases of hypertension the cause can be identified and they are grouped under this heading. The causes include *renal disease, disorders of adrenal medulla, other endocrine abnormalities and genetic disorders.*

In *pregnant women* hypertension may be due to *pressor peptide secreted by placenta.*

Hypertension is a prominent feature of hyperaldosteronism.

It may occur in Cushings' syndrome

Pheochromocytomas, the tumors of adrenal medulla produce hypertension.

Oral contraceptives containing estrogen produce significant hypertension in some women.

Renal hypertension is due to narrowing of the renal arteries and other diseases of the kidney.

Pulmonary hypertension is unrelated to systemic hypertension also occurs as a disease. The pressure in the pulmonary artery is relatively independent of the systemic arteries.

Malignant Hypertension

Chronic hypertension can enter into malignant phase in which necrosis of arterioles takes place resulting in changes in eyes, cerebral symptoms and progressive renal failure, with rapid downhill course and without treatment results in death in few years.

Heart Failure

Chronic hypertension increases the load on the myocardium of the left ventricle and so also in a number of other diseases. The response of the myocardial muscle cells is activation of genes that make myocytes hypertrophy. In some cases there is ventricular remodeling in response to distortions produced by the disease processes. Initially these changes are compensatory but the heart failure may take place when the oxygen supply to the muscle becomes inadequate. The heart fails to put out enough blood to maintain tissue perfusion. At first cardiac output is only decreased during exercise and remains normal at rest but with continued progression of disease it may result in; *systolic heart failure* in which stroke volume is reduced because the ventricular contractions are weak; *diastolic heart failure* in which elasticity of the heart is reduced, hindering cardiac filling.

Systolic weakness increases end-diastolic ventricular volume and reduces ejection fraction. Ejection fraction may fall as low to 20%. Normal ejection fraction is about 65%. Ejection fraction is a valuable index of ventricular function.

Heart failure can be primarily of the right ventricle (**corpulmonale**); more commonly involves left ventricle. Right heart failure may follow left heart failure.

Corpulmonale is a heart condition secondary to pulmonary disorder with increased pulmonary resistance. The lung disease may causes pulmonary hypertension, increased workload of right heart, right ventricular hypertrophy and finally right ventricular failure.

The manifestations of heart failure may be sudden death (e.g. in ventricular fibrillation or air embolism), or cardiogenic shock or chronic congestive heart failure, depending upon the rapidly with which it develops and the degree of circulatory inadequacy. The principal symptoms and signs of chronic **congestive heart failure** include cardiac enlargement and signs and symptoms as listed in the table (Table 6.7).

Corpulmonale with body fluid retention (increased ECF volume) is demonstrated by a raised jugular venous pressure and ankle edema.

Ischemic Heart Disease

When blood flow through a coronary artery is reduced to a point that the myocardium becomes hypoxic (O_2 insufficiency to the muscle) "P" factor accumulates producing pain (angina pectoris).

Many individuals have angina only on exertion and blood flow is adequate for the requirements of the heart at rest. Some may have more severe restriction of blood flow and have angina pain even at rest. Partially occluded coronary arteries can be constricted further by vasospasm.

The pain in angina may be felt in the chest, may also radiate to the arm, neck and jaw. Other factors which may precipitate angina include;

- Cold weather
- Exertion after heavy meal
- Strong emotions

A narrowed coronary artery may be able to supply the needs of myocardium during rest but when greatly increased cardiac output is needed, e.g. during exercise, the atherosclerotic artery wall is narrow and also unable to dilate to supply the increased demands of more active myocardium.

Table 6.7: Symptoms of congestive heart failure with pathology

Abnormality	*Cause*
Weakness, exercise intolerance	"Forward failure" of left ventricle; cardiac output inadequate to perfuse muscles; especially, failure of output to rise with exercise.
Ankle, sacral edema	"Backward failure"! increased peripheral venous pressure! increased fluid transudation.
Hepatomegaly	Increased peripheral venous pressure! increased resistance to portal flow.
Pulmonary congestion	"Backward failure"! increased pulmonary venous pressure! pulmonary venous distention and transudation of fluid into air spaces.
Dyspnea on exertion	Failure of left ventricular output to rise during exercise! increased pulmonary venous pressure.
Paroxysmal dyspnea, pulmonary edema	Probably sudden failure of left heart output to keep up with right heart output! acute rise in pulmonary venous and capillary pressure! transudation of fluid into air spaces.
Orthopnea	Normal pooling of blood in lungs in supine position added to already congested pulmonary vascular system; increased venous return not put by left ventricle (relieved by sitting up, raising head of bed, lying on extra pillows)
Cardiac dilation	Greater ventricular end-diastolic volume

In early stages of development when the output returns to resting level the pain stops.

Cardiac Arrhythmias

Disease processes affecting the sinus node lead to marked bradycardia accompanied by dizziness and syncope (fainting), this is called sick sinus syndrome.

Abnormal Pacemakers

If SA node is depressed the AV node may take over the function of impulse formation, it generates the impulse at a slower rate.

When conduction from the atria to the ventricles is completely interrupted, complete or third degree heart block results and ventricles beat at a lower rate (idioventricular rhythm), independently of the atrial rhythm which beat at normal rate (there may be brief period of a minute or so before the ventricles start beating, leading to an attack of fainting that is called Stokes-Adams Syndrome). The block may be due to disease at AV node (AV nodal block) or in the conducting system below the node (infranodal block). The rate of idioventricular rhythm is approximately 45 beats/min but may be lower.

Implantations of Pacemakers

When there is marked bradycardia in patients with sick sinus syndrome; or in cases of third degree heart block an electronic pacemaker is frequently implanted.

Myocardial Infarction

An infarct is an area of tissue that has died because if lack of oxygen. The commonest cause is obstruction in blood supply caused by atherosclerotic plaque complicated by thrombosis. The damage is permanent because cardiac muscle cannot regenerate and the tissue is replaced by non functional fibrous tissue.

Speedy restorations of blood flow through the blocked artery using clot-dissolving (thrombolytic) drugs can greatly reduce the extent of permanent damage and improve prognosis, but the treatment must be started within a few hours of infarction (cutting off blood supply).

Myocardial infarction is usually accompanied by very severe crushing chest pain behind the sternum, which continues even when the individual resting.

When the myocardial cells die they leak enzymes into the circulation and measuring the rise of **serum enzymes** and isoenzymes produced by infarcted myocardial cells this plays an important role in the diagnosis. The enzymes most commonly measured are the MB isomer of **creatine kinase (CK-MB), troponin T, troponin I.**

Asystole

This occurs when there is no electrical activity in the ventricles and therefore no cardiac output. The ECG shows flat line. Ventricular fibrillation and asystole cause sudden cardiac arrest and death.

Edema

There is excess fluid in the tissues spaces. Causes that can lead to it are:

- Increased venous hydrostatic pressure.
- Congestion of venous circulation, e.g. in heart failure, increases the venous hydrostatic pressure

reducing the effect of osmotic pressure at the venous end of the capillary to reabsorbs fluid into the circulation.

- Decreased colloidal osmotic pressure due to decrease in the concentration of plasma proteins especially the albumin fraction as occurs in some kidney diseases.
- Impaired lymphatic drainage when there is blockage in the lymphatic system as in malignancy of lymph nodes, surgical removal of lymph nodes or chronic inflammation of lymph nodes.
- Increased capillary permeability as in some allergic conditions where histamine is released causing increased capillary permeability leading to leakage of plasma proteins in the tissue fluid that draws fluid out of the capillary and the reabsorption is affected.

The causes are summed up in Table 6.8.

Ascites: It means excess accumulation of fluid in the peritoneal cavity.

Cause can be liver disease or obstruction of lymph vessels in the abdomen, etc.

Varicose Veins

A varicosed vein is one which is so dilated that the valves do not close to prevent backward flow of blood. Such veins loose elasticity and become elongated and tortuous and fibrous tissue replaces the tunica media.

Predisposing Factors

- Heredity as gender females are affected more than males especially following pregnancy.
- Age as progressive loss of elasticity in the vein walls with increasing age so that the elastic recoil is less efficient.
- Obesity as excessive fat does not provide enough support for the veins.
- Gravity as standing for long periods with little movement.

Table 6.8: Causes of edema

Causes of edema
Increased filtration pressure
Venular constriction
Increased venous pressure (heart failure, incompetent valves, venous obstruction, effect of gravity, etc.)
Decreased osmotic pressure gradient across capillary
Decreased plasma protein level
Increased capillary permeability
Histamine and related substances
Inadequate lymph flow

Common Terms used in CVS

Arteriosclerosis: It means hardening of artery due to degenerative changes limiting blood flow through it.

Atherosclerosis: It is narrowing of artery due to deposition of cholesterol and lipids.

Aneurysm: It is a localized weakness in the wall of an artery, which may dilate or rupture causing hemorrhage.

Thrombosis: Formation of clot in a vessel is called thrombosis, commonly it occurs in venous circulation in the leg veins after operation or delivery because slow flow of blood permits accumulation of activated clotting factors instead being washed away. It also occurs in coronary or cerebral vessels at the endothelial damaged site.

If the clot breaks up and travels to another part of the circulation where it lodges this is called **embolus**. It obstructs the blood supply of the organ and causes damage, e.g. obstruction of pulmonary artery or its branches by thrombi from leg veins (pulmonary embolism).

Valvular heart disease. Any of the valves of the heart may be narrowed so that there is restriction of blood flows through them; or the valves may become incompetent causing back flow of blood producing various effects on heart. The various murmurs heard on auscultation over the heart lead to diagnosis.

Congenital abnormalities of the heart Patent ductus arteriosus; atrial septal defects; Fallot's tetralogy; coarctation of aorta are the abnormalities that may occur.

IMPLICATIONS AND APPLICATIONS

- Feel the pulse at the wrist at elbow, neck, abdomen, dorsum of foot and behind the medial malleolus.
- Take blood pressure in upper limb and lower limb.
- Know various sites of intravenous injection.
- Take a sample of blood from any superficial vein.
- Test blood group and Rh.
- Read electrocardiogram (ECG).
- Procedure to resuscitate a person.

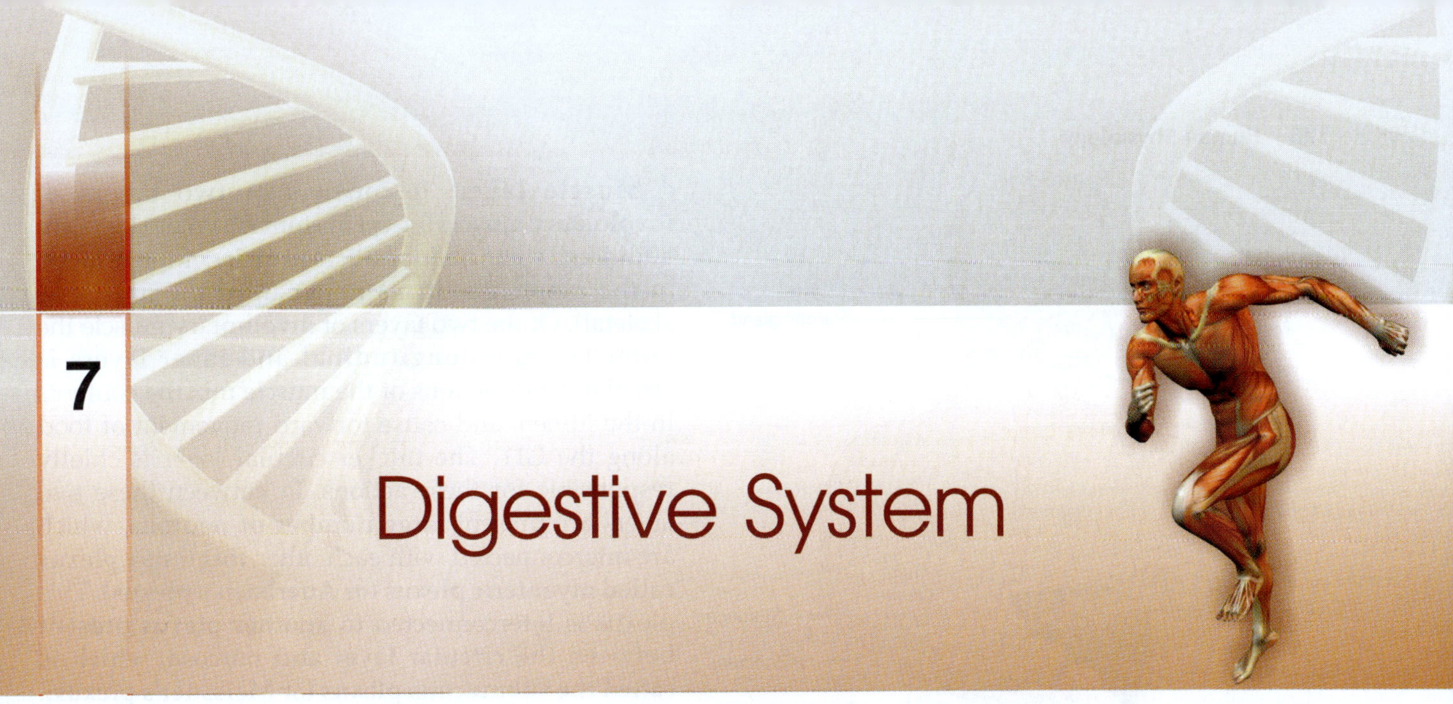

7 Digestive System

Eating is **vital** and for many people it provides pleasure. It serves the requirements of: *metabolic functions; growth* and *development; turnover of tissue protein; pregnancy* and *lactation*.

The food is subjected to the process of digestion, whereby the **carbohydrates, fats** and **proteins** are broken down into smaller particles capable of being absorbed from the gastrointestinal tract into the blood or the lymphatic vessels that are present there. The **minerals** and **vitamins** liberated from the food during digestion and **water** present in the *diet and that of digestive juices*, are absorbed. Most of the absorption takes place in small intestine though *still further* absorption of electrolytes and water also takes place in the large intestine. Nonabsorbed residues of food are thrown out as feces. Digestion of the food stuffs is a process involving the action of a large number of digestive enzymes, secreted by **associated glands** and produced by lining cells; all *working without conscious control*.

The food provides:

- **Carbohydrates:** The dietary carbohydrates are polysaccharides, disaccharides and monosaccharides. Starch and their derivates are the polysaccharides digested in human intestine. Cellulose is not digested. The disaccharides lactose (milk sugar), sucrose (table sugar) also is ingested. Monosaccharides fructose and glucose may be ingested.
- **Lipids:** Mainly are triglycerides (triacylglycerol) and there are phospholipids, cholesterol and essential fatty acids
- Proteins
- **Minerals**
- **Vitamins**
- **Water** or fluids are ingested.

The digestive system begins in the mouth, passes through the thorax, abdomen and pelvis and ends at the anus. The system has general features common to all parts and there are some modifications at different regions for specific functions.

The parts of digestive system (Fig. 7.1) are:

- Mouth and 3 pairs of salivary glands.
- Pharynx
- Esophagus
- Stomach
- Small intestine (duodenum, jejunum ileum), the associated; pancreas, liver, and the gallbladder
- Large intestine (cecum, ascending colon, transverse colon, descending colon) and including rectum and anal canal.

The organs and associated glands are linked together in a long tubular arrangement, where digestion takes place by the enzymes present in the mouth, stomach and intestine (here they are also poured from pancreas via its duct and bile enters from liver via common bile duct) as the food passes along gastrointestinal tract (GIT). The different enzymes are present for action on different components of food, and optimum pH is provided for their action in parts of GIT.

The layers of walls of GIT follow almost a common pattern from the stomach till the end of the tract, with some modifications of structure associated with special functions of that part. The basic structure of the wall is formed of 4 layers (Fig. 7.2), as follows:

- Outer covering of adventitia or serosa

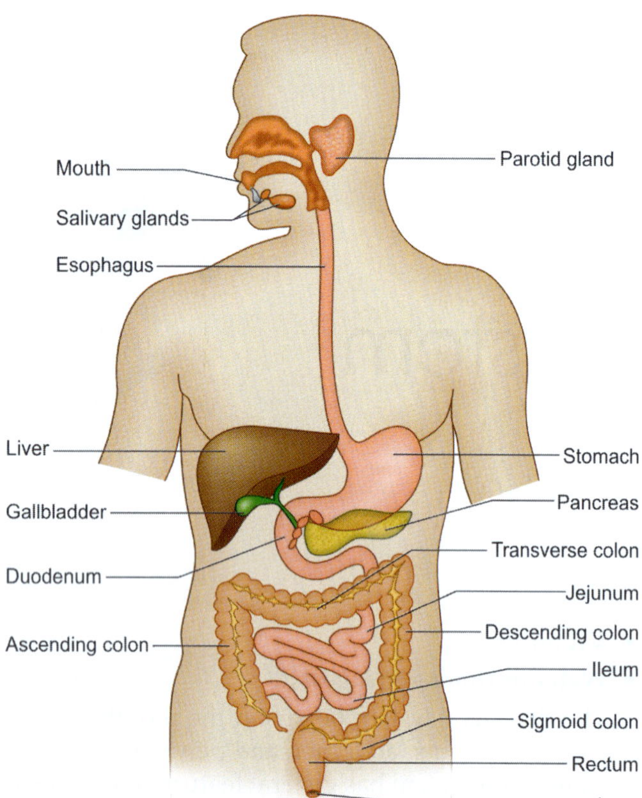

Fig. 7.1: Gastrointestinal tract

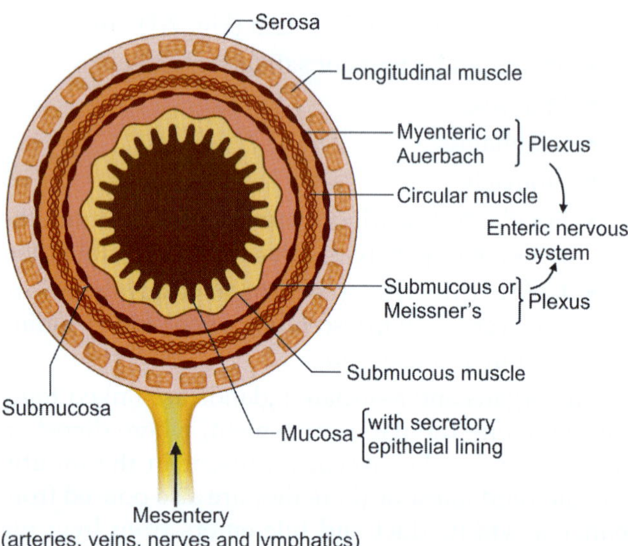

Fig. 7.2: Representation of the layers of the stomach, small intestine, and colon

- Muscle layer consisting of two layers except in stomach where 3 layers are present.
- Submucosal layer
- Mucosa, the inner lining layer.

Adventitia: In the thorax it consists of fibrous tissue and in the abdomen it is formed by covering of serous membrane, the peritoneum.

Muscle layer: It consists of two layers of **involuntary muscle** (*except* in stomach where there are additional some oblique fibers in an incomplete layer; in the esophagus in its upper third the muscle is skeletal). Of the two layers of involuntary muscle the outer layers is **longitudinal** and inner layers is **circular.** Contractions of the muscle mix the contents in the lumen, and cause forward movement of food along the GIT. The thicker circular layer is chiefly responsible for these actions. In between these two layers are present **large number of neurons**, which are interconnected with each other **forming a plexus called myenteric plexus (or Auerbach's plexus).** This plexus is interconnected to **another plexus present between the circular layer and mucosa, which is called the submucous plexus (or Meissner's plexus)**. The two plexuses together are called the **enteric nervous system**. The neurons present are *sensory neurons, interneurons* and *motor neurons*. This system is concerned with regulating the movements and secretions of GIT. Though it is connected with CNS by autonomic nerves; it can function independently without these connections; though normally the autonomic nerves modify their activity (Fig. 7.3). The myenteric plexus functions mainly for control of movements and its motor nerve fibers innervate both the layers of muscle fibers; the submucous plexus innervates the gland cells, and intestinal endocrine cells; and is primarily involved in control of secretions. *Of the extrinsic nerves parasympathetic supply increases the secretion and motility of the tract, whereas the sympathetic nerve activity decreases the motility and causes contraction of sphincters*. The parasympathetic fibers come from **vagal** nerves and **sacral spinal cord**, they are preganglionic fibers which relay on the neurons in myenteric and submucous plexuses. The sympathetic fibers are postganglionic and many of them end on postganglionic parasympathetic neurons and decrease their activity, other sympathetic fibers end directly on the muscle cells, some others on blood vessels where they cause vasoconstriction. The enteric nervous system itself releases some neurotransmitters including acetylcholine, norepinephrine, serotonin GABA, ATP, NO, CO. Many peptides produce

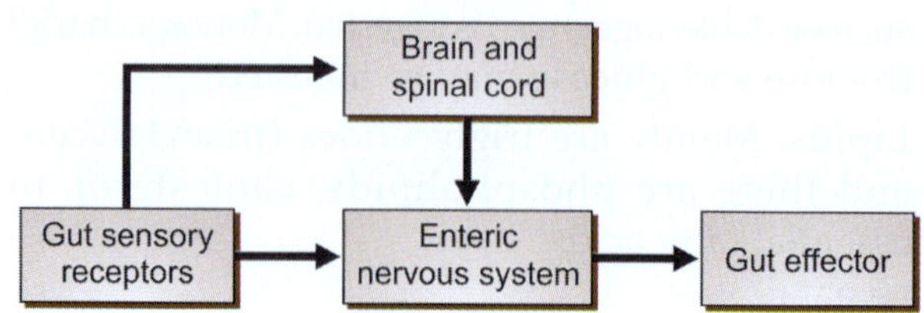

Fig. 7.3: Connections of enteric nervous system

vasodilation of blood vessels. **Peristalsis** is the *movement* by which the food moves along the GIT, from the esophagus till the rectum. The *distension* of the walls due to contents in the lumen stimulates the reflex in the enteric nervous system, *which causes contraction of muscle behind the stimulus and relaxation in front of it. The wave of contraction moves in oral to caudal direction; and is due to integrated activity of the enteric nervous system;* the extrinsic nerves are not essential, though the nerves can modify the activity. This is responsible for movements occurring in any part of GIT.

Control of Gastrointestinal Motor Activities

Control of contractile functions of GIT involves *CNS*, the *intrinsic plexuses* (enteric nervous system), *humoral factors, and electrical coupling among muscle fibers* (smooth muscle).

Submucosa: It consists of loose connective tissue with collagen and elastin fibers and some smooth muscle fibers that is muscularis mucosae; in some regions glands are present; the larger blood vessels travel in the submucosa.

Mucosa: It consists of an epithelium, with some connective tissue, the lamina propria that is rich in glands and contains lymph nodules and capillaries. The nature of epithelium varies in different parts.

MOUTH

Salivary secretions are composed of *water, electrolytes,* enzymes (*amylase, lysozyme*), *mucin, immune globulin IgA, lactoferrin* which is bacteriostatic, and *proline rich proteins* that protect teeth enamel and bind toxic tannins. About **1500 mL of saliva is secreted per day,** from three pairs of salivary glands. The pH of the saliva varies from *7.0 to 8.0.* 99.5% saliva is water (Table 7.1 gives the broad functions of saliva and Table 7.2 the characteristics of three pairs of salivary glands). Figure 7.4, shows histological features of mixed salivary gland.

Table 7.1: Summary of functions of saliva

Salivary secretion		
Source	Parotid, submandibular, and sublingual glands.	Salivary secretion is stimulated by both parasympathetic and sympathetic nerves
Function	1. Alpha-amylase (ptyalin) begins starch digestion 2. Neutralizes oral contents, maintains dental health 3. Mucins (glycoproteins) lubricate food	

Table 7.2: Characteristics of salivary glands

Gland	*Histologic type*
Parotid	Serous
Submandibular (submaxillary)	Mixed
Sublingual	Mucous

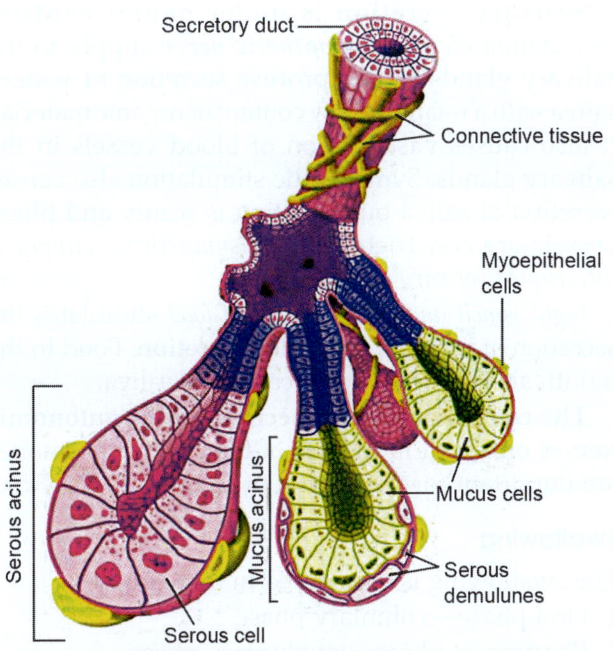

Fig. 7.4: Diagrammatic representation of the secretory and duct system of the submandibular gland. This is a mixed gland containing both serous and mucous cells

In the mouth secretion of saliva keeps the mouth *moist;* facilitating *speech* and sensation of *thirst*; acts solvent for sensation of *taste*; has *cleaning action in* the mouth and teeth to *prevent dental caries;* salivary **amylase** initiates carbohydrate digestion; **lingual lipase** secreted by glands on the tongue is for fat digestion. Saliva helps to clear the esophagus of refluxed gastric secretions. The **mucins** lubricate the food facilitating swallowing, bind bacteria and protect the oral mucosa; secretory immunoglobulin **IgA, lysozyme** attacks the wall of bacteria. When the food is chewed it is mixed with saliva and is broken down to form a soft mass called *bolus*. (Though large food particles can be digested, but they cause strong contractions of the esophageal muscle that are painful).

The saliva contains the enzyme α *amylase* called *ptyalin*. The enzyme hydrolyses starch to maltose or other small polymers of glucose containing three to nine glucose molecules (matotriose and α limit dextrins). The food remains in the mouth only for a short time and only a small part of hydrolysis takes place during this time. The process continues in the bolus, in the stomach till the acid pH of the stomach brings an end to the action of the enzyme. But on an average before the food becomes completely mixed with gastric secretions as much as *30–40% of the starch is hydrolysed*.

Salivary secretion is under **neural control**, stimulation of ***parasympathetic nerve*** supply to the salivary glands causes profuse secretion of watery saliva with a relatively low content of organic material. It also causes vasodilation of blood vessels in the salivary glands. Sympathetic stimulation also causes secretion of saliva but secretion is scanty and blood vessels are constricted. *If parasympathetic supply is interrupted salivary glands atrophy*.

Sight, smell and even thought of food stimulates the secretion of saliva, it is a **reflex secretion**. Food in the mouth also causes reflex secretion of saliva.

The control of salivary secretion is by autonomic nerves only; but in the rest of the GIT the hormones are important for the control of secretions (Fig. 7.5).

Swallowing

The swallowing is considered in three phases:

1. Oral phase—voluntary phase
2. Pharyngeal phase—involuntary phase
3. Esophageal phase—involuntary phase

Swallowing is ***initiated by voluntary action*** but ***after that*** it is a ***reflex response***. The afferent limb of the reflex response begins with tactile receptors near the opening of the pharynx and the impulses are transmitted to areas in medulla; these are integrated in the **Swallowing center** situated in the medulla and lower pons (the areas are together called Swallowing center). From the center motor impulses travel to the muscles of the pharynx and upper esophagus via various cranial nerves. Hence, *Swallowing reflex is orderly sequence of events that result in propulsion of food from mouth to stomach, at the same time preventing reflux into nasopharynx; inhibiting respiration and preventing entry of food into trachea.*

When the bolus collects on the tongue, by voluntary action the bolus is propelled backwards into the pharynx. This is ***oral or voluntary phase***. It is followed by ***pharyngeal phase*** involving a sequence of events: *preventing reflux of food into nasopharynx*, as soft palate is pulled upwards and palatopharyngeal folds move *inwards towards each other; preventing entry of food into trachea, respiration is inhibited*, the vocal cords are pulled together, epiglottis covers the opening of larynx, the larynx moves upwards against the epiglottis hence *glottis is closed* so that food is prevented from entering into the trachea; the *upper esophageal sphincter relaxes* to receive the bolus of food; a wave of involuntary contraction in the pharyngeal muscles is set up that *pushes the material into the esophagus*. Then in the ***esophageal phase*** *peristaltic wave* carries the food down in the esophagus. This phase of swallowing is only partially controlled by swallowing center. The primary peristalsis is set up if

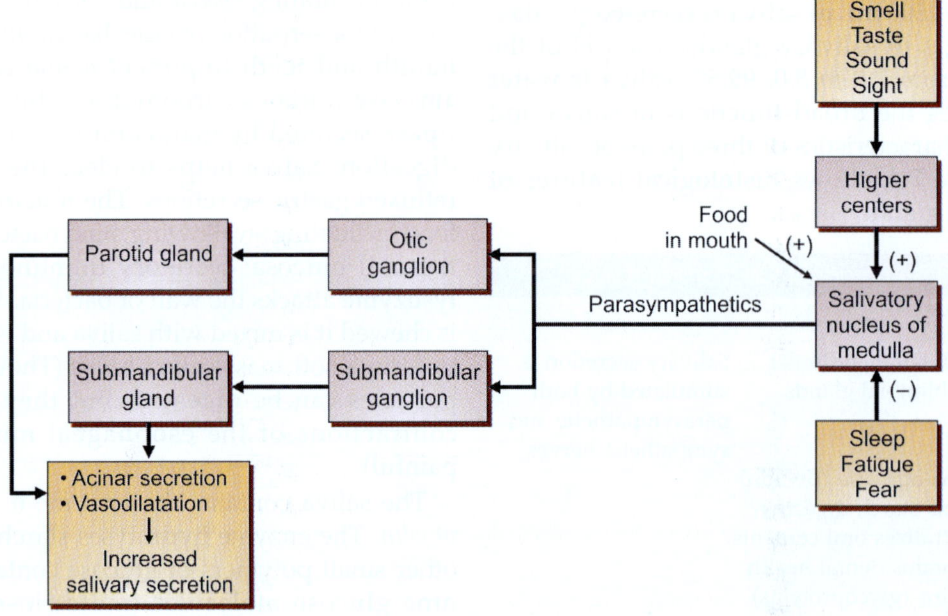

Fig. 7.5: Nervous control of salivary secretion

it fails to clear the esophagus of food, the distension of that region in the esophagus sets up secondary peristalsis that carry the food down the esophagus, this function is brought about by the activity of enteric nervous system.

Swallowing is *difficult* when the mouth is open. At the lower end of the esophagus at the gastro-esophageal junction (***lower esophageal sphincter, LES***) the muscle remains in a state of tonic contraction and relaxes only when the peristaltic wave reaches this region during swallowing. It prevents reflux of gastric contents into the esophagus; it acts as an *intrinsic sphincter*. Fibers of the *crural portion of the diaphragm*, a skeletal muscle, surround the esophagus at this point (*extrinsic sphincter*) and this and the *oblique fibers of the stomach wall* form a flap valve that close off the esophagogastric junction and prevent regurgitation when the intragastric pressure rises. *The tone of LES is under neural control. Enteric nervous system* plays an important role in regulating the function of LES. Release of acetylcholine from vagal endings causes the intrinsic sphincter to contract; and release of NO (nitric oxide) and VIP from interneurons innervated by other vagal fibers cause it to relax. Contraction of the crural portion of the diaphragm, innervated by phrenic nerves is coordinated with respiration. Hence, the intrinsic and extrinsic sphincters operate together to prevent orderly flow of food into the stomach and prevent reflux of gastric contents, into the esophagus. The reflux would cause esophagitis and sensation of heart burn.

Esophagus

It functions as a passage for food from the pharynx to the stomach. It also functions to prevent the air from entering at the upper end of the esophagus; and prevents corrosive gastric contents from re-fluxing back into the esophagus at the lower end. The upper and lower ends function as sphincters to prevent these effects.

The structure of the esophagus follows the general pattern except that in the upper third, both inner circular and outer longitudinal muscle layers are composed of skeletal (striated) muscle fibers.

The upper esophageal sphincter is formed by thickening of circular layer of striated muscle fibers; the sphincter consists of cricopharyngeal muscle and thyropharyngeus part of inferior pharyngeal constrictor.

The esophageal muscle both striated and smooth is supplied mainly by branches of vagal nerves.

Clinical Significance

Reflux esophagitis. It is a common cause of indigestion, caused by regurgitation of acid gastric juice into the esophagus, causing irritation and painful ulceration in chronic cases. Hemorrhage occurs when blood vessels are eroded.

Achalasia. During swallowing in some individuals the lower esophageal sphincter (LES) fails to relax sufficiently to allow food to enter the stomach, this condition is called **achalasia.**

Diffuse esophageal spasm in this condition there are prolonged and painful contractions of the lower end of the esophagus after swallowing instead of normal peristaltic wave.

The ***incompetence of lower esophageal sphincter***, which permits reflux of gastric contents; ***achalasia;*** and ***diffuse esophageal spasm***, are **the common disturbances of dysfunction at this region.**

STOMACH

Functions

The stomach acts as a temporary **storage organ** for the food. The food taken during a meal collects in the stomach. Here it is *churned by the movements* of the stomach, mixed with mucus and pepsin and forms into semi-liquid called **chyme** which passes at a *controlled rate* into the duodenum; the *emptying of stomach* is in small amounts.

In the stomach the **pepsin** and **HCl** present in the gastric juice act on the proteins in the food to initiate digestion. **Mucus** protects the stomach wall, from digestion by HCl.

The cells of the gastric gland secrete about **2500 mL of gastric juice daily.** Gastric juice is thin, colorless liquid with acidic **pH of 2.0.** Some amount of gastric juice is always present in the stomach, but the secretion is stimulated on ingestion of food; the quality of juice depends upon the amount and type of food ingested. The juice contains (Table 7.3) enzymes **Pepsinogen** and **Lipase;** also present are **mucus** and **intrinsic factor** (intrinsic factor is necessary for absorption of vitamin B_{12} as it combines with B_{12} preventing destruction in the stomach and B_{12} is absorbed further down in the terminal portion small intestine). Enzymes and HCl are secreted by the **mucosal cells in the body of the stomach** (Fig. 7.6). Gastrin is secreted by 'G' cells in mucosa of pyloric antrum.

Pepsinogen Secretion

The **chief cells** (Fig. 7.7) in the stomach form enzyme pepsinogen which in itself is inactive but is converted into active form **pepsin** by the HCL in the stomach.

Table 7.3: Secretions of stomach glands with functions

Stomach	*Functions*	*Source secretions*
Mucus	Lubricant, protects surface from H^+	Mucous cell cardiac, pyloric region and surface mucosa
Intrinsic factor	Vitamin B_{12} absorption (in small intestine)	Parietal cell Body region
H^+	Kills bacteria, breaks down food, activates pepsinogen to pepsin	Parietal cell Body region
Pepsinogen	Broken down to pepsin (a protease). Protein digestion	Chief cell Body region
Gastrin	Stimulates acid secretion	G cell Antral mucosa

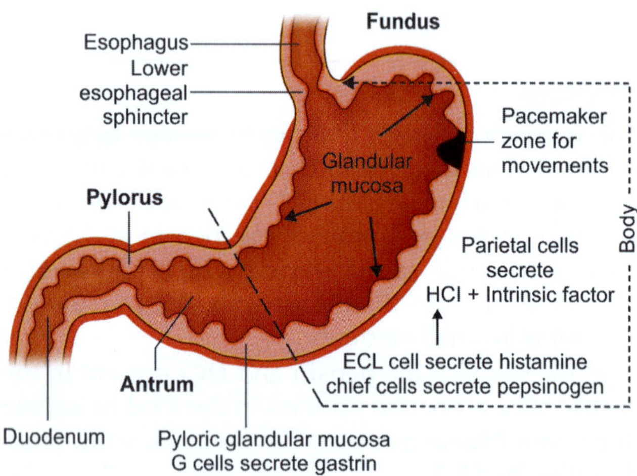

Fig. 7.6: The anatomical divisions of the stomach and secretion from the cells in the mucosa

Pepsin acts on proteins and polypeptides to break them into smaller polypeptides.

Hydrochloric Acid (HCl) Secretion

It is secreted by parietal cells (also called oxyntic cells) (Fig. 7.7). It activates pepsinogen.

HCl also helps to *kill bacteria* present in the food. It provides the *necessary pH for pepsin* to start protein digestion and on entering the duodenum *stimulate the flow of bile.*

Intrinsic factor is also formed by the oxyntic cells in the stomach, the cells which form HCl.

Gastric lipase acts on triglycerides to convert it into fatty acids and glycerol. The gastric lipase is of little importance but lingual lipase is active in stomach and can digest 30% of dietary triglyceride. Both these lipases become important in deficiency of pancreatic lipase.

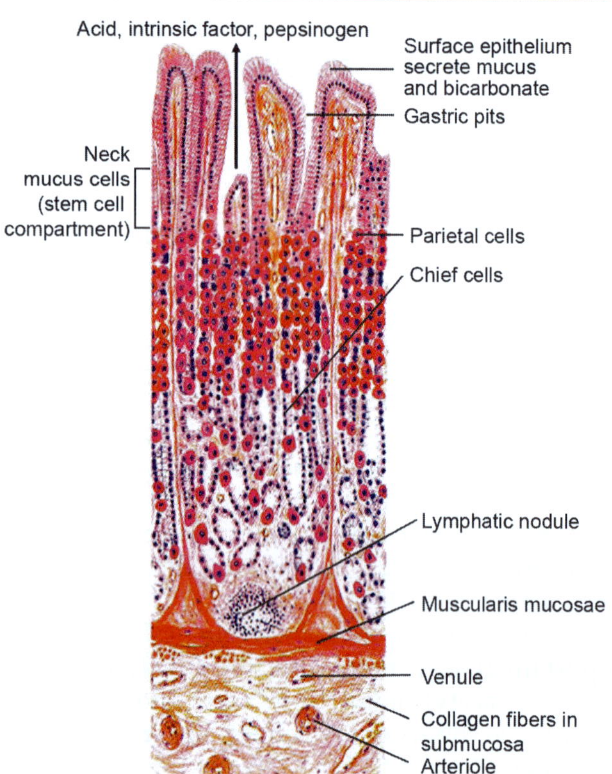

Fig. 7.7: Mucosa of the body of the stomach showing secreting cells

Mucus is secreted by cells in the *neck of glands* and by *surface epithelial cells*. Which also **secrete HCO_3^-**.

Mucosal Barrier

The acid in the stomach would cause tissue damage, but is prevented by mucosal barrier produced by ***mucus and*** **HCO_3^-** secreted by surface mucosal cells, HCl secreted by the parietal cells in the gastric glands crosses this barrier in finger like channels leaving the rest of the gel coating of mucosa intact.

Mucus and HCO_3^- secreted by mucosal cells also plays an important role in **protecting the duodenum** form damage when the acid rich chyme reaches the duodenum. **Prostaglandins** stimulate mucus and HCO_3^- secretion. **Local reflexes** also have a role in HCO_3^- secretion.

Formation and secretion of HCl by Parietal cells.

Carbonic anhydrase enzyme is present in the parietal cells and it catalyzes the hydration of CO_2 resulting in formation of $H_2CO_3^-$ which dissociates into H^+ and HCO_3^- ions. H^+ is actively secreted into the ducts of the gastric glands by H^+K^+ ATPase (Fig. 7.8). There is H^+K^+ ATPase in the apical membrane of parietal cells that pumps H^+ against concentration gradient. The HCO_3^- ions from the parietal cells enter the bloodstream and urine may

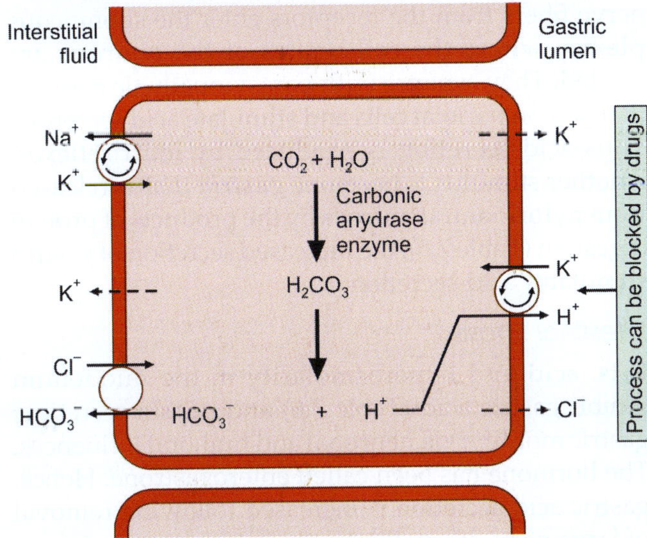

Fig. 7.8: HCl secretion by parietal cells. H^+ is secreted into the gastric lumen in exchange for K^+ by H^+K^+ ATPase. HCO_3^- is exchanged for Cl^- in the interstitial fluid by an antiport protein transporter. Dashed arrows indicate diffusion

become alkaline when H^+ secretion is increased after a meal (postprandial alkaline tide).

Acid secretion by parietal cells is stimulated by **histamine via H_2** receptors; by **acetylcholine** via H_3 muscarinic receptors; and **gastrin** stimulates HCl secretion by direct action on parietal cells as well as via ECL (enterochromaffin like cells), the cells which release histamine, which acts via H_2 receptors to stimulate the secretion of HCl. Prostaglandins particularly of the E series inhibit acid secretion (Fig. 7.9).

If any of the stimuli for secretion is inhibited by drugs stimulatory effects of other stimuli also decrease.

ECL cells (Enterochromaffin-like cells). Present in the mucosa secrete histamine. Gastrin also acts by stimulating the secretion of histamine from ECL cells. Gastrin is inhibited by somatostatin secreted by D cells in GIT, acts in paracrine fashion. Somatostatin secretion is stimulated by acid in lumen.

Gastric Motility and Emptying

When the food enters the stomach, fundus and upper portion of the body (Fig. 7.6) relax (receptive relexation) and accommodate the food. It is a reflex via vagus nerve. Peristalsis then begins in the lower portion of the body; to cause mixing and grinding of the food; by relaxing the pyloric sphincter to permit small semi-liquid portions of chyme to pass through pylorus to enter duodenum. Normally regurgitation from the duodenum does not occur because the contraction of the pyloric segment tends to persist

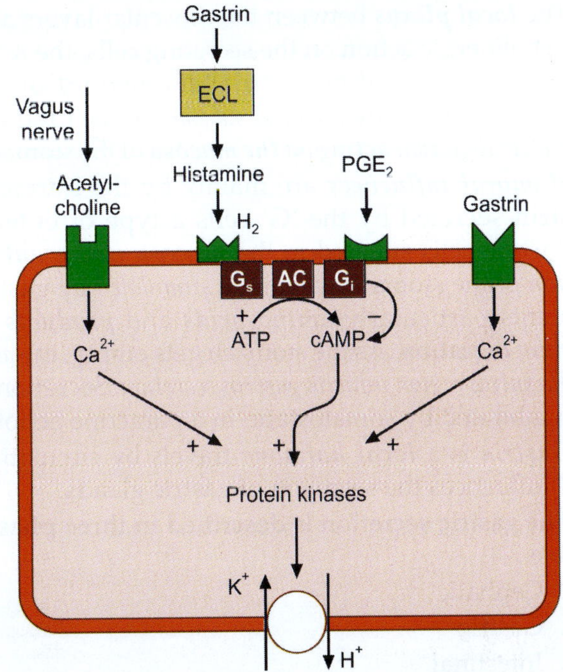

Fig. 7.9: Gastric acid secretion by the parietal cell. Acid secretion is increased by acetylcholine acting on muscarinic receptors and by gastrin acting on gastrin receptors. In addition, gastrin stimulates histamine secretion by enterochromaffin like (ECL) cells. Histamine binds to H_2 receptors. PGE_2 acts via G_i (inhibitory 'G' protein) to decrease HCl secretion. AC is adenylylcyclase, activity increased by histamine and decreased by PGE_2 via Gs and Gi proteins respectively, i.e. stimulatory and inhibitory 'G' proteins

longer than that of duodenum as the contraction waves passes through this region. (Regulation of gastric emptying is described later).

Hunger Contractions

Gastric contractions between meals can sometimes be felt and may even be painful initially. These hunger contractions are associated with sensation of hunger.

Regulation of Gastric Secretion

There is also basal rate of secretion of HCl maximum at night lowest in the morning.

Gastric secretion and motility are regulated by (1) ***neural*** (2) ***humoral*** influences. Nervous influences are by parasympathetic ***vagal nerves*** and parasympathetic postganglionic neurons situated in the enteric nervous plexuses which respond to local influences due to reflexes from the stomach itself.

Vagal stimulation increases acid and pepsin secretion by direct action on the secreting cells. Vagal stimulation also increases secretion of hormone gastrin, from antral region of the stomach, the transmitter being gastrin releasing peptide not acetylcholine.

The ***local plexus*** between the muscular layers also has cholinergic action on the secreting cells, the *reflex action is stimulated* by *stretch* (***distension)*** of the stomach wall and by *chemical substances* like products of *protein digestion* ***acting on the mucosa*** of the stomach.

Humoral influences are mainly by the hormone **gastrin** secreted by the 'G' cells a type of entero-endocrine cells situated in the mucosa of the ***antral region*** of the stomach which are *stimulated* by gastric contents particularly ***amino acids*** and ***products of protein digestion***. As the stomach gets empty, the *acid in the antral region inhibits gastrin secretion*. Secretion is also inhibited by somatostatin in a paracrine action.

Gastrin is a ***local hormone*** travels by circulation and influences the secretion of gastric glands.

The gastric secretion is described in three phases (Table 7.4):

i. Cephalic
ii. Gastric
iii. Intestinal

Cephalic Phase

The presence of *food in the mouth* (even when food has not entered the stomach), stimulates the gastric secretion via the vagal nerves. The *sight, smell* or *thought* of food also stimulates the gastric secretion via the vagal nerves. Anger or hostility cause hyper-secretion, fear and depression decrease gastric secretion. The cephalic phase depends entirely on the ***vagal nerves*** *which also produce* secretion of hormone gastrin from pyloric antral mucosa as mentioned already.

Gastric Phase

Food in the stomach further produces increase in gastric secretion. Receptors in the wall of stomach and mucosa respond to ***stretch*** and ***chemical stimuli of amino acids*** and related products in the stomach. The nerve fibers from the receptors enter the submucous plexus, where the cell bodies of the neurons are located. They synapse with parasympathetic neurons that end on parietal cells and stimulate acid secretion. Thus acid secretion is produced by local reflexes. Another stimulus is hormone ***gastrin*** that is released from **pyloric antral mucosa** by the products of protein digestion (Table 7.5); the increased secretion of gastrin stimulates acid secretion.

Intestinal Phase

Fats, acid and hyperosmolarity in the duodenum inhibit gastric acid (Table 7.6) and pepsin secretion; gastric motility; via neuronal and humoral influences. The hormone has been called enterogastrone. Hence, gastric acid secretion is increased following removal of large parts of small intestines.

Other Influences

Hypoglycemia acts via the nervous system and then the vagal nerves to stimulate acid and pepsin secretion. Alcohol or caffeine act directly on mucosa to increase gastric secretion.

Regulation of Gastric Motility and Emptying

Food remains in the stomach for a time period dependent upon the ***type of food*** and affected by the ***mental state*** of the individual. Also the ***duodenum factors*** may influence the emptying of stomach.

Table 7.4: Mechanisms for stimulation of gastric acid secretion

Phase	*Stimulus*	*Pathway*
Cephalic	Chewing, swallowing, etc.	Vagus nerve to: 1. Parietal cells 2. G. cells
Gastric	Gastric distension	Local and vagovagal reflexes to: 1. Parietal cells 2. G. cells
Intestinal	Protein digestion products in duodenum	1. Intestinal G. cells 2. Intestinal endocrine cells

Table 7.5: Stimuli that affect gastrin secretion

Stimuli that increase gastrin secretion from antrum
Luminal
• Peptides and amino acids
• Distention
Neural
• Increased vagal discharge
Stimuli that inhibit gastrin secretion
Luminal
• Acid
• Somatostatin

Table 7.6: Mechanisms for inhibition of gastric acid secretion

Region	*Stimulus*	*Inhibit gastrin release*	*Inhibit acid secretion*
Antrum	Acid (pH < 3.0)	+	+
Duodenum	Acid	+	+
Duodenum and jejunum	Hyperosmotic solutions, fatty acid, monoglycerides	+	+

Food rich in *carbohydrates leaves the stomach in a few hours* and emptying is *slowest with fatty meal*.

The rate of emptying also depends upon the ***osmotic pressure*** of the material entering the duodenum. *Hyperosmolality* of the duodenal contents slows *gastric emptying*. *Products of protein digestion* and *hydrogen ions* on *the duodenal mucosa*, decrease the rate of gastric emptying due to enterogastric reflex. This gives time for the products to be processed before more enter the duodenum.

Excitement tends to hasten gastric emptying and *fear to slow* it.

Since fats are effective in inhibiting gastric emptying, some people drink olive oil, cream or milk before a cocktail party so that alcohol enters slowly into intestine to be absorbed into blood thus preventing sudden high concentration in the blood to a level that may cause embarrassing intoxication.

Vagotomy may cause relatively severe loss of gastric tone with distension.

Clinical Significance

Cyanocobalamin (vitamin B_{12}) deficiency is produced by:

i. Gastrectomy with removal of the secreting tissue for the intrinsic factor
ii. Pernicious anemia a disease in which there is autoimmune destruction of the parietal cells
iii. Vitamin B_{12} deficiency is also produced with surgical removal of distal ileum or with diseases of distal ileum. Vitamin B_{12} is absorbed in distal ileum.

Deficiency of **vitamin B_{12}** causes megaloblastic anemia and deterioration of certain sensory pathways in CNS.

Dumping syndrome

It is a distressing syndrome that develops in patients in whom portions of stomach have been removed. For the loss of the part producing intrinsic factor vitamin B_{12} *required to be given by injections*. Protein digestion remains normal in the absence of pepsin and nutrition can be maintained. But the patients are prone to develop iron deficiency anemia and other abnormalities, and required to *eat small frequent meals*. The glucose is likely to be absorbed rapidly from the intestines with the resultant hyperglycemia, that result in sudden rise in insulin secretion, hence the patients sometimes develop *hypoglycemic symptoms (weakness, dizziness and sweating) about 2 hours after meals*.

Another cause of symptoms is rapid entry of *hypertonic meals* into intestine that produce movement of water into the gut from the circulating blood (in the gut the water moves along osmotic gradient in either direction) resulting in *significant decrease in blood volume and hypotension*.

Peptic ulcer

Gastric and duodenal ulceration can occur if there is break down of the barrier that normally prevents irritation and auto-digestion of the mucosa by the gastric secretion. Infection with the bacterium Helicobacter pylori disrupts this barrior; also aspirin and other nonsteroidal anti-inflammatory drugs (NSAIDS), as they inhibit the production of prostaglandins resulting in decreased mucus and HCO_3^- secretion.

Another cause of ulceration is *gastrinomas*, tumors which cause excess production of gastrin and hence prolonged excess secretion of acid. Gastric and duodenal ulcers are treated by drugs that produce inhibition of secretion of acid, such as cimetidine that blocks H_2 histamine receptors on parietal cells or omeprazole like drugs that inhibit H^+K^+ ATPase. *Gastrinomas can be treated by surgical removal.*

Vomiting

It is expulsion of gastric contents (sometimes duodenal also) from the mouth. The events during vomiting are controlled by **vomiting center in the medulla**. Vomiting is a reflex action. Usually it is preceded by salivation, nausea, rapid or irregular heart beat, sweating and pallor. *Retching is sensation due to contents entering into esophagus but not entering into pharynx*. Sensory impulses come from irritation of mucosa of the upper digestive tract (Fig. 7.10) and the impulses reach the NTS by IX or X cranial nerves; or when substances present in the blood stimulate an area called **chemoreceptor trigger zone** present in the medulla in the region of area postrema (which is outside blood brain barrier hence accessible to activation by blood borne substances). This area then triggers vomiting center. Other receptors present in different parts of the body also have connections with vomiting center. Ticking of back of throat, distension of stomach can produce vomiting. Some others stimuli can be from genitourinary system.

Events in vomiting reflex are: a wave of *reverse peristalsis* that passes from middle of small intestine to duodenum. *Pyloric sphincter and stomach relax* to receive intestinal contents; forced inspiration occurs against a closed glottis; this decreases intragastric pressure and with *decent of diaphragm there is rise in intra-abdominal pressure and contraction of abdominal muscles push the gastric contents into esophagus*; respiration is inhibited, vocal cords approximate glottis is closed **(preventing entry into trachea);** the lower *esophageal sphincter relaxes* to expel the contents; pylorus and antrum contract reflexly. There is reflex relaxation of upper esophageal sphincter.

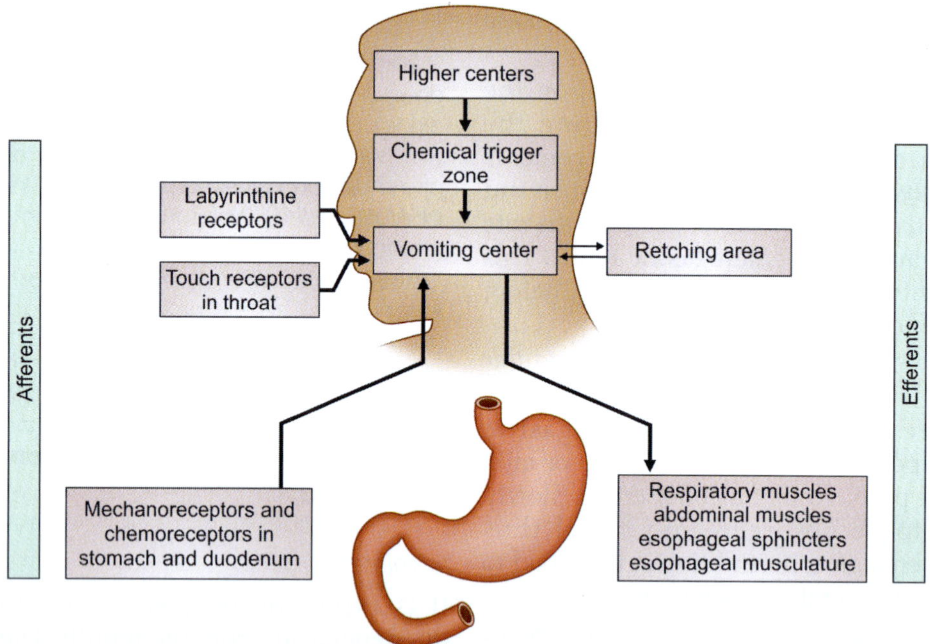

Fig. 7.10: The vomiting reflex

All events are controlled by vomiting center. When a person retches the upper esophageal sphincter remains closed.

SMALL INTESTINE

When the food enters the small intestine it is acted upon by pancreatic juice, bile and intestinal secretions. Most of the digestion and absorption of food takes place in the small intestine. The first 25 cm (10 in) forms duodenum, followed by jejunum and then ileum. In the ***duodenum the ducts from the liver and pancreas open.*** Both these organs produce secretions essential for digestion. The small intestine has an **important role in absorbing nutrients.** The luminal surface of the small intestine is thrown into small finger like projections called villi (Fig. 7.11), which increases the surface area of the lining of the intestine; further the cells lining the villi have minute projections called microvilli, which further increase the surface area for functions of secretion and absorption.

The products absorbed into bloodstream, in the portal vein pass through the liver. Fats are absorbed into lymphatic vessels from where they enter the thoracic duct (left lymphatic duct) which empties into venous system.

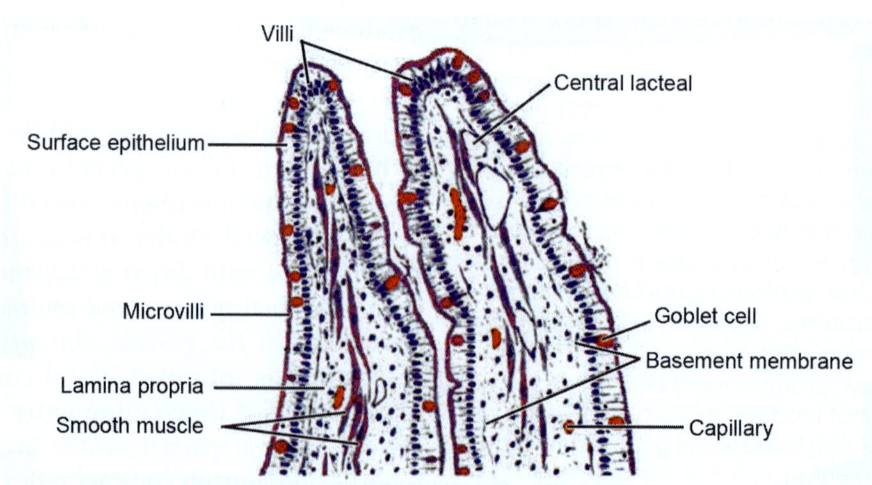

Fig. 7.11: Villi of small intestine

Digestion in Small Intestine

Pancreatic Secretion

Pancreas has two main parts. The exocrine portion secretes pancreatic juice which has role in digestion; contains enzymes that breakdown proteins, carbohydrates and fats and the juice enters the duodenum via a duct. The other part is endocrine portion which forms two important hormones, insulin and glucagon which control the level of blood sugar, and which are poured into the blood directly being ductless secretions.

Exocrine Portion of the Pancreas

The pancreatic juice contains enzymes that are of major importance in digestion. The juice enters the duodenum at the ampulla via pancreatic duct.

Pancreatic juice consists of:

- Water
- Enzymes
- Mineral salts

The pH of pancreatic juice (Table 7.7) is alkaline (**pH8**), as it contains large qualities of bicarbonate ions. When the acid contents of the stomach enter the duodenum they are mixed with pancreatic juice and bile and pH is raised to between 6 to 8. At this pH the pancreatic enzymes act effectively. **About 1500 mL of pancreatic juice is secreted per day.**

Enzymes

For Protein Digestion

Trypsinogen

It is secreted as an inactive enzyme trypsinogen and is activated to active enzyme trypsin by another enzyme present in the duodenum called ***enteropeptidase*** previously called ***enterokinase.*** Trypsin that is formed can also activate trypsinogen.

Trypsin is the chief protein digesting enzyme in the pancreatic juice and breaks the protein units into their smaller components, polypeptides and then peptides and even small amounts aminoacids are formed.

Chymotrypsinogens the other inactive protein digesting enzymes, are activated in the duodenum to form active **chymotrypsins** by the trypsin itself that is produced. The actions of chymotrypsins are also on proteins, to break it down in the same manner as trypsin. ***Procarboxypeptidases*** also secreted by pancreas are inactive and are converted into active enzymes, **carboxypeptidases** by trypsin.

All these enzymes being produced in inactive form and activated in the duodenum (Fig. 7.12) is important as otherwise they would digest the pancreas. The pancreas normally also contains a ***trypsin inhibitor***.

Table 7.7: Composition of pancreatic juice

Cations	:	Na^+, K^+, Ca^{2+}, Mg^{2+} (pH approximately 8.0)
Anions	:	HCO_3^-, Cl^-, SO_4^{2-}, HPO_4^{2-}
Digestive enzymes		

For Carbohydrate Digestion

Pancreas also secretes large amounts of enzyme **amylase** (that is also present in saliva) which reduces ***starch*** into ***maltose***, ***maltotriose*** and alpha ***dextrins.*** But amylase from the pancreas is stronger than that in the saliva, being able to digest uncooked starch.

For fat Digestion

Lipase in the pancreatic juice acts on ***fats*** which have been ***emulsified*** by the ***bile salts*** (present in the bile) and breaks it into their components. Most of the fat digestion begins in the upper intestine, pancreatic lipase being the most important enzyme for fat digestion. The enzyme is most active at 1 and 3 bonds of triglycerides but acts on the 2-bond at a very slow rate, so that the main products formed are ***free fatty acids*** and ***monoglycerides***, some ***glycerol*** may be formed. The activity of this enzyme is facilitated by ***colipase*** (Table 7.8), a protein secreted by pancreas in its inactive form, and activated by trypsin in the intestinal lumen.

Most of the dietary cholesterol is the form of *cholesteryl esters* and *cholesteryl ester hydrolase* (present in pancreatic secretion) also hydrolyzes these esters in the intestinal lumen.

Fats are finely ***emulsified*** in the small intestines by the detergent action of ***bile salts, lecithin*** and ***monoglycerides.***

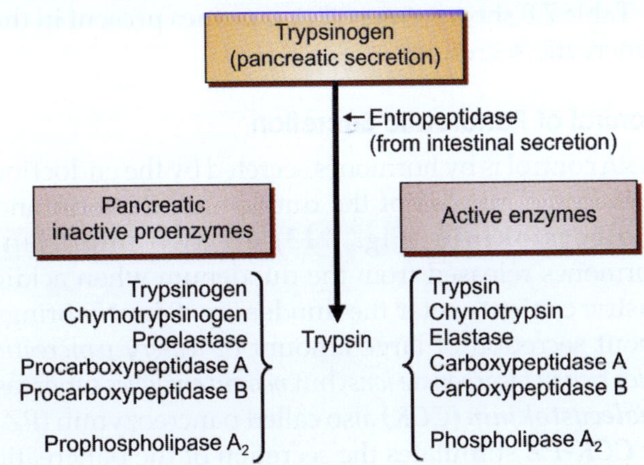

Fig. 7.12: Inactive enzymes of pancreatic secretion activated in intestinal lumen

Table 7.8: Digestive enzymes/proenzymes in the pancreatic juice

Proteolytic enzymes	*Lipolytic enzymes*
Trypsinogen	Lipase
Chymotrypsiongen	Prophospholipase A2
Proelastase	Nonspecific esterase
Procaboxypeptidase A	
Procarboxypeptidase B	
Amylolytic enzymes	*Nucleases*
a-Amylase	Deoxyribonuclease
	Ribonuclease
	Others
	Procolipase
	Trypsin inhibitor

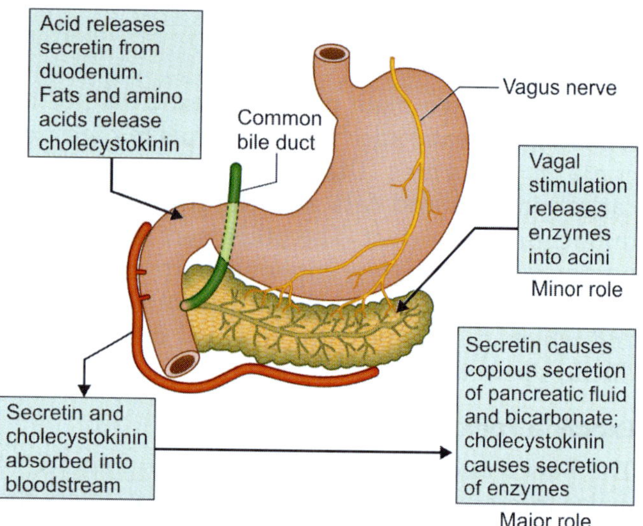

Fig. 7.13: Regulation of pancreatic secretion

Another enzyme secreted by pancreas in inactive form is **phospholipaseA2**, which is also *activated by trypsin* (Fig. 7.12). This active enzyme splits lecithin to form fatty acid and lysolecithin.

The **pancreatic lipase** is found in high concentrations in the pancreatic juice and is **highly efficient**, and only in severe pancreatic deficiency, such as seen in cystic fibrosis there is significant fat malabsorption. Digestion of fat begins in *the stomach, by the acid stable lipase secreted by glands at the back of the tongue (lingual lipase). Triglycerides, especially those that contain fatty acids of short or medium chain length, less than 10 carbon atoms as are found in milk fat, are specially attacked by this enzyme. They are also attacked by gastric lipase. Hence, these enzymes are especially important in newborn.* They are also important in pancreatic insufficiency, such as that present in cystic fibrosis when some digestion of fats can take place even in the complete absence of pancreatic lipase.

Table 7.8 shows some other enzymes present in the pancreatic secretions.

Control of Pancreatic Secretion

Main control is by hormones secreted by the endocrine cells in the mucosa of the duodenum. **Secretin** and **cholecystokinin** (Fig. 7.13) are two important hormones released from the duodenum when acidic gastric contents enter the duodenum. ***Secretin*** brings about secretion of large amount of *watery pancreatic juice rich in bicarbonate ions*, but *poor in enzymes* whereas ***cholecystokinin (CCK)*** also called pancreozymin (PZ) or ***CCK-PZ*** stimulates the secretion of the pancreatic *juice rich in enzymes, but low in volume*. These two hormones, secretin and CCK augment the actions of each other. The hormones released from mucosa travel via blood circulation to reach the secreting cells (Secretin also stimulates secretion of bile by the liver). Cholecystokinin is called so as it causes contraction of gallbladder to release bile into intestine as described later.

Small amount of pancreatic secretion is also produced by nervous stimulation by ***vagal nerves***. This is cephalic phase of secretion stimulated by sight, smell and taste of food. But the hormones from the duodenum have more important role in stimulating pancreatic secretion.

Clinical Significance

Enteropeptidase deficiency may occurs as congenital abnormality and leads to protein malnutrition.

The digestive enzymes do not leak into circulation but in acute pancreatitis, the circulating levels of digestive enzymes rise markedly. Measurement of plasma amylase or lipase concentration is of value in diagnosis of disease.

BILE

The liver produces bile, about **500 mL per day**, a thick green liquid which is stored and *concentrated in gallbladder between meals*.

Bile is rich in bicarbonates and contains **bile salts**, **bile pigment**, **lecithin**, **cholesterol** and some other constituents (Table 7.9). Bile pigments are excretory products and give color to the bile. Bile contains no digestive enzymes but the ***bile salts have important role in digestion and absorption of fat.*** In the intestine bile salts ***emulsify fat*** into small particles that increases the surface area for the *action of the enzyme, pancreatic lipase*. As the chyme enters small intestine, ***hormone***

Table 7.9: Composition of human hepatic duct bile

Water	Bile salts
Bile pigments	Cholesterol
Inorganic salts	Fatty acids
Lecithin	Fat
Alkaline phosphatase	

CCK is secreted by the duodenal mucosal cells; ***it stimulates the contraction of gallbladder*** and relaxation of the sphincter of oddi; enabling the bile juice to flow into the duodenum; and a high fat content of *chyme causes powerful contraction of gallbladder. Since the bile and pancreatic juice that enter the duodenum in response to CCK result in digestion of fat and protein, the products of this digestion stimulate further CCK secretion. This is an example of positive feedback mechanism.*

The bile salts also function to aid ***absorption of fat*** as they form **micelles** *with fat digestion products in the intestine*; the micelles *facilitate the movement* (Fig. 7.14) of hydrophobic fat digestion *products to the mucosa for fat absorption.*

In the distal intestines the **bile salts** are reabsorbed about 95% into portal blood and in the liver secreted again into bile; this is enterohepatic circulation of bile salts (Fig. 7.15). Bile salts in the portal circulation are powerful stimulant for the liver cells to secrete bile salts. (Hence bile salts are called choleretics, the substances that increase the secretion of bile by the liver).

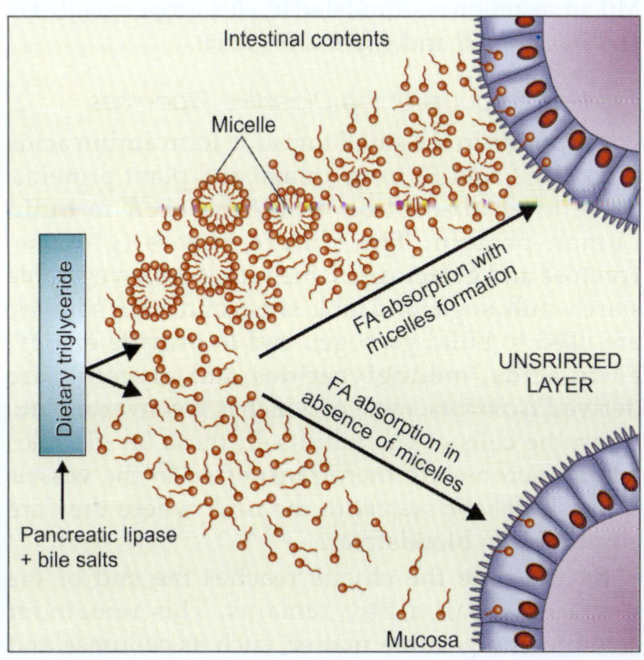

Fig. 7.14: Fat absorption with micelles formation

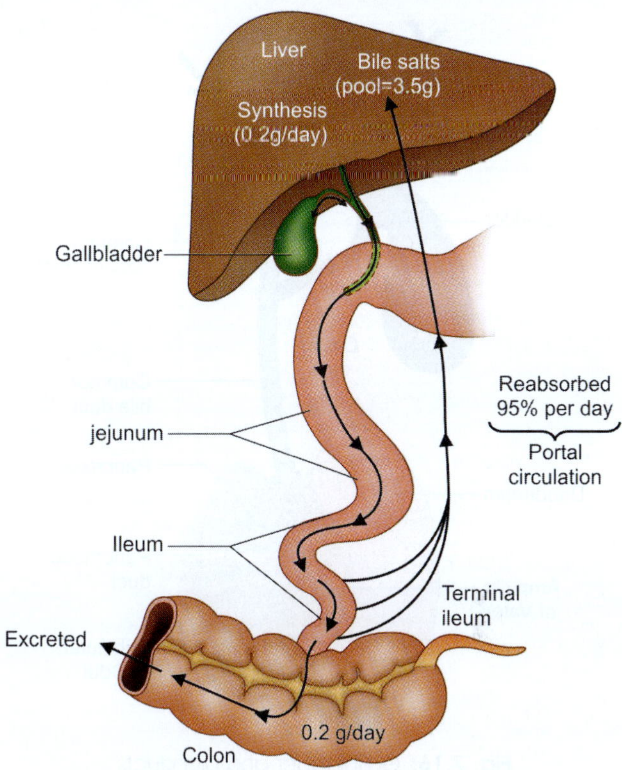

Fig. 7.15: Enterohepatic circulation of bile salts. Small amounts excreted are formed by liver

The small quantities of bile salts that are lost in the passage through the intestine are formed by the liver from cholesterol.

Hormone ***secretin*** stimulates watery ***secretion of bile by the liver***, it is called hydrocholeretic substance.

Functions of Gallbladder

In between meals the bile is stored, as it flows into the gallbladder, sphincter of Oddi (the opening of common bile duct into duodenum) being closed (Fig. 7.16). In the gallbladder the bile is concentrated by absorption of water; some bicarbonate ions are also reabsorbed lowering its pH (Table 7.10). **Bile is discharged into intestine when food enters intestine mainly due to the secretion of hormone cholecystokinin from the duodenum.** It causes contraction of gallbladder and relaxation of sphincter of oddi. Hence, CCK is a cholagogue substance (substances that cause contraction of gallbladder are called cholagogues).

Even as the food enters the mouth the tone of the sphincter of oddi decreases due to reflex action; the efferent nerve being vagal nerve.

In some mammals, such as rat and horse a gallbladder is not present. In some animals, such as rabbit and guinea pig the common bile duct enters the second

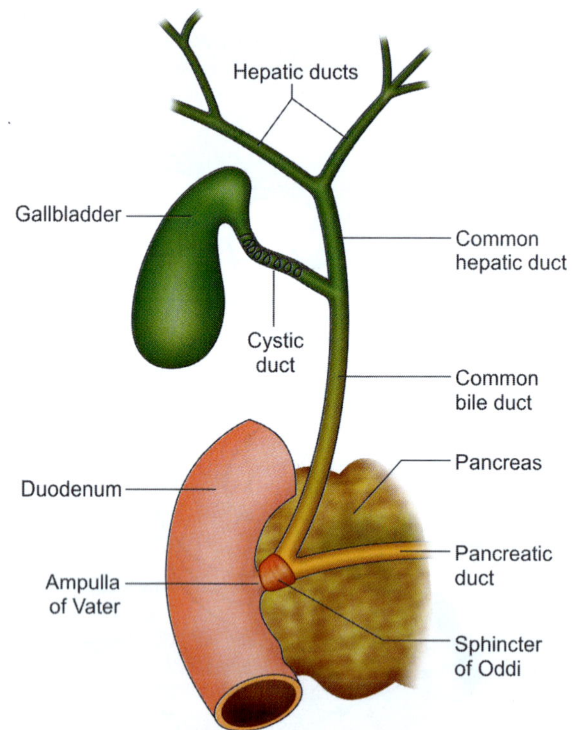

Fig. 7.16: Gallbladder and bile ducts

Table 7.10: Comparison of hepatic duct bile (a) and gallbladder bile (b)

	(a)	*(b)*
Percentage of solids	2–4	10–12
Bile salts (mmol/L)	10–20	50–200
pH	7.8–8.6	7.0–7.4

part of duodenum, whereas the pancreatic duct enters the third portion of duodenum.

Effects of Cholecystectomy

Cholecystectomized persons maintain good health as there remains constant slow flow of bile into the duodenum; also gradually the bile duct becomes dilated to some extent; resulting in more bile to enter after meals than at other times. Such individuals can eat fried food but should avoid foods that are rich in fats.

Intestinal Secretions

Alkaline intestinal juice (pH 7.8 to 8) assists in raising the pH of the intestinal contents to between 6.5 and 7.5.

The main constituents of intestinal secretions are:

- Water
- Mucus
- Mineral salts
- Enzyme, enteropeptidase (enterokinase)

Most of the **digestive enzymes** in the small intestines remain in the cells of the villi. *Digestion of carbohydrate, protein and fat is completed within the cells.*

The enzymes involved in completion of digestion in the cells of the villi are **peptidases, sucrase, maltase** and ***lactase. Enteropeptidase*** (enterokinase) ***is the enzyme present in intestinal secretions and*** it activates pancreatic enzyme trypsin which in turn activates other proteolytic enzymes for the action on protein digestion, that results in formation of smaller peptides and some amino acids (Figs 7.17A and B). The smaller peptides, the ***dipeptides*** are broken down by the *peptidases into amino acids and this action* takes place inside the enterocytes (intestinal mucosal cells) (Fig. 7.17A). Similarly ***disaccharidases*** are present in the brush border, i.e. the membrane of the microvilli of the cells; and these complete the digestion of carbohydrates. These enzymes are ***sucrase, maltase*** and ***lactase*** that split disaccharides, forming **monosaccharides**. ***Sucrose*** (common sugar) is digested into ***glucose*** and ***fructose*** by *sucrase enzyme; maltose* breaks down into ***glucose*** and ***glucose*** by enzyme *maltase*; and ***lactose*** (milk sugar) into ***glucose*** and ***galactose*** by enzyme *lactase*.

Intestinal Mucus

Mucus is secreted by surface epithelial cells throughout the gastrointestinal tract; by Brunner's gland in the duodenum; and by goblet cells in the small and large intestines. Mucus protects mucosa and lubricates food and holds immunoglobulins in place. Mucin secretion is stimulated by *cholinergic stimulation* and by *chemical* and *physical irritation*.

The End Products of the Digestive Processes

For proteins in the small intestine form **amino acids** (Fig. 7.17A and B) from animal and plant proteins; these after absorption would be used to build human protein. **The simple sugars (glucose, fructose** and **galactose**), which come from vegetable starch, milk sugar and table sugar and other sources, are used to build glycogen and to provide energy. **Fatty acids, monoglycerides** and **glycerol**, are derived from fats, most of which is reconverted into fat in the cells of the villi itself; these fat globules (chylomicrons) are then transported in the vessels of the *lymphatic system* to the neck where they are emptied into bloodstream.

By the time the chyme reaches the end of the ileum only half a litre remains. This remainder contains indigestible matter, such as cellulose and fiber.

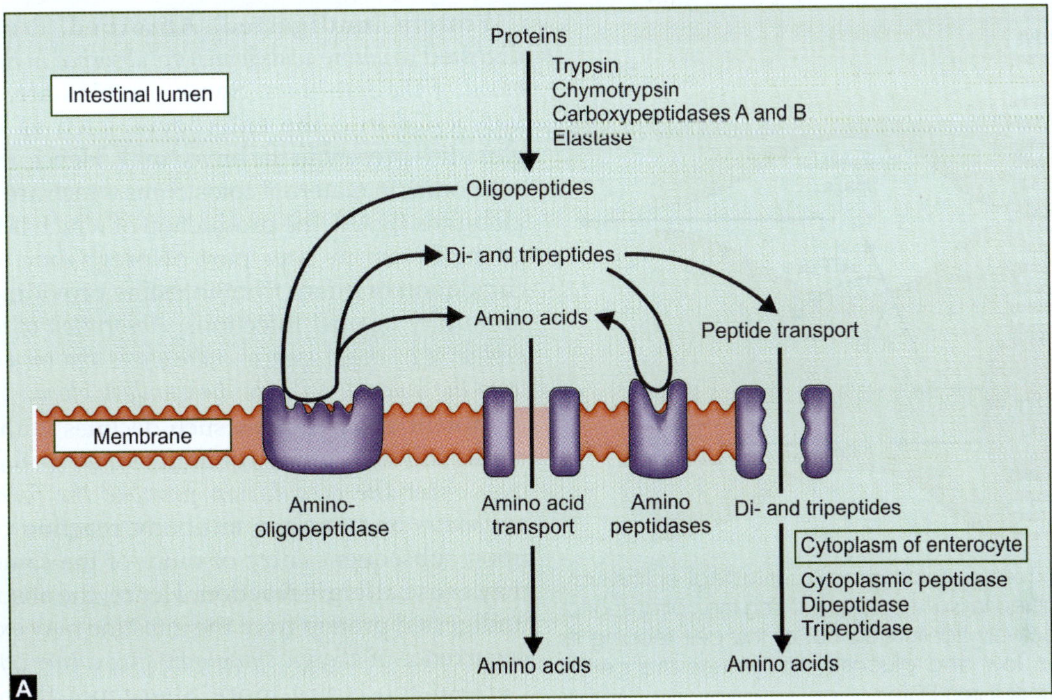

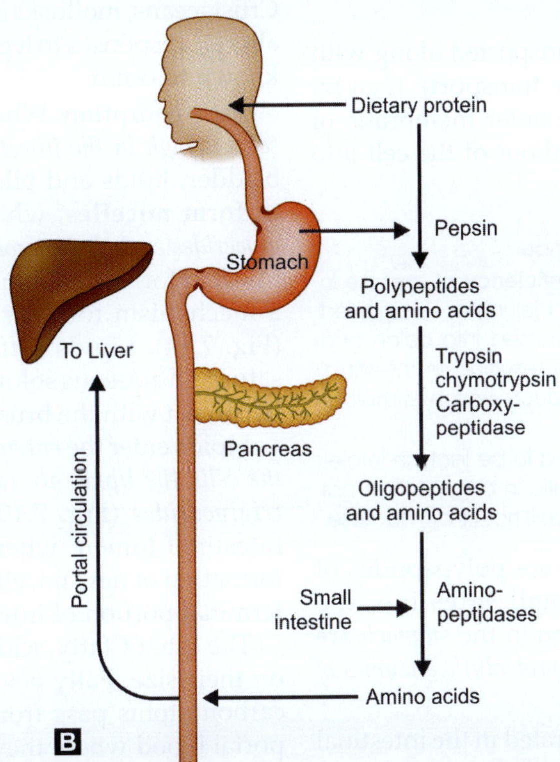

Figs 7.17A and B: (A) Protein digestion in lumen, mucosa, and cytoplasm of the intestinal cell, and (B) Digestion of dietary proteins by the proteolytic enzymes of the gastrointestinal tract

ABSORPTION OF NUTRIENTS

Glucose absorption in the small intestine is by a **secondary active transport process,** which is dependent upon a carrier (Fig. 7.18), a cotransporter, in the luminal membrane which combines with both glucose and sodium; and as sodium is pulled into the cell by its concentration gradient its concentration being low inside the cell; maintained by Na^+ K^+ ATPase, the

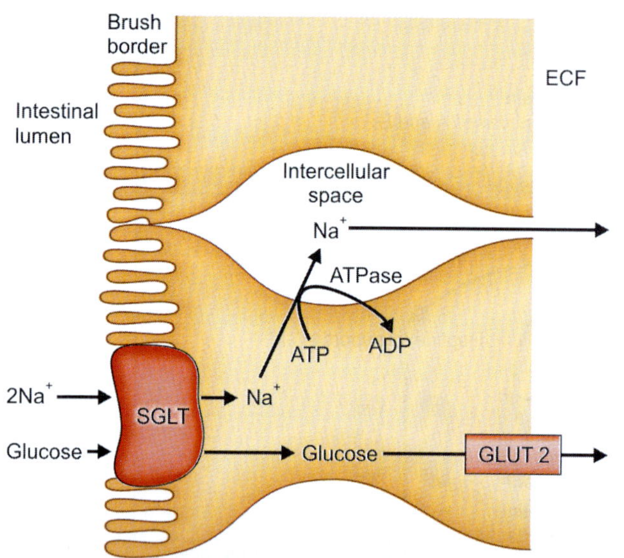

Fig. 7.18: Glucose absorption across intestinal epithelium. Glucose is coupled to Na^+ transport, utilizing the cotransporter SGLT. Na^+ is actively transported out of the cell keeping its concentration low and glucose that enters the cell is transported out of it into ECF

active process; the glucose is transported along with it into the cell (secondary active transport); then by means of another carrier in the outer membrane of enterocyte glucose is transported out of the cell into the capillary blood.

Lactose Intolerance

This disorder occurs when there is **deficiency of lactase** in the brush border of duodenum and jejunum. Undigested lactose cannot be absorbed. It is passed into colon and the colonic bacteria produce gas resulting in intestinal distension and the metabolic products which stimulate colonic motility, producing diarrhea.

Individuals with this disorder are said to be lactose intolerant. The condition is probably genetic in origin. Milk is not tolerated but curd is better tolerated as it has its own lactase.

Products of peptic digestion are polypeptides of very diverse sizes. In the small intestine, the polypeptides formed by digestion in the *stomach* are further digested by the *powerful proteolytic enzymes of the pancreas and intestinal mucosa*.

Some free amino acids are liberated in the intestinal lumen, but others are liberated by enzymes at the cell surface brush border of the enterocytes. Some di and tripeptides are actively transported into the intestinal cell and hydrolysed by intracellular peptidases with the *amino acids entering the bloodstream* (Fig. 7.17A).

Thus the final digestion to amino acids occurs in three locations: in the intestinal lumen; the brush border; in the cytoplasm of the mucosal cells (Fig. 7.17A).

Protein (undigested) Absorbed. Proteins are digested to *amino acids which are absorbed in the capillary blood of the intestines.* Some proteins are absorbed *undigested* into the enterocyte, such as immunoglobulins present in the breast milk. Hence, the protein antibodies in maternal colostrums which are immunoglobulins (IgAs), the production of which is increased in the breast in later part of pregnancy, enter the circulation of infant from intestine providing passive immunity against infections. *Absorption of undigested protein is by the process of endocytosis and then exocytosis from the mucosal cell into the capillary blood.*

Protein absorption as such declines with age, but adults still absorb small quantities. *Foreign proteins that may enter the circulation provoke the formation of antibodies* and antigen antibody reaction occurring upon subsequent entry of more of the same protein may cause **allergic reaction.** Hence, the absorption of undigested protein from the intestine may explain the occurrence of *allergic symptoms after eating certain food.* Certain foods are more allergenic than others. Crustaceans, mollusks and fish are such offenders and allergic responses to legumes, cow's milk, and egg are known to occur.

Fat Absorption. When the concentration of the *bile salts is high in the intestines*, after contraction of gallbladder, lipids and bile salts interact spontaneously to **form micelles**; which contain *fatty acids, monoglycerides* and *cholesterol* in their hydrophobic centers. Micellar formation solubilizes the lipids and provides a mechanism for *their transport* to the enterocytes (Fig. 7.14). Lipids diffuse out of the micelles as a saturated aqueous solution of the lipids is maintained in contact with the brush border of the mucosal cells.

Lipids enter the *enterocytes by passive diffusion. Inside the cells the lipids are rapidly esterified*, i.e. they *form triglycerides* (Fig. 7.19). The bile salts remain in intestinal lumen, where they are available for the formation of new micelles and are finally absorbed in terminal portion of intestine.

The fate of fatty acids in the enterocytes depends on their size. Fatty acids containing less than 10–12 carbon atoms pass from mucosal cells directly into portal blood where they are transported as free fatty acids. The fatty acids containing more than 10–12 carbon atoms re-esterified to triglycerides in the mucosal cells. Some of the absorbed cholesterol is esterified. The triglycerides and cholesterol esters are then coated with a layer of protein, cholesterol and phospholipids to form chylomicrons (Fig. 7.20). These leave the mucosal cell and enter lymphatics and then through the thoracic duct enter the venous circulation.

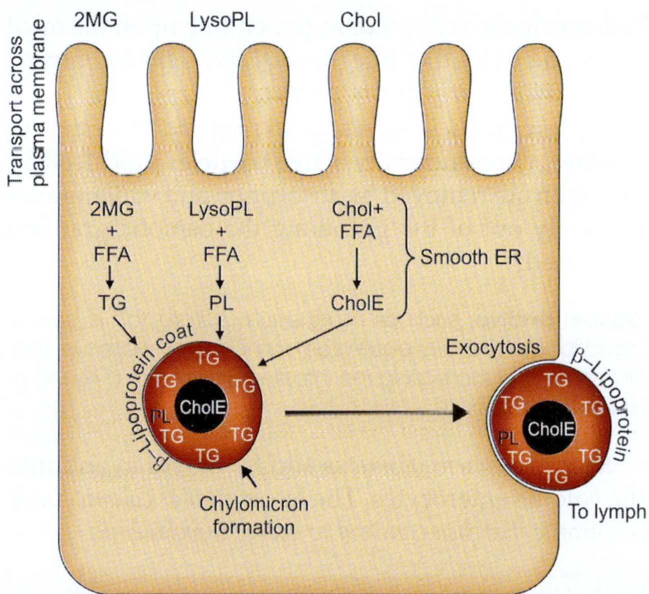

Fig. 7.19: Lipid absorption. Triglycerides are resynthesized in the mucosal cells from monoglycerides and fatty acids; are then converted to chylomicrons and released by exocytosis (MG=monoglycerides; TG=triglycerides; Chol E=cholestrol esters)

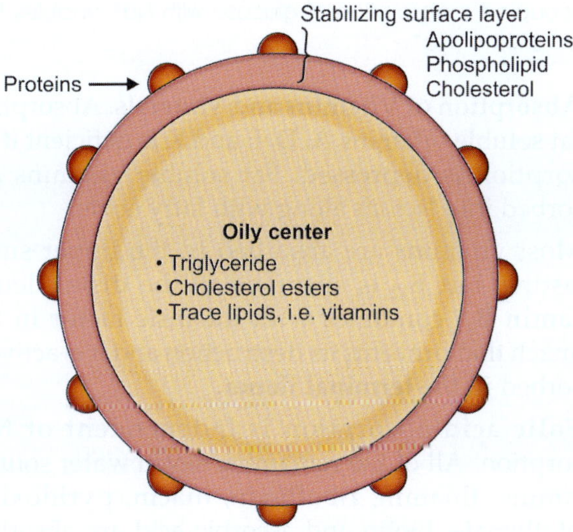

Fig. 7.20: Structure of chylomicrons

Normally with fat intake about 95% or more of the fat is absorbed in the intestine.

> The processes involved in fat absorption are not fully mature at birth, and the infants fail to absorb 10–15% of ingested fat. Hence, they are more susceptible to ill effects of disease processes that reduce fat absorption.

Absorption of Cholesterol and other Sterols. Cholesterol is readily absorbed from the small intestine if bile, fatty acids and pancreatic juice are present, while closely related sterols of plant origin are poorly absorbed. Almost all the absorbed cholesterol is incorporated into chylomicrons that enter the circulation via lymphatics.

Plant sterols, such as those found in soyabeans reduce the *absorption of cholesterol, probably* by **competing with cholesterol** for *esterification with fatty acids.*

> **STEATORRHEA**
>
> Patients with diseases that destroy the exocrine portion of the pancreas have bulky, clay colored, foul smelling and greasy stools with high fat content (steatorrhea) because of impaired digestion and absorption of fat. The steatorrhea is due to lipase deficiency but because of absence of bicarbonate from pancreas relatively acidic pH in the duodenum precipitates some bile salts, impairing their action on fat digestion and absorption.
>
> Acid also inhibits pancreatic lipase and in patients having gastrinoma because of excess secretion of gastric acid and a consequent low duodenal pH, may develop steatorrhea.
>
> *Another cause of steatorrhea is defective reabsorption of bile salts in distal ileum creating a low concentration of bile salts in bile as liver may be unable to form at a rapid rate to make-up with losses.*

Figure 7.21 *describes the possible causes of steatorrhea.*

Absorption of Water and Electrolytes. The intestine are presented each day with about 2000 mL of ingested fluid plus 7000 mL of secretions from the

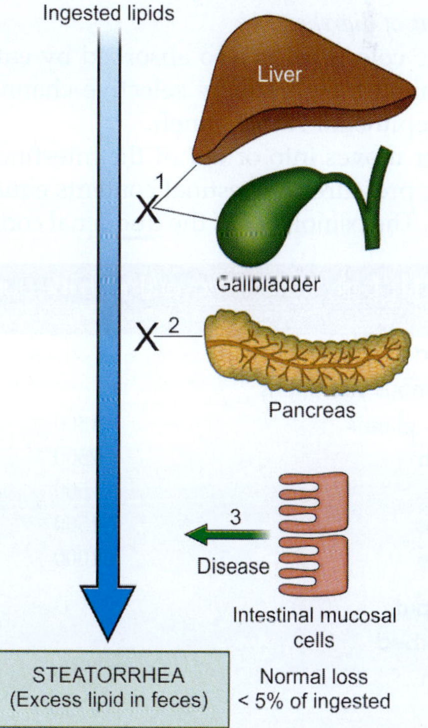

Fig. 7.21: Possible causes of steatorrhea (X^1 and X^2 indicate faulty function

mucosa of the gastrointestinal tract and associated glands (Table 7.11). 98% of this is reabsorbed, with daily fluid loss of only 200 mL in the stools. Only a small amounts of water moves across the gastric mucosa, but water moves in both directions across the mucosa of the small intestine and large intestines in response to osmotic gradients.

The luminal membranes of all enterocytes in the small intestine and colon are permeable to Na^+ and their basolateral membranes contain Na^+K^+ ATPase, which keep the Na^+ concentration low in the cell. Na^+ enters the cells because of concentration gradient and the permeability of the luminal membrane to it.

Sodium is absorbed along the entire length of intestine Na^+ crosses the brush border membrane down the electrochemical gradient and actively extruded from epithelial cells by Na^+ K^+ ATPase. Hence, absorption is active process throughout.

In the jejunum active transport of Na^+ is important in bringing about absorption of glucose, some amino acids and other substances. Conversely the presence of glucose in the intestinal lumen facilitates the *absorption of Na^+. This is physiological basis* for the *treatment of Na^+ and water loss in diarrhea by oral administration of solutions containing NaCl and glucose (rehydration therapy).* This type of treatment has proved to be *beneficial in cholera.*

Cereals containing carbohydrates are also useful in the treatment of diarrhea.

In the colon Na^+ is also absorbed by entry across the luminal membrane by selective channels called ENaC (epithelial Na^+ channel).

Water moves into or out of the intestine until the osmotic pressure of intestinal contents equals that of plasma. The osmolality of the duodenal contents may be hypertonic or hypotonic, depending upon the meal ingested but by the time *the meal enters the jejunum its osmolality is nearly that of plasma.*

This osmolality is maintained throughout the rest of the intestine, the osmotically active particles produced by digestion are removed by absorption and water moves passively out of the gut along the osmotic gradient generated.

Table 7.11: Daily water turnover (mL) in the gastrointestinal tract

Ingested		**2000**
Endogenous secretions		**7000**
Salivary glands	1500	
Stomach	2500	
Bile	500	
Pancreas	1500	
Intestine	1000	
Total input		**9000**
Reabsorbed		**8800**
Jejunum	5500	
Ileum	2000	
Colon	1300	
Balance in stool		200

Saline laxative, such as *magnesium sulfate salt* is *poorly absorbed, it retain equivalent amount of water in the intestine, thus increasing the intestinal volume and exerting a laxative effect.*

K^+ is component of mucus and K^+ moves in and into the colonic enterocytes. The *loss of ileal or colonic fluids in chronic diarrhea can lead to severe hypokalemia.*

CHOLERA

In cholera the chloride secretion from the enterocyte into the luminal fluid is increased and in addition the function of mucosal carrier for Na^+ is reduced, reducing NaCl absorption, resulting in increased electrolyte and water content in the intestinal contents causing diarrhea. But Na^+K^+ATPase and Na^+ glucose cotransport are unaffected so coupled reabsorption of glucose with Na^+ enables the absorption of Na^+.

Absorption of Vitamins and Minerals. Absorption of fat soluble vitamins A, D, E and K is deficient if fat absorption is depressed. Fat soluble vitamins are absorbed into *lacteals* along with fatty acids.

Most vitamins are absorbed in the upper small intestine, but B_{12} is absorbed in the distal ileum. **Vitamin B_{12}** combines with intrinsic factor in the stomach that prevents its destruction and it is actively absorbed in the **terminal ileum**.

Folic acid absorption is independent of Na^+ absorption. All of the remaining seven water soluble vitamins, thiamin, riboflavin, niacin, pyridoxine, pentothenate, biotin and ascorbic acid are absorbed by carriers that are Na^+ cotransporters.

Calcium absorption. From 30 to 80% of ingested calcium is absorbed. The absorptive process is related to 1, 25 dihydroxycholecalciferol (active form of vitamin D). Through this Ca^{2+} absorption is adjusted to body needs, absorption is increased in the presence of Ca^{2+} deficiency and decreased in the presence of Ca^{2+} excess. *Calcium absorption is facilitated by protein.* It is *inhibited by phosphates and oxalates in the diet* as they form insoluble salts with Ca^{2+}.

Iron absorption: In adults iron loss from the body is relatively small. The losses are unregulated and total body stores depend on the changes in the rate at which it is absorbed from the intestine.

Women have larger loss of iron from the body than adult men because of additional loss of blood during menstruation. The average daily intake is about 20 mg, but the amount absorbed is equal to the losses, it ranges about 3 to 6% of the amount ingested. *Phytic acid found in cereals and phosphates and oxalates inhibit the absorption.*

Most of the iron in the diet is in the ferric (Fe^{3+}) form, but it is the ferrous (Fe^{2+}) form that is absorbed. There is Fe^{3+} reductase activity associated with the iron transporter in the brush border of enterocytes.

Only a trace of iron is absorbed in the stomach, but the gastric secretions dissolve the iron and enable it to *form soluble complexes with ascorbic acid and other substances and thus its reduction to the Fe^{2+} form.* Almost all iron absorption occurs in the duodenum. After transport into the enterocyte, some is stored in ferritin in the enterocyte and remainder is transported out of enterocyte. That which is stored as ferritin is lost from the body when the enterocyte is shed off. In the plasma Fe^{2+} is converted to Fe^{3+} and bound to iron transport protein transferrin (Fig. 7.22).

Seventy-five percent iron in the body is in hemoglobin, 3% in myoglobin and the rest in ferritin which is present in many cells besides the enterocytes. Apoferritin is a globular protein which with iron forms ferritin. Ferritin molecules in lysosomal membranes may aggregate in deposits that contain iron. These deposits are called **hemosiderin.**

Intestinal absorption of iron is regulated by three factors. dietary intake of iron; the state of iron stores; the rate of erythropoiesis in the bone marrow. How the absorptive process is adjusted according to the demands is not understood.

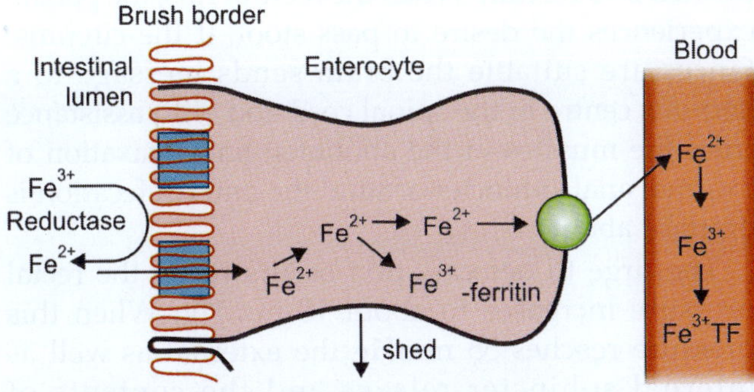

Fig. 7.22: Absorption of iron in intestine (TF = Transferrin)

Iron Excess

Iron deficiency causes anemia. Conversely iron overload causes hemosiderin to accumulate in the tissues, producing hemosiderosis. Large amounts of hemosiderin can damage tissues causing hemochromatosis. This syndrome is characterized by pigmentation of the skin, pancreatic damage with diabetes, cirrhosis of the liver, a high incidence of hepatic carcinoma and gonadal atrophy. Hemochromatosis may be hereditary or acquired.

Acquired hemochromatosis occurs when the iron regulating system is upset by excess iron load due to *chronic destruction of red blood cells, liver disease or repeated transfusions* in disease, such as intractable anemia.

DISORDERS OF ABSORPTIVE FUNCTION

Malabsorption Syndrome

The digestive and absorptive functions of small intestine are essential for life. Removal of short segments of the jejunum or ileum does not cause severe symptoms and there is compensatory hypertrophy and hyperplasia of the remaining mucosa. *If more than 50% of the small intestine is removed or bypassed the absorption of nutrient and vitamins is affected and malnutrition and wasting is likely to occur.*

Various diseases also impair absorption. The deficiencies that result are called malabsorption syndrome (Table 7.12). If there is deficient absorption of amino acids, body wasting occurs and gradually hypoproteinemia and edema would develop. Carbohydrate and fat absorption also get depressed with those diseases; and with defective fat absorption, the fat soluble vitamins (vitamin A, D, E and K) are not absorbed in adequate amounts. The amount of fat and protein in the stools is increased, and the stools become bulky, foul smelling and greasy; condition is called steatorrhea.

INTESTINAL MOTILITY

There are three types of smooth muscle contractions, peristaltic contractions, segmentation contractions and tonic contractions.

Table 7.12: Disease processes associated with malabsorption

Abnormalities of digestion in the intestinal lumen
Glucose/galactose malabsorption Inadequate lipolysis due to pancreatic insufficiency or decreased bile salts (e.g. due to ileal resection or bacterial overgrowth)
Abnormalities of mucosal cell transport
Nonspecific (due to tropical sprue, celiac disease, etc.) Specific (due to deficiency of various disaccharidases, etc.)

Peristalsis ***propels*** intestinal contents (chyme) towards large intestines. The waves pass regularly in ***oral-caudal direction;*** short peristaltic waves occur in small intestine involving usually only a small length of intestine. Very intense peristaltic waves called peristaltic rushes are not seen in normal individuals but they occur when intestine is obstructed.

Segmentation contractions are ring like contractions that appear at regular intervals and then disappear and are replaced by another set of ring contractions in the segments between the previous contractions (Fig. 7.23). They move the ***chyme to and fro*** and thus helps in ***absorptive process*** by bringing fresh surface in contact with chyme and mixing contents with juices.

Tonic contractions are relatively prolonged contractions and isolate one segment of intestine from another. These contractions and segmentation contractions slow the transit time in intestine and thus ***aid in absorptive process.***

The movements are controlled locally but influenced by higher nervous system (Fig. 7.24).

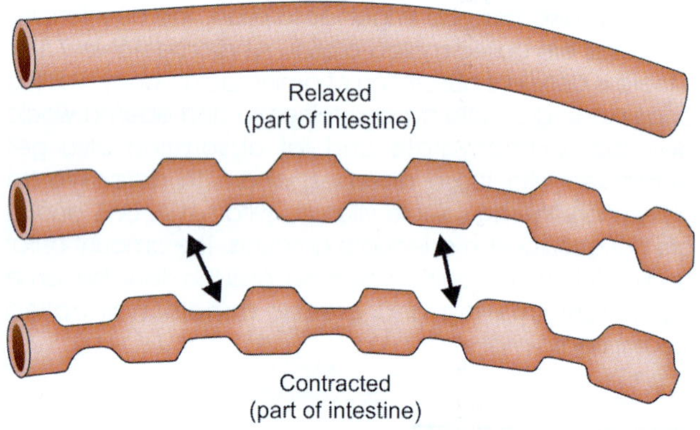

Fig. 7.23: Diagram of segmentation contractions of the intestine

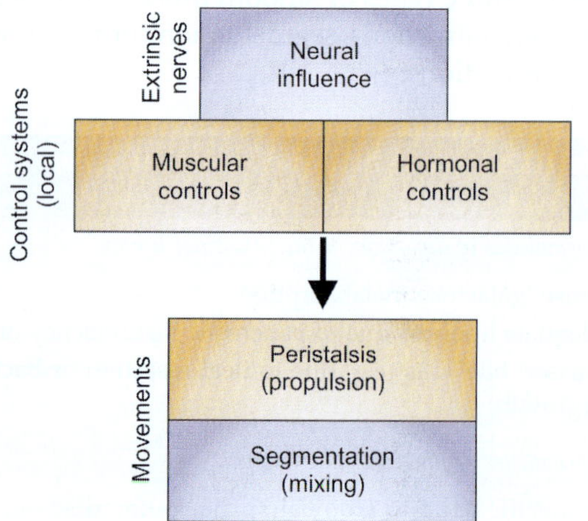

Fig. 7.24: Control of movements of intestine

Adynamic ileus

If intestine are *traumatized* there is inhibition of smooth muscle, which causes decrease in intestinal motility. Also with *irritation of peritoneum* there is inhibition of motility. Both types of inhibition cause paralytic ileus after abdominal operations. Because of diffuse decrease in peristaltic activity in the small intestine, its contents are not propelled into colon, and it becomes distended by gas and fluid. Intestinal peristalsis returns by 6–8 hours, followed by gastric peristalsis but colonic activity takes 2–3 days to return after surgical procedure.

FUNCTIONS OF COLON

No enzymes are secreted by colon. In the colon *absorption of water and* Na^+ *and other minerals* takes place. Na^+ is actively absorbed and osmotic gradient so created results in water reabsorption. Normally there is net *secretion of* K^+ *and* HCO_3^- *into colon. Certain drugs can be absorbed* from colon and in children this route is sometimes used, i.e. sedatives, tranquilizers are absorbed rapidly by this route. *Some of the water in enema* is absorbed and if volume of enema is very large absorption may be rapid enough to cause water intoxication.

Short Chain Fatty Acids (SCFA)

Short chain fatty acids are produced in the colon and are absorbed from there. They are 2–10 carbon weak acids produced by action of bacteria on complex carbohydrates, resistant starches, dietary fiber, that have escaped digestion in the upper GIT. They have *trophic influence on the colonic epithelium and combat inflammation and some exchange of H ions* occurs with their absorption, helps to maintain H ion concenration in the body.

Colonic Movements

In the colon mass movements propel food towards the anus. These movements are stimulated by distension by food residues. In this way the feces are pushed into rectum. When the rectum fills, the person experiences the desire to pass stool. If the circumstances are suitable the brain sends message to a nervous centre in the spinal cord and with assistance from the muscles in the abdomen and relaxation of external anal sphincter around the anus defecation is brought about.

The urge to defecate first occurs when the rectal pressure increases to about 18 mmHg. When this pressure reaches 55 mmHg the external as well as internal sphincter relaxes and the contents of the rectum are expelled. Subjects with spinal cord transaction the reflex evacuation of the rectum is produced in this way.

Defecation can be initiated voluntarily by relaxing the external anal sphincter and contracting the abdominal muscles before that pressure is reached.

Defecation is therefore *a spinal reflex* that can be *voluntarily inhibited* by keeping the external sphincter contracted or *facilitated* by relaxing the sphincter and contracting the abdominal muscles.

Distention of the stomach by food initiates contraction of rectum and frequently a desire to defecate. The response is called gastrocolic reflex.

Defecation involves both reflex and voluntary actions. The *integrating center for reflex action is in the spinal cord, it is modulated by higher centers. The main efferent pathways are cholinergic parasympathetic fibers in the pelvic nerves*. The role of sympathetic pathway is not significant in normal defecation.

Voluntary actions are also important in defecation. The external anal sphincter is voluntarily held in the relaxed state, intra-abdominal pressure is elevated to aid expulsion of feces. There is deep breath which moves the diaphragm downwards. Glottis then closes and contraction of respiratory muscles on full lung volume elevate both intrathoracic and intra-abdominal pressures. Contraction of abdominal wall muscles further increase intra-abdominal pressure which may be as high 200 cm of H_2O. The muscles of the pelvic floor relax allowing floor to drop, this helps to straighten out the rectum and prevent rectal prolapse.

The **feces** are ejected from the body. The waste products are discharged in the feces which average about 100 g a day; are three-quarter water and one quarter solids; later consisting of dead bacteria, fat, protein and undigested roughage (Table 7.13); organic acids formed from carbohydrates by bacteria are responsible for slight acidic reaction of stools (pH 5.0–7.0).

Table 7.13: Approximate composition of feces on an average diet

Component	*Percentage of weight*
Water	75
Solids	25

- Cellulose and other indigestible fiber, bacteria.
- Inorganic material (mostly calcium and phosphates).
- Fat and fat derivative 5% of ingested.
- Also desquamated mucosal cells, mucus, and small amounts of digestive enzymes.

Intestinal Flora

Millions of bacteria are always present in the intestine and are most dense in transverse colon. They cause no harm and in many ways are useful. They can *produce vitamins* K and a *number of B complex vitamins* and digest small amounts of cellulose which comes from plant cells.

Aerophagia and Intestinal Gas

Some air is swallowed during eating and drinking (aerophagia). Some of it is regurgitated (belching) and some is absorbed but much of it passes into the colon. Here some oxygen is absorbed; hydrogen, hydrogen sulfide, carbon dioxide and methane formed by the colonic bacteria from carbohydrates and other substances are added to it.

It is then expelled as flatus. The smell is largely due to sulfides. The volume of gas normally found in human gastrointestinal tract is about 200 mL and the daily production is 500–1500 mL. In some individuals gas in the intestines causes cramps, borborygmi (rumbling noises) and abdominal discomfort.

FUNCTIONS OF THE LIVER

The liver is an important organ for *fat digestion* and *processing of absorbed material*. It has two set of blood supply; one from hepatic artery which supplies oxygen to the liver; and the other from portal vein which brings blood from the spleen, stomach and intestine and it carries the absorbed products; some of these are stored in the liver for future use. Hence, functions can be grouped as follows:

Carbohydrate metabolism: Liver has a role to maintain normal blood glucose level. Liver receives glucose and other monosaccharide absorbed after digestion of food that are converted into glycogen in the liver which is stored and is broken down to release glucose when the level tends to fall in order to maintain the blood sugar level. Muscles produce glycogen from blood glucose and store it for energy purposes. Excess glucose in the blood is stored as fat in fat depots.

Protein metabolism: The amino acids absorbed in the portal blood can pass through the liver and transported in the blood to other organs to build proteins. But proteins that are part of the blood, such as ***albumin, fibrinogen, prothrombin and some clotting factors are synthesized by the liver*** using amino acids. Hepatocytes also remove amino group, NH_2 from amino acids so that remaining part can be used for energy purposes or converted into carbohydrates or fats. NH_2 is used for synthesis of non essential amino acids in the liver and the remaining amount of NH_2 is ***converted into less toxic compound urea*** in the liver. Urea is excreted by the kidneys.

Lipid metabolism: Liver also has an important role in lipid metabolism which is dealt in chapter on metabolism.

Liver forms bile that has role in ***fat digestion*** and in ***excretion of bile pigments.*** The cells in the liver form bile salts. Liver cells congugate bilirubin with glucuronic acid and excrete it into bile canaliculi which join up to form bile ducts (Fig. 7.25). These in turn join the common bile duct, which pours bile into duodenum.

Detoxification: Liver has role in *detoxification* of harmfull substances which include *alcohol* and *toxins from microbes and inactivation of hormones* so that they can be excreted. The hormones included are insulin, glucagons, cortisol, aldosterone, thyroid and sex hormones.

Storage of vitamins and minerals: In addition to storage of **glycogen** liver stores **iron**, **copper** and fat soluble *vitamins A, D, K, E* and water soluble *vitamin* B_{12}. These are released when required by the body. Some other vitamins of B complex are also stored to some extent.

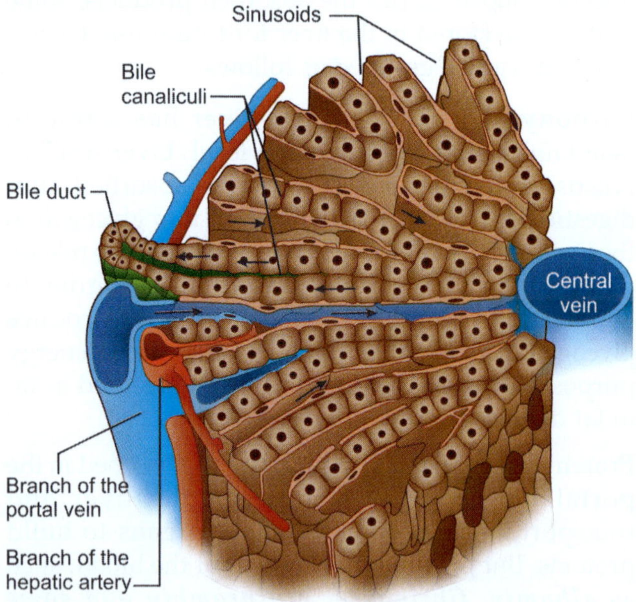

Fig. 7.25: Plates of liver cells. Sinusoids and bile ducts in a liver lobule. Blood flows in sinusoids towards the center of lobule (central vein) and bile in opposite direction in bile ducts

Activation of vitamin D: Liver and kidneys have a role in forming active form of vitamin D.

Phagocytosis: Kuffer cells of the liver remove agile red cells and bacteria from circulation.

Synthesis of vitamin A from carotene: Carotene found in carrots and green leafy vegatables is converted to vitamin A in the liver.

SUMMARY

Tables 7.14 and 7.15, sum up the functions of liver.

Figure 7.26 discusses the causes of gallstones.

Figure 7.27 Tabulates the process of lipid digestion and absorption.

Table 7.16 Tabulates various enzymes of the gastrointestinal tract and their functions.

Table 7.14: Principal functions of the liver

Formation and secretion of bile
Nutrient and vitamin metabolism
• Glucose and other sugars
• Amino acids
• Lipids:
– Fatty acids
– Cholesterol
– Lipoproteins
• Fat-soluble vitamins
• Water-soluble vitamins
Inactivation of various substances
• Toxins
• Steroids
• Other hormones
Synthesis of plasma proteins (*see* Table 7.15)
• Acute-phase proteins
• Albumin
• Clotting factors
• Steroid-binding and other hormone-binding proteins
Immunity
• Kupffer cells

AGE RELATED CHANGES IN GIT FUNCTIONS

- A mild loss of saliva production
- Effects on oropharyngeal and upper esophageal motility, colonic function, gastrointestinal immunity.
- Constipation viewed as functional change.

IMPLICATIONS AND APPLICATIONS

- See the colour, roughness or any ulcer on the tongue. Look for tonsils in a person with mouth wide open.
- To be familiar with endoscopy technique.
- To be able to read Barium meal and Barium enema X-rays.
- Important to know about vomiting.

Table 7.15: Some of the proteins formed by the liver: Physiological functions and properties

Name	*Principal function*	*Binding characteristics*	*Serum or plasma concentration*
Albumin	Binding and carrier protein; osmotic pressure regulator	Hormones, amino, acids, steroids, vitamins, fatty acids	4500–5000 mg/dL
Fibrinogen	Precursor to fibrin in hemostasis		200–450 mg/dL
Proteins, coagulation factors II, VII, IX, X	Blood clotting		
Antithrombin-III	Protease inhibitor of intrinsic coagulation system	1:1 binding to proteases	17–30 mg/dL
Antithrombin C, Protein C	Inhibition of blood clotting		
Insulin-like growth factor I	Mediator of anabolic effects of growth hormone	IGF-I receptor	
Angiotensinogen	Precursor to pressor peptide angiotensin II		
Transferrin	Transport of iron	Two atoms iron/mol	3.0-6.5 mg/dL
Apolipoprotein B	Assembly of lipoprotein particles	Lipid carrier	
Ceruloplasmin	Transport of copper	Six atoms copper/mol	15–60 mg/dL
C-reactive protein	Uncertain; has role in tissue inflammation	Complement C1q	<1 mg/dL; rises in inflammation
Steroid hormone-binding globulin	Carrier protein for steroids in bloodstream	Steroid hormones	3.3 mg/dL
Thyroxine-binding globulin	Carrier protein for thyroid hormone in bloodstream	Thyroid hormones	1.5 mg/dL
Transthyretin (thyroid-binding prealbumin)	Carrier protein for thyroid hormone in bloodstream	Thyroid hormones	25 mg/dL
Haptoglobin	Binding, transport of cell-free hemoglobin	Hemoglobin 1:1 binding	40–180 mg/dL

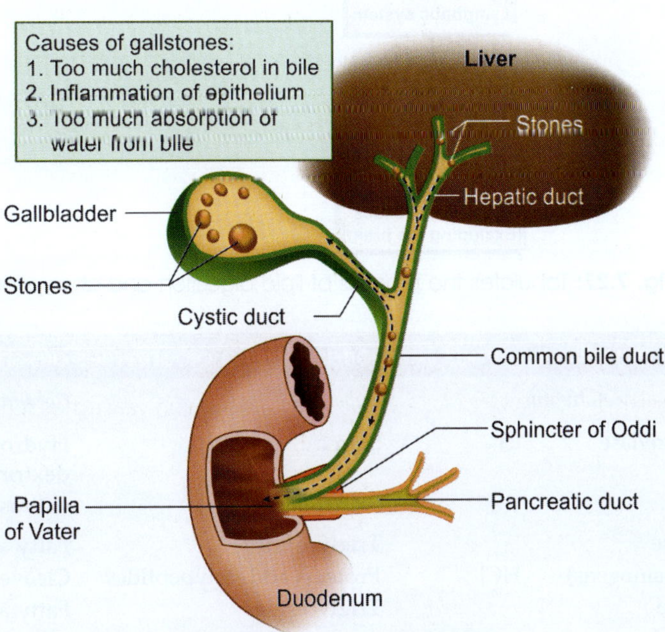

Fig. 7.26: Causes for gallstones

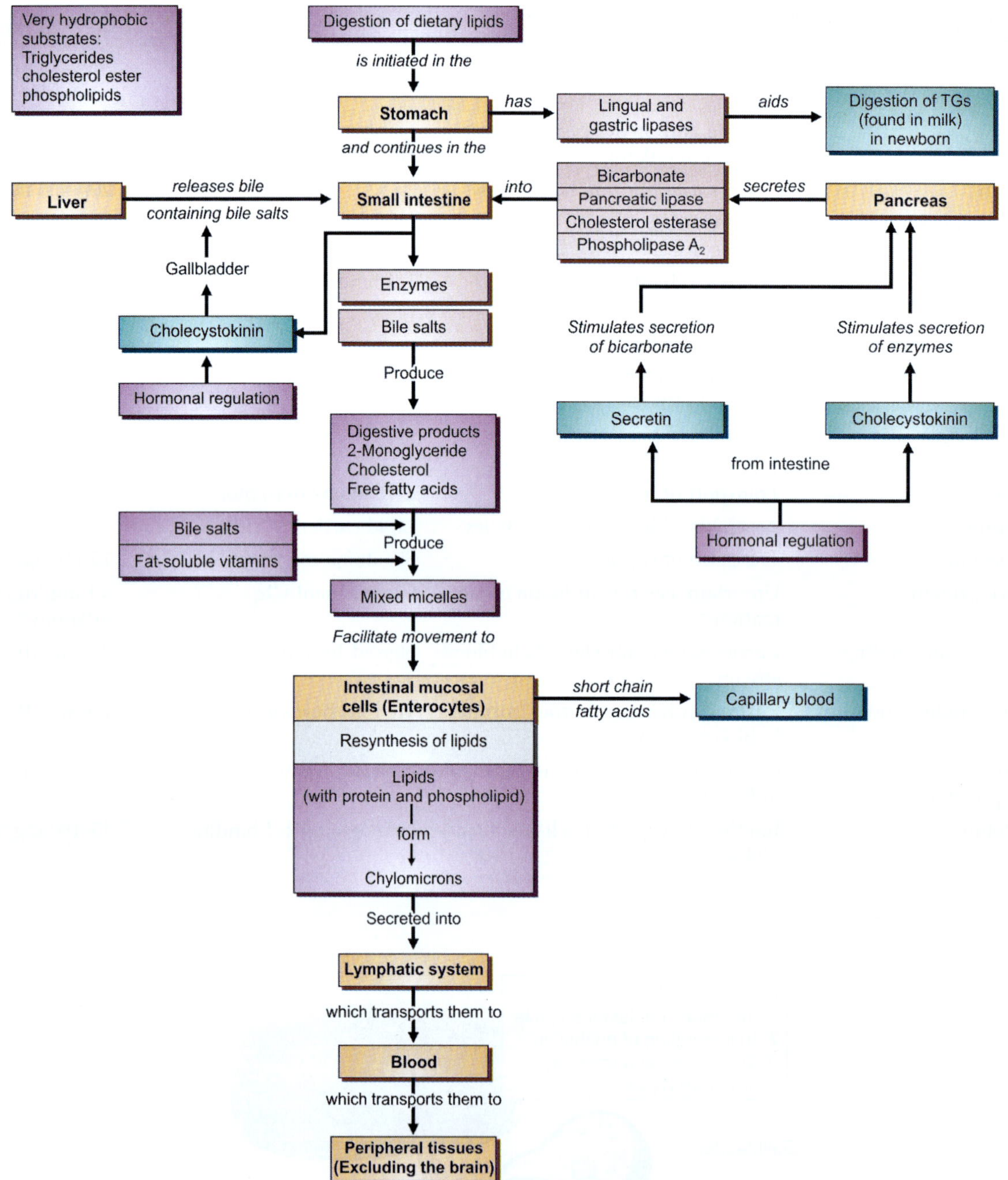

Fig. 7.27: Tabulates the process of lipid digestion and absorption

Table 7.16: Principal digestive enzymes. The corresponding proenzymes are shown in parentheses

Source	*Enzyme*	*Activator*	*Substrate*	*Catalytic function or products*
Salivary glands	Salivary α-amylase	Cl^-	Starch	Hydrolyzes producing α-limit dextrins, maltotriose, and maltose
Lingual glands	Lingual lipase		Triglycerides	Fatty acids plus 1, 2-diacylglycerols
Stomach	Pepsins (pepsinogens)	HCl	Proteins and Polypeptides	Cleave peptide bonds
	Gastric lipase		Triglycerides	Fatty acids and glycerol

(Contd.)

Table 7.16: Principal digestive enzymes. The corresponding proenzymes are shown in parentheses *(Contd.)*

Source	*Enzyme*	*Activator*	*Substrate*	*Catalytic function or products*
Exocrine pancreas	Trypsin (trypsinogen)	Enteropeptidase	Proteins and polypeptides	Cleave peptide bonds
	Chymotrypsins (chymotrypsinogens)	Trypsin	Proteins and polypeptides	Cleaves peptide bonds
	Elastase (proelastase)	Trypsin	Elastin, some other proteins	Cleaves bonds
	Carboxypeptidase A (procarboxypeptidase A)	Trypsin	Proteins and polypeptides	Cleaves carboxyl terminal amino acids
	Carboxypeptidase B (procarboxypeptidase B)	Trypsin	Proteins and polypeptides	Cleaves carboxyl terminal amino acids
	Colipase (procolipase)	Trypsin	Fat droplets	Facilitates exposure of active site of pancreatic lipase
	Pancreatic lipase	—	Triglycerides	Monoglycerides and fatty acids
	Cholesteryl ester hydrolase	—	Cholesteryl esters	Cholesterol
	Pancreatic α-amylase	Cl^-	Starch	Same as salivary α-amylase
	Ribonuclease	—	RNA	Nucleotides
	Deoxyribonuclease	—	DNA	Nucleotides
	Phospholipase A2 (prophospholipase A2)	Trypsin	Phospholipids	Fatty acids, lysophospholipids
Intestinal mucosa	Enteropeptidase	—	Trypsinogen	Trypsin
	Aminopeptidases	—	Polypeptides	Cleave amino terminal amino acid from peptide
	Carboxypeptidases	—	Polypeptides	Cleave carboxyl terminal amino acid form peptide
	Endopeptidases	—	Polypeptides	Cleave in midportion of peptide
	Dipeptidases	—	Dipeptides	Two amino acids
	Maltase	—	Maltose, maltotriose, α-dextrins	Glucose
Intestinal mucosa (continued)	Lactase	—	Lactose	Galactose and glucose
	Sucrase	—	Sucrose;	Fructose and glucose
	α-Dextrinase1	—	α-Dextrins, maltose, maltotriose	Glucose
	Nuclease and related enzymes	—	Nucleic acids	Pentoses and purine and pyrimidine bases
Cytoplasm of mucosal cells	Various peptidases	—	Di-, tri-, and tetrapeptides	Amino acids

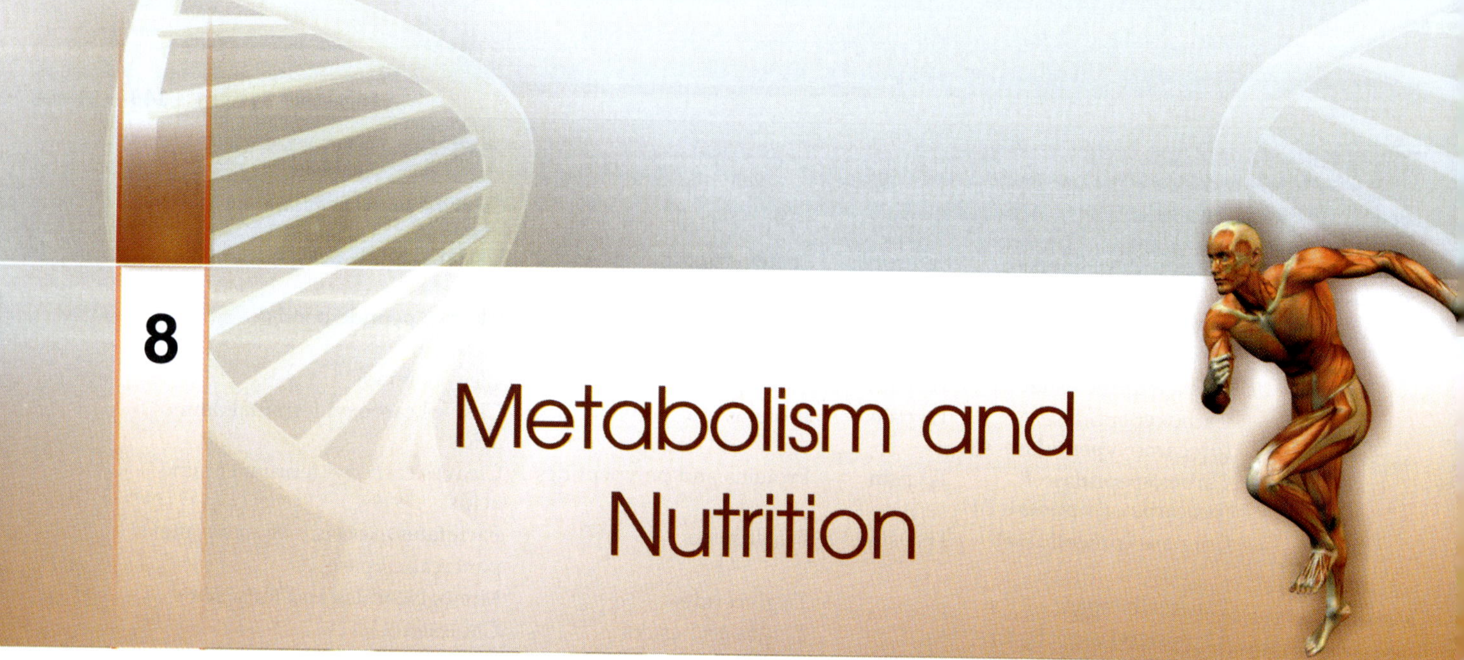

8 Metabolism and Nutrition

METABOLISM

CARBOHYDRATES

There are three groups of carbohydrates. The simplest to more complex form are:

- **Monosaccharides:** The carbohydrates which can not be hydrolysed to simplier carbohydrates. The sugar units which have six carbon atoms are called hexoses, those that have five carbon atoms are called pentoses, e.g. *hexoses* are; glucose, fructose, galactose, and *pentoses* are; ribose, deoxyribose.
- **Disaccharides:** Contain two units of monosaccharides, e.g. *sucrose, lactose* and *maltose.*

  Sucrose is table sugar formed of one unit of glucose and other of fructose.

  Lactose is milk sugar formed of one unit of glucose and other of galactose.

  Maltose is formed of two units of glucose.
- **Oligosaccharides:** Condensation products of two to ten monosaccharides, e.g. maltotriose.
- **Polysaccharides:** Contain many units of monosaccharides, more than ten units, e.g. *glycogen, starch and cellulose.*

Monosaccharide can exist as single units, e.g. glucose. When two monosaccharide molecules are linked together by glycosidic linkage with loss of water molecule they form disaccharides and if many molecules are linked together by such linkages to form long chains, the complex carbohydrates, they are called **polysaccharides**, e.g. starch, glycogen (Fig. 8.1).

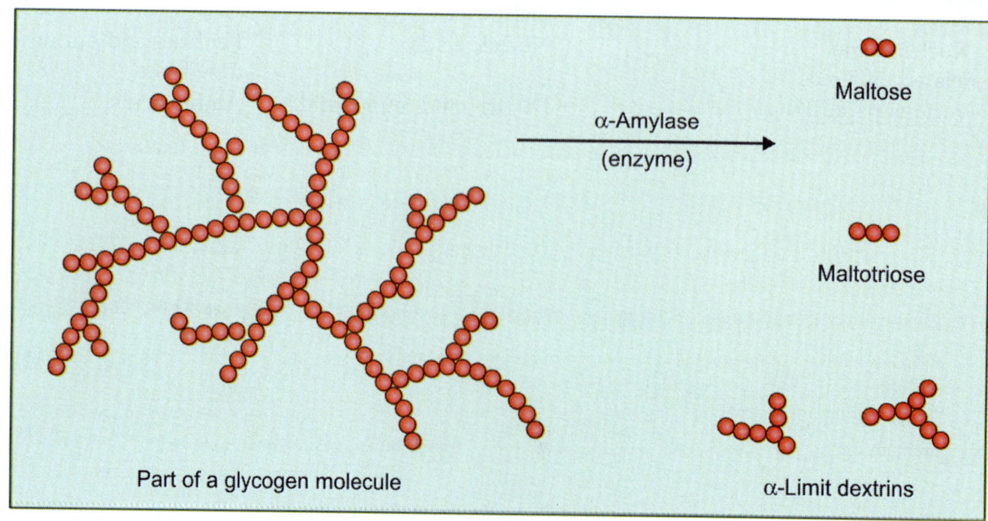

Fig. 8.1: Carbohydrates of varying chains

Disaccharides that are taken in the diet, i.e. sucrose, and lactose are broken down to monosaccharides in the intestine by enzymes (Fig. 8.2); all sugars are absorbed into bloodstream as monosaccharides. *Sucrose* which is table sugar, is broken into glucose and fructose molecules by enzyme *sucrase*. *Lactose* which is milk sugar is hydrolyzed by enzyme *lactase* into glucose and galactose molecules. *Maltose* (the disaccharide), which is formed by hydrolysis of starch by the action of salivary and pancreatic enzymes is hydrolyzed by *maltase* in the intestine into two units of glucose.

Polysaccharides: *Glycogen* is the storage product of carbohydrates in humans (and in all animals) and is stored in the liver and muscle.

Starch is the stored form of carbohydrates in plants and is the main carbohydrate in the food. It is hydrolyzed by enzymes (amylases) in the saliva and pancreatic juice and further digested in intestine (Fig. 8.2) to form monosaccharides.

Cellulose is a part of the cell structure in plants. It is not digested in humans but it is a dietary fiber which stimulates intestinal movements and possibly has some other positive roles in the intestine.

Dietary carbohydrates after digestion are broken down and are absorbed into blood as monosaccharides, most of which is glucose. Glucose is the main sugar in the blood. The other monosaccharides absorbed in the blood are converted into glucose by the liver (Table 8.1, Table also gives clinical significance of different hexoses).

Carbohydrates serve as **energy sources** for the body. Glucose is metabolized in the body either in the presence of oxygen, i.e. by aerobic reactions or in the absence of oxygen by anaerobic reactions. The aerobic metabolism yields much more energy than anaerobic metabolism.

Carbohydrates also form **body components,** e.g. (1) DNA, has deoxyribose; (2) RNA has ribose; (3) glycolipids; (5) glycoproteins are parts of basement membrane collagen; (6) nerve cell myelin; (7) mucopolysaccharides; (8) hormones; and (9) hormone receptors.

Glucose is the precursor for the synthesis of other carbohydrates in the body: glycogen for storage; ribose and deoxyribose in nucleic acids; galactose for lactose in the milk, in glycolipids and glycoproteins.

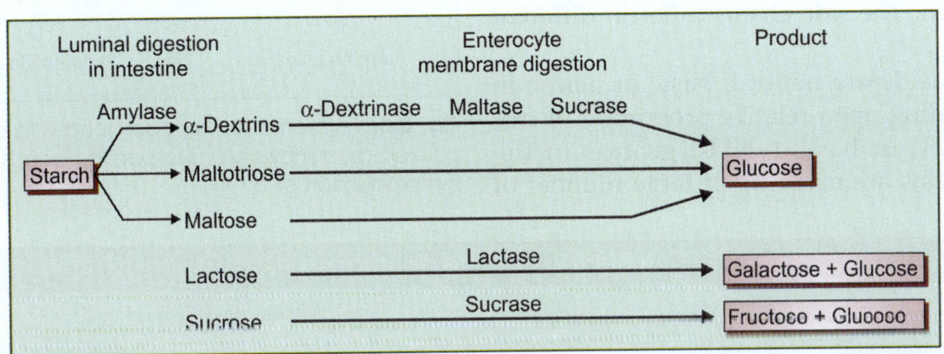

Fig. 8.2: Enzymes involved in carbohydrate digestion, and hexoses final products

Table 8.1: Hexose of physiologic importance

	Source	*Importance*	*Clinical significance*
Glucose	Fruit juices, hydrolysis of starch, cane sugar, maltose, and lactose.	The "sugar" of the body. The sugar carried by blood, the principal one used by the tissues.	Present in the urine (glycosuria) in diabetes mellitus owing to raised blood glucose (hyperglycemia).
Fructose	Fruit juices, honey, hydrolysis of cane sugar	Can be changed to glucose in the liver and so used in the body.	Hereditary fructose intolerance leads to fructose accumulation and hypoglycemia.
Galactose	Hydrolysis of lactose.	Can be changed to glucose in the liver and metabolized. Synthesized in the mammary gland to make the lactose of milk. A constituent of glycolipids and glycoproteins.	Failure to be metabolized leads to galactosemia and cataract.

All sugars are metabolized through glucose pathway. The glucose is transported across the cell membrane to be metabolized in the cell; as it is a large molecule the transport is by the process of facilitated diffusion which requires transporter protein in the cell membrane. There are a number of glucose transporters present in different cell membranes (Table 8.2). The GLUT-1 transporter is for glucose transport across all cells for energy generation. GLUT-4 is the transporter in skeletal, cardiac muscles and adipose tissue and is dependent on insulin for glucose transport across the cell membrane.

Basal plasma glucose levels are regulated and maintained within the range of 70 to 110 mg per dl. *When the plasma glucose level falls below 60 mg per dl, brain uptake of glucose and oxygen decreases; CNS function becomes impaired; if it continues to fall death may result.*

PROTEINS

Proteins are made-up of large number of amino acids. Amino acids contain nitrogen in addition to carbon hydrogen and oxygen which are contained in carbohydrates. Many amino acids also contain sulfur. The units contained in each amino acid are NH_2 (basic amino group) and COOH group (acid carboxyl group) and a side chain. The side chains differ in different amino acids.

The amino acids are neutral, basic or acidic in reaction depending upon relative proportion of free acidic (–COOH) or basic (–NH_2) groups in the molecule. Proteins are made-up of large number of amino acids linked by peptide bonds formed by linkage of amino group of one amino acid to the carboxyl group of the next with elimination of one molecule of water (Fig. 8.3). When two amino acids combine dipeptide results, with three amino acids tripeptide results with further addition of amino acids it results in formation of a chain called polypeptide. The boundaries between peptides, polypeptides are not well defined. Usually the chains containing 2–10 amino acids are called peptides, chains containing more than 10 but less than 100 amino acids are called polypeptides, may be called small proteins if as many as at least 50 amino acids are present in the chain. When 100 or more amino acids are present it is called a protein.

Proteins have hundred or thousands of amino acids and many consist of two or more peptide chains folded together.

The human body is formed *from 20 amino acids, about half of which are called essential amino acids* (*Table 8.3*) *as they cannot be synthesized in the body* (*or are not*

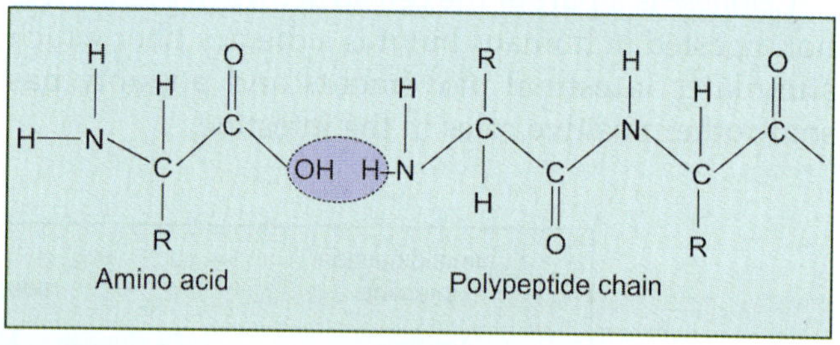

Fig. 8.3: Formation of peptide bond with amino acids. The colored area shows how the peptide bonds are formed, with the production of H_2O

Table 8.2: Glucose transporters

Glucose transporter	*Function*	*Major sites of expression*
Secondary active transport (Na$^+$-glucose cotransport)		
SGLT	Absorption of glucose	Small intestine, renal tubules
Facilitated diffusion		
GLUT-1	Basal glucose uptake	Placenta, blood brain barrier, brain, red cells, kidneys, colon, many other organs
GLUT-2	B cell glucose sensor; transport out of intestinal and renal epithelial cells	B cells of islets, liver, epithelial cells of small intestine, kidneys.
GLUT-3	Basal glucose uptake	Brain, placenta, kidneys, many others organs
GLUT-4	Insulin-stimulated glucose uptake	Skeletal and cardiac muscle, adipose tissue, other tissues
GLUT-5	Fructose transport	Jejunum, sperm
GLUT-6	None	
GLUT-7	Glucose 6-phosphate transporter in endoplasmic reticulum	Liver, may be other tissues

GLUT-4, the major insulin responsive glucose transporter.

Table 8.3: Amino acid requirements of humans

Nutritionally essential	*Nutritionally nonessential*
Arginine[1]	Alanine
Histidine	Asparagine
Isoleucine	Aspartate
Leucine	Cysteine
Lysine	Glutamate
Methonine	Glutamine
Phenylalanine	Glycine
Threonine	Serine
Tryptophan	Tyrosine
Valine	Proline

[1]"Nutritionally semiessential". Synthesized at rates inadequate to support growth of children.

synthesized in amounts required by the body) and must be taken in the diet in the protein that is ingested. The essential amino acids are threonine, methionine, valine, leucine, isoleucine, phenylalanine, lysine, tryptophan and in children arginine, and histidine also. The arginine amino acids can be synthesized in the body but not in amounts enough for growing children.

Within the body the dietary nonessential amino acids are as important metabolically and structurally as are the essential ones. If they are not provided in the diet they must be *synthesized from other nitrogen compounds. For maximum growth, all amino acids are required simultaneously and in appropriate ratios, as well as in sufficient amounts.*

Amino acids are building units of all *tissue proteins, enzymes* and *many hormones*, and have a role as other body components, e.g. *glycine is a neurotransmitter*, arginine is responsible for *urea formation, histidine is precursor of histamine.*

PROTEIN METABOLISM

Proteins are digested in the gastrointestinal tract and absorbed as amino acids. Small amounts of protein, and some peptides may also be absorbed but most proteins are digested to amino acids which are absorbed as such. The amino acids are synthesized into proteins in the body. The amino acids formed from endogenous protein breakdown are identical to those derived from ingested protein and they together form ***common amino acid pool*** that supplies the needs of the body (Fig. 8.4). At all ages small amount of protein is lost as hair (Fig. 8.5) and in women small amounts are lost in menstrual blood loss; small amounts of proteins of digestive secretions that are not reabsorbed in the intestine, are also lost and loss has to be made-up by synthesis of protein. *All essential amino acids are required for normal protein synthesis; deficiency of even one essential amino acid affects the process even though all others may be present.*

Protein requirement for the body is dependent on *total protein content* in the diet as well as *biological effectiveness;* which depends on the ratio of essential to nonessential amino acids present in the diet. **Milk** and **egg** and all **animal protein** are of the *highest quality.*

Positive nitrogen balance. In growing children with gain in body mass, urinary nitrogen excretion is less than intake of protein nitrogen. The individual is said to be in *positive nitrogen balance.*

Negative nitrogen balance. When protein breakdown is greatly accelerated by tissue trauma or disease, urinary urea plus ammonia nitrogen may be more than the protein nitrogen intake such individual is said to be *negative nitrogen balance.*

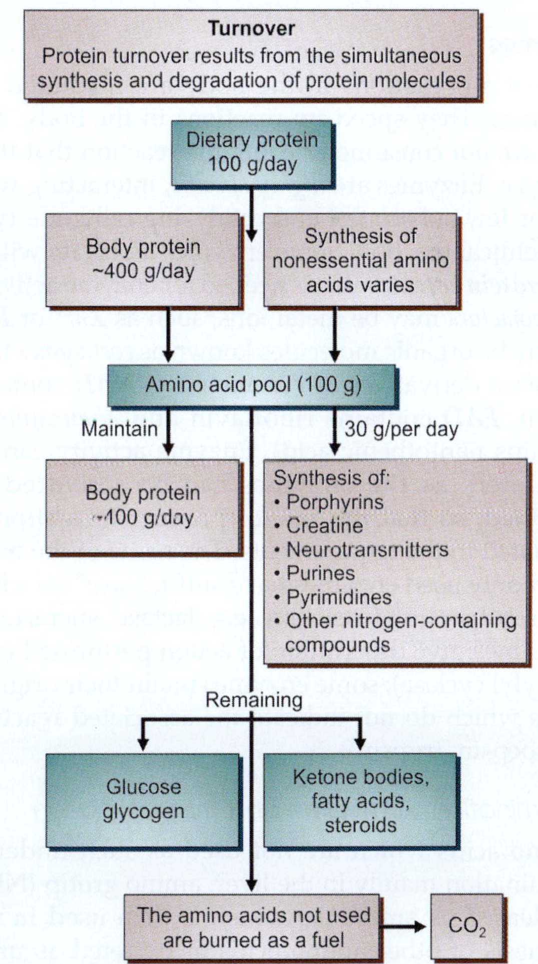

Fig. 8.4: Sources and fates of amino acids. The total amount of protein in the body remains constant

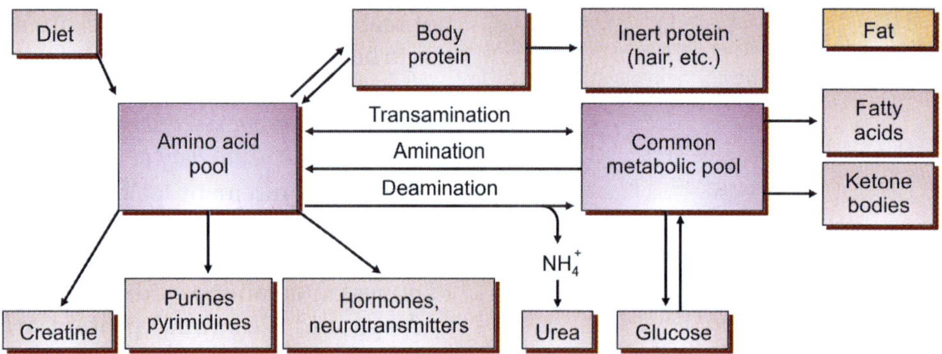

Fig. 8.5: Amino acid metabolism

Proteins have many *roles* in the body. They are responsible for the **structure** of body tissues. **Enzymes** are also proteins. Muscles have **proteins** which produce **contraction** of the muscles. **Plasma albumin** has many important functions. **Antibodies** are also proteins and they defend against in invading micro-organisms. **Some of the hormones** are protein in nature, e.g. insulin.

Enzymes

Almost all reactions in the body are mediated by enzymes. They speed up reactions in the body. But they are not consumed during the reaction that they catalyze. Enzymes are *highly specific*, interacting with one or few substrates, and catalyzing only one type of chemical reaction. Some enzymes associate with a ***nonprotein cofactor*** that is needed for enzyme activity. The *cofactors* may be metal ions, such as Zn^{2+} or Fe^{2+} or may be organic molecules known as *coenzymes* that are often derivatives of vitamins (e.g. *NAD* contains niacin, *FAD* contains riboflavin and ***coenzyme A*** contains pantothenic acid). Enzyme activity can be regulated, as the enzymes can be activated or inhibited, so that the rate of product formation is regulated to the requirements. The name of the most commonly used enzymes have suffix "***-ase***" attached to the substrate of reaction (e.g. lactase, sucrase) or the names give description of action performed (e.g. adenylyl cyclase); some enzymes retain their original name which do not indicate the associated reaction (e.g. pepsin, trypsin).

Deamination, Amination and Transamination

Amino acids which are not used as such undergo deamination mainly in the liver; amino group (NH_2) is released as ammonia; which is then used in the synthesis of other amino acids or excreted as urea. The non-nitrogenous residues after transformation enter the citric acid cycle and are either completely dissimilated or are converted into glucose, fat, ketone bodies or other amino acids (Fig. 8.5).

Urea Formation

Most of the ammonia formed by deamination of amino acids in the liver is converted to urea (Fig. 8.6), and the urea is excreted in the urine. *Most of the urea is formed in the liver and in severe liver disease the urea level in blood falls and blood NH_3 rises.*

Nucleic Acids

These are large molecules in the body and are built up from nucleotides. Nucleotides consist of three parts:

- Sugar unit
- Base
- Phosphate group/groups

The **bases** are classified as purines and pyrimidines. Adenine and guanine are purine bases. Cystosine, uracil and thymine are pyrimidine bases. The physiological important purines and pyrimidines are shown in Fig. 8.7. The compounds containing them in Table 8.4.

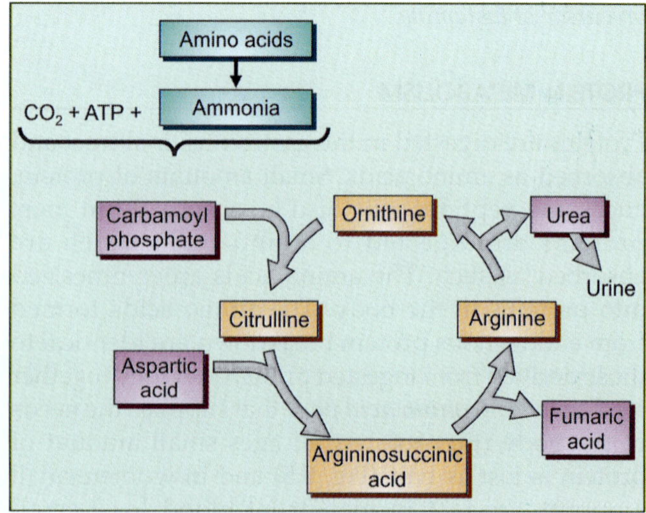

Fig. 8.6: Urea cycle converts ammonia to urea

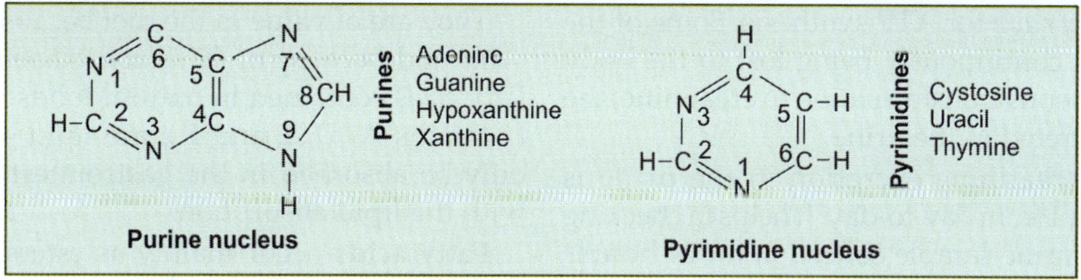

Fig. 8.7: Principal physiologically important purines and pyrimidines

Table 8.4: Purine and pyrimidine containing compounds

Type of compound	*Components*
Nucleoside	Purine or pyrimidine plus ribose or 2-deoxyribose
Nucleotide (mononucleotide)	Nucleoside plus phosphoric acid residue
Nucleic acid	Many nucleotides forming polynucleotide chains.
Nucleoprotein	Nucleic acid and one or more simple basic proteins
Contain ribose (sugar)	Ribonucleic acids (RNA)
Contain 2-deoxyribose (sugar)	Deoxyribonucleic acids (DNA)

Deoxyribonucleic Acid (DNA)

It is present in the nucleus in the chromosomes. Genes, which determine the inherited characteristics in an individual, are parts of DNA in the chromosomes. DNA is a double strand of nucleotides (Fig. 8.8).

The nucleotides in DNA consist of deoxyribose the sugar, phosphate group and one of the four bases (adenine, thymine, guanine and cytosine).

Ribonucleic Acid (RNA)

It is the other type of nucleic acid. It relays instructions from the genes in DNA to guide the synthesis of proteins in the cytoplasm in the ribosomes.

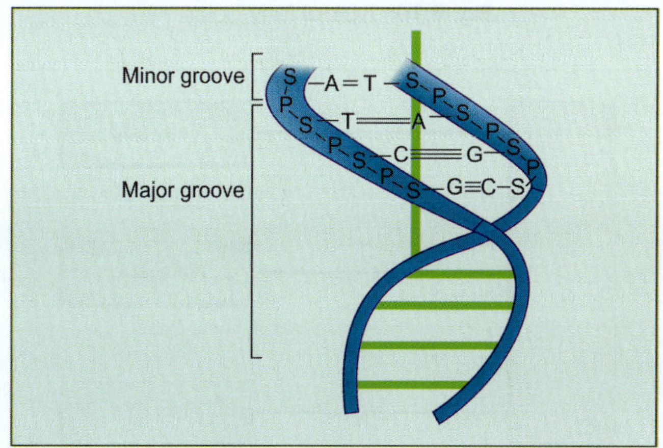

Fig. 8.8: Double-helical structure of DNA, with adenine (A) binding to thymine (T) and cytosine (C) to guanine (G)

RNA is made-up of nucleotides but it is a single strand. The sugar in the nucleotides is ribose instead of deoxyribose and the bases, three of them the same as in DNA (i.e. adenine, guanine, cytosine), except one which is uracil instead of thymine.

Metabolism of Nucleic Acids

In the diet nucleic acids are digested and their constituent bases are absorbed, but most of the purines and pyrimidines are synthesized from amino acids mainly in the liver. The purines and pyrimidines released by breakdown of nucleotides may be reused or catabolized. ***The pyrimidines are catabolized to CO_2 and water and purines are converted to uric acid. Uric acid is also synthesized.*** **Uric acid** *is excreted in urine, but in other mammals uric acid is oxidized to allantoin before excretion. The normal blood level in humans is approximately 4 mg/dL.* The uric acid excretion on purine free diet is 0.5 gm/day and on a regular diet about 1 gm/day.

In the kidney uric acid is filtered, reabsorbed and secreted.

Adenosine Triphosphate (ATP)

It is a nucleotide which contains ribose (the sugar unit) adenine (the base) and three phosphate groups. Many of the reactions in the body release energy, e.g. breakdown of sugars and fats, released energy is used to make ATP from adenosine diphosphate (ADP). When the body needs chemical energy for activities, e.g. *muscular activity*; for the functions of *pumps* to transport substances across cell membranes; and for building *biological molecules*; energy from ATP is utilized by splitting the high energy phosphate bond and ADP is again formed as a result. ADP also contains one more high energy bond.

Creatine and Creatinine

Creatine is synthesized in the **liver**, from methionine, glycine and arginine. It is discharged into the blood and taken up by the muscle as required. In the skeletal muscle it is phosphorylated by ATP to form **phosphorylcreatine** (creatine phosphate). This is important *energy store* for ATP synthesis. Some of the creatine store is continuously being lost to the body by slow spontaneous transformation to creatinine; the creatinine is excreted in the urine.

The rate of creatinine excretion in the urine is relatively constant from day-to-day. It helps in checking the accuracy of urine sample collection for 24 hours.

LIPIDS

Lipids are made-up of carbon, hydrogen and oxygen atoms. Lipids are strongly hydrophobic (water hating) and so the lipids do not mix with water. They provide more than twice the amount of energy per gram as do carbohydrates and proteins.

Sources of fat in the body are from diet; and formed from carbohydrates in the body (Fig. 8.9).

Excess dietary carbohydrates, proteins, fats and oils are deposited in adipose tissue as triglycerides. Lipids are heterogeneous group of compounds that include **fats, oils, steroids**, waxes and related compounds. Oils are fat in liquid state. Lipids have a common property of being relatively insoluble in water and soluble in non-polar solvents, such as ether and chloroform.

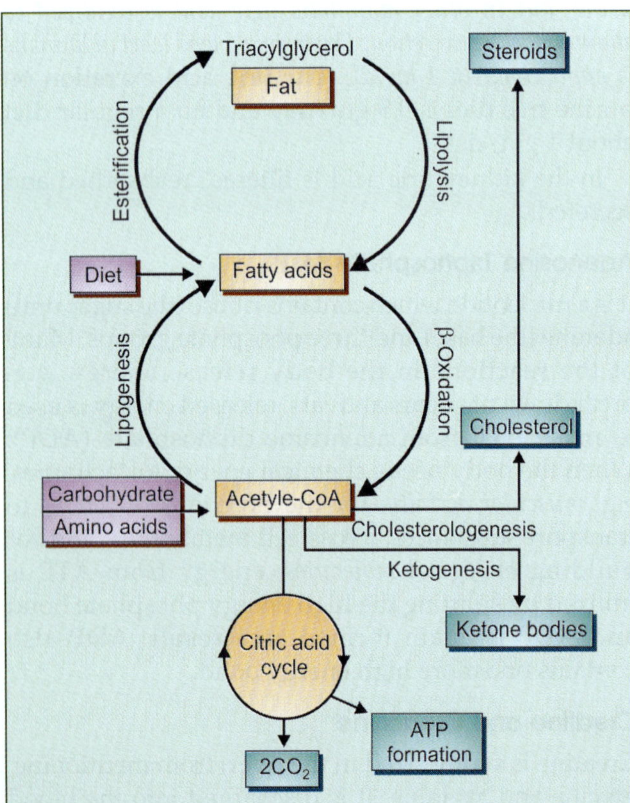

Fig. 8.9: Overview of fatty acid metabolism showing the major pathways and end products. Ketone bodies comprise the substances acetoacetate, â-hydroxy- butyrate, and acetone

They are of value in the diet because of *high energy value* and because of *fat soluble vitamins* and *essential fatty acids* contained in natural foods. Some vitamins (vitamins A, D, E and K), are lipid soluble and can only be absorbed in the gastrointestinal tract along with the lipid absorption.

Fatty acids occur mainly as esters in natural fats and oils; but in plasma do occur in the unesterified form as **free fatty acids**, a transport form. Fatty acids that occur in natural fats are usually straight-chain derivatives that contain an even number of carbon atoms. The chain may be saturated (containing no double bond) or unsaturated (Fig. 8.10) (containing one or more double bonds).

Major components of lipids in the diet consists of **triglycerides**; formed by three long chain fatty acids each linked to glycerol molecule (Fig. 8.11). The fatty acids may be **saturated** (palmitic, stearic) or unsaturated with double bonds (monounsaturated, oleic acid) (Fig. 8.10).

Triglycerides in the diet are absorbed as chylomicrons.

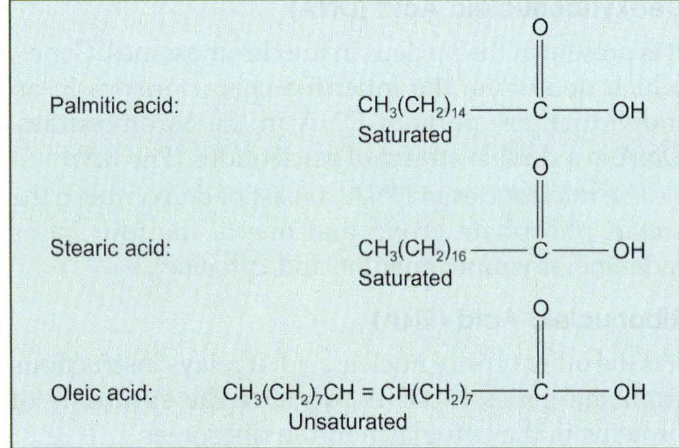

Fig. 8.10: Typical fatty acids

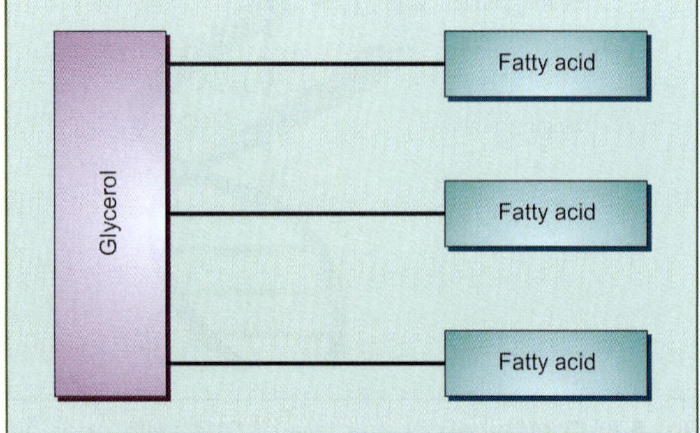

Fig. 8.11: Basic structure of triglycerides

The fat stored in fat depots in the body is also in the form of triglyceride. Fat stored in the subcutaneous tissue and around certain organs also acts as a *thermal insulator*.

The other lipids (Table 8.5) are the **phospholipids** (which form a part of the cell membrane) and **cholesterol**. *Cholesterol is both ingested and synthesized in the body.* The steroid molecule of cholesterol has number of functions: functions in membranes; is a precursor of bile acids and steroid hormones.

Steroids have four rings of carbon atom (Fig. 8.12); differ in structure from the triglycerides.

The steroid hormones are the hormones of adrenal cortex and the main hormones of sex glands. The active derivatives of vitamin D are also steroids.

The smallest lipids (some fatty acids) are only lipids that can dissolve in watery plasma. To become more soluble in plasma, other lipid molecules form complexes with hydrophilic protein molecules. These lipid protein complexes are called **lipoproteins.**

Lipoproteins are also important cellular constituents, occurring in cell membrane and in mitochondria.

The fatty acids can be synthesized in the body, in the liver and adipose tissue, no strict dietary requirements for fat exists. But some of the fatty acids are polyunsaturated and cannot be synthesized in the body. These are termed **essential fatty acids** (*linoleic, linolenic* and *arachidonic*) and they are required for certain membrane phospholipids and glycolipid substances; and for important intracellular mediators, the prostaglandins.

Table 8.5: Lipids
Typical fatty acids:
Palmitic acid:
Stearic acid:
Oleic acid:
Triglycerides (triacylglycerols): Esters of glycerol and three fatty acids.
Phospholipids:
A. Esters of glycerol, two fatty acids, and
1. Phosphate = phosphatidic acid
2. Phosphate plus inositol = phosphatidylinositol
3. Phosphate plus choline = phosphatidylcholine (lecithin)
4. Phosphate plus ethanolamine = phosphatidylethanolamine (cephalin)
5. Phosphate plus serine = phosphatidylserine
B. Other phosphate containing derivatives of glycerol
C. Sphingomyelins containing phosphate, choline, and the amino alcohol sphingosine.
Cerebrosides: Compounds containing galactose, fatty acid, and sphingosine.
Sterols: Cholesterol and its derivatives, (steroid hormones, bile acids, and vitamins).

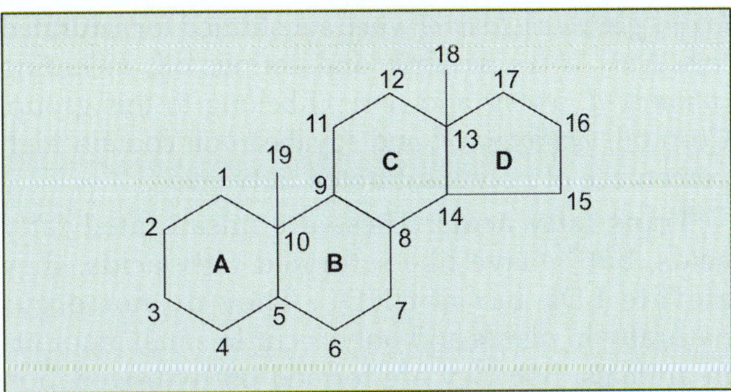

Fig. 8.12: The steroid nucleus

Thus, the **lipid family** includes **triglycerides** (*fats and oils*), **phospholipids** (lipids that contain phosphorus) **steroids** (lipids that contain rings of carbon atoms), **prostaglandins/eicosanoids** (20 carbon lipids) and a variety of other lipids, including **fatty acids,** and **lipoproteins**. **Fat soluble vitamins** are vitamin A, D, E and K.

Saturated fats are triglycerides that contain only single covalent bonds between carbon atoms of fatty acids. Because they lack double bonds, each carbon atom is saturated with hydrogen atom. Triglycerides with mainly saturated fatty acids usually are solid at room temperature.

Although saturated fats occur mostly in animal tissues, they are also found in many plant products, such as palm oil and coconut oil.

Monounsaturated fats contain primarily fatty acids with one double bond. Unsaturated fatty acids are generally derived from *vegetables* and *fish*. When substituted for saturated fatty acids in the diet monounsaturated fats *lower both total plasma cholesterol and LDL cholesterol* but increase useful cholesterol, the HDL. *Olive oil* and *peanut oil* are rich in triglycerides with monounsaturated fatty acids.

Polyunsaturated fat containing primarily fatty acids with more than one double bond are called polyunsaturated fats. Their effect on cardiovascular disease is influenced by the location of the double bonds within the molecule. **Omega 6** fatty acids are long chain, polyunsaturated fatty acids (with the first double bond beginning at the sixth carbon atom, when counting from methyl end of the fatty acid molecule) hence they are called omega 6 fatty acids. Consumption of these fatty acids obtained from vegetable oils, *lowers plasma cholesterol* when substituted for saturated fats. *Nuts, olives, soyabean* and various oils including *cotton seed, sesame* and *corn oil* belong to this group. Corn oil, *sunflower oil* and soyabean oil contain high percentage of polyunsaturated fatty acids.

Trans fatty acids: These are unsaturated fatty acids, but behave like saturated fatty acids, they elevate LDL but not HDL. They do not occur naturally in plants and only occur in small amounts in animals. But they are formed on hydrogenation of liquid vegetable oils, e.g. in the manufacture of margarine.

Eicosanoids are derivatives of 20 carbon polyunsaturated fatty acids and comprise the leukotrienes (LTs), and lipoxins (LXs), prostaglandins (PGs), prostacyclines (PGIs) and thromboxanes (TXs) (Fig. 8.13). The two principal subclasses of eicosonoids are **prostaglandins** and **leukotrienes. Prostaglandins** have a wide variety of functions. They *modify responses to hormones, contribute to inflammatory responses, prevent stomach ulcers, dilate airways to the lungs, influence body temperature and many other functions including reproduction*; thromboxanes are involved *blood coagulation.* Nonsteroid anti-inflammatory drugs act by inhibiting prostaglandins synthesis.

Leukotrienes *participate in allergic and inflammatory responses, causes bronchoconstriction* and have role in asthma.

Fatty acids: Body lipids also include fatty acids; which can undergo either hydrolysis to provide *ATP* or are used to synthesize triglycerides or phospholipids.

Fat soluble vitamins, such as beta-carotenes (yellow-orange pigment in egg yolk, carrots, and tomatoes that are converted to vitamin A) are lipids.

Lipids in the Diet

Mainly are triglycerides, that are hydrolysed to monoglycerides and fatty acids in the small intestine; cholesterol esters are hydrolysed to cholesterol though most of the cholesterol is present in free form in the diet; products are absorbed, and then again esterified in the intestinal mucosal cells, where they are packed with protein to form chylomicrons which are secreted into lymphatic system and reach bloodstream as large lipoproteins. Chylomicrons also contain other lipids, and fat soluble vitamins.

Chylomicrons are first metabolized by tissues that have lipoprotein lipase, which hydrolyzes the triacylglycerol, releasing fatty acids that are taken up into tissue lipids or oxidized as fuel (Fig. 8.14).

The chylomicron remnants (containing cholesteryl esters, phospholipids, apolipoproteins, and some triacylglycerol) bind to receptors in the liver and are endocytosed. The remnants are hydrolysed to component parts, i.e. free cholesterol, fatty acids and amino acids.

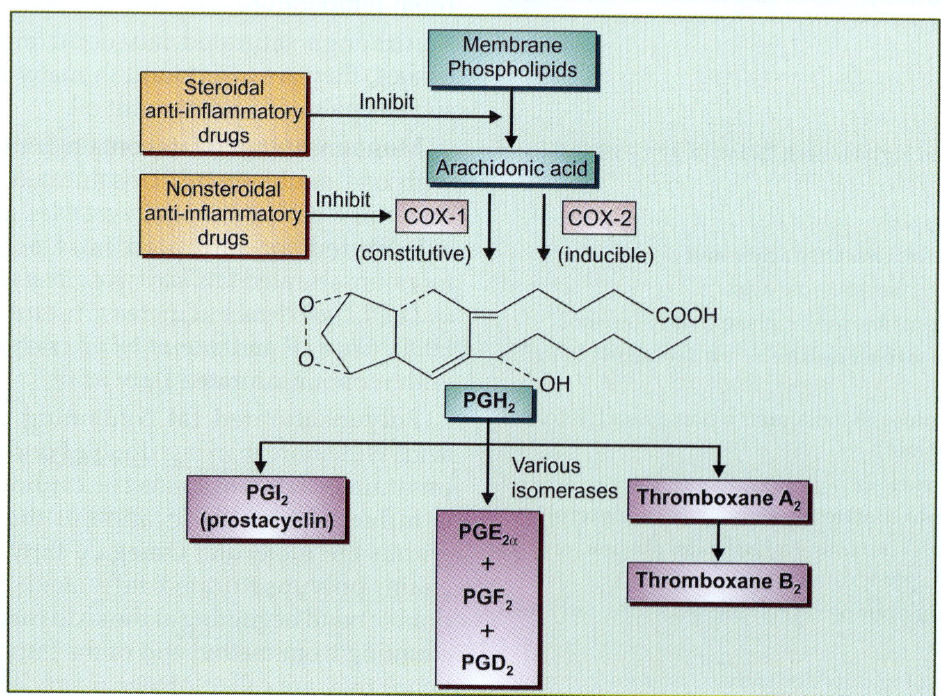

Fig. 8.13: Formation of prostaglandins and thromboxanes from membrane phospholipids and action of some drugs

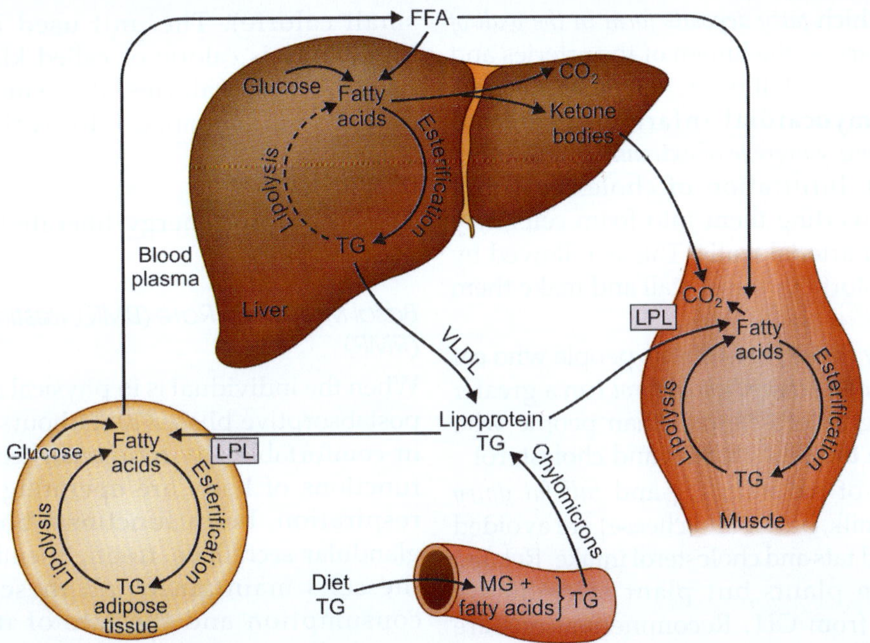

Fig. 8.14: Transport and fate of major lipid substrates and metabolites. (FFA, free fatty acids; LPL, lipoprotein lipase; MG, monoacylglycerol; TG, triacylglycerol; VLDL, very low density lipoprotein)

Lipogenesis

The other major source of long chain fatty acid is carbohydrate mainly in adipose tissue and liver, i.e. synthesis.

Adipose Tissue

It is the main fuel reserve of the body. On hydrolysis (lipolysis), free fatty acids are released into circulation. These are taken up by most tissues; but not brain or red cells; and esterfied to acylglycerol or oxidized as fuel.

In the liver triacylglycerol arising from lipogenesis, free fatty acids and chylomicron remnants is secreted into circulation as very low density lipoprotein (VLDL), which has same fate as chylomicrons. They are composed mainly of triacylglycerol and their function is to carry this lipid from the liver to the peripheral tissues. There triacylglycerol is degraded by lipoprotein lipase, causing VLDL to decrease in size and become denser. Finally triacylglycerol are transferred from VLDL to HDL in an exchange reaction that transfers cholesteryl esters from HDL to VLDL, hence VLDL is converted to LDL. LDL particles have high concentration of cholesterol and cholesterol esters than their VLDL predecessors.

Figure 8.15 shows the sources of liver cholesterol and routes of leaving the liver.

Atherosclerosis

Saturated fats, cholesterol and atherosclerosis. There is role of **cholesterol** in **atherosclerosis.** Atherosclerosis

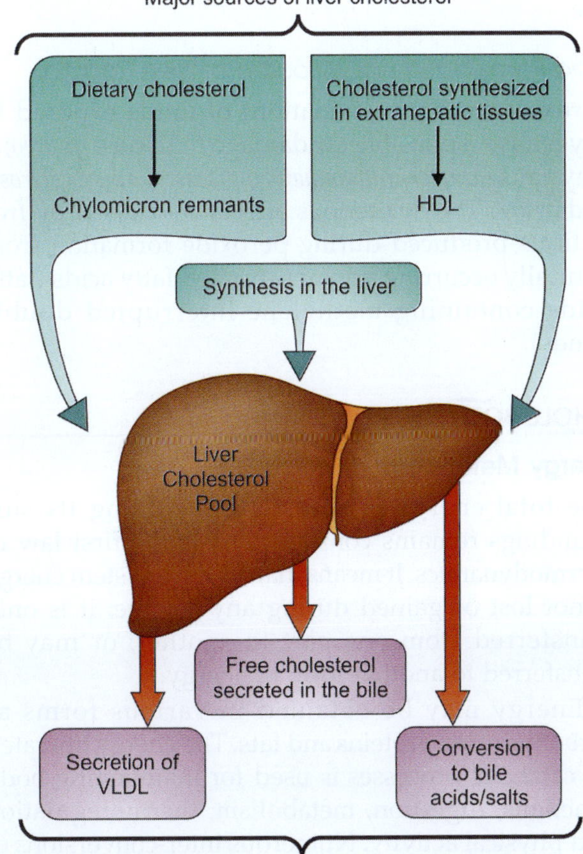

Fig. 8.15: Sources of liver cholesterol and routes by which cholesterol leaves the liver

is a disorder in which *fatty deposits form in the wall of the arteries*, they narrow the lumen of the arteries and the blood flow in limited. It **is a widespread disease, predisposes to myocardial infarction, cerebral thrombosis,** *ischemic gangrene of extremities* and other serious illnesses. Infiltration of cholesterol into macrophages, converting them into foam cells may occur in lesions of arterial walls. This is followed by changes which distort the vessel wall and make them rigid.

Although many factors contribute, people who eat a diet *high in saturated fats and cholesterol* run a greater risk of developing atherosclerosis than people who eat a diet lower in the saturated fat and cholesterol.

Dietary intake of *red meat, egg* and *full fat dairy* products (whole milk, butter and cheese) are avoided to reduce saturated fats and cholesterol intake. Related steroids occur in plants but plant steroids are poorly absorbed from GIT. Recommendations are (1) selection of diet, (2) weight control, (3) no smoking and (4) regular exercises to lessen the risk of cardiovascular diseases. The individuals with genetic predisposition should be more careful from earlier age.

Lipid Peroxidation as a Source of Free Radical

Peroxidation (auto-oxidation) of lipids exposed to oxygen is responsible for damage to tissues *in vivo*; it may cause *cancer, inflammatory diseases, atherosclerosis* and *aging*. The deleterious effects are caused by free radicals produced during peroxide formation from naturally occurring polyunsaturated fatty acids (fatty acids containing methylene-interrupted double bonds).

WHOLE BODY METABOLISM

Energy Metabolism

The total energy of a system, including its surroundings remains constant; this is the first law of thermodynamics. It means that within a system energy is not lost or gained during any change; it is only transferred from one part to another; or may be transferred to another form of energy.

Energy may be obtained in various forms as carbohydrates, proteins and fats. The energy liberated by catabolic processes is used for maintaining body functions, digestion, metabolism, thermoregulation and physical activity. Numerous inter-conversions of chemical, mechanical and thermal energy are possible. It is converted to *external work, heat* and *energy storage*. The standard unit of heat energy is calorie (cal or c or small calorie). The unit used in medicine and physiology is calorie or called kilocalorie which is equal to 1000 calories, it is simply written as C (C written in capital). C = 1000 calories.

Metabolic Rate

The amount of energy liberated per unit time is metabolic rate.

Basal Metabolic Rate (BMR)/Resting Metabolic Rate (RMR)

When the individual is in physical and mental rest, in postabsorptive phase (10–14 hours after a meal) and in comfortable environmental temperature certain functions of body are operating (like heart beat, respiration, brain functions, body temperature, glandular secretions, resting membrane potential in the cells maintained) all these require energy consumption and the rate of it is called **basal metabolic rate.** *It is also called resting metabolic rate (RMR).* BMR amounts to on an average daily expenditure of about 20 to 25 calories/kg of body weight. In other words in an adult, the RMR requires about 1800 C/day for a man of 70 kg weight and 1300 C/day for a woman of 50 kg weight.

BMR of an individual depends on (1) *age*, (2) *sex*, (3) *body surface area*; it decreases with age, it is more in males, more with higher surface area. During sleep BMR falls by 10–15%. **BMR increases in hyperthyroidism**, and decreases in hypothyroidism.

Clinically BMR is expressed as a percentage above or below the accepted normal standard for an individual, taking into account his age, sex, height and weight; BMR of +40 would mean it is 40% above normal average for that person.

Physical activity, ingestion of food further increase the metabolic rate over and above BMR.

Respiratory Quotient/RQ

RQ = CO_2 output/O_2 consumption

During metabolism the proportion of carbon dioxide produced to oxygen used varies according to the substances being used as fuel, the ratio is known as respiratory quotient. The ratio is 0.8 when mixed substances are being used as fuel, 1 if mainly carbohydrates are being used and 0.7 when mainly fat is the fuel.

Currency of Energy

The chemical currency of energy in all living cells is two high energy phosphate bonds contained in **ATP (adenosine triphosphate)**. To a lesser extent, other similar compounds (guanosine triphosphate, cytosine triphosphate, etc.) also serve as energy sources after the energy from ATP is transferred to them. In muscle, **creatine phosphate (CrP/phosphorylcreatine)** is a high energy molecule of importance.

The two terminal bonds of ATP each contain about 12 kcal of potential energy per mole under physiological conditions.

Intermediate Metabolism

The citric acid cycle is a series of reactions **in mitochondria** that oxidize acetyl residues (**acetyl-CoA**); that produce reduced form of coenzymes which upon re-oxidation are **linked to formation of ATP.**

The citric acid cycle is the ***common pathway for the oxidation of carbohydrate, lipid, and protein*** because glucose, fatty acids and some amino acids are metabolized to acetyl-CoA (Fig. 8.16) *or in the case of number of amino acids to* intermediates of the cycle. It has a central role in ***gluconeogenesis*** (formation of glucose from non carbohydrate sources), ***lipogenesis*** (Fig. 8.17) and ***interconversion of amino acids***. *Many* of these processes occur in most tissues, but liver is the only tissue in which *all occur* to a significant extent.

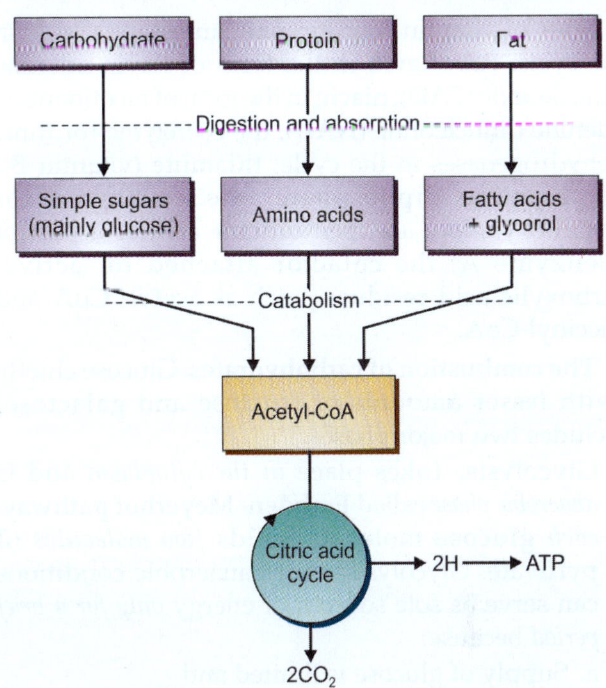

Fig. 8.16: Outline of the pathways for the catabolism of dietary carbohydrate, protein, and fat. All the pathways lead to the production of acetyl-CoA, which is oxidized in the citric acid cycle, ultimately yielding ATP in the process of oxidative phosphorylation

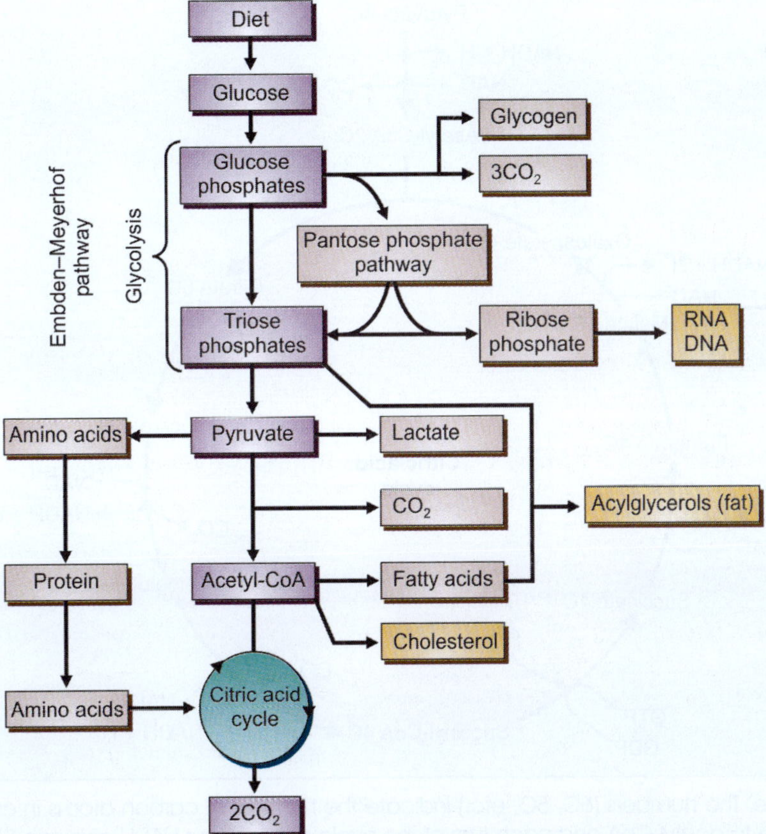

Fig. 8.17: Overview of carbohydrate metabolism showing the major pathways and end products

Four of vitamin B group play an essential role in the cycle. **Riboflavin** in the form of flavin adenine dinucleotide (FAD); **niacin** in the form of nicotinamide adenine dinucleotide (NAD), the coenzyme for three dehydrogenases in the cycle; **thiamine** (vitamin B_1) as thiamine diphosphate, the coenzyme for decarboxylation; and **pentothenic acid** as a part of coenzyme A, the cofactor attached to 'active' carboxylic acid residues, such as acetyl- CoA and succinyl-CoA.

The combustion of carbohydrates: Glucose chiefly (with lesser amounts of fructose and galactose) includes two major phases.

1. Glycolysis: Takes place *in the cytoplasm* and is *anaerobic phase* called **Embden- Meyerhof pathway**, *each* **glucose** molecule yields *two molecules* of pyruvate. Glycolysis under anaerobic conditions can serve as sole sources of energy *only for a brief period* because:
   a. Supply of glucose is limited and
   b. Accumulated pyruvate must be converted into lactate a product that is harmful.
2. **Krebs cycle/tricarboxylic acid cycle/citric acid cycle**. The two molecules of pyruvate are oxidized to CO_2 by the **citric acid cycle** in the **mitochondria, it requires oxygen**, is the aerobic phase and the remaining energy is liberated. In this pathway acetyl coenzyme A (acetyl-CoA, i.e. acetic acid bound to coenzyme A) initially formed by oxidative decarboxylation of pyruvate is condensed with oxaloacetate to form citrate (Fig. 8.18), and through a cyclic series of reactions the carbons of acetyl-CoA form CO_2 and oxaloacetate is regenerated (Fig. 8.18). (In neoglucogenesis, substrates, such as lactate and pyruvate which are formed in the cytoplasm enter the mitochondria to form oxaloacetate before forming glucose).

The combustion of fatty acids, the major energy components of fats, takes place in the mitochondria through a repetitive biochemical process known as β-oxidation. This process releases two carbons at a time in the form of acetyl-CoA until the entire fatty acid molecule is broken down. The acetyl-CoA is used up in the citric acid cycle.

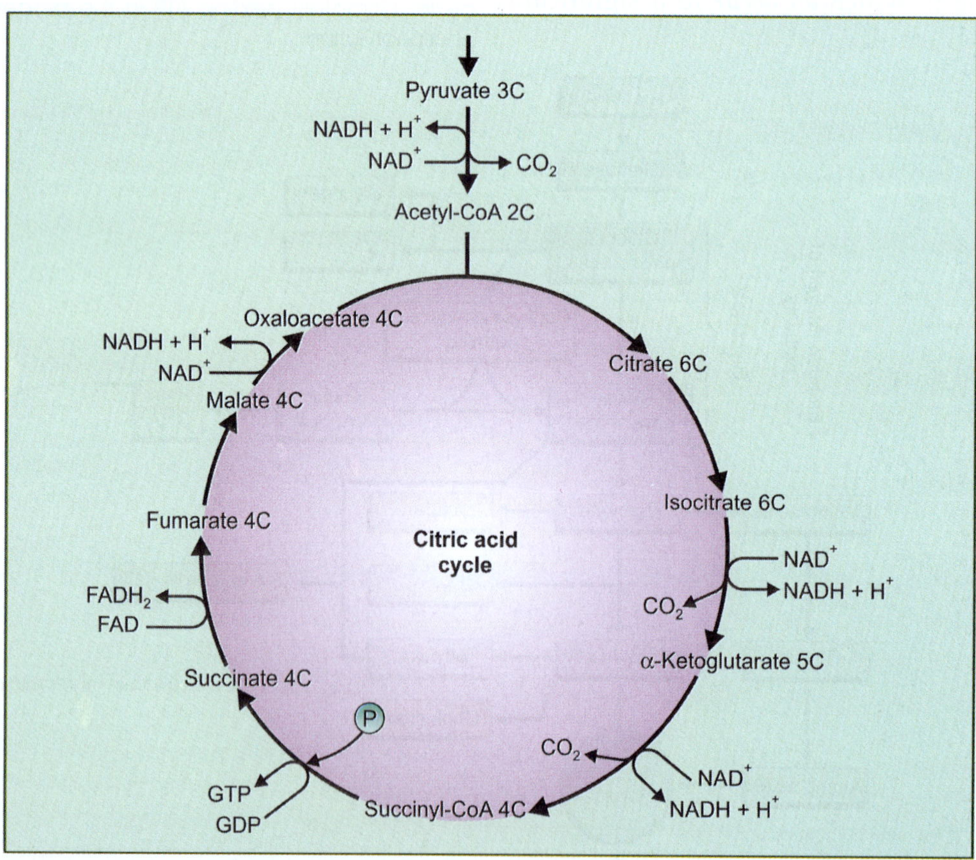

Fig. 8.18: Citric acid cycle. The numbers (6C, 5C, etc.) indicate the number of carbon atoms in each of the intermediates. The conversion of pyruvate to acetyl-CoA and each turn of the cycle provide four NADH and one FADH2 for oxidation via the flavoprotein-cytochrome chain plus formation of one GTP that is readily converted to ATP

A variable portion of fatty acid oxidation in the ***liver*** forms four carbon units (two fragments of acetyl CoA are recombined to form these) to yield **ketoacids,** i.e. **acetoacetate** and **β-hydroxybutyrate**. The production of these is because of an *imbalance,* between the flow of fatty acids into the liver mitochondria and the activity of the Krebs cycle. The water soluble ketoacids are released by the liver to be oxidized in other tissues as additional energy substances. Concentration of ketoacids is very low in the blood normally. Aceto-acetate can undergoes decarboxylation to produce **acetone** which along with the two ketoacids as above (hydroxybutyrate, acetoacetate) are all three called **ketone bodies;** the formation of which may increase in ***starvation*** and in ***diabetes mellitus*** with dearrange-ment of fat metabolism.

The **combustion of protein** first requires hydrolysis to its component **amino acids**. Each of these undergoes degradation by individual pathways, which ultimately lead to intermediate compounds of the citric acid cycle and then to acetyl-CoA and CO_2.

The citric acid cycle is the common pathway for oxidation to CO_2 and H_2O of carbohydrates, fats and some amino acids. The major entry into it is through acetyl-CoA, but a number of amino acids can be converted into citric acid cycle intermediates by deamination.

The combustion of all foods stuffs yields a large number of hydrogen atoms. These hydrogen atoms are oxidized to H_2O in the mitochondria in linkage with phosphorylation of ADP to ATP (storage of energy). In this process, three high-energy phosphate bonds are formed for each atom of oxygen used.

The citric acid cycle requires O_2 and does not func-tion under anaerobic conditions.

Energy Production

The net production of energy rich phosphate com-pounds via Embden-Meyerhof pathway, *4 molecules of ATP generated per molecule of glucose metabolized to pyruvate, reactions occur in the absence of oxygen and represent anaerobic production of energy*. Some energy is consumed in formation of products, the net gain if starting from glucose molecules is 2 molecules of ATP, and 3 molecules if starting from glycogen. Since it is anaerobic pathway the pyruvate is converted into lactate if oxygen is not available hence energy production can continue only for a while. *The lactate formed reconverts to pyruvate when oxygen becomes available.*

In this pathway NAD^+ enzyme is necessary for the conversion of phosphoglyceraldehyde to phosphglycerate. Under anaerobic conditions a block of glycolysis at the phosphoglyceraldehye conversion would occur when the NAD^+ is all converted to NADH. But pyruvate can accept H^+ from NADH to form lactate and convert it back to NAD^+ (Fig. 8.19), so the metabolism can continue for limited time in the absence of oxygen.

During muscular activity if muscular activity exceeds certain intensity and oxygen becomes limiting relative to the demand, some lactic acid can be formed under aerobic conditions; hence lactic acid can form under both aerobic and anaerobic conditions of activity.

During aerobic conditions the net production of energy (ATP) is much more; as 2 ATPs are formed under anaerobic conditions and total **of 38 ATPs are formed during aerobic conditions via both Embden-Meyerhof pathway, and citric acid cycle.** The net production of ATP per molecule of blood glucose in addition to 2 metabolized is 38.

Hexose monophosphate shunt (HMP/pentose phosphate pathway). Another pathway of glucose utilization is hexose monophosphate shunt that provides pentoses. It is direct oxidative pathway that takes place in the cytoplasm (Fig. 8.19).

Interconversions between carbohydrates, fats, and protein include conversions of a number of amino acids with carbon skeleton resembling intermediates in the Embden-Meyerhof pathway, and citric acid cycle to the intermediates by deamination. In this way; *and* by conversion of lactate to glucose; nonglucose molecules (Fig. 8.20) can be converted to glucose or glycogen **(gluconeogenesis)**. Glucose can be converted to fats (Fig. 8.17) via acetyl- CoA, but fats cannot be converted to glucose via this pathway (because the conversion of pyrauvate to acetyl-CoA is irreversible reaction), except for minor production from glycerol. Glucose can also be formed from parts of the carbon skeleton of amino acids in protein except leucine and lysine.

The **phospholipids** are constituents of cell memb-ranes and provide ***intracellular and intercellular signalling molecules.*** Fatty acids are important source of energy. For example, 1 mol of six-carbon fatty acid through citric acid cycle generates 44 mols of ATP. Compared with 38 mols generated by six-carbon of carbohydrates.

Energy Storage and Transfers

The organism has mechanisms of storage of energy for future use. The greatest part of energy reserves is in the form of fat as triglyceride, stored in adipose

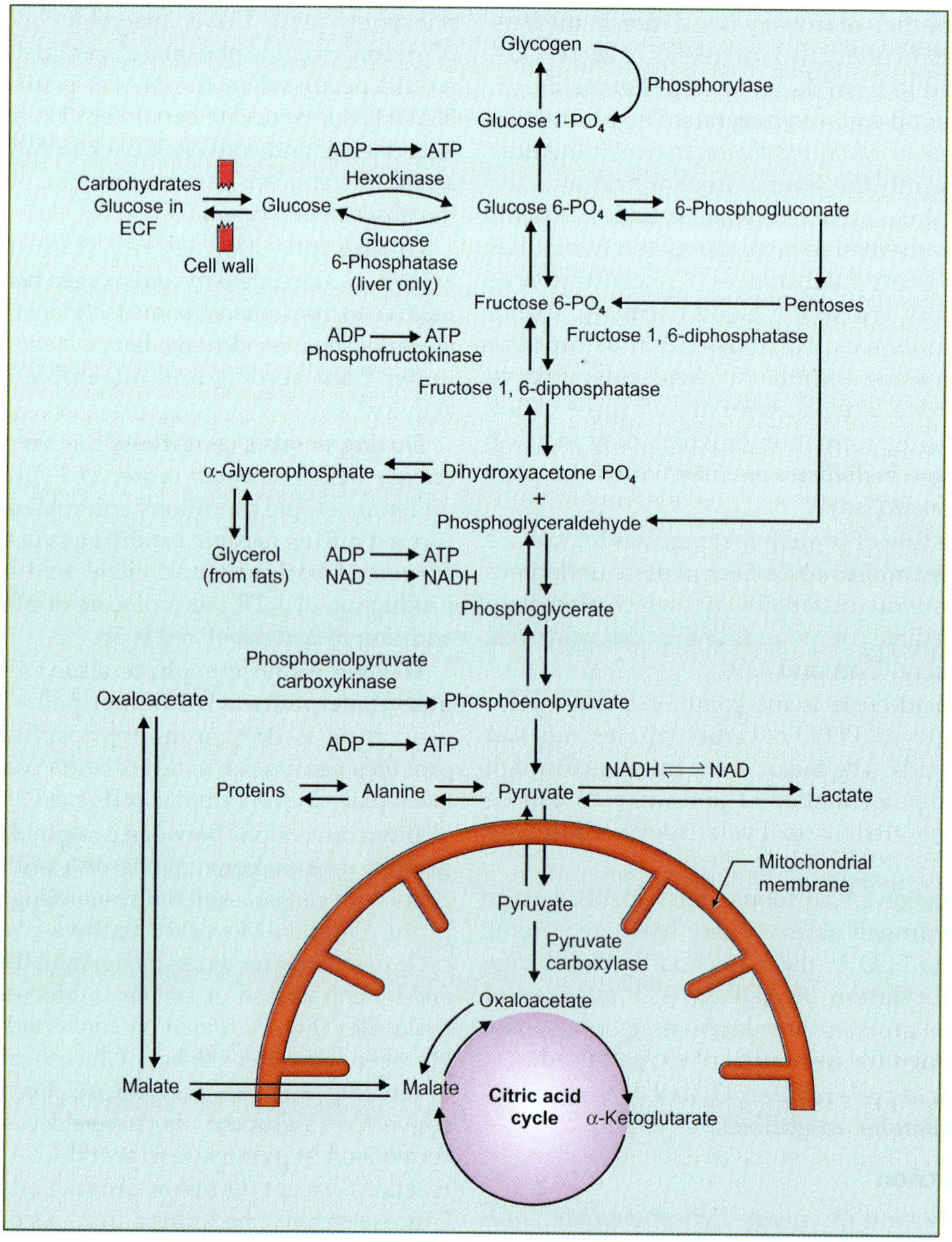

Fig. 8.19: Outline of the metabolism of carbohydrate in cells

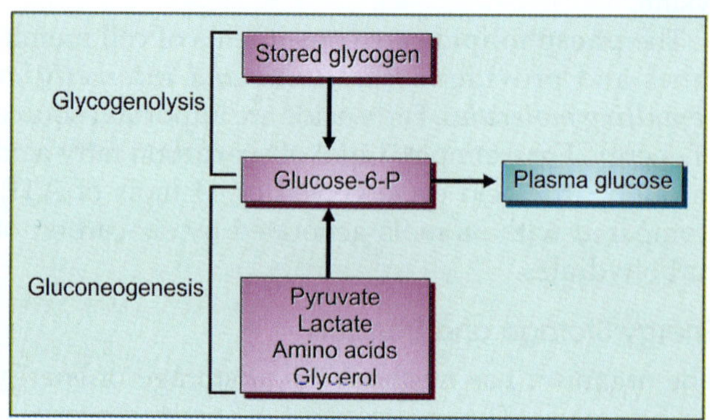

Fig. 8.20: Hepatic contribution to plasma glucose

tissue. Proportion of carbohydrate stores are trivial relative to fat store (Fig. 8.21).

In normal weight human fat constitutes 10–30% of body weight but can reach 80% in very obese individuals.

Fat is particularly efficient storage fuel (Table 8.6) because of high energy caloric density kcal/g and because of little water content. Its stores can supply energy needs of up to 2 months in totally fasted individuals of normal weight.

Triglycerides are formed by esterification of free fatty acids, mainly derived from the diet, with a

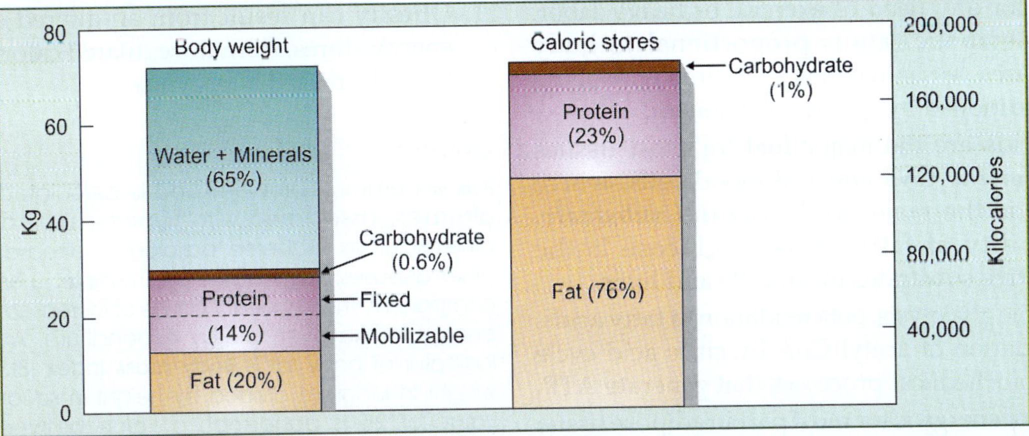

Fig. 8.21: The composition of an average 70 kg human shown in terms of weight (left) and caloric stores (right). The trivial proportion of carbohydrate stores relative to fat stores

Table 8.6: Energy equivalents of foodstuffs

	Kilocalories produced per gram	*Respiratory quotient*
Carbohydrate	4.2	1.00
Fat	9.4	0.70
Protein	4.3	0.80
Typical fuel mix	—	0.85

glycerol phosphate. But free fatty acids can also be synthesized from acetyl CoA derived from oxidation of glucose; thus carbohydrates can be converted to fat in the liver and adipose tissue and its energy stored in the adipose tissue and the energy stored in more efficient form. Fatty acid synthesis (Fig. 8.17) occurs in the cytoplasm.

Protein (4 kcal/g) constitutes almost 25% of potential energy reserves and the component amino acids can contribute to the glucose supply. As all proteins serve some vital structural and functional role, therefore their use as a major source of energy is the last resort before death from fasting.

Carbohydrates (4 kcal/gm) in the form of glucose polymer, glycogen, forms less than 1% of total energy reserves. But this portion is vital for support of **central nervous system** metabolism and for short bursts of intense muscle work. Approximately one fourth of glycogen stores (75 to 100 g) is in the liver and about three fourth (300 to 400 g) in the muscle mass.

Liver glycogen can be made available to other tissues by process of glycogenolysis and glucose release (Fig. 8.20). Muscle glycogen can only be used by muscle, since it lacks glucose 6 phosphatase, which is required for release of glucose from glycogen into bloodstream.

Glycogen can be formed from three major dietary sugars. In addition, in the liver glucose itself can also be synthesized *de novo* from three carbon precursor pyruvate, lactate and glycerol and from parts of the carbon skeleton of all 20 amino acids in protein except leucine and lysine.

The process of energy storage and transfer, themselves expends energy. This partly accounts for the stimulation of oxygen use after a meal (i.e. diet induced thermogenesis).

Because glucose and fatty acids are alternatives for competing energy substrates, some relationship between their use and their synthesis and storage within the cells exists. *Under circumstances in which fatty acids supply and plasma free fatty acids levels are increased, glucose uptake by cells is decreased.* Also intermediates of fatty acid oxidation retard glycolysis.

Conversely when dietary glucose is plentiful, glycolysis is augmented, more acetyl CoA is generated from pyruvate and more citrate is formed in the mitochondria. The citrate diffuses into cytoplasm where it is potent activator of the first step in the synthesis of fatty acids. Thus when supply of glucose is plentiful, there is net conversion of glucose carbon to fatty acid carbon. The combination of increased fatty acid synthesis and glycerol phosphate availability results in increased synthesis of triglycerides and reduced oxidation of fat. Thus increased carbohydrate utilization shifts fat metabolism from oxidation to storage.

SUMMARY

1. Energy intake is from carbohydrate, fat and protein. The expenditure is for basal metabolism, diet induced thermogenesis, sedentary activity,

further for any need of exercise or heavy labor. Basal metabolic rate is proportional to body surface area, lesser in females, declines with aging and conditioned by genetic component.

2. Fatty acids are the major fuel for most tissues ***except for the CNS*** and red blood cells, where ***glucose*** is the major and ***essential substrate***. Availability of fatty acids or glucose is the competitive substrates for muscle and liver.
3. Anaerobic glycolysis, beta oxidation of fatty acids, and oxidation of acetyl CoA by citric acid cycle are the biochemical processes that generate ATP.
4. Storage of energy is for most part in adipose tissue as triglycerides; lesser amounts as protein. Carbohydrate stores are small, hence there is need for glucose production by the liver, i.e. gluconeogenesis to maintain plasma glucose level as the need arises.
5. During long-term fasting, gluconeogenesis from amino acids, glycerol and lactate is required to maintain vital functions of metabolism of CNS and others dependent on glucose. Muscle glycogen cannot be converted into glucose, but lactate formed from it can be converted to glucose by the liver by pathway of gluconeogenesis.
6. Greater use of fatty acids during fasting greatly increases production of the ketoacids; acetone, β-hydroxybutyrate and acetoacetate.
7. Endogenous protein turnover makes it necessary a daily ingestion of protein, in particular the essential amino acids. These amino acids are irreversibly degraded and their carbon skeleton cannot be synthesized in the body.
8. Fat metabolism involves a variety of circulating lipoprotein particles that transfer triglycerides and cholesterol either originating in the diet or from synthesis in the liver; to and from various tissues. **Low density lipoprotein particles (LDL)** ***rich in cholesterol, play a role in development of atherosclerosis, whereas*** **high density lipoprotein particles (HDL)** *have a protective effect*.
9. Energy needs during exercise are met in succession by stored muscle creatine phosphate and ATP, muscle glycogen, anaerobic glycolysis and finally aerobic oxidation of glucose and then fatty acids taken up from plasma. These substances are supplied by hepatic glycogenolysis and gluconeogenesis and adipose tissue lipolysis.
10. Link of energy intake and expenditure with energy stores is not well understood process, probably controlled by hypothalamus.
11. **Obesity** can result from an altered set point of energy stores, from unregulated caloric intake, or from decreased energy use.

Obesity

It is a common problem and is associated with many diseases; associated with hypertension, accelerated atherosclerosis, diabetes, gallbladder diseases and many other diseases. The causes are multiple. There is genetic component. The important cause of increased fat is excess energy intake over energy expenditure. A convenient indicator of body fat is **Body mass index** (BMI), i.e. body weight in kilogram divided by height in square meters. A value of 25 is abnormal, a value between 25–30 is overweight and value above 35 is obese.

Hormones Related to Obesity

Leptin and Ghrelin

Intake of food is under control involving signals from periphery and central nervous system.

Leptin and ghrelin are peripheral factors that act reciprocally on food intake. Both activate their receptors on the hypothalamus.

Leptin is a satiety-producing hormone secreted by fat cells in the body.

Ghrelin is secreted by stomach and appears to play an important role in control of food intake, it stimulates food intake.

Ghrelin is **orexin** affects via actions on hypothalamus, increases synthesis and release of central orexins, suppresses the ability of leptin to stimulate anorexingenic factors in the hypothalamus. Leptin produced by adipose tissue signals the status of fat stores. As adipocytes increase in size they increase the release of leptin and this tends to decrease food intake. Leptin also stimulates the metabolic rate.

Ghrelin is fast acting and stimulates food intake. It is believed to be involved in meal initiation and unlike long acting effects of leptin, though it also acts at the hypothalamus.

CCK by 'I' cells in the intestine or released in the brain by nerve endings inhibits food intake and is a satiety factor (anorexin).

Other possible explanation to obesity occurrence. Resistance to leptin could be a factor causing obesity. Ability of leptin to reduce ghrelin secretion may be lost in obesity.

Loss of activity of ghrelin may be partly responsible for effectiveness of gastric bypass procedures for obesity.

METABOLIC ADAPTATIONS

Fasting

In fasting state individual depends on endogenous substates for energy. Mobilization of glucose provides essential fuel for the CNS, release of free fatty acids provides for needs of other tissues. During long-term fasting gluconeogenesis from amino acids, glycerol, lactate is required to sustain CNS metabolism and other critical functions dependent on glucose. Increased use of fatty acids during fasting greatly increases production of the ketoacids, β-hydroxybutyrate and acetoacetate.

NUTRITION

The aim of nutrition is to determine the food substances that promote health and well-being. It must have energy value sufficient to provide for: the requirements of BMR; diet induced thermogenesis; varying needs of muscular and external work; in children growing tissue needs; special needs of menstruation, pregnancy, lactation, illness and old age must be taken into account. It includes the problem of undernutrition and overnutrition.

Essential Dietary Nutrients

Diet should include adequate amount of *water, adequate calories, protein, fat, minerals and vitamins.*

Calorie intake. Intake must balance the output, if body weight is to be kept constant. **About 2000 Calories a day are required for Basal metabolic rate and thermogenic effect of food in an adult; 500–2500 C** more may be required depending on the amount of **physical activity** carried on daily.

The absolute minimal energy expenditure, i.e. basal metabolic rate (BMR) amounts to on an average daily expenditure of about 20 to 25 Calories/kg of body weight.

Ingestion of food causes a small increase in energy expenditure called **diet induced thermogenesis**. It is due to increased rate of reactions involved in deposition of the ingested calories, like storage of glucose as glycogen or degradation of amino acids to urea.

Additional energy is used in **occupational and purposeful exercise**, it varies in individuals. During short periods of occupational or recreational exercise energy expenditure can increase more than tenfold over basal levels.

The distribution of calories among carbohydrate, protein and fat is determined by physiological and economic factors and the taste requirements When calculating dietary needs, **protein requirement** is first calculated; daily intake of 1 gm of protein per kg body weight is enough to supply **essential amino acids** and other requirements. The source of protein is also important. **Grade I proteins**, the animal proteins of meat, fish, egg, contain amino acids adequate for protein synthesis and other uses; **grade II proteins** from vegetable sources, because they lack in one or the other **essential amino acid**, the intake should be from variable sources and in large amounts. Some vegetable proteins like those from **soyabean** flour are often classified as grade I proteins. Pregnant and lactating women require more protein about 1.5–2 gm/kg of body weight.

Fats are expensive and low fat intake adequate to provide **essential fatty acids and fat soluble vitamins** is recommended; with ***high ratio of unsaturated to saturated fat***. In cold climates where calorie need is high or for physical work; the bulk of meal can be reduced by including more fat in food as they provide more calories per gm of weight. ***Animal fats are rich source of vitamin A and D. Vegetable fats are effective*** in providing calories but ***deficient in vitamins except vitamin E.***

Carbohydrates are cheap source of calorie requirements and at least 50% Calorie needs can be met by taking them, 15% can come from protein and 35% from fat.

Vitamins are defined as substances necessary for life, health and growth that do not function for supply for energy. Required for health and inadequate intake leads to diseases as tabulated (Table 8.7). They are divided into two groups; fat soluble which are vitamin A, D, E, K, these are fat soluble and present in fats; water soluble vitamins are **vitamin C and B complex.** B complex is a group which includes—**Thiamine, riboflavin, nicotinic acid, pyridoxine, biotin, pantothenic acid, folic acid, vitamin B_{12}.** The water soluble vitamins are easily absorbed; fat soluble vitamins suffer absorption if fats are poorly absorbed. Very large doses of fat soluble are toxic.

Vitamins A: Sources include liver fat, egg and milk fat. Beta carotene is provitamin, which is converted into vitamin A in the body. It is derived from green vegetables and carrots and fruits. Vitamin A maintains helath of epithelial cells; it is essential constituent of pigment in rods and cones (the visual receptors); essential for fetal development and cell development throughout life. Both Vitamin A and carotene are stable and can withstand ordinary process of cooking.

Vitamins D: It is fomed in the skin by sunlight which converts 7- dehydrocholesterol to cholecalciferol

Table 8.7: Diseases resulting from vitamin deficiency

Vitamin	*Deficiency disease*
Water soluble vitamins	
Thiamine	Leads to beriberi, GI disturbances, skeletal muscle paralysis, congestive heart failure and polyneuropathy (due to degeneration of myelin sheath), poor appetite and impaired growth
Riboflavin	Angular fissures in the lips (cheilosis), angular stomatitis, poor growth, dermatitis, and cataract
Cyanocobalamin (B)	*Decreased RBC count* and hemoglobin leading to pernicious anaemia, *neurological lesions* leading to ataxia, memory loss, mood changes
Pyridoxine (B)	Dermatitis of eye, nose and mouth, growth retardation
Pantothenic acid	Fatigue, muscle spasms, vomiting, deficient production of adrenal steroids
Biotin	Depression, dermatitis, muscular pain, fatigue
Folic acid	*Megaloblastic anaemia,* decreased hemoglobin, gastrointestinal lesions
Niacin	Inflammation of tongue, lips, dry skin, diarrhoea, irritability, dementia, anxiety (pellagra)
Vitamin C	*Bleeding spongy gums,* loose teeth leading to scurvy, *decreased immunity,* patient is prone to infections, poor wound healing
Fat soluble vitamins	
Vitamin A	Dry skin, hair and cornea; *increased incidence of infection; night blindness;* faulty development of bone and teeth; conjunctival ulceration
Vitamin D	Rickets in children and osteomalacia in adults due to *defective utilization of calcium*
Vitamin E	Hemolytic anaemia, abnormal function of mitochondria and lysosomes, ataxia
Vitamin K	Excessive bleeding due to *increased clotting time*

which is activated in the liver and kidney. Dietary sources include fish liver oils, egg yolk and fat of the milk. It is essential for absorption of calcium and phosphorus from GI tract and helps to maintain calcium balancce in the body.

Vitamins E: Sources include milk, eggs, meat, fresh nuts, wheat grain and green leafy vegetables.

Vitamins K is produced by intestinal bacteria. Dietary sources are spinach, cauliflower, cabbage and liver. It is required for formation of clotting factors in the liver.

B group vitamins: Sources include yeast, fermented foods, milk, liver, green vegetables, pulses and cereals.

The vitamin group has role as coenzymes in the metabolism of protein, carbohydrates, fat and in hemopoiesis.

Vitamins C (Ascorbic acid): Citrus fruits are rich sources, other fruits and green leafy vegetables also supply the vitamin. It is required for the maintenance of healthy gums, skin, protection against infection. It promotes collagen synthesis and wound healing.

Vitamins B_6, B_{12}, and folate: An elevated level of homocysteine is associated with increased cardiovascular risk. Homocysteine which is thought to be toxic to vascular endothelium is converted to harmless amino acids by the action of enzymes that require the B vitamins; foliate, B_6 (pyridoxine), and B_{12} (cobalamine). Foliate and B_6 are found in leafy green vegetables, whole grains, some fruits. B_{12} is found in animal food, meat, fish and eggs.

Minerals also form an important requirement in the diet. A number of minerals must be ingested in the diet daily (Table 8.8), besides some trace elements (iodine for thyroid function, zinc is a part of many enzymes, carbonic anhydrase and some peptidases for protein digestion in GIT, etc.) should be included. Trace elements are defined as those present in tissues in small amounts.

Calcium absorption is influenced by **vitamin D** and adequate intake of it should be especially important in growing children, pregnant and lactating mothers. Iron requirement is to be taken care, especially important in growing children, pregnant and lactating women. **Iron deficiency** results in anemia. Cobalt is a part of **vitamin B_{12}** and deficiency of this vitamin results in megaloblastic anemia. Iodine deficiency causes thyroid disorders. Zinc deficiency causes skin ulcers, depressed immune responses, and hypogonadal dwarfism. Copper deficiency causes anemia and changes in ossification. Chromium deficiency causes insulin resistance. Fluorine deficiency causes increased incidence of dental caries.

Dietary fiber, is the nondigestable carbohydrates and lignin (a complex polymer of phenylpropanoid subunits) present in plants. Dietary fiber does not provide energy but has many other functions. It adds bulk to the diet, absorbs water, drawing fluid into the lumen of intestine and increases bowl motility, also results in delays absorption of glucose to reduce peaks. LDL level is reduced due to reduced absorption of bile in the intestine. Constipation, hemorrhoids risk, diverticulosis and colon cancer risk is reduced.

Calorie requirements decrease in **old age** due to decrease in BMR and physical activity.

Table 8.8: Nutrients and their source

Essential nutrients	*Nature of nutrient*	*Source*
Amino acids	Essential amino acids viz. methionine, tryptophan, threonine, valine, leucine, isoleucine, phenylalanine and lysine	Soya beans, milk, fish meat and eggs
Fatty acids	Polyunsaturated fatty acids (PUFA) viz. linoleic acid and arachidonic acid	All vegetables oils
Water soluble vitamins	B group vitamins and vitamin C	Milk, liver green vegetables, yeast and citrus fruits
Fat soluble vitamins	A, D, E, K	Milk, fish, liver oil, cooking oils, green vegetables, carrots, etc.
Energy foods	Carbohydrates, fats and proteins	Rice, wheat, cooking oils, butter, pulses, meat, fish and eggs
Fibre	Undigestible plant material like cellulose, gums, pectins, lignins	Husk of cereals, whole wheat flour, vegetables, salads and fruits
Water	Critical component of diet	Drinking water, all vegetables and fruits
Iodine	Sea fish, onion, iodised salt	Thyroid hormones require iodine for their synthesis
Iron	Meat, fish, dark green vegetables, soya bean, spinach	Forms essential part of hemoglobin, constituent of many enzymes in carbohydrate metabolism
Calcium	Eggs, milk, cheese, green vegetables, soya beans and lentils	It is needed for teeth and bone formation, coagulation of blood, muscle contraction and enzyme activity, release of hormones and neurotransmitters
Phosphorus	Eggs, milk, cheese, liver, green vegetables, wheat, maize, soya beans and nuts	Teeth and bone formation, salts of it act as blood buffers and energy rich biomolecules (ATP), role in muscle contraction and nerve activity
Sodium	Table salt, found in all types of food	It plays a role in neuronal transmission, role in nerve and muscle action potential, maintenance of electrolyte balance
Potassium	Found in all foods	Required in muscle contraction and neve transmission, maintenance of electrolyte balance
Fluorine	Drinking water, tea and fish	Fluorine in tooth helps in maintaining dental enamel. It prevents caries
Magnesium	Seafood, cereals, green leafy vegetables	Role in functioning of muscle and nervous tissue, bone formation, constituent of many coenzymes

The Table 8.9, gives the recommended dietary allowances for different age groups.

Hypervitaminosis

Large doses of the fat soluble vitamins are toxic. **Hypervitaminosis A** is characterized by anorexia, headache, hepatosplenomegaly, irritability, scaly dermatitus patchy loss of hair, bone pain, and hyperostosis. Acute vitamin A intoxication with headache, diarrhea, and dizziness. **Hypervitaminosis D** is associated weight loss, calcification of many soft tissues, and renal failure. **Hypervitaminosis K** is characterized by gastrointestinal disturbances and anemia. Large doses of water soluble vitamins are less likely to cause problems because they can be rapidly cleared from the body. But ingestion of mega dose of pyridoxine (vitamin B_6) can produce peripheral neuropathy.

Inadequate nutrition in **children** can lead to **marasmus** due to deficient calorie and protein intake and or to **Kwashiorkor** due to deficient protein intake.

MARASMUS

It occurs when calorie deprivation is relatively greater than the reduction in protein. It occurs in children younger than one year of age when the breast milk is supplemented with thin watery cereals. There is stunned growth, extreme muscle wasting, weakness and anemia, but there is no edema.

KWASHIORKOR

It occurs when protein deprivation is relatively greater than reduction in total calories. There is severe loss of visceral protein. It is often seen in children after weaning at about one year of age, when the diet consists predominantly of carbohydrates. Symptoms include stunted growth, edema, skin lesions, anorexia, and enlarged fatty liver. The child shows big belly due to edema.

Table 8.9: Recommended dietary allowance (RDA) for Indian population (Indian Council of Medical Research, 1922)

	Energy (kcal)	*Protein (g)*	*Calcium (mg)*	*Iron (mg)*	*Vit. A (μg)*	*Vit. C (mg)*	*Folic acid (μg)*	*Vit. B_{12} (μg)*
Men (adult)	2875	60	400	28	600	40	100	1.0
Women (adult)	2225	50	400	30	600	40	100	1.0
Pregnancy	2525	65	1000	38	600	40	400	1.0
Lactation	2775	75	1000	30	950	80	150	1.5
Infants								
0–6 months	108 kcal/kg	2.05 g/kg	500	—	350	25	25	0.2
6–12 months	98 kcal/kg	1.65 g/kg	500	—	350	25	25	0.2
Children								
1–3 years	1240	22	400	12	400	40	30	1.0
3–6 years	1690	30	400	18	400	40	40	1.0
6–9 years	1950	41	400	26	600	40	60	1.0
Boys								
10–12 years	2190	54	600	19	600	40	70	1.0
13–15 years	2450	70	600	28	600	40	100	1.0
16–18 years	2640	78	500	30	600	40	100	1.0
Girls								
10–12 years	1970	57	600	34	600	40	70	1.0
13–15 years	2060	65	600	41	600	40	100	1.0
16–18 years	2060	63	500	50	600	40	100	1.0

Table 8.10: Lipid profile

LDL cholesterol	<100	Optimal
	100–129	Near or above normal
	130–159	Borderline high
	160–189	High
	>190	Very high
Total cholesterol	<200	Desirable
	200–239	Borderling high
	>240	High
HDL cholesterol	<40	Low
	>60	High

Table 8.11: Proportion of types of fat in different oils

Oils	*Saturated*	*Mono-unsaturated*	*Poly-unsaturated*	*Trans*
Olive	13	72	8	0
Mustard	7	58	29	0
Safflower	9	12	74	0
Sunflower	10	20	66	0
Soyabean	16	44	37	0
Peanut	17	49	32	0
Palm	50	37	10	0
Coconut	87	6	2	0
Dalda (lard)	39	44	11	1
Butter	60	26	5	5
Shortening	22	2	29	18

IMPLICATIONS AND APPLICATIONS

- Understand the requirement of the essential constituents of a balanced diet; the special requirements during pregnancy, lactation and for a growing child.
- Recommend the diet to prevent cardiovascular diseases, diabetes and obesity. Refer to Tables 8.10 and 8.11.

Four major groups of plasma lipoproteins identified

- Because fat is less dense than water, the density of a lipoprotein decreases as the proportion of lipid to protein increases. In addition to FFA, four major groups of lipoproteins are identified, important physiologically and in clinical diagnosis. These are:
  1. **Chylomicrons**, from intestinal absorption of triacylglycerol and other lipids.
  2. **Very low density lipoproteins** (VLDL), derived from the liver for the export of triacylglycerol.
  3. **Low-density lipoproteins** (LDL), representing a final stage in the catabolism of VLDL.
  4. **High-density lipoproteins** (HDL), involved in VLDL and chylomicron metabolism and also in cholesterol transport. Triacylglycerol is the predominent lipid in chylomicrons and VLDL, whereas cholesterol and phospholipid are the predominent lipids in LDL and HDL, respectively.

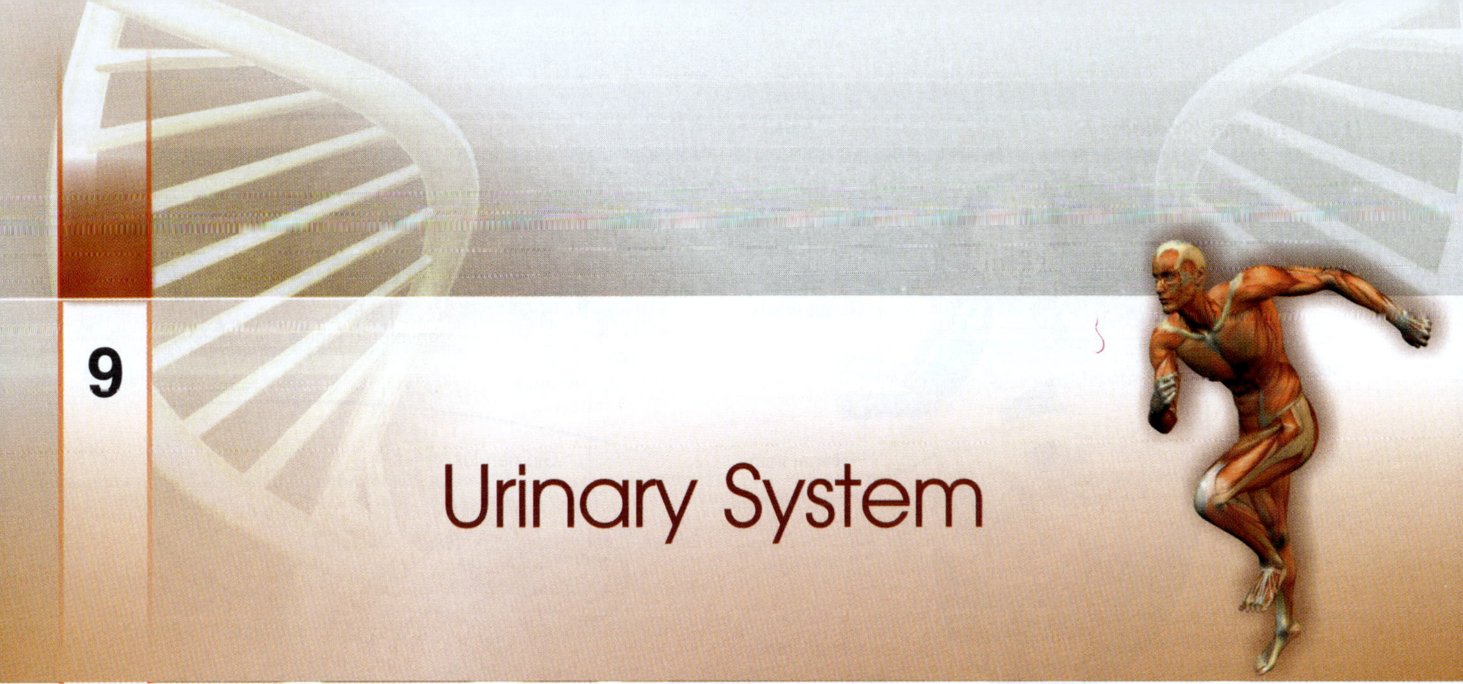

9 Urinary System

The urinary system is essentially an excretory system. But, the kidneys also have a role in the formation of some hormones.

The urinary system consists of:

- Two kidneys which form urine; two ureters, one from each kidney through which urine passes from the kidney to the urinary bladder (Fig. 9.1).
- One urinary bladder where the urine collects to be stored temporarily.

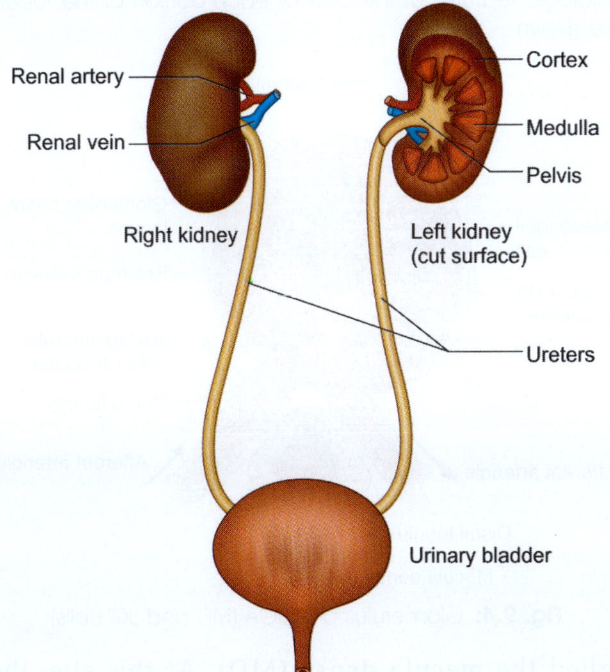

Fig. 9.1: Kidneys with parts of the urinary system. Cut section of kidney on the left

- One urethra through which the urine is voided from the bladder to the exterior by the process of micturition.

The functions of kidneys are:

- Maintain homeostasis of water and electrolyte concentrations, hence maintains body fluid osmolality and volume.
- Excrete metabolic waste products, e.g. urea, uric acid, and foreign substances, etc.
- Maintain pH of blood by excreting acidic or alkaline urine.
- Form erythropoietin, a hormone which has an important role in erythropoiesis.
- Produce renin which has a role in the regulation of blood pressure.
- Form ***active*** vitamin D_3 (calcitriol).

ANATOMICAL POSITION

The kidneys lie in the posterior abdominal wall, one on each side of vertebral column with right kidney being slightly lower than left, embedded in fat, behind the peritoneum (retroperitoneal position). A thin capsule covers each kidney. Adrenal glands are at the upper part of kidneys on each side.

GROSS STRUCTURE

Below the capsule of the kidney seen on cut section is the outer part cortex and in inner part the medulla (Fig. 9.1). The medulla is made-up of 15 or 16 medullary pyramids, the apex of which open into calyces, which communicate with the pelvis of the kidney from where the ureter arises on each side (Fig. 9.2).

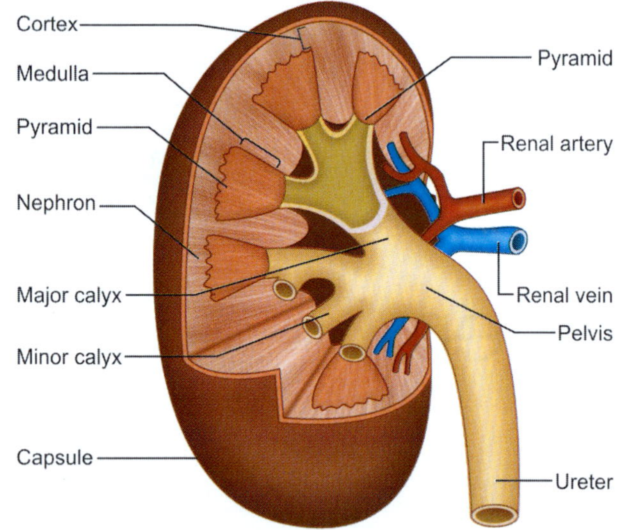

Fig. 9.2: Structure of the kidney, cut open (posterior view) parts of capsule seen

MICROSCOPIC STRUCTURE

The functional unit of kidney is a nephron and each kidney contains over a million nephrons.

The nephron is a tubule which is closed at one end where it engulfs a tuft of intercommunicating capillaries, the glomerulus (Fig. 9.3). The capillaries are surrounded by the closed end of nephron forming Bowman's capsule, with two layers, the inner one surrounds the capillaries and the outer one is continuous with the next part of the nephron called the proximal convoluted tubule (Figs 9.4 and 9.5). The two layers enclose a space where filtered fluid is formed.

The afferent arteriole brings blood into the glomerular capillaries and capillaries unite to form efferent arteriole which leaves the capillary tuft. Hence, the glomerular capillaries are present between two sets of arterioles (Fig. 9.4) unlike at other sites where capillaries drain into venules. As a result, the hydrostatic pressure is higher in glomerular capillaries than elsewhere in capillaries.

The proximal convoluted tubule (PCT) is highly convoluted and is present in the cortex. It continues as the descending limb of loop of Henle which dips down into the medulla of the kidney then forms the ascending limb (AL) of the loop of Henle which ascends to reach the cortex at a place between the afferent and the efferent arterioles of its own glomerulus; where it forms the distal convoluted tubule (DCT) which is present in the cortex of the kidney. At the formation of DCT, the epithelial cells of the AL are closely packed together. This region is

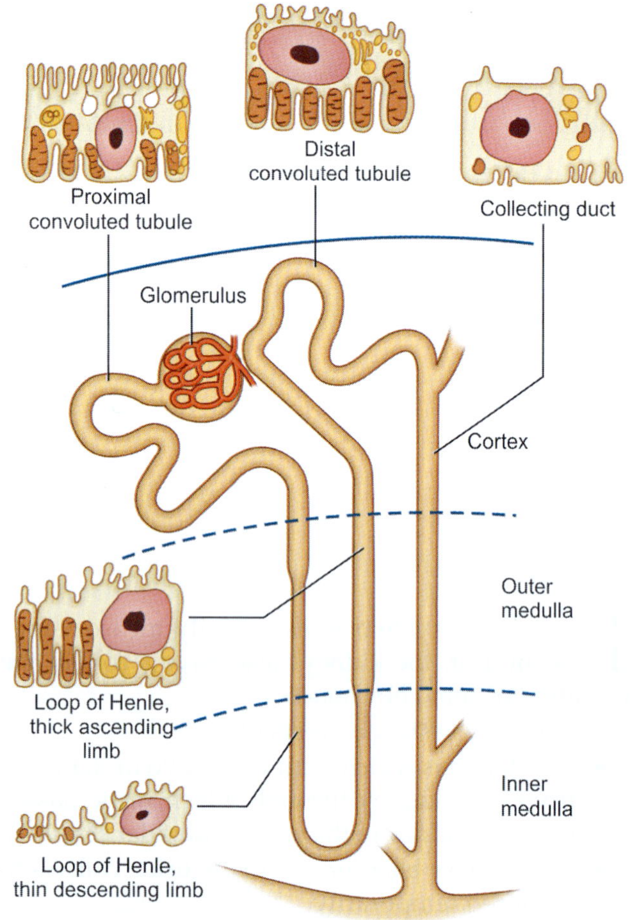

Fig. 9.3: Diagram of a nephron (juxtamedullary). The main histologic features of the cells of each portion of the tubule are shown

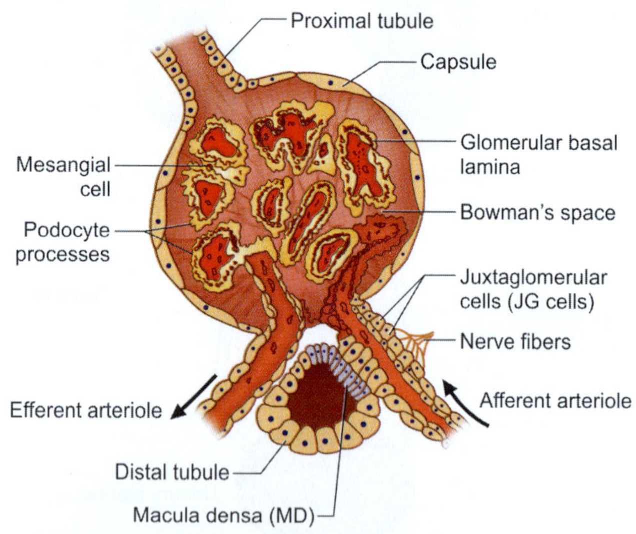

Fig. 9.4: Glomerulus and JGA (MD and JG cells)

called the **macula densa (MD).** At this site, the adjoining afferent arteriole in its media contains cells, the **juxtaglomerular (JG) cells** which secrete renin.

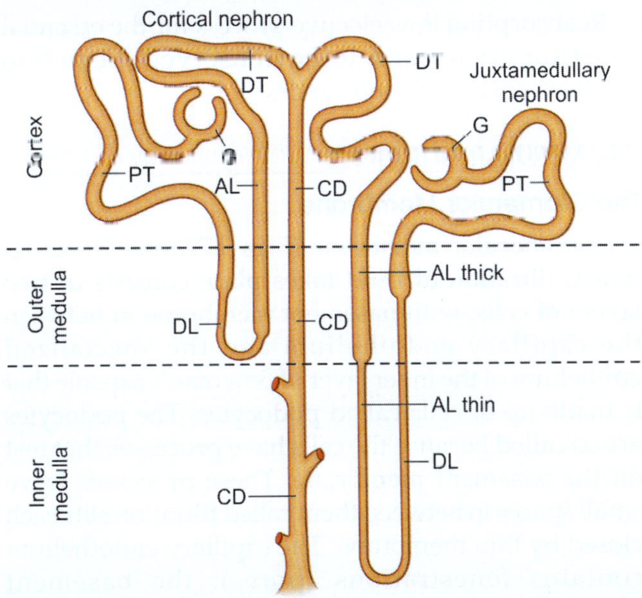

Fig. 9.5: Nephrons of cortical and juxtamedullary types: G–glomerulus, PT–proximal tubule, DT–distal tubule, DL–descending limb, AL–ascending limb, CD–collecting duct

The JG cells and the MD cells (Fig. 9.4) and some lacis cells in between them, all three structures are called the **Juxtaglomerular apparatus (JGA).** JGA has a role in the regulation of renin secretion. MD has a role in sensing some constituents of filtrate and the stimulus is transmitted to the JG cells for the secretion of renin which regulates glomerular filtration rate (GFR).

The glomeruli are present only in the cortex of the kidney. Those glomeruli which are present in the superficial region of the cortex have short loops of Henle. Other glomeruli that are present deep in the cortex at the junction of the cortex with medulla, the nephrons are called **juxtamedullary nephrons** and have long loops of Henle (Fig. 9.5) and the ascending limb of the loop of Henle has long thick portion after the thin portion. The absorption of ions in this thick portion contributes to the urinary dilution. Hence, these nephrons have an important role in the formation of very dilute or concentrated urine. The juxtamedullary nephrons form 15% of the total nephron population.

The distal convoluted tubule opens into a collecting duct. The kidney tubules are thin tubules consisting of single layer of epithelium. The collecting ducts pass through the cortex and then through the medulla to open into the pelvis of the kidney at the medullary pyramids.

The renal artery enters the kidney at the hilum and divides into smaller branches which give rise to an afferent arteriole for each glomerulus. It breaks into glomerular capillary network that rejoins to form the efferent arteriole which again breaks up into another set of capillaries which surround the tubules of nephrons. The efferent arteriole from the juxtamedullary nephrons forms long straight vessels (vasa recta) that descend deep down into medulla (Figs 9.6A and B) and ascend up again along with the long loops of

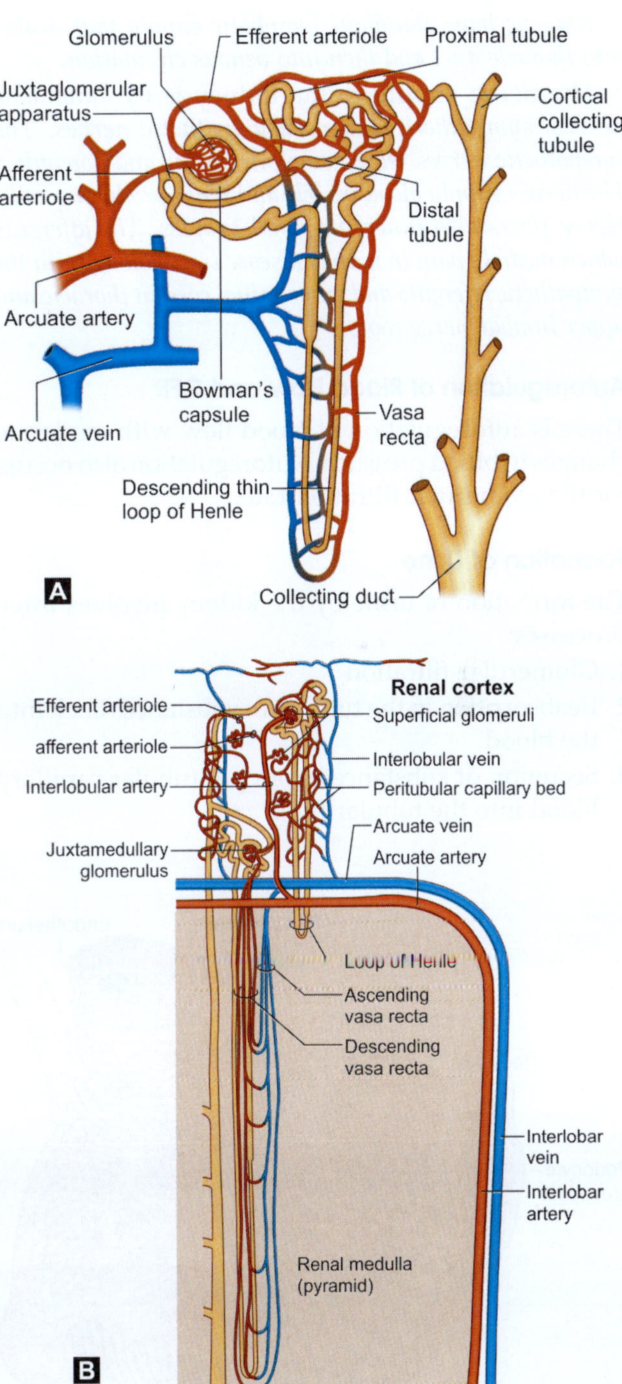

Figs 9.6A and B: (A) Enlarged juxtamedullary nephron with vasa recta. (B) Glomerular capillaries and blood vessels

Henle of these nephrons. These long straight vessels have important role in the concentration of urine, in association with long loops of Henle. The blood finally drains into the renal vein which leaves the kidney to open into inferior vena cava.

The total renal blood flow to the kidneys is approximately 1,300 mL/min (25% of the resting cardiac output).

Kidneys have abundant lymphatic supply that drains into thoracic duct and then into venous circulation.

The nerve supply to the kidney is by *autonomic nerves, sympathetic and parasympathetic nerves. The sympathetic nerves release norepinephrine and dopamine. The nerves supply blood vessels and renin producing cells. Nerve fibers also innervate renal tubules. The afferents which mediate pain in kidney disease travel along with the sympathetic efferents and enter spinal cord in thoracic and upper lumbar nerve roots.*

Autoregulation of Blood Flow and GFR

There is autoregulation of blood flow with moderate changes in blood pressure. Autoregulation also occurs for the glomerular filtration rate.

Formation of Urine

The formation of urine by the kidney involves three processes:

1. Glomerular filtration
2. Reabsorption in the tubules of substances back into the blood.
3. Secretion of substances from peritubular capillary blood into the tubular fluid.

Reabsorption is a selective process for the essential constituents needed to be conserved. Secretion involves only some substances.

GLOMERULAR FILTRATION

The Glomerular Membrane

The glomerular membrane (Figs 9.7A and B) across which filtration of fluid takes place consists of two layers of cells, with basement membrane in between the capillary endothelium and the specialized epithelium of the inner layer of Bowman's capsule that is made-up of cells called podocytes. The podocytes are so called because the cells have processes that rest on the basement membrane. These processes leave small spaces in between them called filtration slits each closed by thin membrane. The capillary endothelium contains fenestrations (pores); the basement membrane is complete with no pores. This structure of the glomerular membrane does not permit the blood cells or plasma proteins to pass through it, because of their large size; and there are negative charges on the membrane which repel the negatively charged proteins in the blood. There are cells called mesangial cells that are located in between the basement membrane and the capillary endothelium (Fig. 9.8). They are contractile in function and play a role in regulation of GFR.

Filtration takes place from the glomerular capillaries, ultrafiltrate of plasma (plasma minus proteins) is formed into the Bowman's capsular space, and there are no cells that pass into the capsular fluid. The rate of filtration of glomerular fluid taking place

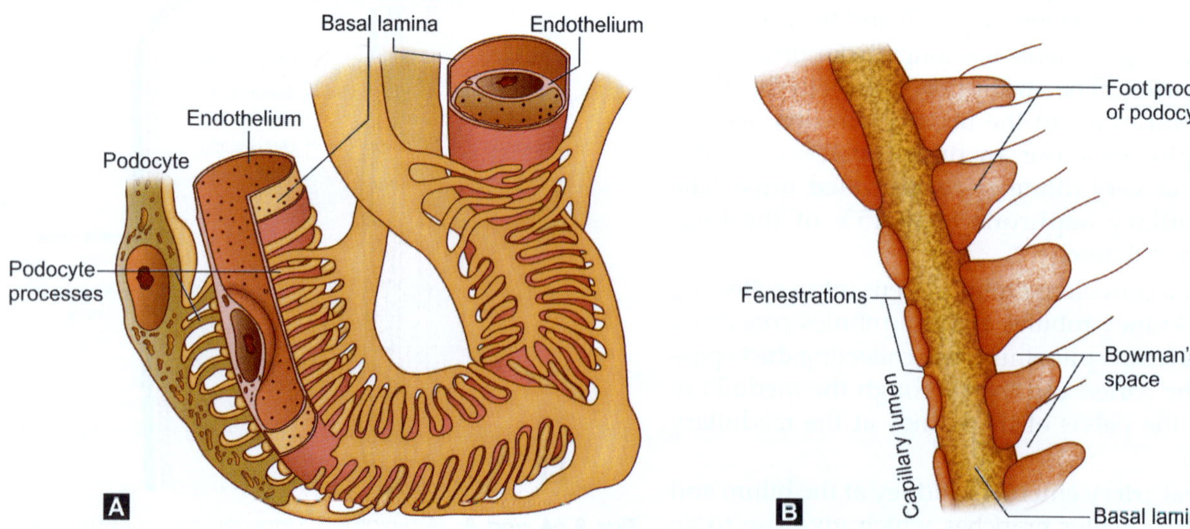

Figs 9.7A and B: (A) Podocyte processes lining capillary wall (B) The filtration membrane

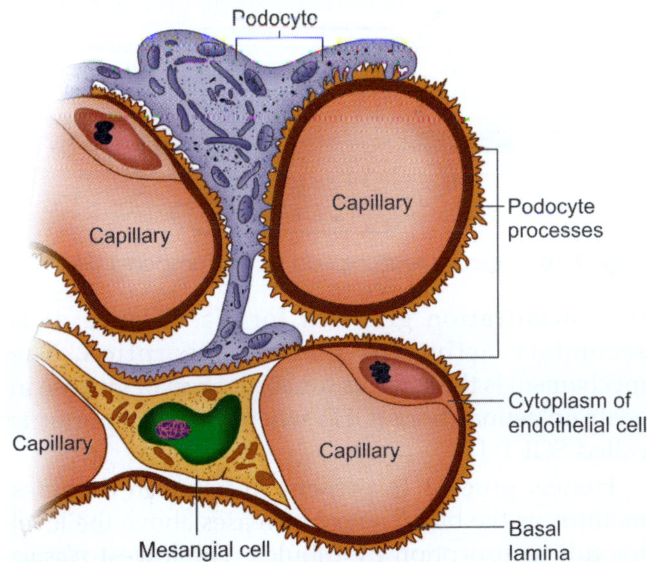

Fig. 9.8: Mesangial cell and its relation to glomerular capillaries

in all the glomeruli of both the kidneys is called **GFR.** This is approximately ***125 mL/min in an adult***.

The rate is dependent upon the (1) filtration *pressure in the glomeruli* and (2) the *rate of blood flow through the kidney*. The other factors that remain constant except in pathological conditions are (1) the total area of glomerular membrane available for filtration and (2) the permeability of the membrane.

The filtration pressure which determines the GFR is dependent on *net hydrostatic* and *net osmotic pressures*.

Glomerular Pressures

Hydrostatic pressure of blood in the glomerular capillaries minus the hydrostatic pressure in Bowman's capsule is the net hydrostatic pressure which promotes filtration by forcing water and solutes of plasma through the filtration membrane. Plasma proteins are unable to pass through the filtration membrane. There are normally no proteins in the Bowman's capsular fluid and the osmotic pressure of plasma proteins of 25–30 mmHg is the net oncotic pressure which opposes filtration and it tends to retain fluid in the capillaries. The balance is in favor of filtration as the net hydrostatic pressure exceeds by about 10–15 mmHg, the net oncotic pressure of plasma proteins (Fig. 9.9), filtration is caused by this pressure difference.

Hence the:

$$GFR = K_f\,[(P_{GC} - P_T) - (\pi_{GC} - \pi_T)]$$

K_f is glomerular ultrafiltration coefficient, is a product of the glomerular capillary wall permeability and the effective filtration surface area. P_{GC} is the mean hydrostatic pressure in the glomerular capillaries. π_{GC} is the oncotic pressure of the plasma in the glomerular capillaries and P_T is the hydrostic pressure in tubule in Bowman's space and π_T is the oncotic pressure of the filtrate in Bowman's space.

The GFR is about 125 mL per minute, resulting GFR per day (in 24 hours) is about 180 liters formed by both the kidneys. Most of this, filtered fluid is reabsorbed in the tubules of the kidney and the urine formed per day by an adult is about 1–1.5 liters. It may vary depending upon intake of fluids and output of water from other routes in the body. Kidneys maintain the homeostasis of water balance. Table 9.1 shows other routes of water loss.

The minimum excretion of urine in an adult can not decrease to less than 500 mL. This volume is necessary for excretion of solutes, and this urine volume is called ***volume obligatoire***.

Filtration Fraction

The ratio of the **GFR** to the renal plasma flow (**RPF**) is filtration fraction. It is normally between 0.16 and 0.20 (GFR = 125/RPF = 700). When there is fall in systemic blood pressure, the GFR falls less than RBF because of constriction of efferent arterioles due to sympathetic discharge.

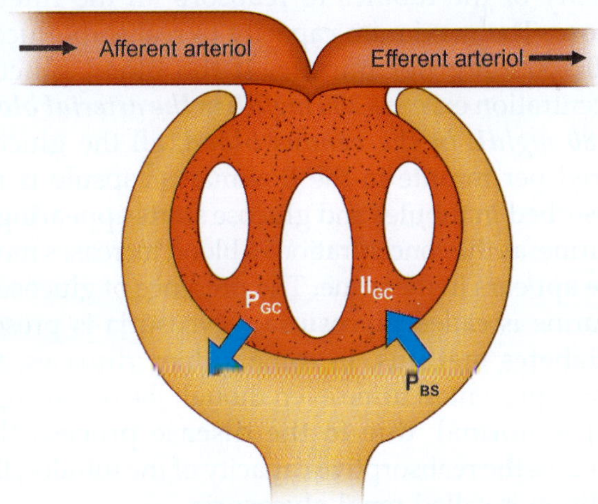

Fig. 9.9: Glomerular pressures

Glomerular capillary (P_{GC}) hydrostatic pressure—45 mmHg; Bowman's space (P_{BS}) hydrostatic pressure—10 mmHg — Net hydrostatic pressure 35 mmHg

Glomerular capillary oncotic (π_{GC}) pressure—25 mmHg; Bowman's space oncotic pressure—0 mm Hg — Net oncotic pressure 25 mmHg

Net filtration pressure = 35–25 = 10 mmHg

Table 9.1: Daily loss of water (in milliliters)

	Normal temperature	*Hot weather*	*Prolonged heavy exercise*
Insensible loss			
• Skin	350	350	350
• Respiratory tract	350	250	650
Urine	1,400	1,200	500
Sweat	100	1,400	5,000
Feces	100	100	100
Total	**2,300**	**3,300**	**6,600**

The final composition of the urine differs from that of plasma because of the selective process of reabsorption and secretion in the tubules involving different components of the filtrate.

Reabsorption

There is selective reabsorption as follows:

Glucose

Normally, all the glucose filtered in the glomerular fluid is reabsorbed in the PCT. Hence, there is no glucose in the urine in normal individuals. This holds true till the filtered glucose does not exceed the capacity of the tubules to reabsorb all the filtered glucose. The maximum capacity to reabsorb glucose is 300–375 mg per minute. If the blood glucose concentration exceeds ***200 mg/dL in the arterial blood or 180 mg/dL in the venous blood,*** all the glucose filtered per minute in the Bowman's capsule is not reabsorbed in tubules and glucose starts appearing in the urine; as the concentration in blood increases more, more appears in the urine. The presence of glucose in the urine is called **glycosuria**. Glycosuria is present in **diabetes mellitus**. In some kidney diseases, the sugar is present in urine even though the blood sugar level is normal, due to the disease process that decreases the reabsorptive capacity of the tubules, this condition is called **renal glycosuria**.

The mechanism for glucose reabsorption in the proximal tubule involves a carrier protein in the membrane of the tubular cells, called glucose transporter, SGLT-2. It is a cotransporter (Fig. 9.10) which requires presence of sodium ions for transport of glucose across the membrane, and the process is secondary active since it depends on active transport of sodium ions across the basolateral membrane, that creates a low concentration of sodium in the cell; that draws the glucose along with sodium into the cell due

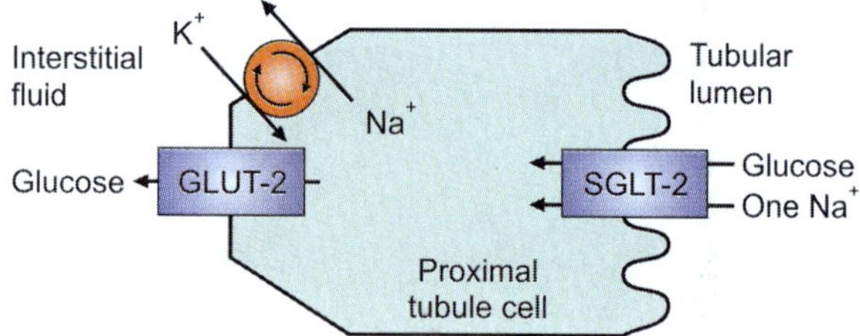

Fig. 9.10: Glucose reabsorption via cotransporter (SGLT-2)

to concentration gradient for Na^+. Hence, it is secondary active for glucose absorption. The mechanism is the same as for absorption of glucose in gastrointestinal tract (GIT) where the transporter is called SGLT-1.

Hence, glucose is present in urine in diabetes mellitus as the blood sugar increases above the level for full reabsorption by tubules. The lowest *plasma glucose* level at which the glucose first appears in the urine is called **renal threshold for glucose. Renal threshold for glucose is 200 mg/dL for arterial blood or 180 mg/dL for venous blood.**

Amino Acids

Amino acids are also completely reabsorbed in the proximal tubules and no loss takes place in the urine with normal kidney function. The reabsorption involves cotransporter in the membrane which combines with sodium and amino acids for transport across the membrane. Mechanism is also secondary active transport and energy is required for sodium transport at the basolateral margin of the cell.

Sodium and Chloride

The reabsorption of these ions plays a major role in electrolyte and water homeostasis of extracellular fluid (ECF) volume. Sodium and chloride are reabsorbed from the filtrate in all parts of the nephron. Most of the sodium is reabsorbed in the *proximal tubules,* about *60–70% of the filtered amount.* Sodium reabsorption is an *active process,* requires energy from ATP. Sodium reabsorption results in passive reabsorption of water due to osmotic gradient created by sodium reabsorption.

The sodium is further reabsorbed in the loop of Henle.

In the distal parts of the nephron, aldosterone hormone of the adrenal cortex acts on the collecting duct to increase the reabsorption of sodium and increases the excretion of potassium. The aldosterone regulates the reabsorption to maintain homeostasis of sodium balance. Regulation in this part of the nephron where bulk already has been reduced with the reabsorption taken place in proximal parts, enables finer regulation to be carried by the hormones to maintain the concentration of these electrolytes in the body.

Normally, a total of 96–99% of the filtered sodium is reabsorbed from the total filtered. Most of the sodium ion that is reabsorbed is accompanied by chloride ion reabsorption, but some accompanied by bicarbonate ion and some in the process of exchange with H^+ ion or potassium ion.

Calcium

Calcium is reabsorbed from PCT and thick AL. The hormones; parathyroid hormone and calcitonin regulate reabsorption from kidney. Approximately, 98% of filtered Ca^{++} is reabsorbed.

Reabsorption of Water

In the proximal tubule, water reabsorption depends upon the active reabsorption of Na^+ and water reabsorption is passive depending upon the osmotic gradient created. As about 65% of filtered sodium is reabsorbed in this segment, the reabsorption of 65% filtered water results and tubular fluid remains isotonic in the proximal tubule. Antidiuretic hormone (ADH) has no role in water reabsorption by PCT. ADH regulates the reabsorption of water from the collecting ducts.

Nitrogenous Waste

Urea and **uric acid** are reabsorbed to some extent in the tubules. Urea reabsorption is about 50% of that filtered.

Secretion

In the tubules, the secretion is less important and involves some substances. Some foreign materials, drugs like penicillin are secreted in the tubules. Secretion of H^+ is described later.

WATER EXCRETION

GFR of approximately 127/min has the same composition as that of plasma except that no plasma proteins are present. **In the proximal tubules,** 65% of the filtered Na^+ is reabsorbed by active process. The reabsorption results in reabsorption of **65% of filtered water** which is a passive process dependent upon sodium reabsorption which tends to make filtrate hypotonic; but water reabsorption takes place due to the permeability of the tubule to water and due to the osmotic pressure gradient created. Hence, fluid in the proximal tubule remains isotonic; the osmolality of about 300 mosm/kg of water, the same as that of plasma.

As the filtrate passes through the **loop of Henle, about 15% of the filtered water is further reabsorbed.** The descending limb of the loop of Henle is permeable to water due to presence of aquaporin 1 (water channels). The medullary interstitial fluid is hypertonic and water is reabsorbed in this part of the loop of Henle. It is permeable to water and the tubular fluid becomes hypertonic (as the surroundings are hypertonic and water reabsorption regulated by osmotic pressure gradient). Further the **thick ascending limb of loop of Henle,** is **impermable to water,** sodium is reabsorbed by a carrier (Fig. 9.11) which cotransports Na^+, Cl^- and K^+ ions, the process is secondary active transport as it is dependent on active transport of Na^+ at the basolateral margin of the cell where ATP is required. ***But as the thick ascending limb of loop of Henle is impermeable to water*** *the sodium reabsorption is not followed by reabsorption of water in this part of the nephron.* As a result, the tubular fluid in the **ascending limb of loop of Henle becomes hypotonic** (osmolality of about 150 mosm/kg of H_2O) and **the medullary interstitium becomes hypertonic** (Fig. 9.12), as sodium passes into it, but water does not follow it. This produces the hypertonicity of the renal medulla, and there is graded increase towards the depth of medulla. Graded increase is due to the countercurrent multiplier mechanism which operates in the long loops of Henle due to inflow of tubular fluid (in descending limb) in parallel to the outflow (in ascending limb) for some distance in the long loops of Henle. Urea in the medullary interstitium also contributes to the hyperosmolality. The longer the length of the loop, the

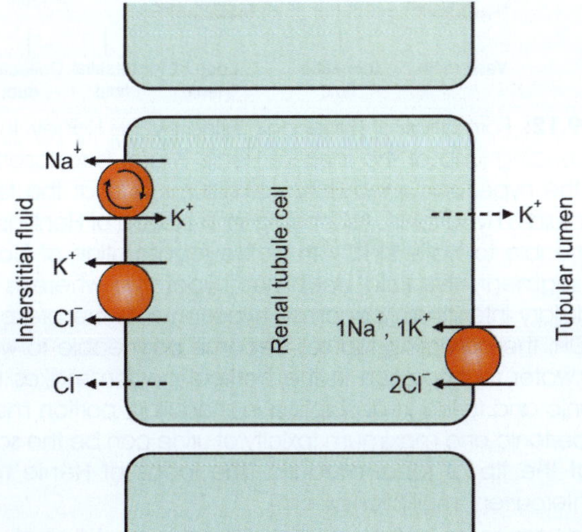

Fig. 9.11: Cells of the thick ascending limb of loop of Henle cotransport of Na^+, K^+ and Cl^- by secondary active transport mechanism

greater the hypertonicity. The blood vessels of the medulla (vasa recta) help to maintain the hypertonicity by forming counter current exchanger system (Fig. 9.12).

The solutes diffuse into vessels descending into pyramid and diffuse out of the vessels conducting blood towards cortex. Also water diffuses out of the descending vessels and into the ascending vessels. Hence, solutes tend to recirculate in medulla and water tends to bypass, maintaining hypertonicity of medulla.

In the **distal tubules** there is about 5% further reabsorption of water. Tubular fluid osmolality reaches 100 mos of H_2O and about 16 mL/min of water (15% of GFR) reaches the collecting ducts from the distal tubules. **In the collecting ducts** the water reabsorption **depends upon the presence of ADH** and the urine volume excreted and concentration of urine depends upon the presence or absence of hormone ADH. In the complete absence of ADH, the collecting tubules are completely impermeable to water and about 15 mL/min of dilute urine is excreted. The urine is dilute because it was made hypotonic in the loop of Henle and with further Na^+ reabsorption in distal tubules (Fig. 9.13). In the other extreme situation, i.e. in the presence of maximal ADH secretion, the urine volume is reduced to a fraction of a mL in 1 min and the urine is maximally concentrated as the collecting ducts become permeable to water and passing through cortex, the water is reabsorbed from tubules due to osmotic gradient; fluid being hypotonic to the surrounding tissue fluid which is isotonic; and further passing through medulla the surrounding interstitium is hypertonic, tubules permeable to water due to ADH, water is lost to the surroundings (and from there reabsorbed into the blood).

Concentration of urine takes place in the medullary portion of the collecting ducts as the environment is hypertonic and with ADH the tubules permeable to water that permits reabsorption under the osmotic pressure gradient (Fig. 9.12).

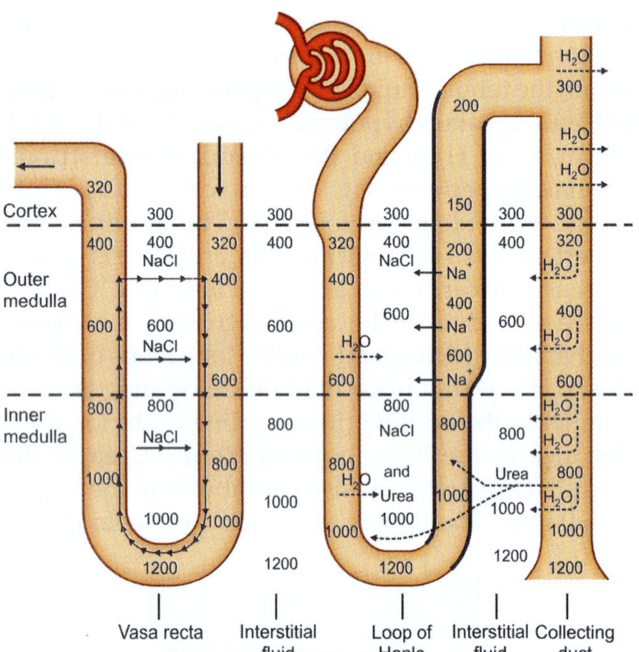

Fig. 9.12: Formation of hypertonic urine by the kidney. In the descending limb of the loop of Henle, water is reabsorbed into the hypertonic medullary interstitiums and at the tip of loop fluid is hypertonic. Ascending limb of loop of Henle is not permeable to water and with active reabsorption of Na^+ in this segment, the fluid becomes hypotonic whereas the medullary interstitium becomes hypertonic. In the presence of ADH, the collecting tubules become permeable to water and water reabsorption in the cortical portion makes fluid isotonic and further reabsorption in medullary portion makes it hypertonic and maximum toxicity of urine can be the same as at the tip of renal medulla (the loops of Henle form countercurrent multiplier system).

The vasa recta as they descend into the medulla gain salt from the surroundings and again passing up loose salt to medulla; as a result, the hypertoxicity of medulla is maintained (they form countercurrent exchanger system)

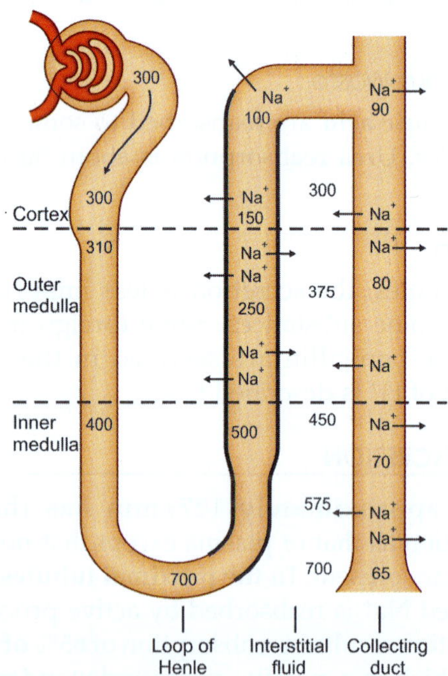

Fig. 9.13: Formation of dilute urine. As a result of active reabsorption of sodium in the thick-ascending limb of loop of Henle, which is impermeable to water the fluid which leaves the ascending limb of loop of Henle is hypotonic; and in the absence of ADH, the collecting ducts are impermeable to water not allowing water reabsorption, further reabsorption of sodium results in formation of hypotonic urine

Between the two situations described and depending upon the amount of ADH secreted the volume and osmolality of the urine are regulated. When urine is hypotonic, the osmolality may decrease to about 50 mosm/kg of H_2O. If it is maximally concentrated, it may rise to 1,200 mosm/kg of H_2O.

Diabetes insipidus is due to complete lack of ADH or when ADH is ineffective due to its nonresponsive receptors (due to mutation in their gene) the urine volume of 12–15 mL per minute may remain throughout the day, about 23 liters of urine would be excreted per day. Sense of thirst is then aroused and necessitates ingestion of water which is essential to prevent dehydration.

Regulation of ADH Hormone

Water is lost from the body from several routes (Table 9.1); that lost from lungs during respiration is called insensible loss; from skin by perspiration, part of it is also insensible loss, and the rest is variable during the day that depends upon the need of maintaining body temperature; some is lost in feces and there is loss in urine. Of these losses, that from kidney is important as renal water losses are regulated to maintain the osmolality of body fluids.

> Disorders of water balance are manifested by alterations in osmolality of plasma. The osmolality is mainly dependent on Na^+. These disorders alter the plasma Na^+ concentration. On the other hand, if the sodium balance is primarily upset, it alters the volume of extracellular fluid and not its osmolality.

Antidiuretic hormone is secreted by posterior pituitary and secretion is regulated to maintain the **osmotic pressure of the ECF**, and **the volume of the ECF.** When the osmotic pressure of the plasma increases, the osmoreceptors situated in the hypothalamus sense the stimulus, and posterior pituitary is stimulated to increase the secretion of ADH therein greater reabsorption of water from the collecting ducts (water excretion is decreased, the urine is concentrated) that regulate the osmotic pressure of plasma and ECF. When the osmotic pressure of plasma decreases, the stimulus from osmoreceptors to the posterior pituitary is inhibited and ADH secretion is decreased, water reabsorption is decreased, water excretion is increased and urine becomes hypotonic (water in excess of solutes is excreted), osmotic pressure of plasma and ECF is regulated.

Another stimulus which regulates the ADH secretion and so excretion of water is the **volume of ECF**. When the volume of ECF increases, the volume receptors situated in the great veins, right and left atria, pulmonary vessels get stimulated and the stimulus inhibits the secretion of ADH, the increased excretion of water regulates the ECF volume.

Hence, the volume of urine excreted per day is regulated to maintain ECF osmolality and volume of ECF.

*If there is lesion of the posterior pituitary with total loss of ADH secretion, the volume of urine can reach up to 23 liters/day and this disease is called diabetes insipidus. The diabetes insipidus can also result when there are nonresponsive ADH receptors in the kidney (**nephrogenic diabetes insipidus**). There is diuresis (excessive urine volume), but no sugar in the urine and so it is different from diabetes mellitus. As the loss of water is excessive there is great increase in the thirst sensation and water is drunk in equal amounts to the losses. Person is constantly shifting between tap and toilet.*

***Osmotic diuresis:** It differs from diuresis due to lack of ADH, as ADH only influences reabsorption of water from collecting ducts, and osmotic diuretic substances affect reabsorption even in the proximal tubules and all along in the nephron segments. Osmotic diuresis takes place in uncontrolled diabetes mellitus when sugar remains in tubular fluid and is not completely reabsorbed in the proximal tubules. It exerts an osmotic pressure which decreases water reabsorption in the proximal tubules and in the rest of the tubules of the nephron. More water is retained in the tubules and excreted in the urine. This is the cause of polyuria in diabetes mellitus.*

Presence of nonabsorbable substances like mannitol by holding water in PCT decrease water reabsorption in this part of the nephron where it is dependent upon osmotic gradient and cause osmotic diuresis.

Regulation of Electrolyte Balance

Sodium is the most common electrolyte in the extracellular fluid and potassium is the most common electrolyte in the intracellular fluid.

Sodium is the constituent of almost all foods and it is added to the diet during cooking. Hence, it is eaten in excess of body needs and is lost in urine and sweat. The amount lost in the sweat is variable and depends upon the amount of sweat produced. Hence, the kidneys regulate the excretion to maintain homeostasis.

As already pointed out the bulk of sodium is reabsorbed in the proximal tubules which is mostly independent of hormones except that angiotensin II and sympathetic nerve activity stimulates the reabsorption. The main regulation of the amount excreted to maintain homeostasis of sodium balance is achieved in the distal segments of the nephron by the hormone, **aldosterone**.

Aldosterone hormone is secreted by adrenal cortex; its secretion is regulated mainly by angiotensin II, but also by adrenocorticotropic hormone (ACTH) and rise of K^+ level in plasma and to minor degree by fall of Na^+ level in plasma. The hormone has an important role in maintenance of homeostasis of Na^+ balance. There is another hormone called ANP, secreted by atrial muscle of the heart, which has role in sodium excretion (natriuresis) (Table 9.2).

Hormonal Regulation for Reabsorption

The tubules reabsorb substances which need to be conserved in the body and regulate the excretion of others to maintain homeostasis. The regulation involves water balance regulated by hormone ADH, Na^+ balance regulation by hormone aldosterone. Some other factors like atrial natriuretic peptide (ANP), angiotensin II, PGE_2 are also involved; have role in sodium reabsorption or excretion of sodium. The Na^+ reabsorption by aldosterone results in excretion of K^+ ions by the kidney.

Natriuretic hormones, are secreted by the heart muscles in the atria to a lesser extent in ventricles, are stimulated by expansion of ECF volume, the hormones cause natriuresis (excretion of Na^+) followed by water excretion. Angiotensin II formed by renin stimules Na^+ reabsorption in PCT.

Renin Angiotensin System

When the *blood volume is low* or the *arterial blood pressure falls, renin is released* from the afferent arteriole of the kidney, renin acts on a protein, angiotensinogen produced by the liver and converts it into angiotensin I; another enzyme called angiotensin-converting enzyme (ACE), produced mainly by lungs, but also by other tissues of the body converts angiotensin I to angiotensin II. Angiotensin I is inactive. ***Angiotensin II*** is a powerful ***vasoconstrictor***, it constricts arterioles; and also ***stimulates the secretion of aldosterone*** by the adrenal cortex (Fig. 9.14) which stimulates sodium reabsorption in the kidney. Angiotensin II also stimulates ***thirst sensation***. The mechanisms which increase sodium reabsorption raise the ECF volume as increased sodium reabsorption is followed by water reabsorption to maintain osmotic pressure of ECF. Hence, these homeostatic mechanisms tend to restore the blood volume or blood pressure.

Similarly, renin is released when there is constriction of one renal artery, and it results in hypertension (renal hypertension).

In the treatment of clinical hypertension drugs which inhibit the formation of angiotensin II (inhibiting the converting enzyme) are used. Similar effect is also achieved by blocking the receptors for angiotensin II.

Function of Kidney in the Maintenance of pH of Blood

H^+ ions are secreted in all parts of the nephron and excretion is regulated to maintain the pH of the blood.

The diet produces variable amounts of acidic or basic radicals and to maintain the pH of blood kidney has an important role. Buffers in the blood mop-up the excess acid or base produced by the metabolism of foodstuffs. But the extra acidic or basic radicals have to be excreted from the body, in order that the buffer store is replenished.

All segments of kidney tubules secrete H^+ ions. In the proximal tubules, carbonic anhydrase enzyme hydrates CO_2 to form carbonic acid which disassociates into H^+ and bicarbonate ions. H^+ ions are secreted into tubular fluid and bicarbonate ions are absorbed into the blood (Fig. 9.15). When one H^+

Table 9.2: Hormones that regulate NaCl and H_2O reabsorption

Hormone	*Major stimulus*	*Nephron site of action*	*Effect on transport*
Angiotensin II	↑Renin	PT	↑NaCl and H_2O reabsorption
Aldosterone	↑Angiotensin II, ↑$[K^+]_P$	TAL, DT/CD	↑NaCl and H_2O reabsorption*
ANP	↑ECV	CD	↓H_2O and NaCl reabsorption
Sympathetic nerves	↓ECV	PT, TAL, DT/CD	↑NaCl and H_2O reabsorption*
Dopamine	↑ECV	PT	↓H_2O and NaCl reabsorption
ADH	↑P_{osm}, ↓ECV	DT/CD	↑H_2O reabsorption*

Hormones listed act within minutes except its action on NaCl reabsorption with a delay of 1 hour. PT—proximal tubule; TAL—thick-ascending limb; DT/CD—distal tubule and collecting duct; ECV—effective circulating volume; $[K^+]_p$—plasma concentration K^+; P_{osm}—plasma osmolality. The * indicates that the effect on H_2O reabsorption does not inculde the TAL. ↓indicates a decrease and ↑indicates an increase.

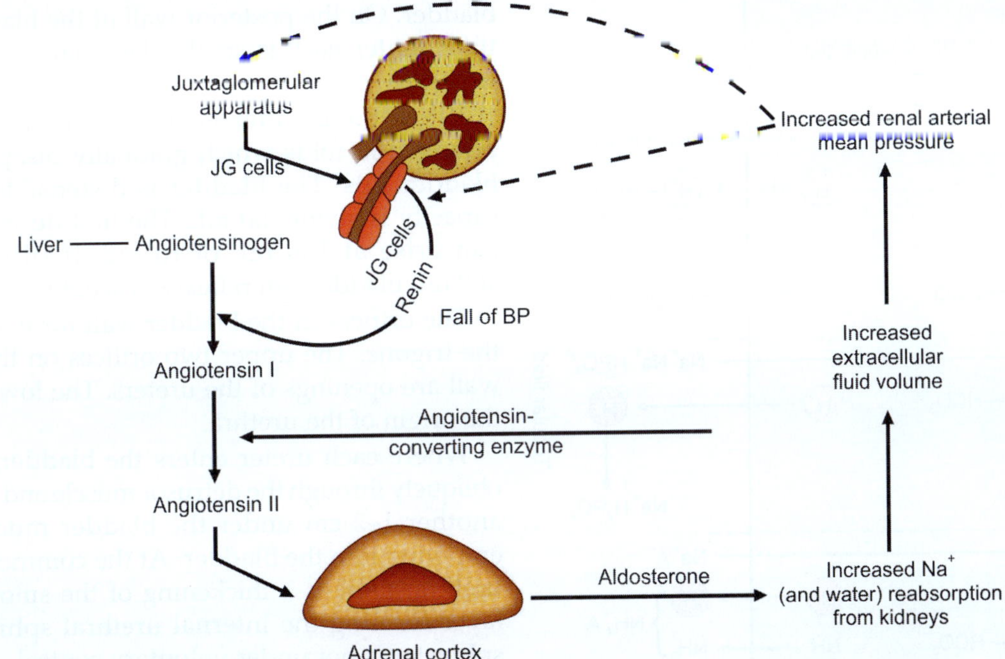

Fig. 9.14: Feedback mechanism regulating aldosterone secretion. The dashed arrows indicates inhibition

ion is secreted into tubular fluid, one HCO_3^- ion is reabsorbed into blood. The H^+ ions secreted into the tubular fluid combine with the buffers present in the filtrate which mop-up the H^+ ions, so that more H^+ ion can be secreted in the tubular fluid. The urine cannot be more acidic than pH 4.5 (this is called the limiting pH of the urine), and if there were no buffers in the filtrate, this limiting pH would be reached too soon; and not permit the normal excretion of H^+ ions. The buffers present in the filtrate help in the adequate excretion of H^+. There are three buffer systems in the filtrate which mop-up the H^+ ions to permit adequate excretion (Fig. 9.16).

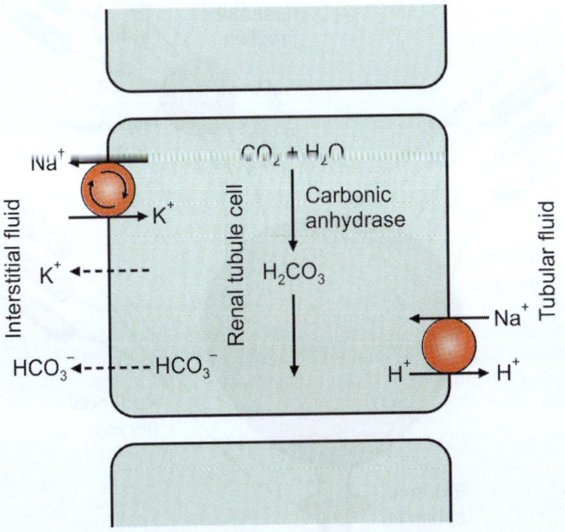

Fig. 9.15: Secretion of acid by proximal tubular cells in the kidney. H^+ is transported into the tubular lumen, HCO_3^- diffuses into the interstitial fluid and absorbed into the blood

1. Bicarbonate buffer when H^+ enters to filtrate it and forms carbonic acid with the bicarbonate ions present in the tubular fluid. The carbonic acid formed dissociates to carbon dioxide and water.

$$HCO_3^- + H^+ = H_2CO_3 = CO_2 + H_2O$$
(CO_2 diffuses into the cell)

   This mechanism is responsible for reabsorption of bicarbonate ions in PCT.

2. Hydrogen phosphate in the tubular fluid combines with H^+ ions secreted into tubular fluid, forming dihydrogen phosphate mopping hydrogen ions.

$$HPO_4^{2-} + H^+ = H_2PO_4^-$$

   This mechanism operates in more distal segments of tubules because of increase in concentration of phosphate buffer with reabsorption of water in PCT.

3. Ammonia formed by the kidney cells and secreted into tubular fluid combines with H^+ forming ammonium ions.

$$NH_3 + H^+ = NH_4^+$$

   Ammonia is formed in the kidney by the tubular cells and secreted into the tubular fluid in all segments of tubules. In chronic acidosis NH_4^+ excreted at any urine pH increases the cause is not clear.

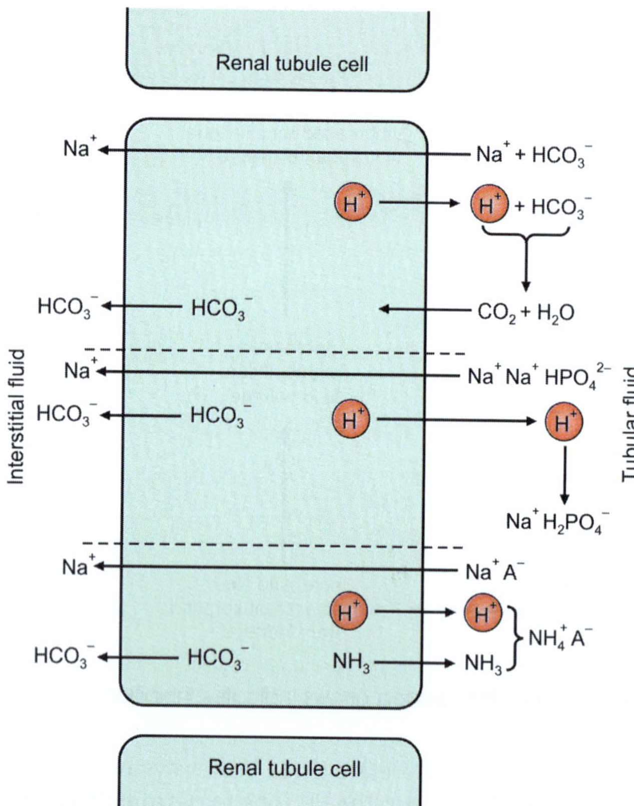

Fig. 9.16: Fate of H^+ secreted into a tubule and it exchanges for Na^+

The normal pH of the urine varies between pH 4.5–8; average is 6.5, i.e. acidic.

When food contains more basic ions, the urine becomes alkaline. If the acid products produced by the body exceed the capacity of the kidney to excrete H^+, acidosis results. The condition may occur in uncontrolled diabetes mellitus. At high altitude, the urine is alkaline as the respiration is stimulated due to hypoxia and CO_2 tension is reduced in the blood, shifting blood pH towards alkaline side that results in the formation of alkaline urine.

URETERS

The ureters propel the urine from the kidneys into the bladder by peristaltic contractions which are not controlled by autonomic nerves. The waves send little spurts of urine into bladder.

URINARY BLADDER

It is a reservoir of urine. It lies in the pelvic cavity, when distended rises into the abdominal cavity.

The muscle in the bladder is called the detrusor muscle. It is the detrusor muscle which empties the bladder. On the posterior wall of the bladder, above the bladder neck is small triangular area called the trigone.

When the bladder is empty, the inner lining is arranged in folds which gradually disappear as the bladder fills. The bladder is distensible. The total capacity is about 600 mL. The first desire to urinate can arise at 150 mL of filling, if filling reaches 400 mL bladder can reflexly evacuate.

The orifices in the bladder wall form a triangle in the trigone. The upper two orifices on the posterior wall are openings of the ureters. The lower orifice is the origin of the urethra.

Where each ureter enters the bladder, it courses obliquely through the detrusor muscle and then passes another 1–2 cm under the bladder mucosa before emptying into the bladder. At the commencement of urethra, there is a thickening of the smooth muscle layer forming the internal urethral sphincter. This sphincter is not under voluntary control.

Innervation of the Bladder

The main nerve supply of the bladder is by pelvic nerves through the sacral plexus connecting with the sacral segments of spinal cord (Fig. 9.17). Through the pelvic nerves pass the sensory and motor nerve fibers. The sensory nerves detect the stretch of the bladder wall. The motor fibers are parasympathetic fibers which have ganglia in the bladder wall and innervate detrusor muscle. The pudendal nerves innervate the

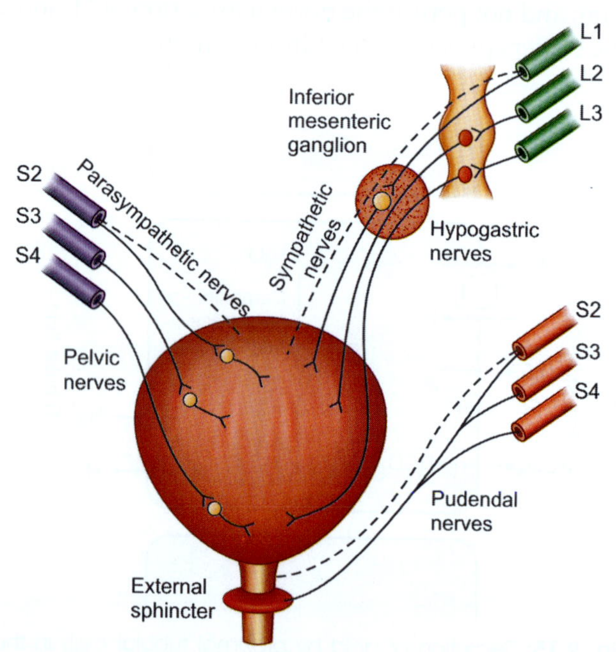

Fig. 9.17: Innervation of the bladder. Dashed lines indicate sensory nerves

external sphincter, these being somatic nerves have voluntary control over sphincter. Bladder receives sympathetic innervation through sympathetic chain and hypogastric nerves. These nerves mainly stimulate the muscle of blood vessels and have very little effect on bladder, are located mainy in the bladder neck and the urethra. Some sensory fibers pass via sympathetic nerves and may be important for sensation of fullness and pain in some cases.

URETHRA

It leads from the neck of the bladder to the exterior, at the external urethral orifice. Its length differs in the male and the female. Female urethra is about 4 cm long and runs downwards and forwards behind the pubic symphysis to open at the external urethral orifice above vagina.

The external urethral orifice is guarded by the external urethral sphincter which is under voluntary control.

Male urethra is 15–20 cm long and has three parts: (1) the prostatic as it courses through prostate gland (2) membranous surrounded by sphincter urethra and (3) a spongy part passing through the middle of corpus spongiosum of penis to open at external urethral orifice at the tip of the glans penis.

The male urethra forms a common passage for both the urine and the semen.

Micturition

The urinary bladder is stimulated due to stretch of the wall. Afferent impulses travel to the spinal cord and to the brain to raise awareness of bladder filling. The reflex can be inhibited by higher centers for sometime. But with the desire to pass urine, the impulses travel via parasympathetic nerves from the micturition center in the spinal cord to cause the contraction of the detrusor muscle and relaxation of the internal sphincter, making voiding possible, and the external sphincter is relaxed by voluntary activity. If the bladder fills to 400 mL and the urine is not passed voluntarily, the reflex evacuation of urine can takes place if there is no obstruction to the urinary pathway.

Fibers in the pelvic nerves are the afferent limb of the voiding reflex (the fibers convey the desire to evacuate) and the parasympathetic fibers to the bladder constitute the efferent limb and travel in the same nerves. The reflex is integrated in the sacral portion of the spinal cord. Micturition is basically a spinal reflex, facilitated and inhibited by higher centers in the brain. This gives voluntary control.

Urine enters the bladder without producing much increase in the pressure until it is well-filled. A plot of intravesical pressure against the fluid in the bladder is called cystometrogram (Fig. 9.18).

During micturition, the perineal muscles and external urethral sphincter are relaxed.

Water Intoxication

Normally, the maximum urine flow that can be produced with rapid ingestion of water is about 15 mL/ min. If water is ingested at a higher rate for any length of time, it causes dilution of the ECF, i.e. hypotonicity of ECF results. This causes swelling of the cells which take up water due to osmotic gradient; this may become severe and the symptoms of water intoxication may develop.

Swelling of cells in the brain (neurons) results in convulsions and coma and eventually leads to death. Water intoxication also occurs when water intake is not reduced after administration of exogenous vasopressin or secretion of endogenous vasopressin in response to nonosmotic stimuli, such as surgical trauma or stress; as stress can stimulate the secretion of ADH.

Normal Urine

Urine is yellow-colored liquid with faint odor. On average 96% formed of water and remainder consists of dissolved waste products, consists of urea, uric acid, sodium chloride, phosphates, ammonia, creatinine, potassium, etc. The color of urine is darker when urine is concentrated and it is paler when large amount of water is drunk.

Very dark urine can be abnormal. Blood in the urine can give it a dark reddish-brown color. In jaundice,

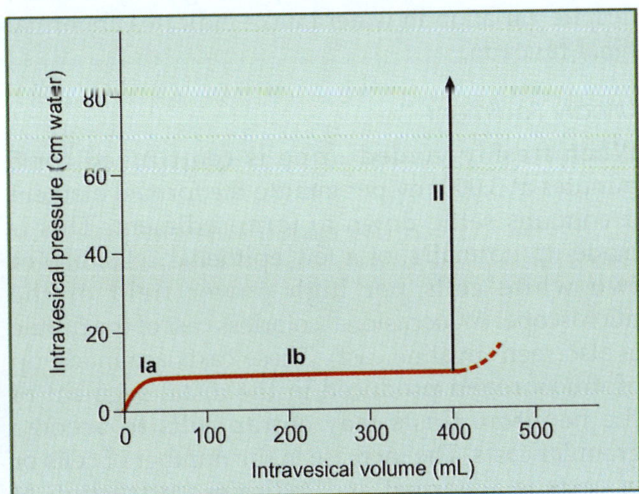

Fig. 9.18: Cystometrogram in a normal bladder

the urine may be dark, may be with orange tinge. Black urine may be due to malaria or other rare diseases. Medicines may give color to the urine; eating beet root may color the urine.

In a healthy person, the urine is sterile, i.e. it is germ free.

Tests for the presence of protein (albumin) and glucose in the urine can be done easily. Albumin appears in the urine in a number of conditions particularly kidney disease and toxemia of pregnancy.

The detection of glucose in the urine forms a screening test for diabetes.

Renal Function Tests

Urine Volume

The volume of urine formed in a healthy adult depends upon the water intake, solute excretion and water lost in sweat (water also lost from the lungs during breathing although this amount remains fairly constant). Normally, the urine volume remains within 1–2 liters in a day.

Oliguria is a reduction in the volume of urine voided and is pathological, if it continues despite variation in salt and water intake. **Polyuria** is the state where more urine is voided than normal and is significant, if persists. **Anuria** means no urine formation.

The specific gravity of the urine may vary from 1,001 to 1,034 (usually it remains in the range of 1,020–1,030). If water is not drunk or liquid food is not ingested for 12 hours, the specific gravity should be approximately 1,025. Failure to reach this value indicates abnormal renal function. Persistent production of urine with specific gravity isomolar with plasma (300 mosm/L = specific gravity of 1,007) despite variation in water intake indicates abnormal renal function.

Urinary Sediment

When freshly voided urine is centrifuged for 5 minutes at 3,000 rev per minute the formed element it contains settle down to form sediment. This is made-up normally, of a few epithelial cells, one or two white cells per high power field of the microscope. An occasional colorless cast of the tubule is also seen (hyaline cast). These casts are made-up of mucoprotein produced in the distal segment of the nephron. Casts may entrap cells to become granular casts. The increase in the number of cells or of casts is abnormal and indicates destruction of glomeruli or tubular cells.

Proteinuria

Some proteins mainly albumin is normally filtered in small amount in the glomerulus. This is normally reabsorbed in the proximal tubule. Proteinuria is diagnosed when a patient excretes more than 150 mg of protein per day. It could be due to changes in the permeability of the glomerular membrane or the absorptive process in the tubule. The amount of protein in the urine may be very large especially in nephrosis.

A benign condition of proteinuria when the individual stands up is called orthostatic albuminuria; the cause of it is not understood; the urine formed in lying down condition is protein-free.

Glucose in the Urine

Normally, urine is free of glucose (a very small amount not detected by ordinary tests may be present normally). Glucose in the urine indicates diabetes mellitus or renal glycosuria.

Blood Levels of Urea and Creatinine

Are useful indices of glomerular filtration. An increase in the blood level of urea above normal indicates reduction in the glomerular filtration rate (GFR). The plasma creatinine level, if it is increased, is also an indication of reduction in GFR. The urea level in the blood provides a useful indication of the degree to which a patient is accumulating harmful waste products when the kidneys are not functioning properly. The condition in which there is high level of urea in the blood is called uremia.

Clearance Tests

Clearance value of a plasma constituent is the volume of plasma which contains the same amount of substance which is excreted in the urine in 1 minute. For this test, the plasma concentration is measured and per minute excretion of the substance in the urine. Various clearance tests are used for assessing the functions of the kidneys. **GFR** is best measured by the **inulin clearance test.** Other markers can also be used. A convenient method is **endogenous creatinine clearance** for measurement of GFR.

Hence, Clearance refers to the volume of plasma that would be necessary to supply the amount of substance excreted in the urine per unit time. Stated mathematically,

$$C_x \times P_x = U_x \times V$$

where C_x is the clearance rate of a substance x, P_x is the plasma concentration of the substance, U_x is the urine concentration of that substance, and V is the urine flow rate. Rearranging this equation, clearance can be expressed as

$$C_x = \frac{U_x \times V}{P_x}$$

Thus, renal clearance of a substance is calculated from the urinary excretion rate ($U_x \times V$) of that substance divided by its plasma concentration.

Inulin Clearance can be Used to Estimate GFR

If a substance is freely filtered and is not reabsorbed or secreted by the renal tubules, then the rate at which that substance is excreted in the urine ($U_x \times V$) is equal to the filtration rate of the substance by the kidneys ($GFR \times P_x$).

Thus,

$$GFR \times P_x = U_x \times V$$

The GFR, therefore, can be calculated as the clearance of the substance as follows:

$$GFR = \frac{U_x \times V}{P_x} = C_x$$

A substance that fits these criteria is *inulin,* a polysaccharide molecule with a molecular weight of about 5200. Inulin, which is not produced in the body derived from certain plants and must be administered intravenously to a patient to measure GFR.

Figure 9.19 shows the renal handling of inulin. Inulin clearance is calculated as the urine excretion rate of inulin divided by the plasma concentration.

Inulin is not the only substance that can be used for determining GFR. Other substances that have been used clinically to estimate GFR include *radioactive isotopes* and *creatinine.*

Creatinine Clearance

Creatinine is a by-product of muscle metabolism and is cleared from the body fluids by glomerular filtration only. Therefore, the clearance of creatininie can also be used to assess GFR. Because measurement of creatinine clearance does not require intravenous infusion this method is much more widely used than inulin clearance for estimating GFR. However, creatinine clearance is not a perfect marker of GFR because a small amount of it is secreted by the tubules, so that the amount of creatinine excreted slightly exceeds the amount filtered.

For measuring GFR, the inulin clearance is accurate; but the substance has to be injected whereas creatinine is already present in the plasma; the endogenous clearance is more convenient though not as accurate.

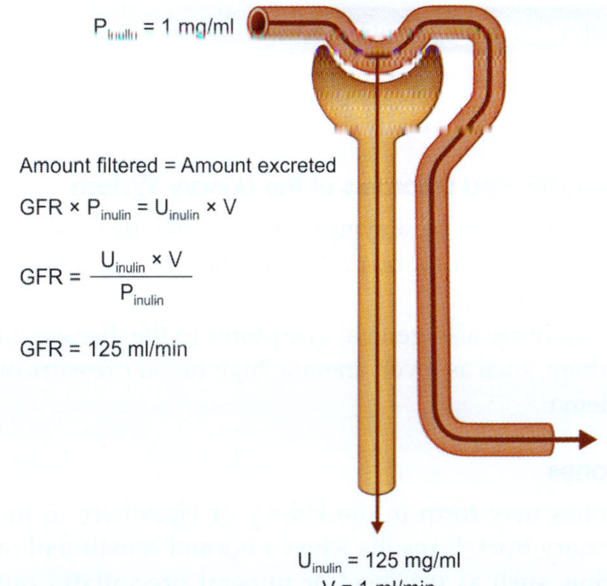

Fig. 9.19: Measurement of glomerular filtration rate (GFR) from the renal clearance of inulin. Inulin is freely filtered by the glomerular capillary is not reabsorbed by the renal tubules. P_{inulin}, plasma inulin concentration U_{inulin}, urine inulin concentration; V urine flow rate

Renal blood flow is measured by clearance of substance p-aminohippuric acid (PAH) which measures plasma flow from which blood flow is calculated by taking into account the hematocrit.

PAH Clearance can be Used to Estimate Renal Plasma Flow

Theoretically, if a substance is *completely* cleared from the plasma in one circulation, the clearance rate of that substance is equal to the total renal plasma flow. The amount of the substance delivered to the kidneys in the blood (renal plasma flow × P_{PAH}) would be equal to the amount excreted in the urine ($U_{PAH} \times V$). Thus, renal plasma flow (RPF) could be calculated as

$$\frac{U_{PAH} \times V}{P_{PAH}} = C_{PAH}$$

Because the GFR is only about 20 percent of the total plasma flow, a substance that is completely cleared from the plasma must be excreted by tubular secretion as well as glomerular filtration. There is no known substance that is *completely* cleared by the kidneys. One substance, PAH, is about 90 percent cleared from the plasma. Therefore, the clearance of PAH can be used as of renal plasma flow. To be more accurate, one can correct for the percentage of PAH still in the blood when it leaves the kidneys.

Clinical Significance

Table 9.3 shows some diuretics used in clinical practice.

Diseases and Disorders of the Urinary System

Back pain can be a symptom of kidney disease and presence of blood or protein in the urine is another important sign.

There are also general symptoms in the diseases of kidney, such as fever, anemia, high blood pressure or edema.

Stones

Stones may form in the kidney or elsewhere in the urinary tract. It results when a normal constituent of urine, such as uric acid or mineral precipitates out of solution and concentrates on a bacteria or speck of protein, then more material collects on it. Why stones form in some people and not in others is not understood. Stones vary in their composition, size, shape and color. Calcium oxalate and calcium phosphate stones are common; uric acid stones are less common.

Symptoms are caused when stones pass from kidney to the ureter, they cause a dull aching pain. Sometimes, a kidney stone passing down the ureter causes renal colic, a very severe pain.

Some Kidney Diseases

Glomerulonephritis

The disease is produced when glomeruli become inflamed, but not directly infected by microorganisms. The condition takes several forms.

In chronic nephritis, the glomeruli become damaged over many years and are replaced by fibrous scars. This affects filtration at the glomeruli, leading to toxemia. The treatment consists of taking preventive measures to stop the progression of the disease.

When the kidney abnormality is associated with raised blood pressure, the condition is called nephrosclerosis.

Nephrotic Syndrome

Nephrotic syndrome is produced by a variety of disorders, characterized by an incraease in the permeability of the glomerular capillaries to proteins. The increased permeability results in an increase in urinary protein excretion (**proteinuria**). Individuals may also develop edema and hypoalbuminemia as a result of proteinuria, liver being unable to produce albumin at an increased rate required.

Signs of Kidney Disease

Analysis of urine can reveal about the disease involving kidneys. Tests for protein and glucose can be done easily.

Small amounts of protein in the urine within normal limit are quite common, but larger amounts suggest disease of the kidney, such as damage to the glomeruli.

Most of the protein is albumin. The great loss of albumin in disease can result in decrease in the concentration of albumin in the plasma, if the liver is unable to synthesize albumin at the rate at which it is being lost in the urine. Decrease in the concentration of plasma albumin results in puffiness of the face and swelling of lower parts of the body, i.e. edema.

Table 9.3: Some diuretics used in clinical practice (diuretics, their mechanisms of action and tubular sites of action)

Class of diuretic	*Mechanism of action*	*Tubular site of action*
1. Osmotic diuretics (mannitol)	Inhibit water and solute reabsorption by increasing osmolaritry to tubular fluid	Mainly proximal tubules
2. Carbonic anhydrase inhibitors (acetazolamide)	Inhibit H^+ secretion and HCO_3^- reabsorption, which reduces Na^+ reabsorption	Proximal tubules
3. Thiazide diuretics (hydrochlorothiazide, chlorthalidone)	Inhibit Na^+–Cl^- cotransport in luminal membrane	Early distal tubules
4. Loop diuretics (furosemide)	Inhibit Na^+–K^+–Cl^- cotransport in luminal membrane	Thick ascending loop of Henle
5. Aldosterone antagonists (spironolactone)	Inhibit action of aldosterone on tubular receptor, decrease Na^+ reabsorption and decrease K^+ secretion	Collecting tubules
6. Sodium channel blockers (amiloride)	Block entry of Na^+ into Na^+ channels of luminal membrane, decrease Na^+ reabsorption and decrease K^+ secretion	Collecting tubules

Filtration and presence of albumin in the Bowman's capsule results in increase in GFR due to osmotic force of the protein in the Bowman's space.

Acute glomerulonephritis usually clears up completely. The chronic form may develop over months or years, if it does not respond to any sort of treatment leads to kidney failure.

Kidney Failure

Renal failure can be acute or chronic. Acute kidney failure is produced by any condition which leads to sudden and *prolonged period* of *low blood pressure*, such as large hemorrhage or acute heart failure.

There are numerous causes of chronic renal failure. An acute renal failure or renal disease may eventually become chronic. In some cases, the cause is not discovered; and the patient may not notice that anything is wrong until the disorder is very advanced.

Chronic Renal Failure

This is reached when irreversible damage of nephrons is so severe that 75% renal function has lost. The main causes are glomerulonephritis, diabetes mellitus, chronic pyelonephritis and hypertension. Symptoms like uremia, polyuria, fixed specific gravity of urine, acidosis, electrolyte imbalance (raised potassium in blood and abnormal retention of sodium), anemia and hypertension, may be present.

Treatment of acute renal failure takes place in specialized renal units. The kidney usually improves after several weeks. With chronic kidney failure where symptoms appear gradually the kidneys become less and less efficient as damage to them increases.

When the kidneys completely fail, the satisfactory form of treatment is either dialysis or kidney transplant.

Hemodialysis/Peritoneal Dialysis

Blood of the patients is cleaned artificially to remove all waste products; depends upon the ability of the machine to do the work of the kidney.

Kidney Transplant

Many people dependent on dialysis prefer a transplant of healthy kidney from either a living or dead donor. After the transplant, the patient is required to take drugs to suppress the immune system to reduce the chances of body's natural defense system to reject the donor kidney. Before the operation, tests are conducted for compatible transplant.

Congenital Abnormalities of the Kidney

Polycystic Kidney

Inherited condition in which the both kidneys are affected. Dilatations (cysts) grow in the kidneys, enlarge and cause ischemia and necrosis of nephrons resulting in their destruction. The disease is progressive and secondary hypertension and chronic renal failure develops.

Tumors of the Kidney

Malignant Tumors

Renal cell carcinoma: It is a tumor of the tubular epithelium; spread involves the renal vein and leads to early blood spread, most commonly to lungs and bones; it is more common after 50 years age. Other tumors are benign.

Cystitis and Urethritis

Inflammation of bladder is called cystitis and that of uretha is called urethritis, usually caused by bacterial infection.

Cystitis and urethritis are more common in women because of shortness of female urethra, close relationship to vagina which makes it highly accessible to bacteria. Contraceptives have been thought to cause cystitis and urethritis because they change the environment in the vagina, and growth of bacteria may invade urinary system.

Cystitis and urethritis in men most often occur as a result of either obstruction to the urethra by the enlarged prostate or an infection of the prostate spreading to bladder and urethra.

Symptoms of both the conditions are frequent passing of urine with intense pain. There may be pain in the lower abdomen and a frequent urgent desire to pass urine.

Urinary Incontinence

In this condition, there is defective voluntary control over external urethral sphincter. The cause can be stress incontinence, retention with overflow or urge incontinence.

Classification of incontinence (Fig. 9.20)

- Urethral sphincter incompetence (urodynamic stress incontinence)
- Detrusor overactivity or the unstable activity—this is either neurogenic or nonneurogenic.

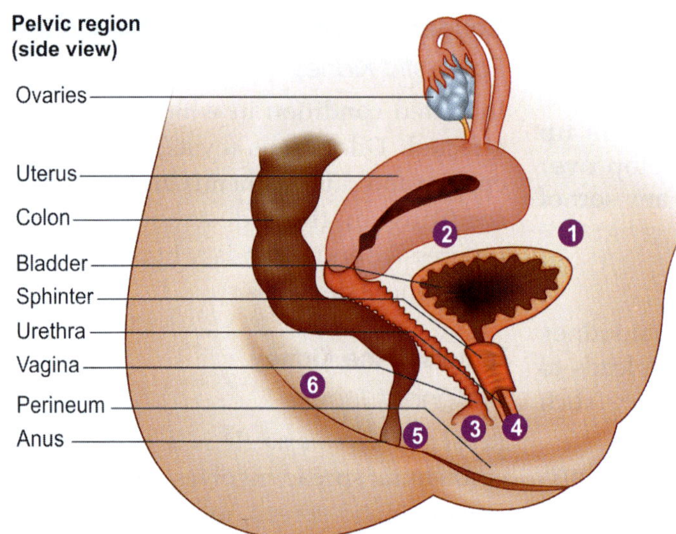

Fig. 9.20: The anatomy of incontinence

- Retention with overflow
- Congenital causes
- Fistula
- Extraurethral causes.

Retention and Overflow Incontinence

This occurs when there is retention of urine due to obstruction of urinary outflow, e.g. enlarged prostate or urethral stricture.

IMPLICATIONS AND APPLICATIONS

- To know the referred pain of kidney or ureter.
- To understand intravenous pyelogram.
- To be able to measure urinary output.
- To be able to put catheter in male or female urethra.

Neurological abnormality may affect nerves involved in micturition, e.g. stroke, spinal cord injury or multiple sclerosis.

10

Reproductive System

DEVELOPMENT OF GONADS

The ovum at the time of fertilization carries haploid number of chromosomes, the number has been reduced from the full number of 46 chromosomes (23 pairs) during the meiotic division to 23 chromosomes of which 22 are somatic chromosomes (autosomes) and one is sex chromosome. The sex chromosome is X chromosome in the ovum. The sperm at the time of fertilization also has haploid number of chromosomes, i.e. 23 of which 22 are somatic, and one is sex chromosome. The sex chromosome is X chromosome in half the sperms and Y in the others. If the ovum gets fertilized with a sperm which carries Y chromosome, testes form in the fetus which results in male sexual development; if it gets fertilized with a sperm having X chromosome ovaries form in the fetus; in the absence of Y chromosome there is female sexual development.

The presence of a single chromosome, the Y chromosome (with its normal genetic material) is responsible for formation of testes in the fetus; and in its absence ovaries form.

In the male during **fetal life** the fetal testes secrete androgens which are responsible for the formation of male internal and external genitalia (Fig. 10.1).

In the female fetus, the ovaries do not secrete any hormones; only the absence of testes results in the development of female internal and external genitalia (Fig. 10.1).

The gonads remain **nonfunctional till the time of puberty**. At this time due to some change at the level of hypothalamus, the hypothalamus starts secretion of gonadotropin-releasing hormone (**GnRH**) that stimulates the pituitary to secrete gonadotropins; the two gonadotropins are follicle-stimulating hormone (FSH) and luteinizing hormone (LH); their action on the gonads results in the gonads to function; the functions are the secretion of sex hormones and the development of gametes. The sex hormones effect the development of internal genitalia. The first meiotic division had started in the oocyte in the prenatal life in ovaries.

In the male, under the influence of LH testes secrete testosterone. Under the influence of follicle-stimulating hormone (FSH), the formation of sperms from the gonads is stimulated.

In the female, the gonadotropins FSH and LH secreted in cyclic manner stimulate the development of graafian follicle and the secretion of estrogen, ovulation from the developed follicle and secretion of progesterone along with estrogen after the formation of corpus luteum. The ovarian hormones have negative and even positive feedback effects on the secretion of gonadotropins and GnRH.

Puberty

There is a transition from nonreproductive to a reproductive state during puberty. Before the child reaches at age of 10 year, the LH and FSH levels are low.

A change at the level of hypothalamus at puberty leads to increased synthesis and release of GnRH. GnRH secretion which is ***pulsatile*** results in secretion of LH and FSH. As the gonads respond to FSH and LH secretions, the final maturation of reproductive system takes place. Testosterone levels increase in males and estrogen levels in females; these hormones

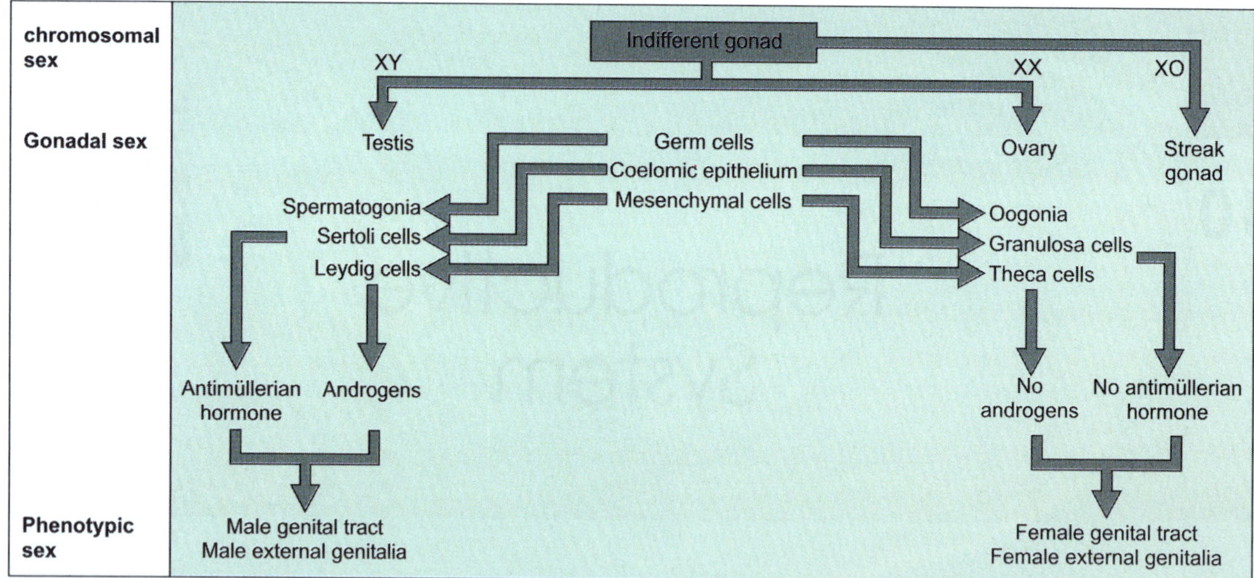

Fig. 10.1: Overview of the development of the cells of the ovary and testis from the primitive indifferent gonad. The hormonal products from the testis and the absence of these products from the ovary result in gender differences in the internal genital tracts and the external genitalia

are responsible for the secondary sex characters that develop at puberty. The period of final maturation is known as adolescence, also called puberty; although puberty stands for the period when the gametogenic functions of the gonads have first developed to the point where reproduction is possible and so it is the end of period of adolescence.

The **secondary sex characteristics** and other changes taking place **in girls at puberty** are: The development of breasts which is the first change, followed by development of axillary and pubic hair and then the first menstrual period (menarche); the maturation involves the uterus and vagina under the influence of estrogen. There is female distribution of fat in the breasts and buttocks, the voice stays high pitched. There is less body hair and more scalp hair; and pubic hair has flat upper border. Axillary hair is due to androgens from adrenal cortex; rather than estrogen. At the time of puberty, there is an increase in the secretion of **adrenal androgens**. The initial menstrual periods are generally anovulatory.

Secondary sex characteristics and other changes that take place **in boys at puberty** are: The penis increases in size and width; scrotum becomes pigmented; internal genitalia mature; voice becomes deeper; hair growth takes place, beard appears, pubic hair grow with male pattern, hair appear in axilla, on chest, general body hair increase; temperament becomes aggressive; predisposition to acne on skin.

The **age at the time of puberty** is variable. It is mostly between 10 years and 13 years in girls, 11 years and 14 years in boys.

The reproductive period in the females lasts from puberty to menopause.

Menopause

It is the time when the ovarian function regresses and oocytes are no longer liberated and so the pregnancy cannot result. Menstruation becomes irregular and cease between 45 years and 55 years. It occurs at average age of 52 years or roughly 50 years.

Changes at Menopause in Females

The ***ovaries become unresponsive to gonadotropins*** with advancing age and their function declines so that sexual cycles disappear. The ovaries no longer secrete progesterone and estrogen in appreciable quantities, and estrogen is made only in small quantities in peripheral tissues.

The uterus and vagina become atrophic due to decreased estrogen level. As a result of lack of negative feedback effects of ovarian hormones on pituitary gonadotropins, the *FSH and LH levels in plasma increase to high levels.*

Sensation of warmth spreading from trunk to face (hot flushes), night sweats and various psychic symptoms are common after ovarian function has ceased. Hot flushes may continue for as long as 40 years. They also occur with early menopause produced by bilateral ovariectomy and they are prevented by estrogen treatment. Their cause is unknown. May be some event in the hypothalamus initiates both release of LH and episode of flushing. The other effects are: Shrinkage of breast; axillary and pubic hair become sparse; episodes of characteristic behavior, sometimes irritability, mood changes; gradual thinning of skin.

In the male, there is no specific menopause and the testicular function continues, though it declines in old age, but since the sperms continue to form, reproductive capacity remains in the male usually up to the eighth decade.

Sex Hormones

The chemical nature of sex hormones: Sex hormones **estrogen, progesterone, testosterone** and other **androgens** are ***steroid hormones***. Ovaries also secrete **relaxin** especially during pregnancy which relaxes the ligaments of pubic symphysis and softens the cervix. It is a ***polypeptide hormone***.

FEMALE REPRODUCTIVE SYSTEM

The organs of reproduction in the female are: Ovary one on each side of the body hence two ovaries (Fig. 10.2).

- Internal genitalia (Fig 10.2): Two uterine (fallopian) tubes, uterus and vagina
- External genitalia: Labia majora, labia minora, clitoris, vestibular glands and hymen.

Ovaries

The ovaries lie in shallow fosse on the lateral walls of the pelvis. Ovary has a hilum for the entry and exit of vessels, nerves and lymphatics. Blood vessels and nerves pass to the ovary through the mesovarium.

The ovaries produce ova and female sex hormones. The sex hormones are estrogen and progesterone. The two hormones are formed and secreted under the control of gonadotropins from the anterior pituitary. Gonadotropins are secreted in a cyclic manner. The female hormones in turn are responsible for changes in the uterus; the changes which are suitable for implantation of the zygote, if the ovum is fertilized, so that the fetus develops in the uterus.

The ovaries have two layers of tissue:

1. **The medulla:** It is the central part and consists of fibrous tissue, blood vessels and nerves.
2. **The cortex:** It is the outer part and consists of connective tissue, the stroma covered by germinal epithelium which has ovarian follicles, each of which contains a flattened oocyte. Before puberty, immature follicles are called primordial follicles *which are present since birth.*

Internal Genitalia

The internal organs in the female reproductive system consists of **two uterine tubes** called **fallopian tubes**, one on each side with its one end near the ovary and the other end opening into uterus; one opening is thereon each side of uterus for two uterine tubes.

The uterus lying in the pelvic cavity is a muscular organ, it has urinary bladder in front and rectum

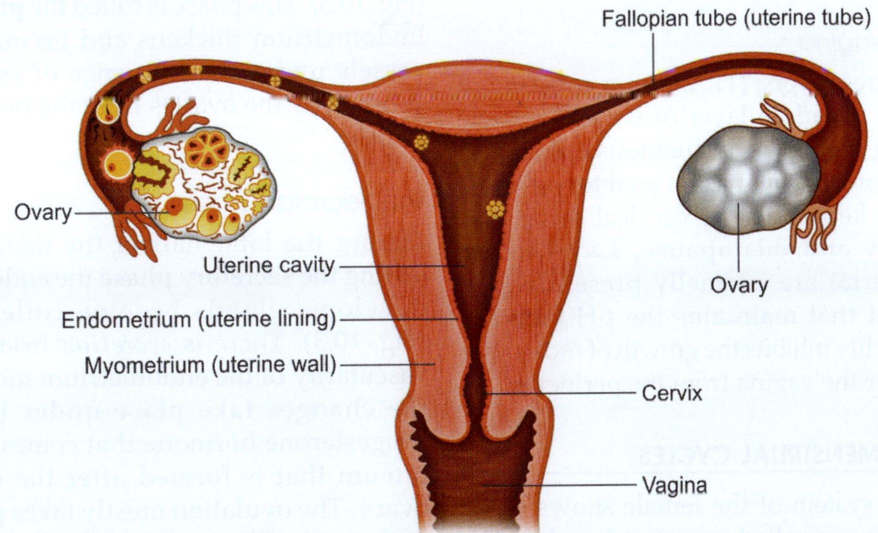

Fig. 10.2: The female reproductive system. The passage of ova has been traced in uterine tube to uterus

behind. Its parts are fundus, body and cervix. The fundus is the upper part above the opening of uterine tubes. The main part is called the body which narrows at internal os, and is continuous with the cervix. The cervix extends down and protrudes in vagina.

The uterus is composed of three layers of tissues: (1) The outermost is perimetrium; (2) the middle is thick smooth muscle the myometrium; and (3) the inner lining of epithelium with glands is the endometrium.

Myometrium is a thick smooth muscle with interlacing blood vessels, nerves and areolar tissue.

Endometrium is the inner lining of columnar epithelium containing large number of mucus-secreting tubular glands. This is divided into two layers: (1) The *functional layer* is the inner layer which shows changes during menstrual cycles and is shed off during menstruation and (2) *the basal layer* lies next to the myometrium and is not lost during menstruation. From this layer, a new functional layer is generated after menstruation (when pregnancy has not occurred).

The upper two-thirds of the cervical canal is lined with this mucous layer; further towards the vagina, the mucosa become stratified squamous epithelium like the lining of vagina.

Vagina

It is the female organ of copulation. It is a muscular tube lying obliquely behind pubic symphysis and in front of rectum and anal canal. The vagina is lined with stratified squamous epithelium. Lower end of vagina opens into perineum.

It provides an elastic passage through which baby passes out during child birth.

Structure of the Vagina

The vagina has three layers: (1) An outer covering of areolar tissue, (2) a middle layer of smooth muscle (3) an inner lining of stratified squamous epithelium that forms ridges or rugae. It has no secretory glands, but the surface is kept moist by cervical secretions. Between puberty and menopause, *Lactobacillus acidophilus* (bacteria) are normally present which secrete lactic acid that maintains the pH between 4.9 and 3.5. The acidity inhibits the growth of most other microbes that enter the vagina from the perineum.

PHYSIOLOGY OF MENSTRUAL CYCLES

The reproductive system of the female shows cyclic changes; the cycles are called **menstrual cycles**. The average duration of a cycle is 28 days, but can vary from 21 to 35 days (depending mostly on the length of the follicular phase). For about the first 4 days, there is bleeding from the vagina, **the menstruation**; the cycle days are numbered from the first day of menstruation. The cycles begin at puberty and continue during the reproductive period to end at menopause with end of reproductive period.

Menstrual Cycle

Its average duration is 28 days. The first day of bleeding is day one. The normal menstrual bleeding is mainly arterial with only about 25% of blood is venous in origin.

The Menstruation

The duration of **menstrual flow** is 3–5 days, but flow as short as 1 day and as long as 8 days can occur in normal women. The amount of blood lost; the average amount is about 30 mL normally; but varies from slight spotting. More than 80 mL is abnormal. Menstrual blood contains tissue debris, prostaglandins, and large amounts of fibrinolysin from the endometrial tissue. The fibrinolysin lyses clot so that menstrual blood does not clot normally.

The Proliferative Phase

There are cyclic changes in the uterus as a result of hormones secreted by ovary. Following the menstruation, there is secretion of estrogens from ovary. Under the influence of this hormone, the uterus shows proliferation of endometrium (its inner lining) from 5th to 14th day (during the first half of menstrual cycle). Uterine glands are drawn out as they lengthen, but they do not become convoluted and do not secrete (Fig. 10.3). This phase is called the **proliferative phase**. Endometrium thickens and becomes rich in blood vessels under the influence of estrogen hormone secreted by the ovaries from the developing graafian follicle.

The Secretory Phase

During the later half of the menstrual cycle, i.e. during the **secretory phase** the endometrium further develops; glands become coiled and tortuous (Fig. 10.3). There is ***secretion*** from the glands, the vascularity of the endometrium increases still more; the changes take place under the influence of progesterone hormone that comes from the corpus luteum that is formed after the ovulation in the ovary. The ovulation mostly takes place on 14th day of the cycle. The oocyte normally enters the uterine tubes.

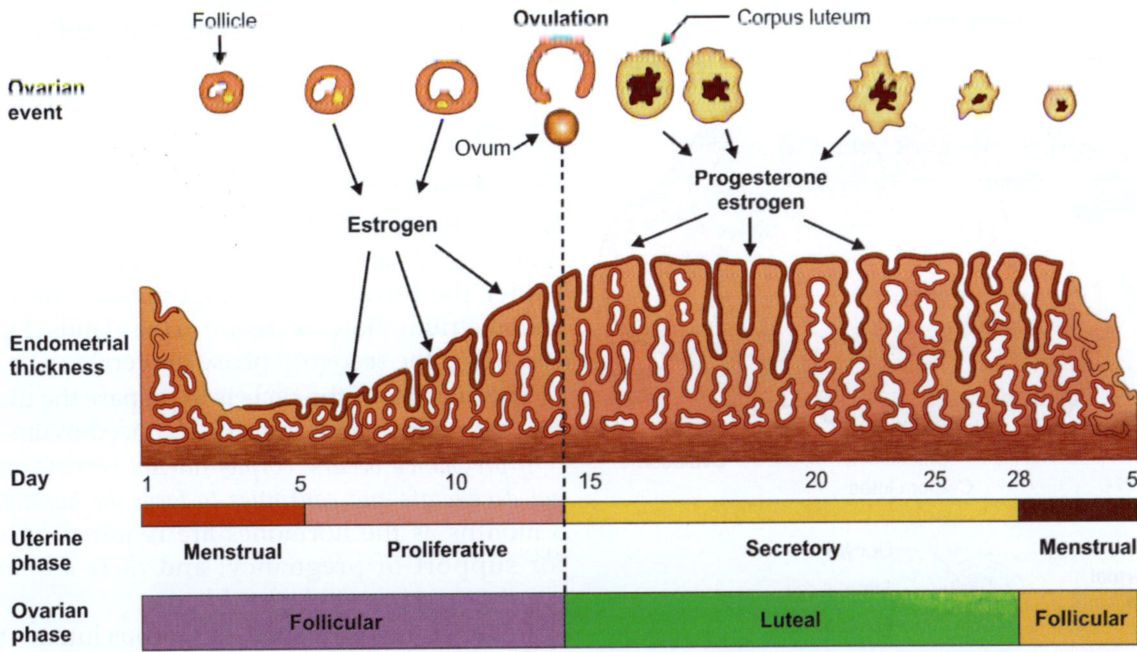

Fig. 10.3: Changes in the endometrium during the menstrual cycle. Relationship with ovarian cycle

The **corpus luteum** is formed in ovary after ovulation and secretes progesterone and estrogen. The progesterone is responsible for secretory changes in the endometrial glands. The **secretory endometrium is an indication that ovulation has occurred** in the ovary; surge in the excretion of pregnanediol, the end product of progesterone metabolism, in urine indicates that ovulation has occurred in the cycle.

The secretory phase is the preparation of the uterus to implant a fertilized ovum. If pregnancy does not result, the endometrial lining is shed off in the **menstruation** after which the next cycle starts. Menstruation occurs when the corpus luteum degenerates and so the hormonal support (of progesterone and estrogen) of the endometrium is withdrawn. Foci of necrosis appear in the endometrium and these coalesce, there is spasm and necrosis of the wall of spiral arteries leading to hemorrhages. The spasm may be produced by locally released prostaglandins. Hence, menstrual cycle has three phases:

1. Menstruation : 1st to 4th day
2. Proliferative phase : 5th to 14th day
3. Secretory phase : 15th to 28th day.

Ovarian Cycle

The Follicular Phase

Under the ovarian epithelium there are primordial follicles (Fig. 10.4A), each contains an oogonia or oocytes which is present from the time of the birth. No ova or follicles are formed after birth. At the start of each menstrual cycle, several of these follicles enlarge and a cavity forms around the oocyte. This cavity is filled with follicular fluid. After about the sixth day, one of the follicles in anyone ovary starts to grow rapidly and becomes the dominant follicle, the others regress, during the **follicular phase** of ovarian cycle. Estrogen is secreted into the circulation and also secreted inside the follicle as is needed for its final maturation.

> **Clinical Significance**
>
> During treatment of infertility, women are given highly purified pituitary gonadotropin preparations by injections; as a result many follicles develop simultaneously.

The structure of the maturing graafian follicle is shown in Figs 10.4A and B. The cells of the theca interna of the follicle are the main source of estrogen in the blood circulation. The follicular fluid has high estrogen content and much of this estrogen comes from the granulosa cells. Under the influence of estrogen in the circulation, the uterine endometrium enlarges and this is the proliferative phase of uterine cycle.

The Ovulation

On about the 14th day of the cycle, the developing follicle ruptures and the secodnary oocyte is released (ovulation) into the abdominal cavity which is picked

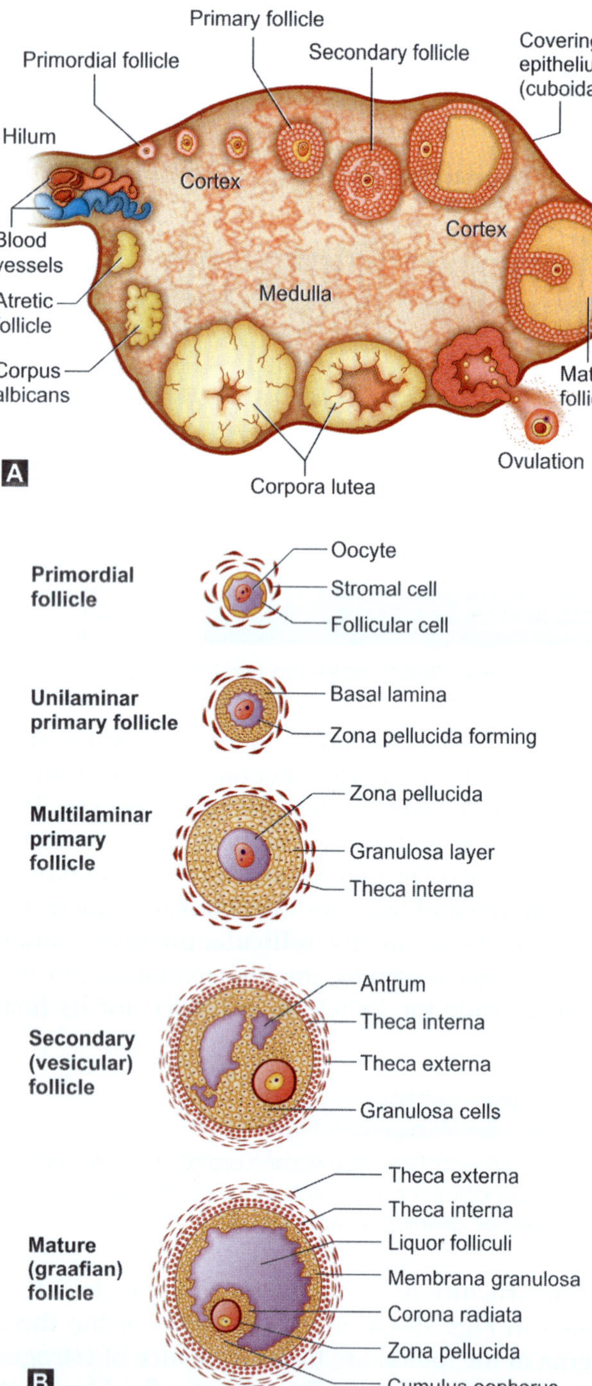

Figs 10.4A and B: (A) Representation of the ovary showing the various stages in the development of the follicle and its successor, the corpus luteum, (B) Details of each stage showing how the oocyte draws successive layers of nutritive, supportive and protective cells around it as it reaches its maximum size in the secondary follicle

up by the fimbriated end of the uterine tube and is transported to the uterus. If **fertilized in the tube,** it implants in the uterus, and if not, it is lost through the vagina. The ruptured follicle gets filled with blood and granulosa and theca cells of the follicle lining begin to proliferate and clotted blood is replaced by yellowish lipid filled luteal cells that form corpus luteum.

The Luteal Phase

Now in the **luteal phase** of ovarian cycle the luteal cells (Fig. 10.4A) secrete estrogen and progesterone. Under the influence of progesterone the uterine endometrium shows secretion in the glands (Fig. 10.5) and this is the secretory phase of uterine cycle.

The purpose of the cycle is to prepare the uterus to receive, nourish and protect a fertilized ovum.

If pregnancy occurs, corpus luteum persists and does not degenerate and continues to form the hormones for 3 months as the hormones are required by uterus for support of pregnancy; and *there are no more menstrual periods until after delivery.*

If there is no pregnancy, the corpus luteum begins to degenerate after it functions for about 12 days, 2 days prior to menstruation on about the 26th day of menstrual cycle. With this degeneration there is no progesterone or estrogen in the circulation (Fig. 10.5), the hormonal support of the endometrium is withdrawn and the endometrium is shed off producing bleeding due to ruptured blood vessels.

The duration of secretory phase remains constant. If there are changes in the duration of the cycle, it is due to changes in the duration of proliferative phase. After the menstrual bleeding normally of 4 days; another cycle starts with the secretion of FSH, as there is no negative feedback effect on it, as there is no estrogen or progesterone secreted by the ovary now. New endometrium regenerates from the basal layer of endometrium.

In each cycle, the reproductive unit in the females is the single ovarian follicle which is composed of one germ cell completely surrounded by group of **endocrine cells**. These function to:

1. Nurture the contained oocyte till ovulation
2. Prepare the fallopian tubes to assist in fertilization
3. Prepare the vagina for sperm survival
4. Prepare the lining of uterus to implant a zygote
5. Maintain hormonal support for pregnancy until placenta takes over.

Control of Ovarian Function

FSH from pituitary is responsible for early maturation of ovarian follicles. FSH and LH together are responsible for the final maturation of one follicle. *A burst of LH secretion* ***(LH surge)*** *is responsible for ovulation*

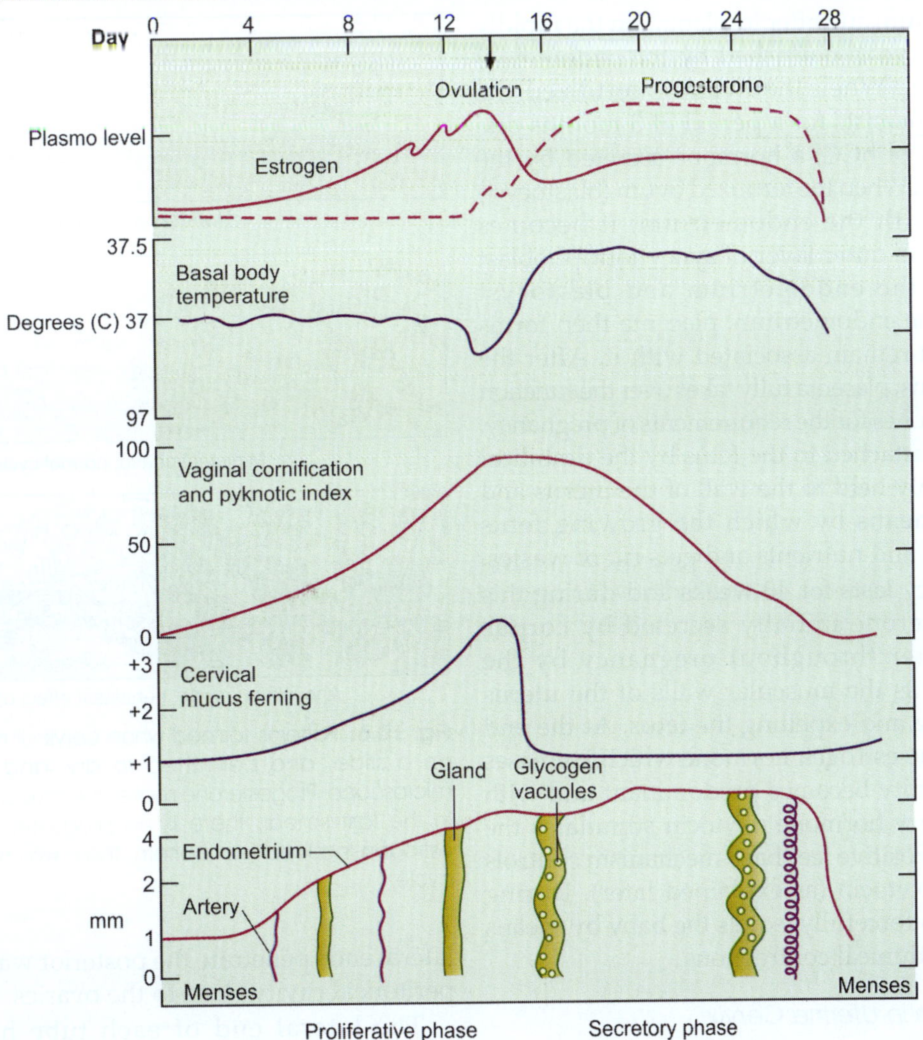

Fig. 10.5: Correlation of biological changes throughout the menstrual cycle with the plasma estradiol and progesterone levels

and initial formation of corpus luteum. FSH and LH stimulate secretion of estrogen and progesterone from the corpus luteum.

The corpus luteum is formed under the influence of the LH of the pituitary. It secretes progesterone and estrogen. The progesterone is responsible for secretory changes in the endometrial glands. As the concentration of hormones increase gonadotropin secretions decrease because of their negative feedback effects on pituitary. The corpus luteum degenerates; its hormones are not produced to support the endometrium and that results in menstruation.

After the menstrual bleeding of normally 4 days; another cycle starts with the secretion of FSH.

If pregnancy takes place, corpus luteum at the time of fertilization fails to regress and instead enlarges in response to stimulation by gonadotropic hormone secreted by placenta. The placental gonadotropin is called human chorionic gonadotropin (hCG). The enlarged corpus luteum secretes estrogen, progesterone, and relaxin. The relaxin helps to maintain pregnancy by inhibiting myometrial contractions. In humans, if ovary is removed during early pregnancy, it leads to abortion, but later in pregnancy the placenta produces sufficient estrogen and progesterone for pregnancy to continue. The corpus luteum normally functions for 3 months during pregnancy after which its function declines.

Functions of Uterus in Pregnancy

If the ovum is fertilized in the uterine tube; the fertilized ovum travels to the uterus and embeds itself in the uterine wall. The uterine muscle grows to accommodate the developing embryo (during its first 8 weeks) and fetus for the remainder of pregnancy. Uterine secretions nourish the ovum before it implants in the endometrium and after implantation the rapidly expanding embryo is nourished by the endometrial cells themselves. When the ovum is fertilized the corpus luteum persists for a period of 3 months due to the secretion of hCG, a hormone secreted by the trophoblast cells. When the fertilized ovum (blastocyst) is in contact with the endometrium, it becomes surrounded by an outer layer of syncytiotrophoblast which erodes the endometrium and blastocyst implants into the endometrium; placenta then forms and trophoblast remain associated with it. After the period of 3 months, placenta fully takes over the function of forming hormones for the requirements of pregnancy. The placenta is attached to the fetus by the umbilical cord and is firmly held to the wall of the uterus and provides the means by which the growing fetus receives oxygen and nutrients and gets rid of wastes.

The pregnancy lasts for 40 weeks and during this period progesterone initially secreted by corpus luteum and later throughout pregnancy by the placenta, prevents the muscular walls of the uterus from contracting and expelling the fetus. At the end of pregnancy, the estrogen hormone which increases uterine contractility becomes predominant and with posterior pituitary hormone oxytocin stimulates the uterine muscle. Positive feedback mechanism controls the release of oxytocin (as explained later). During labor, the uterus forcefully expels the baby by means of powerful rhythmical contractions.

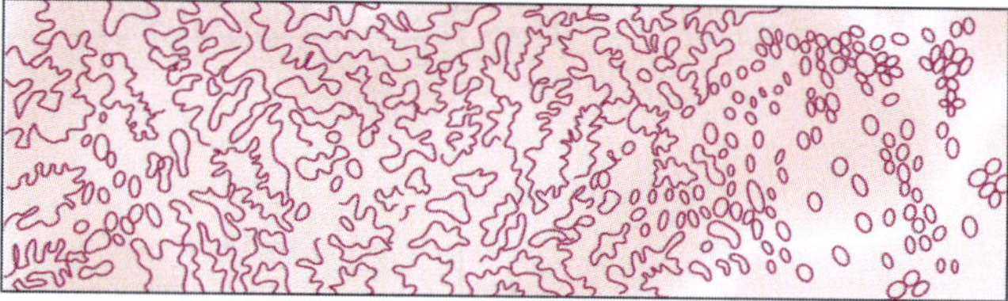

Normal cycle, 14th day

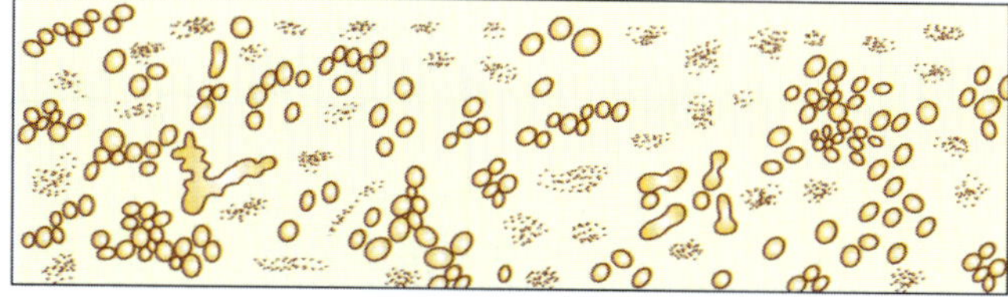

Midluteal phase, normal cycle

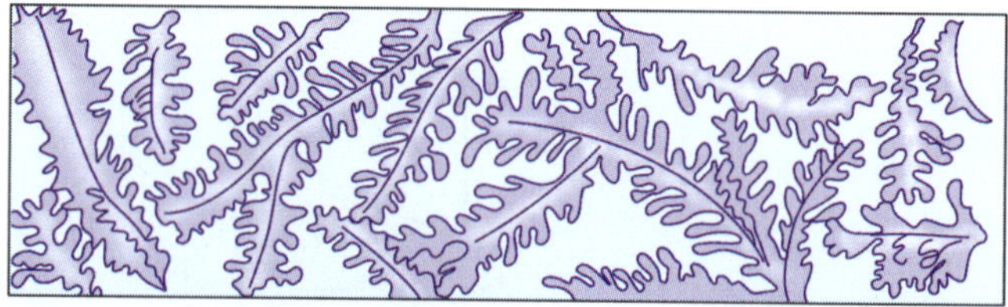

Anovulatory cycle, persistent effect of estrogen

Fig. 10.6: Patterns formed when cervical mucus is smeared on a slide, and permitted to dry, and seen under the microscope. Progesterone makes the mucus thick and cellular. In the last smear, there is no progesterone to inhibit the estrogen-induced fern pattern, there was no ovulation in the cycle

Cyclic Changes in Uterine Cervix

Although it is continuous with the body of the uterus, the cervix of the uterus is different in many ways. The mucosa of the cervix does not undergo similar changes as those in the uterus. But there are regular changes in the cervical mucus with the hormones secreted during the cycle.

Estrogen makes the mucus thinner and more alkaline; these changes promote the survival and transport of sperms; progesterone makes it thick, and cellular. The mucus is thinnest at the time of ovulation and its elasticity increases so that by midcycle a drop of it can be stretched into a long thin thread that may be as long as 8–12 cm; it dries an arborizing fern-like pattern, when a layer is spread on a slide (Fig. 10.6). After ovulation and during pregnancy because of progesterone it becomes thick and fails to form fern pattern.

Uterine Tubes

The uterine tubes extend from the sides of the uterus between the body and the fundus. They lie in the upper free border of the broad ligament and their lateral ends penetrate the posterior wall, opening into peritoneal cavity close to the ovaries.

The lateral end of each tube has finger-like projections called fimbriae. The longest of these is the ovarian fimbria which is in close association with the ovary. The tube consists of four portions, from lateral to medial are infundibulum, ampulla, isthmus and intramural part. The tubes are covered by peritoneum (broad ligament); have a middle coat of smooth muscle; and are lined by ciliated epithelium.

Functions of the Uterine Tubes

The uterine tubes convey the oocyte from the ovary to the uterus by peristalsis and ciliary movements.

The mucus secreted by the lining membrane provides ideal conditions for the movement of oocyte and spermatozoa. Fertilization of the ovum usually takes place in the ampulla of the uterine tube and the zygote is propelled into the uterus for implantation.

During the follicular phase estrogen causes: Increase in the number of cilia and in their rate of beating; and number of actively secreting epithelial cells. Estrogen also stimulates mucoid secretions so that sperms may move efficiently upstream against ciliary beat.

During the luteal phase progesterone increases the secretions for nutrition for the secondary oocyte, and to any incoming sperm and to zygote, if fertilization occurs. With the fertilization there is completion of the second meiotic division, resulting in haploid, 23 chromosomes in ovum and second polar body is discarded.

Hypothalamic Role in Ovarian Cycles

Hypothalamus controls gonadotropin secretions, its effect is exerted by GnRH, secreted into the portal hypophyseal vessels. GnRH stimulates the secretions of FSH and LH.

GnRH is secreted in pulses and not continuously. The pulses are essential for normal secretions of gonadotropins. If GnRH is administered by constant infusion, the GnRH receptors in the anterior pituitary are down regulated and LH secretion declines to zero.

Frequency of pulses is increased by estrogen and decreased by progesterone and testosterone. The frequency increases late in the follicular phase of the cycle, resulting in LH surge. During the secretory phase, the frequency decreases as a result of action of progesterone. But once the estrogen and progesterone secretion decrease at the end of the cycle, the frequency once again increases.

> Constantly elevated levels of GnRH decrease the secretion of LH, this observation has led to the use of long-acting GnRH analogs to inhibit LH secretion in precocious puberty and in cancer of prostate.

Feedback Effects

During the early part of follicular phase inhibin (Fig. 10.7) is an another hormone produced by ovary (it inhibits gonadotropins from pituitary). Its concentration is low and FSH is moderately elevated, resulting in follicular growth. LH secretion is held in check by negative feedback effect of the plasma estrogen level. At 36–48 hours before ovulation, the estrogen concentration becomes high and now the feedback effect becomes positive and this initiates LH secretion, **LH surge** (peak secretion) **occurs that produces ovulation.**

Ovulation occurs a few hours after LH peak. FSH secretion also shows peak, probably because of strong stimulation of gonadotropes by GnRH. During the luteal phase, the secretion of LH and FSH is low because of the feedback effects of elevated levels of estrogen, progesterone and inhibin.

Moderate constant level of estrogen exerts a negative feedback effect on LH secretion whereas

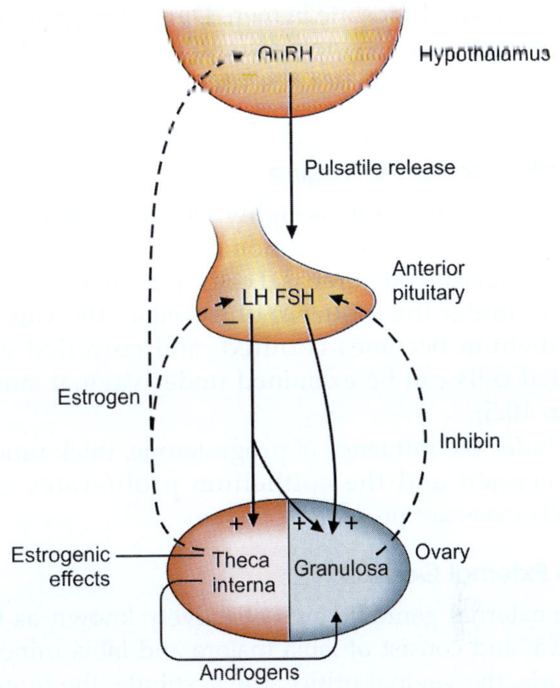

Fig. 10.7: Feedback regulation of ovarian function. The cells of the theca interna provide androgens to the granulosa cells, and theca cells also produce the circulating estrogens that inhibit the secretion of GnRH, LH and FSH. Inhibin from the granulosa cells inhibits FSH secretion. LH regulates the thecal cells whereas the granulosa cells are regulated by both LH and FSH. The dashed arrows indicate inhibitory effects and the solid arrows indicate stimulatory effects. Androgens provided to granulosa cells sustain estrogen secretion

during the cycle an elevated estrogen level exerts a positive feedback effect and stimulates LH secretion.

When the progesterone levels are high, the positive feedback effect of estrogen is inhibited.

The Ovum

The ovum lives for 72 hours after it is extruded from the follicles. But it is fertilizable for a much shorter time than this.

In midcycle, there is increase, in the responsiveness of the pituitary to GnRH and surge in LH secretion takes place. The ovulation takes place and the formation of corpus luteum follows. There is fall in the secretion of estrogen, but progesterone and estrogen levels after that rise, so also the inhibin level. The high levels of these inhibit FSH and LH secretion till luteolysis (degeneration of corpus luteum) takes place and a new cycle starts.

Relaxin

It is a polypeptide hormone that is produced by corpus luteum, also by uterus, placenta and mammary glands in women and prostate in men. During pregnancy, it relaxes the pubic symphysis and other pelvic joints and soften and dilates the uterine cervix. Thus it facilitates delivery.

Cyclic Changes in Vagina

The lining epithelium is highly sensitive to estrogen. In the absence of the hormone, there is only a thin layer of basal and parabasal cells. During menstrual cycles under the influence of estrogen, the vaginal epithelium becomes cornifed, and cornified epithelial cells can be examined under vaginal smear (Fig. 10.5).

Under the influence of progesterone, thick mucus is secreted and the epithelium proliferates and leuckocytes are present.

The External Genitalia

The external genitalia are collectively known as the vulva, and consist of labia majora and labia minora, clitoris, the vaginal orifice, the vestibule, the hymen and the vestibular glands (Bartholin's glands).

CONTRACEPTION

Some sperms can survive in the female genital tract and able to produce fertilization for up to 120 hours, if ovulation occurs during that period, but most fertile period is 48 hours. The ovum lives for 72 hours after it is extruded from the follicles, but it is fertilizable for a much shorter time than this.

The rhythm method of contraception is based on avoiding intercourse during the middle part of menstrual cycle and restricting it to the safe period after and before menstruation. But is not 100% safe, as pregnancy has found to have resulted from isolated intercourse on everyday of the cycle.

Methods commonly used to prevent conception are based on the principle: **Prevent ovulation** from occurring; **prevent the fertilization of ovum**; **prevent embedding of the ovum**, or **by abortion** by giving anti-progestational drugs. If conception has occurred, abortion can be produced by progesterone antagonists.

Methods of Contraception

- **Rhythm method** based on safe period as mentioned above is not very reliable.
- **Withdrawal method:** The penis is withdrawn before ejaculation occurs, i.e. prevent semen to be deposited in the vagina. But this method is also not reliable as some semen may be deposited before full ejaculation occurs.

The other methods are:

- **Intrauterine devices (IUDs): Implantation of a foreign body,** pieces of metal or plastic [intrauterine devices, (IUDs)] in the uterus does not alter the period of menstrual cycle. But it acts as effective contraceptive device. The mechanism of action is not clear; perhaps they prevent the sperm from fertilizing ova. The devices containing copper perhaps have spermicidal action; IUD's that slowly release progesterone (or synthetic progestins) have additional effect on cervical mucus to make it thick so that entry of sperm into uterus is hindered.
- **Barrier methods: Diaphragm** in women and **condom** in males are used; condoms are also there for females though not very popular; condoms are also recommended to prevent transmission of HIV infection to the partner. Spermicidal creams used along with diaphragm are also available.
- **Oral pills:** Women undergoing long-term treatment with **relatively large doses of estrogen do not ovulate** probably due to depressed levels of FSH and multiple irregular peaks of LH secretion. Women treated with similar doses of **estrogen along with progestational** agent (progestin) do not ovulate due to inhibition of both gonadotropins; also progestin makes the cervical mucus thick and unfavorable for sperm movement. Orally active estrogen is often combined with synthetic progestin in **oral pills**. The pills are taken one a day for 21 days, then withdrawn for 5–7 days to permit menstrual flow and started again.

It is also realized that small as well as large doses of estrogen are effective; the use of small doses reduce the risk of venous thromboses or other complications. Progestins alone can be used for contraception although they are not as effective as when combined with estrogen.

- **Implants of progestin inserted under the skin** can prevent pregnancy up to 5 years. They often produce amenorrhea, but otherwise they appear to be effective and well-tolerated.
- **Postcoital "morning after" contraception:** Women are sometimes given large doses of estrogen for 4–6 days to prevent conception following coitus that has been during the fertile period (postcoital "morning after" contraception). Pregnancy is possibly prevented by preventing implantation of a fertilized ovum, if it has been fertilized.

- **Surgical methods of contraception:** Ligation of both uterine tubes (**tubal ligation, tubectomy**) in women or ligations of the vas deferens in males **(vasectomy)** are surgical methods used. Fertility, if it is to be restored in males by recanalization, becomes difficult as in some cases antibodies to sperm are produced after this procedure in males.

Indicators of Ovulation

For infertility or for avoiding conception, it becomes important to know the day, the ovulation occurs in any woman during her menstrual cycle. Though ovulation occurs on the 14th day, it may not be so in all women.

A convenient and fairly reliable method is by recording **basal body temperature (oral or rectal)** before getting out of the bed in the morning with a thermometer that has large graduations. There is a change in body temperature at the time of ovulation and following the ovulation the body temperature remains about 0.5°C higher due to thermogenic effect of progesterone (Fig. 10.5).

Cervical mucus smears made would show changes due to progesterone, if ovulation has taken place in the menstrual cycle. Progestational changes would occur only if ovulation has taken place following which corpus luteum is formed that secretes progesterone.

Urine for surge in excretion of metabolic products of progesterone.

Other Functions of Sex Hormones

Estrogens produce ***duct growth in the breast*** and are largely responsible for breast enlargement at puberty in girls; they have been called growth hormone of the breast. Progesterone causes growth of lobules and alveoli. Breast swelling, tenderness and pain during last 10 days preceding the menstruation are due to distention of the ducts, hyperemia, and edema of the breast. All these changes regress and symptoms regress with menstruation.

Salt and water retention and weight gain before menstruation is due to estrogens. Estrogens **lower plasma cholesterol**; produce vasodilation by increasing local production of nitric oxide (NO). These actions inhibit atherogenesis during reproductive period in women.

Abnormalities of Ovarian Function

Menstrual Abnormalities

Anovulatory cycles: In some cases, ovulation fails to occur during menstrual cycle. Such anovulatory cycles are common for the first 12–18 months after menarche (the first period after puberty) and again before onset of menopause. When ovulation does not occur, corpus luteum is not formed and effects of progesterone on endometrium are absent. Estrogen continues to cause growth of endometrium and proliferative endometrium breaks down and bleeding occurs. The cycle duration may be less than 28 days. The blood loss may be from scanty to profuse.

Amenorrhea is the absence of menstrual periods. If the menstrual bleeding has never occurred, the condition is called *primary amenorrhea*. Cessation of cycles in women after normal periods is called *secondary amenorrhea*.

During pregnancy there is amenorrhea and all amenorrhea should be considered due to pregnancy until proved otherwise. *Other causes of amenorrhea include changes in environment, emotional stimuli and diseased conditions like ovarian pituitary disorders or hypothalamic diseases and even various systemic diseases.*

- Hypomenorrhea refers to scanty periods.
- Menorrhagia refers to profuse periods.
- Metrorrhagia is bleeding from uterus between periods.
- Oligomenorrhea reduced frequency of periods.

Dysmenorrhea is painful menstruation. Sometimes women have severe menstrual cramps during menstruation often disappears after first pregnancy. Most of the symptoms of dysmenorrhea are due to prostaglandins in the uterus which accumulates at this time and relief of symptoms occurs by drugs which are inhibitors of their synthesis.

Premenstrual Syndrome (PMS)

During the last 7–10 days before the periods some women develop symptoms like depression, decreased ability to concentrate, headache, constipation, irritability, bloating, emotional lability. These symptoms of PMS are due to salt and water retention.

Genetic Defects

A number of single gene mutations cause reproductive abnormalities:

1. Kallmann's syndrome, a hypogonadism due to low levels of circulating gonadotropins with partial or complete loss of sense of smell; pubertal maturation of gonads fails to occur.

   This syndrome is more common in men and cause in many cases is mutation of a gene on X chromosome.

2. GnRH resistance, FSH resistance and LH resistance which are due to defects of receptors for corresponding hormones.
3. Enzyme deficiency which prevents formation of estrogen.

These are all caused by loss of function due to genes mutation. A case of gain in function due to gene mutation is seen in McCune-Albright syndrome; abnormalities, include precocious puberty and amenorrhea with galactorrhea.

Structure of the Breast

The Mammary Glands

The two mammary glands lie over pectoralis major and serratus anterior muscles; attached to them by a layer of deep fascia composed of dense connective tissue.

Each breast has a tiny projection, the nipple surrounded by a colored area of skin called areola; areola appears rough because it contains modified sebaceous glands (Montgomery's tubercles); they lubricate the nipple during lactation. Connective tissue strands called the suspensory ligaments run between the skin and the deep fascia and support the breast; these become looser with age. The gland is composed of 15–20 lobes, radiating from nipple. The lactiferous duct from each lobe opens separately on the nipple (Fig. 10.8). Just prior to the opening, the duct is dilated to form lactiferous sinus. Lobules consist of cluster of alveoli which open into small ducts and they unite to form large duct, called lactiferous ducts. The lactiferous ducts converge towards the center of the breast and they form dilatations for reservoirs of milk. Leading from each dilatation is a narrow duct which opens into the surface of the nipple.

Fibrous tissue supports glandular tissue and ducts and fat covers the surface of the gland and is found between the lobes.

The breasts are accessory glands of the female reproductive system. They are rudimentary in males.

In the female, the breasts until puberty are immature and small. There is **growth at puberty** under the influence of estrogens. Further some growth take place with **each menstrual cycle** under the influence of estrogens and progesterone with some **regression at the end** of menstrual cycle. The **estrogens** are responsible for *the proliferation of the ducts in the breast; progesterone causes development of lobules. Glucocorticoids, insulin and growth hormone are probably necessary for mammary development in response to other hormones, but they do not by themselves cause growth of the breast.*

During pregnancy, prolactin levels increase progressively until term and under the influence of this hormone and high levels of estrogen and progesterone full lobuloalveolar development of the breast takes place.

Secretion and Ejection of Milk

In the breast that develops under the influence of estrogen and progesterone, *prolactin causes formation of milk droplets and their secretion into the ducts.*

It is seen that breast growth and lactation can occur in dwarfs with congenital growth hormone deficiency.

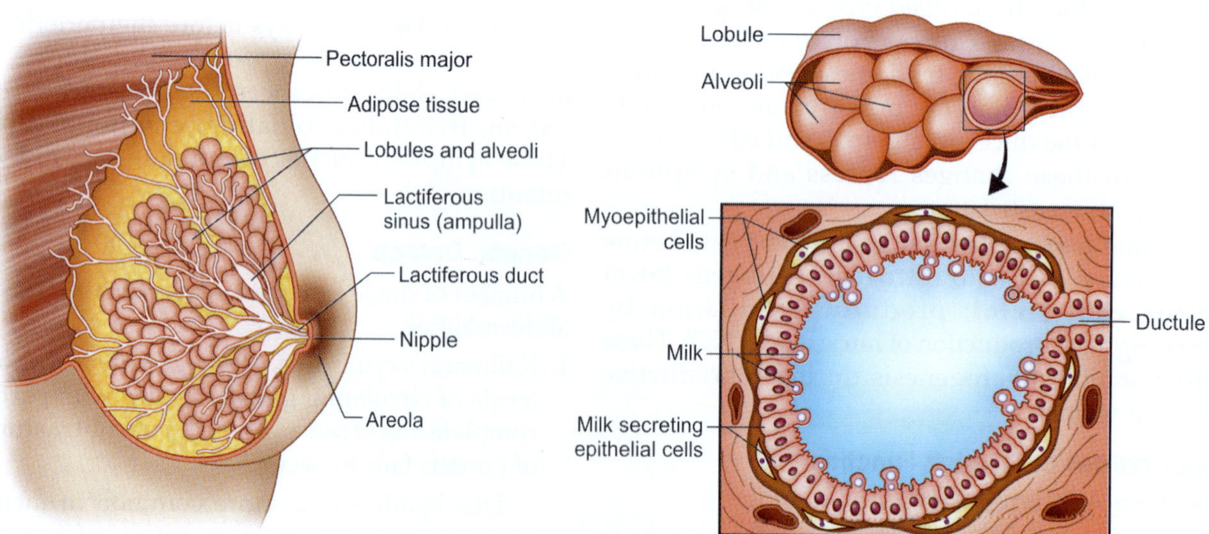

Fig. 10.8: The breast and its mammary gland

Initiation of Lactation after Delivery

The breasts enlarge during pregnancy in response to high circulating levels of estrogen, progesterone, and prolactin.

Some milk is secreted in the ducts about fifth month of pregnancy, but in small amounts. It usually takes 1–3 days for milk to come after delivery; and after that there is surge of milk secretion.

When placenta is expelled at parturition, there is abrupt decline in circulating estrogens and progesterone. Lactation is initiated by the drop in circulating estrogens. Prolactin and estrogen together produce breast growth, but estrogens inhibit the milk producing effect of prolactin.

Oxytocin causes contraction of myoepithelial cells lining the duct walls with resulting ejection of milk through nipple.

The oxytocin is liberated in response to reflex, initiated by touching the nipples and areolas (milk ejection reflex), **oxytocin is essential for milk ejection.** *Antibodies are transferred to the infant by colostrums.*

Table 10.1 gives the composition of milk.

Suckling produces **reflex oxytocin** secretion and **milk ejection; suckling also** influences the **secretion** of milk as it stimulates **prolactin** secretion.

Table 10.1: Composition of colostrum and milk (units are weight per deciliter)

Component	*Human colostrum*	*Human milk*	*Cow's milk*
Water (g)	—	88	88
Lactose (g)	5.3	6.8	5.0
Protein (g)	2.7	1.2	3.3
Casein: Lactalbumin ratio	—	1:2	3:1
Fat (g)	2.9	3.8	3.7
Linoleic acid	—	8.3% of fat	1.6% of fat
Sodium (mg)	92	15	58
Potassium (mg)	55	55	138
Chloride (mg)	117	43	103
Calcium (mg)	31	33	125
Magnesium (mg)	4	4	12
Phosphorus (mg)	14	15	100
Iron (mg)	0.09[2]	0.15[2]	0.10[2]
Vitamin A (µg)	89	53	34
Vitamin D (µg)	—	0.03[2]	0.06[2]
Thiamine (µg)	15	16	42
Riboflavin (µg)	30	43	157
Nicotinic acid (µg)	75	172	85
Ascorbic acid (µg)	4.4[2]	4.3[2]	1.6[2]

[2]Poor source

Effects of Lactation on Menstrual Cycles

Menstrual periods usually return after 6 weeks of delivery in women who do not breastfeed their infants. But with regular breastfeeding, there is amenorrhea for about 25–30 weeks and further about 50% of the cycles in the first 6 months after resumption of menstruation are anovulatory.

Breastfeeding stimulates prolactin secretion and prolactin possibly inhibits secretion of GnRH; inhibits the action of GnRH on the pituitary; and antagonizes the action of gonadotropins on the ovaries. Ovaries are inactive; and ovulation is inhibited; secretion of estrogens and progesterone is low. But 5–10% of women do become pregnant again during suckling period.

MALE REPRODUCTIVE SYSTEM

The male reproductive system consists of following organs (Fig. 10.9):

- *Testis:* One on each side, i.e. two (plural is testes)
- *Epididymis:* One on each side, i.e. two (plural is epididymes)
- *Vas deferens:* One on each side, i.e. two in number
- *Seminal vesicle:* One on each side, i.e. two in number
- *Ejaculatory duct:* One on each side, i.e. two in number
- *Prostate:* One
- *Penis:* One.

Scrotum

It is a pouch with deeply pigmented skin, fibrous and connective tissue and smooth muscle. It is divided partially into two compartments each of which contains one testis, one epididymis and the testicular end of spermatic cord. It lies below the symphysis, pubis and behind the penis.

Testes

They are the reproductive glands of the male and form sperms and male sex hormone, testosterone. During early fetal life testes, develop in the lumbar region of the abdominal cavity, they descend to the scrotum and take with them the covering of peritoneum, blood and lymph vessels, nerves and the vas deferens. The peritoneum then surrounds testis in the scrotum and becomes detached from the abdominal peritoneum. ***Descent of the testes into the scrotum should be completed by the 8th month of fetal life.***

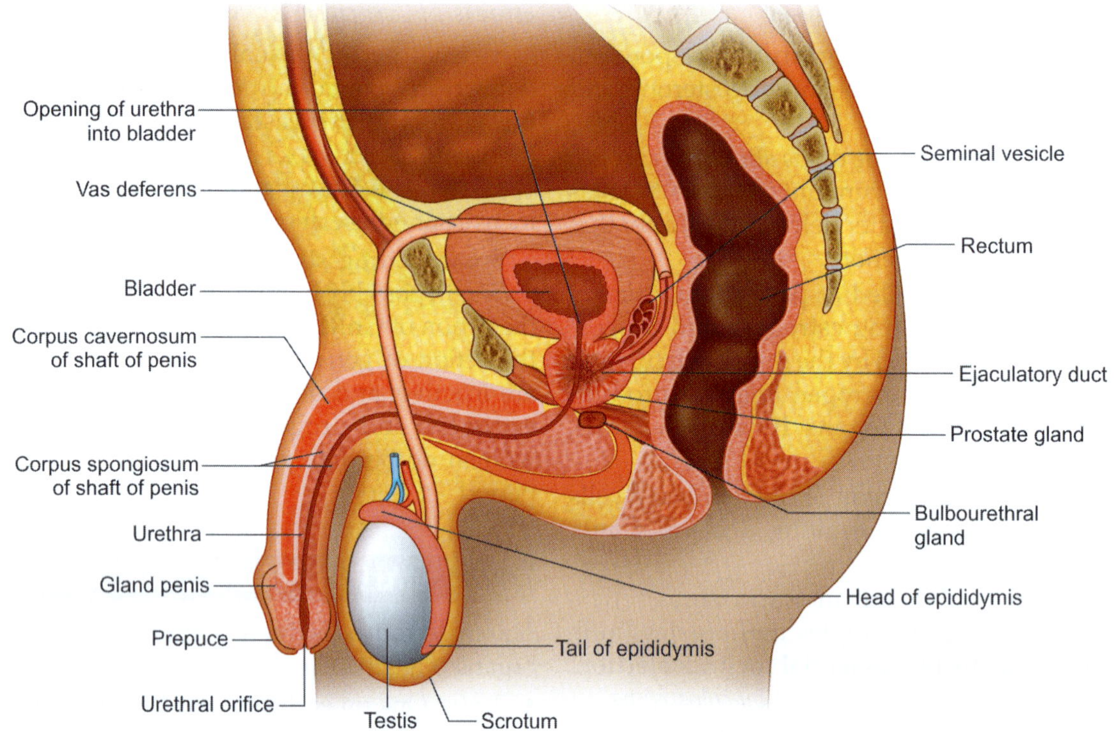

Fig. 10.9: Male genital organs

Structure of the Testes

In each testis there are 200–300 lobules and each lobule has 1–4 seminiferous tubules (Fig. 10.10A). Between the tubules, there are groups of **interstitial cells of Leydig** (Fig. 10.10B); these cells secrete the ***hormone, testosterone*** after puberty.

At the upper pole of the testis, tubules unite to form a single tubule. This tubule is repeatedly folded and tightly packed into the epididymis. It leaves the scrotum as the vas deferens (Fig. 10.9) in the spermatic cord. Blood vessels and lymph vessels pass to the testes in the spermatic cords.

The spermatic arteries to the testes are tortuous and blood in them runs parallel, but in the opposite direction to blood in the plexus of spermatic veins. This anatomical arrangement may permit counter current exchange of heat and testosterone; so that heat from arterial side is passed onto venous side shortcircuiting testes; high levels of testosterone in the venous blood exchange onto arterial blood going to the testes.

Functions of the Testes

In the walls of seminiferous tubules (Fig. 10.10A), spermatozoa (sperms) are formed from the primitive germ cells, the **spermatogonia,** by the process called **spermatogenesis**. Spermatogonia are in the lining of the seminiferous tubules in the outermost part and are supported by cells called **Sertoli cells** (Fig. 10.10B). The sertoli cells are large, contain glycogen and extend from basal lamina of the tubule to the lumen. Germ cells stay in contact with sertoli cells to develop; contact is maintained by bridges of carbohydrate molecules. Tight junctions between the adjacent Sertoli cells near the basal lamina form a **blood-testis barrier** that prevents many large molecules passing from interstitial tissue into the tubular lumen. **Testosterone** hormone which is produced by Leydig cells in the interstitial compartment; being a steroid hormone can pass through; ***the hormone supports spermatogenesis***. The barrier protects the germ cells from blood borne harmful substances (that may enter into the interstitial fluid) from passing into seminiferous tubules; and prevents antigenic products of germ cell division from entering the interstitial compartment to pass into circulation and produce autoimmune responses (antibodies against these substances which are own body substances).

Spermatogenesis begins at adolescence; ***FSH from pituitary stimulates the process***; testosterone secretion under the influence of LH on Leydig cells also has a role in the process.

The **spermatogonia**, which are primitive germ cells, mature into **primary spermatocytes,** which contain

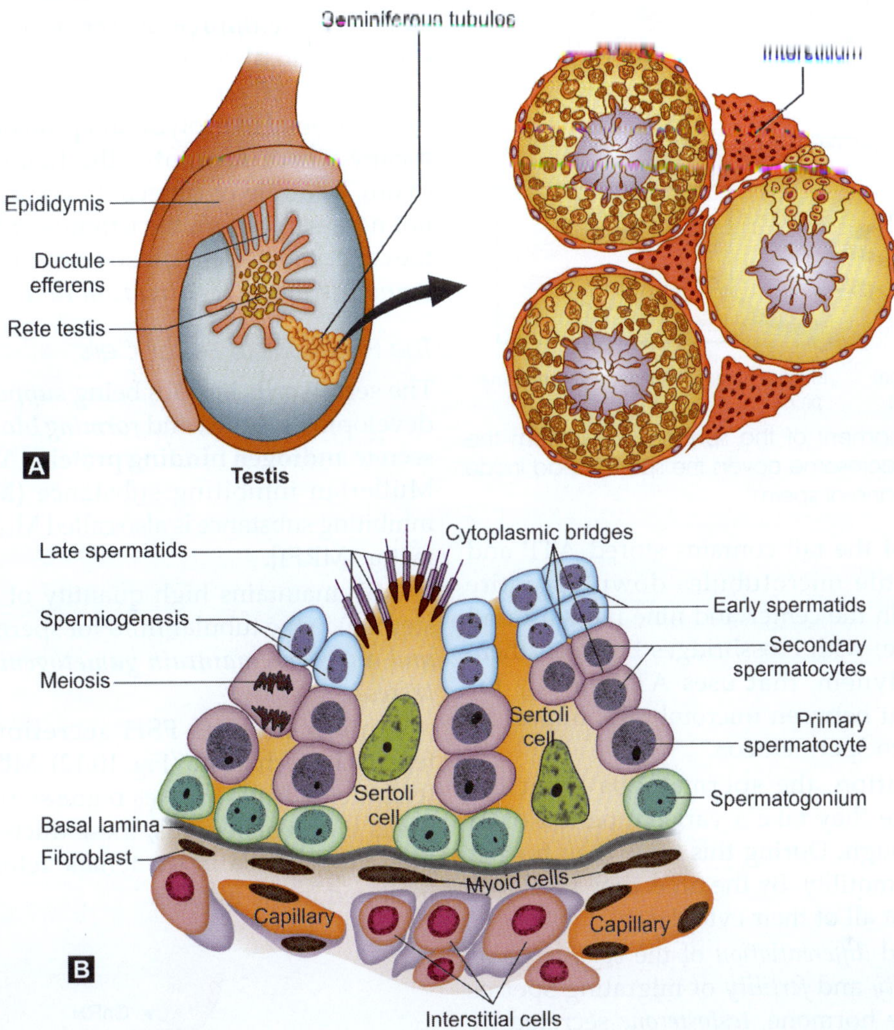

Figs 10.10A and B: (A) Seminiferous tubules, (B) Seminiferous epithelium. The maturing germ cells remain connected by cytoplasmic bridges and these cells are closely invested by Sertoli cell cytoplasm as they move from the basal lamina to the lumen

diploid number of chromosomes. The primary spermatocytes divide to form **secondary spermatocytes** which divide into **spermatids**; during these divisions reduction of chromosomes by 1st and 2nd meiotic divisions takes place; reducing the number of chromosomes in the spermatids, to the *haploid number of* 23 chromosomes, i.e. 22 autosomal chromosomes and one sex chromosome; either X or Y sex chromosome in one spermatid (Fig. 10.16).

The spermatids *mature* into **spermatozoa (sperms)**. This process is called **spermiogenesis**. It includes nuclear condensation, shrinkage of cytoplasm; formation of acrosome and development of a tail.

A number of spermatids is formed from a single spermatogonium. 100 to 200 million sperms approximately are produced per day requiring the spermatogonia to renew by cell division. It is different from female reproductive system where at birth there are fixed number of oocytes with no additions after birth and the number decreases throughout life with the menstrual cycles.

The spermatids lie near the lumen of the seminiferous tubule (Fig. 10.10B). They remain attached to the sertoli cells. The sperms are then extruded into the lumen with most of the cytoplasm remaining embedded in the cytoplasm of a sertoli cell. Hence, the sertoli cells also remove excess cytoplasm of the spermatids.

Once the **sperms** have entered the lumen of the seminiferous tubule they consist of long structure composed of several functional components (Fig. 10.11). The **head contains nucleus**, and covering it like a **cap is acrosome, containing enzymes**, hydrolytic and proteolytic which facilitate *penetration of the sperm into the ovum*. The middle piece or body contains mitochondria which generates energy for motility. The

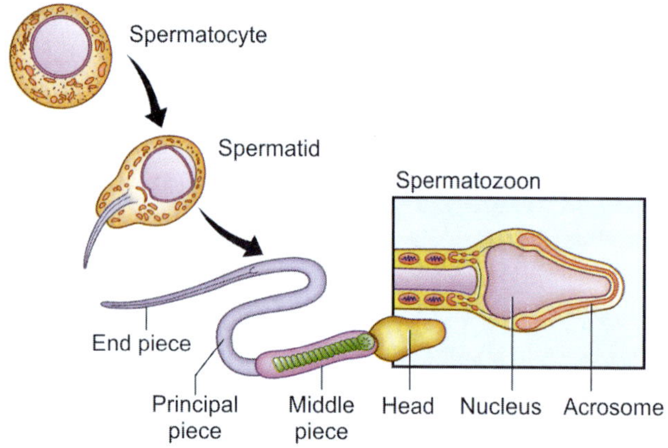

Fig. 10.11: Development of the spermatozoon from the spermatocyte. The acrosome covers the sperm head inside the plasma membrane of sperm

principal piece of the tail contains stored ATP and pairs of contractile microtubules down its entire length, one pair in the center and nine pairs around the circumference; with crossbridges between them which contain dynein, that uses ATP energy for sliding movement between microtubules; imparting flagellar motion to spermatozoa.

After spermiation, the spermatozoa enter the epididymis where they take a variable period of 24 days to pass through. During this time, they further mature and gain motility. By the time, they reach vas deferens have lost all of their cytoplasm.

The *growth* and *differentiation* of the *epididymis* as well as the *motility* and *fertility* of migrating sperms depend upon the hormone, *testosterone* secreted by Leydig cells. Motility of sperms is perhaps an important function of epididymis. *The ability to move forward (progressive motility) is acquired in the epididymis.*

The total amount of sperms stored in the epididymis is about an equivalent of a single ejaculate or single day's production. A number of proteins present in the epididymal fluid and seminiferous tubular fluid bind to the membrane of the sperms and enhance their function.

Delivery of spermatozoa into the female genital tract occurs by ***ejaculation*** which has the contents of vas deferens; to it fluids are added from prostate gland and from the seminal vesicles. Ejaculated sperms cannot immediately fertilize an ovum *in vivo* fertilization takes place only after the sperm has been in the female genital tract for 4–6 hours, process called ***capacitation***. *In vitro* fertilization can take place after spermatozoa are washed-free of seminal fluid; perhaps the materials in the female genital tract remove or neutralize substances on the surface of sperms. With ***capacitation motility becomes whiplike that may enhance penetration of the ovum.*** Capacitation also results in acrosomal reaction, i.e. breakdown of acrosomal membrane through which the acrosomal hydrolytic and proteolytic enzymes can escape which facilitates the fusion of sperm with ovum. The role of capacitation is facilitatory though not necessary. From the isthmus of the uterine tubes, the capacitated spermatozoa move rapidly to the ***tubal ampullas where fertilization takes place.***

The Functions of Sertoli Cells

The sertoli cells besides being ***supporting cells*** to the developing sperms; and ***forming blood-testes barrier***; secrete **androgen binding protein (ABP)**, **inhibin**, and Müllerian inhibiting substance **(MIS).** [Müllerian inhibiting substance is also called Müllerian regression factor (MRF)].

ABP maintains high quantity of androgen (testosterone) in the tubular fluid for spermatogenesis. ***FSH and androgen maintain gametogenic function of the testes.***

Inhibin inhibits FSH secretion in a negative feedback mechanism (Fig. 10.12). MIS secreted during fetal life by testes; causes regression of the Müllerian ducts in the male fetus; these ducts form the female internal genitalia in the female fetus as they are not inhibited in the females.

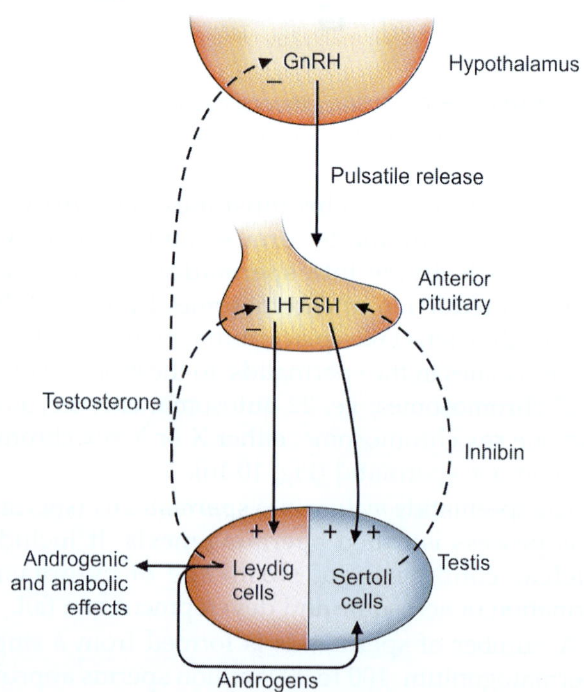

Fig. 10.12: Postulated interrelationships between the hypothalamus, anterior pituitary and testes. Solid arrows indicate excitatory effects; dashed arrows indicate inhibitory effects

Effects of Temperature

The testes normally remain at a temperature lower than that of the body by about 2–4°C. They are kept cool by air circulating around the scrotum and probably by the heat exchange in counter fashion between spermatic arteries and veins.

If the testes do not descend in the scrotum; but remain in the abdomen, degeneration of the germ epithelium and sterility would results.

Seminal Vesicles

They are two small fibromuscular pouches lined with columnar epithelium lying on the posterior aspect of bladder (Fig. 10.9).

At the lower end, each seminal vesicle opens into a short duct which joins with corresponding vas deferens to form an ejaculatory duct (Fig. 10.9).

Functions of Seminal Vesicles

The seminal vesicles contract and expel their stored contents, seminal fluid during ejaculation. The seminal fluid which forms 60% of the bulk of the fluid ejaculated at male orgasm, contains nutrients to support the sperm during their journey through the female reproductive tract.

Prostate Gland

It lies in the pelvic cavity in front of the rectum and behind the symphysis pubis, surrounding the first part (3 cm) of urethra (Fig. 10.9). It consists of an outer fibrous covering, a layer of smooth muscle and glandular substance composed of columnar epithelial cells.

Functions of Prostate Gland

Delivery of spermatozoa into the female genital tract occurs by ejaculation from the vas deferens. To the contents of the vas deferens successive fluids are added. The secretions from the prostate gland contain citrate, calcium, zinc and acid phosphates. The alkalinity of prostatic fluid helps to neutralize acid pH of semen and the vaginal and cervical secretions.

Prostatic secretions also contain a clotting enzyme which thickens semen in the vagina, increasing the likelihood of semen being retained in the vicinity of cervix.

URETHRA AND PENIS

Urethra

The male urethra provides a common passage for the flow of urine and semen. It is about 19–20 cm long and consists of three parts.

1. The prostatic urethra
2. Membranous urethra
3. The penile urethra

There are two urethral sphincters. The internal sphincter consists of smooth muscle fibers at the neck of the bladder above the prostate gland. The external sphincter consists of skeletal muscle fibers surrounding the membranous part.

Delivery of Sperm into Vagina

It requires **penile erection** which is caused by filling of the venous sinuses with blood. This converts the penis into a firm organ for penetration. The venous sinuses are filled by the arteriolar dilatation and venous constriction. **The erection is under impulses from the parasympathetic nervous system**.

Parasympathetic stimulation leads to filling of the spongy erectile tissue with blood due to arteriolar dilatation, and as the erectile tissue fills with blood the veins are compressed, with compression of veins outflow of blood is obstructed, the penis therefore, becomes engorged and erect (**erection**). The *integrating centers are in the* ***lumbar segment of the spinal cord*** that are activated by afferents from genitalia and descending tracts that mediate erection in response to psychic stimuli. The efferent parasympathetic nerves are the nervi erigentes. The fibers presumably release acetylcholine and VIP as neurotransmitters. There are also nonadrenergic, noncholinergic fibers in the nervi erigentes and these contain large amounts of NO synthase, the enzyme that catalyzes the formation of NO, vasodilator substance.

Ejaculation

Ejaculation is effected by sympathetic nervous system.

During ejaculation at the point of male orgasm, spermatozoa are expelled from the vas deferens, the ejaculatory duct and the urethra. The semen is propelled by powerful rhythmical contractions of the smooth muscle in the walls of vas deferens. Muscles in the wall of the seminal vesicles and prostate gland also contract. The force generated by these combined processes leads to emission of the semen through the external urethral sphincter.

Sperm comprises only 10% of the final ejaculate. The remainder is made-up of seminal and prostatic fluids which are added during male orgasm; also the mucus produced in the urethra.

If not ejaculated, the sperms gradually lose their fertility after several months and are reabsorbed by the epididymis. Ejaculation is a two-part spinal reflex that involves **emission,** the movement of semen into urethra; and **ejaculation** proper, the propulsion of semen out of urethra.

The afferent pathways are mostly fibers from touch receptors in the glans penis that reaches the spinal cord through the internal pudendal nerves.

Emission is a sympathetic response integrated in the ***upper lumbar segments of the spinal cord*** and affected by contractions of the smooth muscle of the vasa deferentia and seminal vesicles.

The semen is **propelled out** of urethra by **contraction** of the **bulbocavernosus muscle** (a skeletal muscle). *The spinal reflex centers for this part of the reflex are in the upper sacral and lowest lumbar segments*, the motor pathways transverse the first to third sacral roots and the pudendal nerve. Carbon monoxide (CO) may be involved in control of ejaculation.

Semen

It contains sperms and secretion of the seminal vesicles, prostate, Cowper's glands and probably the urethral glands. The average volume per ejaculate is 2.5–3.5 mL after several days of abstinence. Typical emissions are about 200–400 million spermatozoa in a volume of 3–4 mL.

The volume and the sperm count decrease rapidly with repeated ejaculation. There are normally about 100 million sperms per mL of semen (Table 10.2 also gives the composition of semen).

Table 10.2: Composition of human semen

Color: White, opalescent
Specific gravity: 1.028
pH: 7.35–7.50
Sperm count: Average about 100 million/mL with fewer than 20% abnormal forms

Other components:

Fructose (1.5–6.5 mg/mL) Phosphorylcholine Ergothioneine Ascorbic acid Flavins Prostaglandins	From seminal vesicles
Spermine Citric acid Cholesterol, phospholipids Fibrinolysin, fibrinogenase Zinc Acid phosphatase	From prostate
Phosphatase Bicarbonate Hyaluronidase	Buffers

Fifty percent of men with counts of 20–40 million/mL and all with counts under 20 million/mL are sterile, although it takes only one sperm to fertilize the ovum; the presence of many morphologically abnormal or immotile spermatozoa also correlate with infertility.

Human sperms move at a speed of about 3 mm/min through the female genital tract. Sperms reach the uterine tubes 30–60 minutes after copulation. The life span of sperms in female genital tract is approximately 2 days.

Prostate-specific Antigen

The prostate produces and secretes into the semen and bloodstream is a serine protease called **prostate-specific antigen** (PSA).

PSA hydrolyzes the sperm motility inhibitor semenogelin in semen.

An elevated plasma level occurs in prostate cancer and is used as a test for this disease; though PSA is also elevated in benign prostatic hyperplasia and prostatitis.

Vasectomy

Bilateral ligation of vas deferens (vasectomy) is a safe and convenient contraceptive procedure. But, if the patency has to be restored again for fertility, the success rate is only 50%. Some men also develop antibodies against spermatozoa and this may contribute to the infertility after restoration operation. The antibodies to spermatozoa do not have other harmful effects.

ENDOCRINE FUNCTIONS OF THE TESTES

Testosterone is the principal hormone of the testes. It is steroid in nature. It is synthesized from cholesterol in the Leydig cells and is also formed from androstenedione secreted by the adrenal cortex. Females also form it in small amounts possibly in the adrenal cortex.

The secretion of testosterone is under control of LH.

Functions

Besides its actions during development in the male fetus, Its functions are (Appendix I: Functions of Textosterone):

- Development of secondary sex characteristics; and with some role in their maintenance also.
- Exerting an important protein anabolic, growth promoting effects on the body.

- Along with FSH, it maintains spermatogenesis.
- Inhibitory feedback effect on LH secretion.

Control of Testicular Functions

- FSH is trophic to the sertoli cells.
- FSH and androgens maintain gametogenic function of testes. FSH also stimulates secretion of ABP and inhibin. Inhibin feedbacks to inhibit FSH.
- LH is tropic to Leydig cells and stimulates the secretion of testosterone which feedback to inhibit LH secretion.

Hypothalamic Diseases in Humans

Hypothalamic diseases in humans lead to atrophy of testes and loss of their function.

Abnormalities of Testicular Functions

Testes develop in the abdominal cavity and normally migrate to the scrotum during fetal life. Testicular descent to the inguinal region depends on MIS, and the descent from the inguinal region to the scrotum depends on other factors.

Descend is incomplete in one or less commonly both sides in 10% of newborn males, the testes remain in abdominal cavity or inguinal canal. Gonadotropic hormone treatment speeds descent in some cases or the defect can be corrected surgically.

Spontaneous descent of the testes is the rule, and the proportion of boys with undescended testes (cryptorchidism) falls to 2% at age 1 and 0.3% after puberty.

But early treatment is recommended despite these observations as there is higher incidence of malignant tumors in undescended than in scrotal testes. Beside after puberty, the higher temperature in the abdomen causes irreversible damage to spermatogenic epithelium.

Male Hypogonadism

The depiction depends upon whether testicular deficiency develops before or after puberty. In adults, if it is due to testicular disease, circulating gonadotropin levels are elevated (hypergonadotropic hypogonadism), and if it is secondary to disorders of pituitary or hypothalamus, levels are depressed. When Leydig cell deficiency starts from childhood the clinical picture is that of eunuchoidism, the individuals over the age of 20 are characteristically tall, although not as tall as hyperpituitary giants. They have narrow shoulders and small muscles, a body configuration resembling that of adult female. The genitalia are small and the voice is high pitched. Pubic hair and axillary hair are present, produced by adrenocortical androgen secretion. But the hair is sparse and pubic hair has female pattern.

Androgen-secreting Tumors

Leydig cell tumors are rare and cause detectable endocrine symptoms only in prepubertal boys who develop pseudopuberty.

PREGNANCY

In human, fertilization of the ovum by the sperm usually occurs in the ampulla of the uterine tubes. Fertilization involves:

1. Chemoattraction of the sperm to the ovum by the substance produced by the ovum
2. Adherence to the zona pellucida, the membrane surrounding the ovum.
3. Penetration of the zona pellucida and acrosome reaction
4. Adherence of the sperm head to the cell membrane of the ovum, breakdown of the area of fusion and release of the sperm nucleus into the cytoplasm of the ovum.

Millions of sperms are deposited in the vagina during intercourse. 50–100 sperms reach the ovum and many of them contact zona pellucida. Sperm bind to sperm receptor called ZP3 in the zona and this is followed by acrosomal reaction, i.e. the breakdown of acrosome (Fig. 10.13).

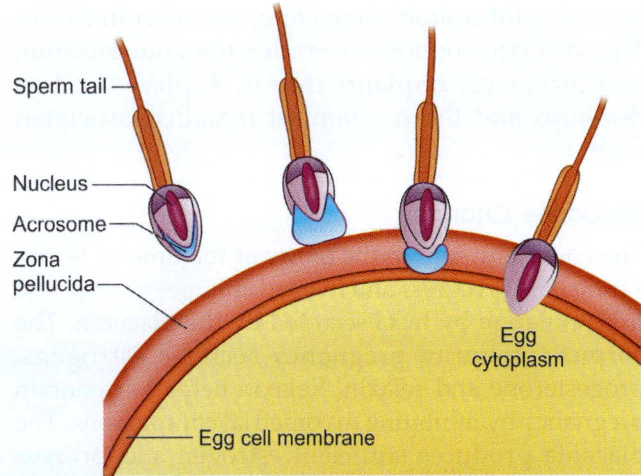

Fig. 10.13: Sequential events in fertilization. Sperms are attached to the ovum, bind to the zona pellucida, release acrosomal enzymes, penetrate the zona pellucida, and fuse with the membrane of the ovum, releasing the sperm nucleus into its cytoplasm

Various enzymes are released, including the trypsin like protease acrosin. Acrosin facilitates for sperm penetration through zona pellucida. When one sperm reaches the membrane of the ovum; fusion to the ovum membrane is mediated by *fertilin* (a protein) on the surface of the sperm head. The fusion provides the signal that initiates development, also starts a reduction in the membrane potential of the ovum that prevents polyspermy (the fertilization of the ovum by more than one sperm). This transient change is followed by structural change in the zona pellucida that provides protection against polyspermy on long-term basis. This zygote is transported in the fallopian tubes. Three to four days are required for passage of the zygote through the tube to the cavity of the uterus. During this time, the survival is dependent on the secretions of the epithelium of the tube. The first series of cellular divisions take place while the ovum is in the tube, so by the time, it enters the uterus and is referred as a *blastocyst*. Shortly after ovulation, the *isthmus* of the fallopian tube becomes tonically contracted, blocking movement between the tubes and uterus. The final entry into the uterus does not take place until the smooth muscle at the isthmus relaxes with the influence of rising levels of progesterone from the corpus luteum. The developing embryo called **blastocyst** moves down the tube into the uterus, the passage of 3 days, during which the blastocyst reaches 8 or 16 cell stage. Once in contact with the endometrium, the blastocyst is surrounded by an outer layer of **syncytiotrophoblas**t, a multinucleate mass with no distinct cell boundaries and an inner layer of **cytotrophoblast** made-up of individual cells. The syncytiotrophoblast erodes the endometrium and blastocyst implants into it. A placenta then develops and the trophoblast remains associated with it.

Endocrine Changes

The corpus luteum in the ovary at the time of fertilization fails to regress and instead enlarges in response to stimulation by hCG secreted by the placenta. The corpus luteum of pregnancy secretes estrogens, progesterone and relaxin. Relaxin helps to maintain pregnancy by inhibiting myometrial contractions. The placenta produces sufficient estrogen and progesterone from maternal and fetal precursors to take over the function of corpus luteum after 9–12 weeks of pregnancy. Ovariectomy seventh or even 12 weeks of pregnency results in abortion. The function of the corpus luteum begins to decline after 10–12 weeks of pregnancy, but it persists throughout pregnancy. hCG secretion decreases after an initial marked rise, but estrogen and progesterone secretion from placenta increase until just before parturition.

hCG

It is a glycoprotein. It is made-up of a and b subunits. The a units are identical to a subunits of LH, FSH and thyroid stimulating hormone (TSH). hCG is primarily luteinizing and luteotropic and has little FSH activity. It can be measured by radioimmunoassay and detected in the blood as early as 9 days of conception **produced by syncytiotrophoblast**. Its presence in the urine in early pregnancy is the basis of laboratory **tests for pregnancy** and it is sometimes detected in urine as early as 14 days after conception. hCG is not absolutely specific for pregnancy. The fetal liver and kidney normally produce small amounts of hCG. Small amounts are secreted by a variety of ***tumors in both sexes***.

Other Placental Hormones

In addition to hCG, progesterone and estrogens; the placenta secretes other hormones. Human chorionic somatomammotropin (hCS) which is protein in nature and secreted by syncytiotrophoblast. It has lactogenic and has small amount of growth-promoting activities.

Fetoplacental Unit

The fetus and placenta interact in the formation of steroid hormones (Fig. 10.14).

PARTURITION

The duration of pregnancy in humans on an average is 270 days from fertilization (284 days from the first day of the last menstrual period). Irregular uterine contractions increase in frequency in the last month of pregnancy.

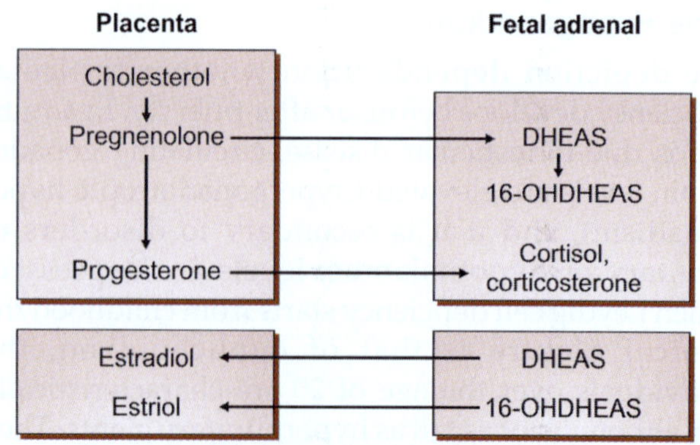

Fig. 10.14: Interactions between placenta and fetal adrenal cortex in the production of steroids

The difference between the body of the uterus and the cervix becomes evident at the time of delivery while the body of the uterus contracts to expel the fetus, the cervix which is firm in nonpregnant state and throughout pregnancy softens and dilates.

There is uncertainty about the mechanisms responsible for the onset of labor. One factor is the increase in the circulating estrogen. This makes the uterus more excitable, and increases the number of gap junctions between myometrial cells and causes production of more prostaglandins which in turn produce uterine contractions. Progesterone has a quieting effect on uterus, however, drop in its level does not occur in humans. In humans, CRH secretion by the fetal hypothalamus increases and is supplemented by increased placental production of corticotropin-releasing hormone (CRH). This increases circulating adrenocorticotropic hormone (ACTH) in the fetus, and resulting increase in cortisol hastens the maturation of respiratory system. Thus, the role of fetus, the fetus picks up the time to be born by increasing CRH secretion.

The number of oxytocin receptors in the myometrium and the decidua (the endometrium of pregnancy) increase during pregnancy and reach a peak during early labor. *Estrogens increase the number of oxytocin receptors late in pregnancy.* In early labor, the oxytocin concentration in maternal plasma is not elevated from prelabor value. It is possible that the marked increase in oxytocin receptors causes the uterus to respond to normal plasma oxytocin concentrations. *Once labor is started, the uterine contractions dilate the cervix and this distention produces signals in afferent nerves that increase oxytocin secretion.* The plasma oxytocin level rises and more oxytocin becomes available to act on the uterus. **A positive feedback loop is established that aids delivery.**

Oxytocin increases uterine contractions in two ways:

1. It acts directly on uterine smooth *muscle cells* to make them *contract*.
2. It stimulates the formation of prostaglandins in the decidua. The *prostaglandins enhance the oxytocin-induced contractions.*

During labor spinal reflexes and voluntary contractions of the abdominal muscles (bearing down) also aid in delivery. But, delivery can occur without bearing down since paraplegic women can go into labor and deliver.

Infertility

In 30% of the cases, the problem is in the man; in 45%, the problem is in the women; in 20% there is problem with both parents; and in 5% no cause can be found. Recent observations have suggested that in 50% of the cases male is responsible.

In vitro fertilization, i.e. removing mature ova, fertilizing them with sperms, and implanting one or more of them in the uterus at four cell stage is of some value in these cases. Chance of producing a live birth is low.

Meiotic Division in Germ Cells

Figure 10.15 shows comparison of male and female gamete production.

Chromosome Abnormalities Resulting in Aberrant Sexual Differentiations

Figure 10.16 sums up the normal basis of genetic sex determination. Figure 10.17 shows how four types of defects are produced due to nondisjunction of sex chromosomes at the time of meiosis.

Hormones and Cancer

About 30% of **carcinomas of breast** in women of child-bearing age are estrogen-dependent; their continued growth depends upon the presence of estrogen in the circulation.

The tumors are not cured by decreasing estrogen secretion, but symptoms are markedly relieved and tumor regresses for months or years before recurring.

Women with estrogen-dependent tumors often have a remission when their ovaries are removed. The incidence of a favorable response is greater when the tumor contains estrogen receptors and greatest when the tumor contains both estrogen and progesterone receptors, because the estrogen stimulates the formation of progesterone receptors and their presence indicates that estrogen is not only binding to, but acting on the tumor cells.

Women with either type of receptors will respond to endocrine therapy. When the disease recurs another remission follows bilateral adrenalectomy. Since ovaries and adrenal estrogen secretions are both inhibited by hypophysectomy, the operation has been performed in some cancer patients.

There some evidences that growth hormone and prolactin stimulate the growth of breast carcinomas; hypophysectomy removes these stimuli.

Some carcinomas of prostate are androgen-dependent and regress temporarily after the removal of testes or treatment with GnRH agonists in high doses that are sufficient to produce down regulation through GnRH receptors on gonadotropes and decrease LH level.

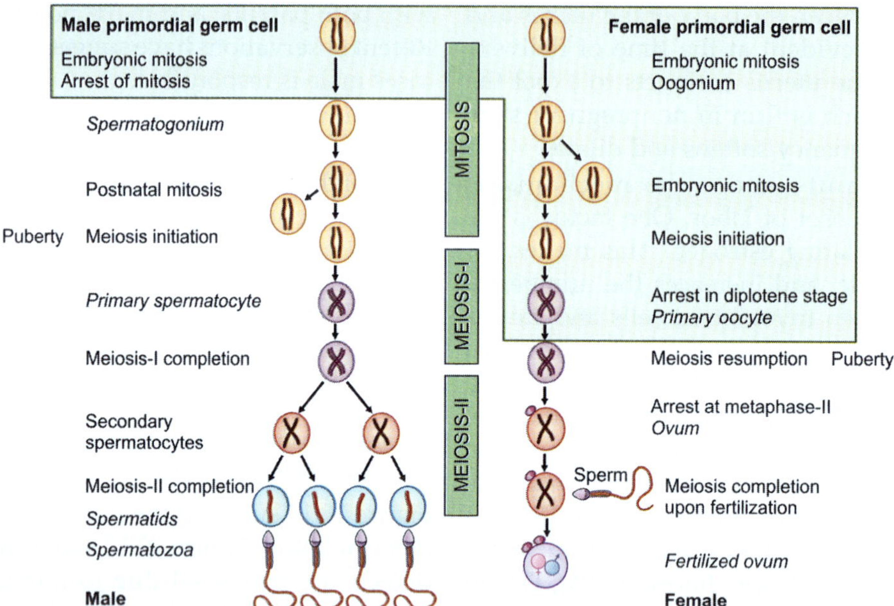

Fig. 10.15: Comparison of male gamete and female gamete production from primitive germ cells. Whereas female germ cells enter meiosis in embryonic life and remain suspended in that state for many years before resuming development after puberty, male germ cells start into meiosis only after puberty. Each female germ cell yields a single ovum, whereas each male germ cell yields many sperm

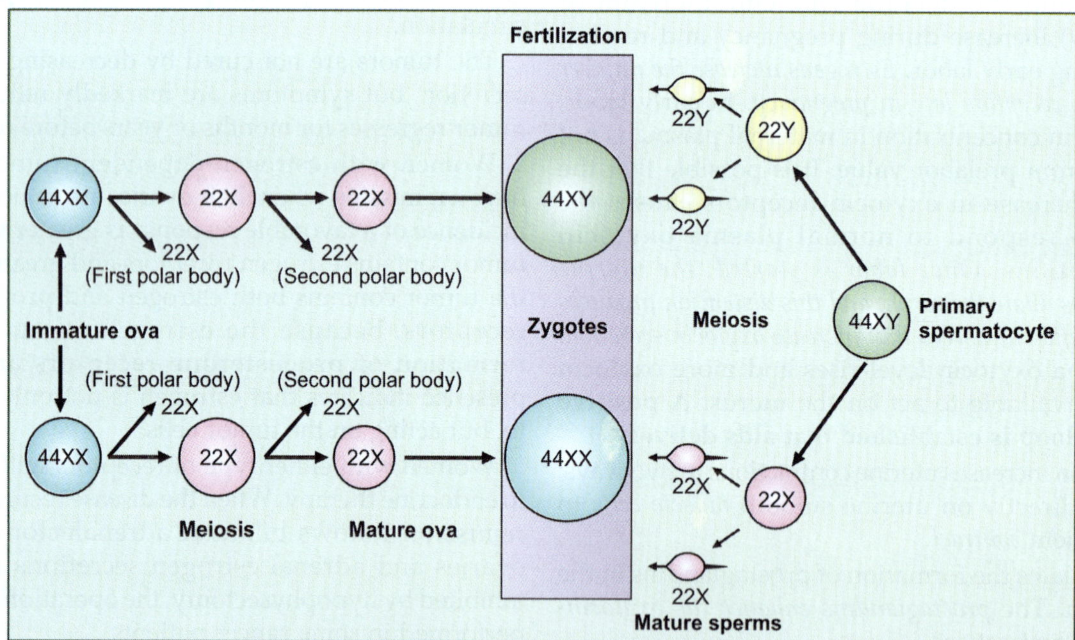

Fig. 10.16: Basis of genetic sex determination. In the two-stage meiotic division in the female, only one cell survives as the mature ovum. In the male, the meiotic division results in the formation of four sperms, two containing the X and two the Y chromosomes. Fertilization thus produces a male zygote with 22 pairs of autosomes plus an XY or a female zygote with 22 pairs of autosomes and two X chromosomes

Functions of Placenta

While the trophoblastic cords from the blastocyst are attaching to the uterus, blood capillaries grow into the cords from the vascular system of the embryo; by 16 days of fertilization blood begins to flow. Simultaneously, blood sinuses supplied by blood from mother develop around the trophoblastic cords. The trophoblast cells send out more and more projections

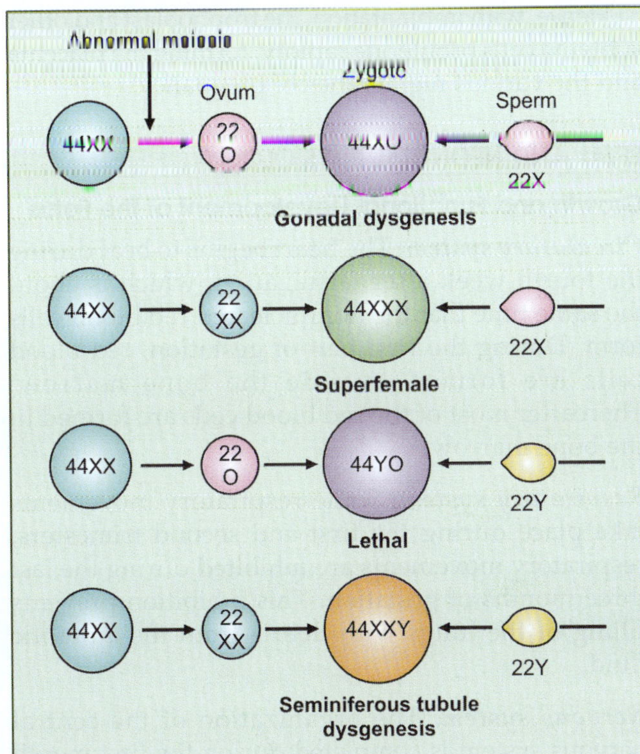

Fig. 10.17: Summary of four possible defects produced by maternal nondisjunction of the sex chromosomes at the time of meiosis. The YO combination is believed to be lethal, and the fetus dies *in utero*

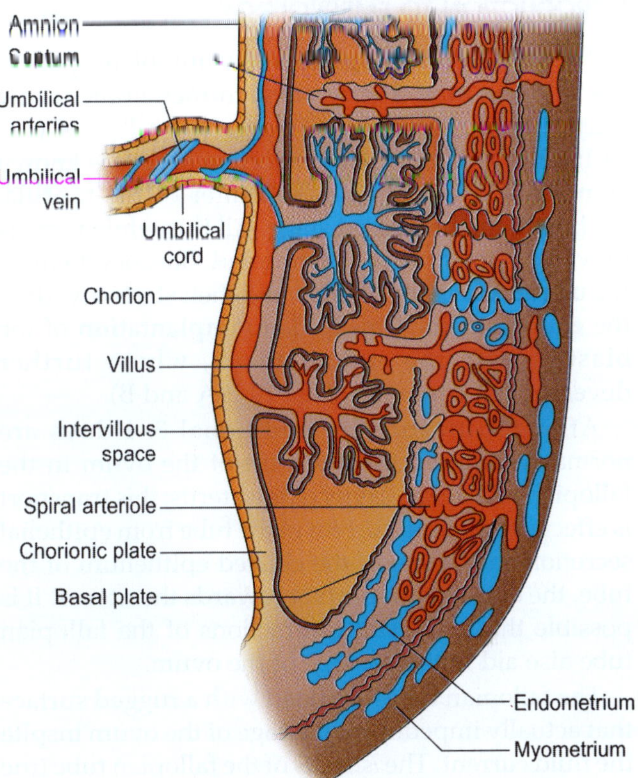

Fig. 10.18: Oxygenation of fetal blood in the placenta

which become placental villi into which capillaries grow. Thus villi carry fetal blood and are surrounded by sinuses containing maternal blood (Fig. 10.18).

The fetal blood flows through two umbilical arteries then to the capillaries of the villi then back to the umbilical vein into the fetus. The mothers blood flows through the uterine arteries into the large maternal sinuses surrounding the villi and back into the uterine veins of the mother. During the first 16 weeks of pregnancy, still another additional layer of cells is present immediately beneath the syncytial trophoblast layer. This layer is composed of distinct cuboidal cells called cytotrophoblast cells or cells of Langerhans.

The major function of the placenta is to provide for diffusion of oxygen and foodstuffs from mother's blood to fetus blood and also diffusion of excretory products from fetus back into the mother.

Diffusion of oxygen through placental membrane: The mean PO_2 in the mother's blood in the maternal sinuses is approximately 50 mmHg, and the mean PO_2 in fetal blood after it becomes oxygenated is about 30 mmHg. There are three factors that help in the transport of enough oxygen to the fetus in spite of low pressure gradient for oxygen diffusion. The presence of fetal Hb which has higher affinity for oxygen, higher concentration of Hb in fetal blood, and Bohr effect (low CO_2 in the fetal blood that increases the affinity of Hb for oxygen). Due to these three factors fetus is capable of receiving enough oxygen in spite of low PO_2 in the blood returning to fetus.

Diffusion of CO_2 Occurs through Placenta

CO_2 diffuses through plecenta from the fetal blood to maternal blood.

Diffusion of food stuffs through placenta: The foodstuffs required by the fetus diffuse through placenta. Glucose diffuses by facilitated diffusion by trophoblasts in the placental membrane; fatty acids diffuse because of their solubility in the cell membranes; substances like ketone bodies and potassium, sodium and chloride ions diffuse from maternal blood to fetal blood.

Excretion through placental membrane: The excretory products diffuse through placental membrane by diffusion and are then excreted through the maternal excretory system.

Placenta forms large quantities of **human chorionic gonadotropin, estrogen, progesterone,** and **human chorionic somatomammotropin,** the first three and possibly fourth are essential for maintenance of pregnancy.

INTRODUCTION TO EMBRYOLOGY

The fertilization takes place in the ampullary part of the fallopian tube. The *zygote* so formed immediately starts dividing into two cell stages → 4 cells → 8 cells → 16 cells → 32 cells. This collection of cells is known as **morula**. Fluid appears in center of the morula, leading to the **blastocyst** stage. All this while there is movement towards the uterine end. Blastocyst enters the uterine cavity by 5th day and then starts invading the **endometrium**. This leads to **implantation** of the blastocyst in the endometrium, where further development continues (Figs 10.19A and B).

After fertilization an additional 3–4 days are normally required for transport of the ovum in the fallopian tube to the cavity of the uterus; this transport is effected by a fluid current in the tube from epithelial secretion and action of the ciliated epithelium of the tube, the cilia always beating towards the uterus. It is possible that the weak contractions of the fallopian tube also aid in the passage of the ovum.

The fallopian tubes are lined with a rugged surface that actually impedes the passage of the ovum inspite the fluid current. The *isthmus* of the fallopian tube (the last 2 cm before the uterus is entered) remains spastically contracted for the first 3 days following ovulation. After this time, the rapidly increasing progesterone first promotes increasing progesterone receptors on the smooth muscle cells and then activates these, exerting a relaxing effect that allows entry of the ovum into the uterus.

The delayed transport of the ovum through the fallopian tube allows several stages of division to occur the *blastocyst* enters the uterus. During this time, large quantities of secretions are formed by secretory cells that alternate with ciliated cells lining the fallopian tube. These secretions are for nutrition of the blastocyst.

Implantation of the Blastocyst in the Uterus

After reaching the uterus, the developing blastocyst usually remains in the uterine cavity, an additional 2–4 days before it implants in the endometium; thus, implantation ordinarily occurs on about the seventh day after ovulation. Before implantation, the blastocyst obtains its nutrition from the endometrial secretions called "uterine milk".

Implantation results from the action of *trophoblast cells* that develop over the surface of the blastocyst (Fig. 10.19B). These cells secrete proteolytic enzymes that digest and liquefy the cells of the endometrium. The fluid and nutrients thus released are transported by the same trophoblast cells into the blastocyst adding still further substance for growth.

Hence, with implantation, the trophoblast and other sublying cells proliferate rapidly, forming the placenta and the various membranes of pregnancy.

FETAL AND NEONATAL PHYSIOLOGY

Growth and Functional Development of the Fetus

Circulatory system: The heart begins to beat during the fourth week after fertilization, which is about the same time that the nonnucleated red blood cells form. During the first half of gestation, red blood cells are formed outside the bone marrow; Thereafter most of the red blood cells are formed in the bone marrow.

Respiratory system: Some respiratory movements take place during the first and second trimesters, respiratory movements are inhibited during the last three months of gestation. This inhibition prevents filling of the lungs with debris from the amniotic fluid.

Nervous system: The organization of the central nervous system is completed during the first month of gestation, but full development and complete myelination takes place until after delivery.

Gastrointestinal tract: By midpregnancy, the fetus ingests amniotic fluid and excretes *meconium* from the gastrointestinal tract. Meconium is composed of residue from amniotic fluid and waste products from the epithelium of the gastrointestinal tract. In the final months of gestation, gastrointestinal tract function approaches maturity.

Kidneys: The fetal kidneys can form urine beginning in the second trimester and urination takes place during the latter half of gestation. The ability of the kidneys to regulate the composition of the extracellular fluid accurately remains poorly-developed until several months after birth.

Adjustments of the Infant to Extrauterine Life

Onset of breathing: Normally, an infant begins to breathe within seconds of delivery. The stimuli for the sudden activation of the respiratory system include hypoxia during delivery and sudden cooling of the face on exposure to outside. A normal pattern of breathing develops within 1 minute of delivery although in some cases the breathing may be delayed. Newborn infants can tolerate 8–10 minutes without breathing before permanent damage occurs; in adults, death or severe damage takes place, if there is interruption for 4–5 minutes.

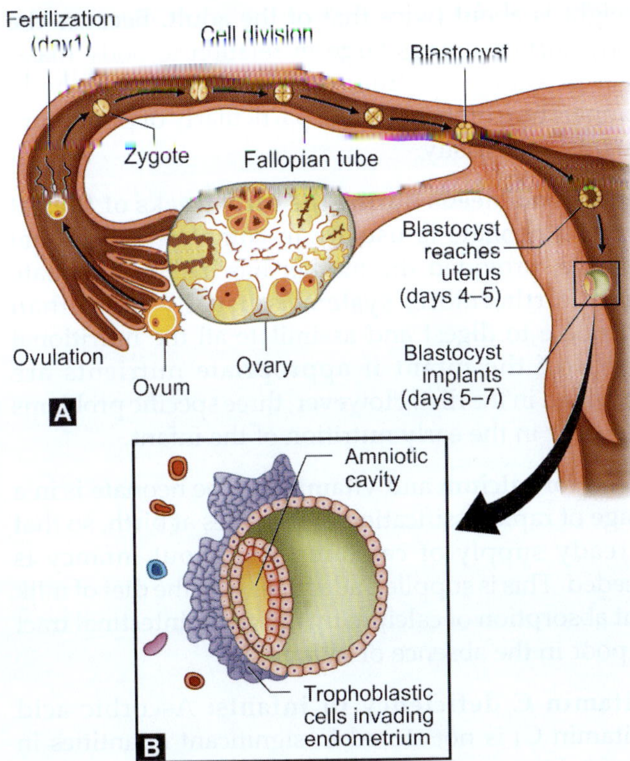

Figs 10.19A and B: (A) Ovulation, fertilization of the ovum in the fallopian tube, and implantation of the blastocyst in the uterus; (B) Action of trophoblast cells during implantation of the blastocyst in the uterine endometrium

Expansion of the lungs at birth: The surface tension of the fluid-filled lungs at birth keeps the alveoli in a collapsed state. With approximately 25 mmHg of negative inspiratory pressure required to overcome the surface tension. At birth, the first inspirations are powerful and generate about 60 mmHg negative intrapleural pressure.

Circulatory Readjustments at Birth

Two primary changes occur in the fetal circulation at birth:

- A *doubling of systemic vascular resistance* due to loss of the placenta which has very low vascular resistance. This increases aortic pressure and left ventricular and left atrial pressures.
- A *fivefold decrease in pulmonary vascular resistance* due expansion of the lungs following the first inspiration. As a result, pulmonary arterial, right ventricular and right atrial pressure decrease.

After these initial changes, other alterations follow:

- The *foramen ovale, which is located between the right and left atria,* closes owing to the pressure in the left side being greater than the pressure in the right.
- The *ductus arteriosus between the pulmonary artery and descending aorta closes.*
- The *ductus venosus closes:* During fetal life, carries blood from the umbilical vein to the fetal portal vein to enter directly to the inferior vena cava, bypassing the fetal liver.

(For details of fetal circulation refer to Chapter 15). With these adjustments, the fetal circulation is transformed within a matter of hours to the neonatal configuration.

Special Problems in the Neonate

In the newborn, most of the cardiovascular, hormonal and neural control systems are poorly developed and are often unstable.

Respiratory system: Because of the relatively small residual capacity (less than one-half the volume per kilogram of body weight than that of adults), relatively high metabolic rate of the newborn and immaturity of the neural components of the respiratory control system, blood gas values fluctuate widely during the first weeks of life.

Circulation: Blood volume at birth is normally about 300 milliliters. If the baby is left attached to the placenta for a few minutes after birth, approximately 75 mL of additional blood can enter the baby's circulatory system, which is equivalent to a transfusion of 25% of the blood volume. This overload could contribute to an elevation of left atrial pressure and a tendency to develop pulmonary edema.

Liver function: Bilirubin formed from the breakdown of hemoglobin from red blood cells is normally excreted by the liver into the bile conjugated with glucuronic acid; however, the neonatal liver has inadequate ability to conjugate bilirubin at the rate it is formed. As a result, the blood concentration of bilirubin rises for the first 3 days after birth and then returns to normal as the capability of the liver increases. This condition is referred to as *physiologic hyperbilirubinemia* and can be seen in some cases as a slight jaundice or yellowish tint in the skin and sclera of the eyes.

In addition to the potential problems associated with bilirubin conjugation, the limited capability of the liver during the first few days of life can lead to difficulty in synthesizing adequate quantities of protein for maintaining colloid osmotic pressure, adequate amounts of glucose and necessary amounts of the factors required for coagulation.

These potential limitations of hepatic function rapidly diminish during the first weeks of postnatal life.

Fluid balance and renal function: On a per kilogram of body weight basis, the neonate takes in seven times as much fluid as an adult. In addition, the metabolic rate per kilogram of body weight of the newborn is twice as great as that of the adult. Other factors including these can contribute to problems in the newborn regarding the regulation of fluid balance, electrolyte concentrations, pH and colloid osmotic pressure.

Digestion and metabolism: The gastrointestinal absorptive capacity and hepatic digestive function of neonates are limited to some extent.

Fluid Balance, Acid-base Balance and Renal Function

The rate of fluid intake and fluid excretion in the newborn infant is seven times as great to weight as in the adult, that even a slight percentage alteration of fluid intake or fluid output can cause rapidly developing abnormalities.

The rate of metabolism in the infant is also twice as great to body mass as in the adult, which means that twice as much acid is normally formed. Functional development of the kidneys is not complete until the end of about the first month of life. Therefore, considering the immaturity of the kidneys, together with the marked fluid turnover in the infant and rapid formation of acid, among the most important problems of infancy are acidosis, dehydration and more rarely, overhydration.

Digestion, Absorption and Metabolism of Energy Foods; and Nutrition

In general, the ability of the newborn to digest, absorb, and metabolize foods is no different from that of the older child, with the following three exceptions.

First, secretion of pancreatic amylase in the neonate is deficient, so that the neonate uses starches less adequately than do older children.

Second, absorption of fats from the gastrointestinal tract is somewhat less than that in the older child. Consequently, milk with a high fat content, such as cow's milk, is frequently inadequately absorbed.

Third liver functions imperfectly during at least the first week of life, the glucose concentration in the blood is unstable and low.

Metabolic rate and body temperature: The normal metabolic rate of the neonate in relation to body weight is about twice that of the adult. Because the body surface area is large in relation to body mass, heat is readily lost from the body. Hence, the body temperature of the neonate, particularly of premature infants, falls easily.

Nutritional needs during the early weeks of life: At birth, a neonate is usually in complete nutritional balance, provided the mother has had an adequate diet. Furthermore, system is usually more than adequate to digest and assimilate all the nutritional needs of the infant if appropriate nutrients are provided in the diet. However, three specific problems do occur in the early nutrition of the infant.

Need for calcium and vitamin D: The neonate is in a stage of rapid ossification of its bones at birth, so that a ready supply of calcium throughout infancy is needed. This is supplied adequately by the diet of milk but absorption of calcium by the gastrointestinal tract is poor in the absence of vitamin D.

Vitamin C deficiency in infants: Ascorbic acid (vitamin C) is not stored in significant quantities in the fetal tissues; it is required for proper formation of cartilage, bone structures of the infant. Furthermore, milk has poor supplies of ascorbic acid, especially cow's milk. For this reason, orange juice or other sources of ascorbic acid are often prescribed by the third week of life.

Immunity

The neonate inherits much immunity from the mother because many protein antibodies diffuse from the mother's blood through the placenta into the fetus. However, the neonate does not form antibodies of its own to a significant extent. Baby's gamma globulins, are decreased, with a decrease in immunity. Thereafter, the baby's own immunity system begins to form antibodies, and the gamma globulin concentration returns essentially to normal by the age of 12 to 20 months.

Despite the decrease in gamma globulins soon after birth, the antibodies inherited from the mother protect the infant for about 6 months against most major childhood infectious diseases.

Allergy: The newborn infant is seldom subject to allergy. Several months later, however, when the infant's own antibodies first begin to form extreme allergic states can develop, eczema, gastrointestinal abnormalities and even anaphylaxis. As the child grows older and still higher degrees of immunity develop, these allergic manifestations usually disappear.

Endocrine Problems

Ordinarily, the endocrine system of the infant is highly developed at birth, and the infant seldom exhibits any immediate endocrine abnormalities.

SUMMARY

Figures 10.20 and 10.21 give functions of testosterone and secretion.

IMPLICATIONS AND APPLICATIONS

- To understand mechanism of labor.
- To know various methods of family welfare in male and female.
- To understand tubectomy and vasectomy
- Advice to pregnant woman about diet, hygeine, etc.
- Role of sex chromosone in determination sex of the fetus.

Functions of Testosterone

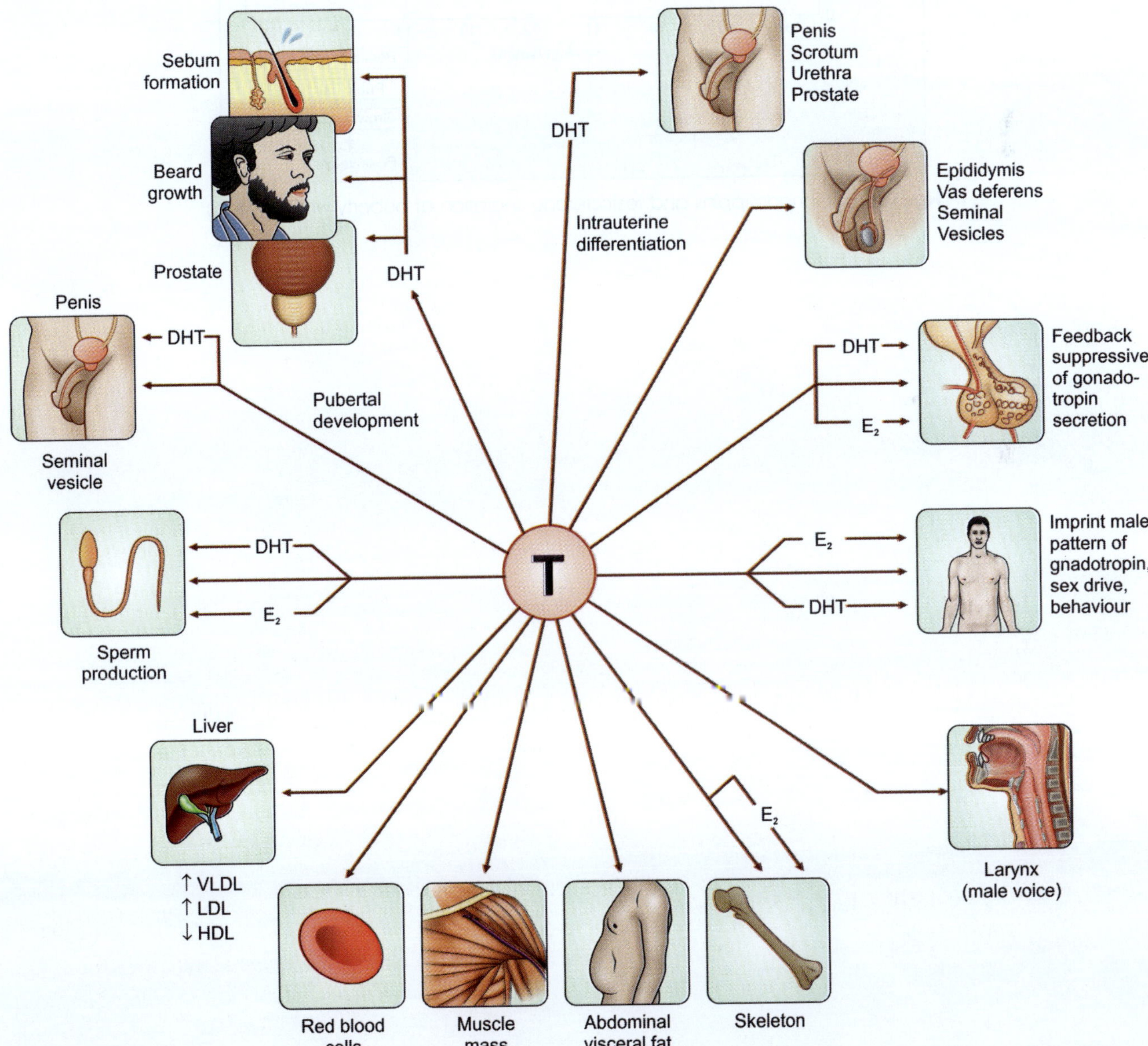

Fig. 10.20: Male sex hormones and their functions. DHT=dihydrotestosterone, E_2=estradiol, both are produced from testosterone; VLDL=very low density-, LDL=low density-, HDL=high density-lipoproteins

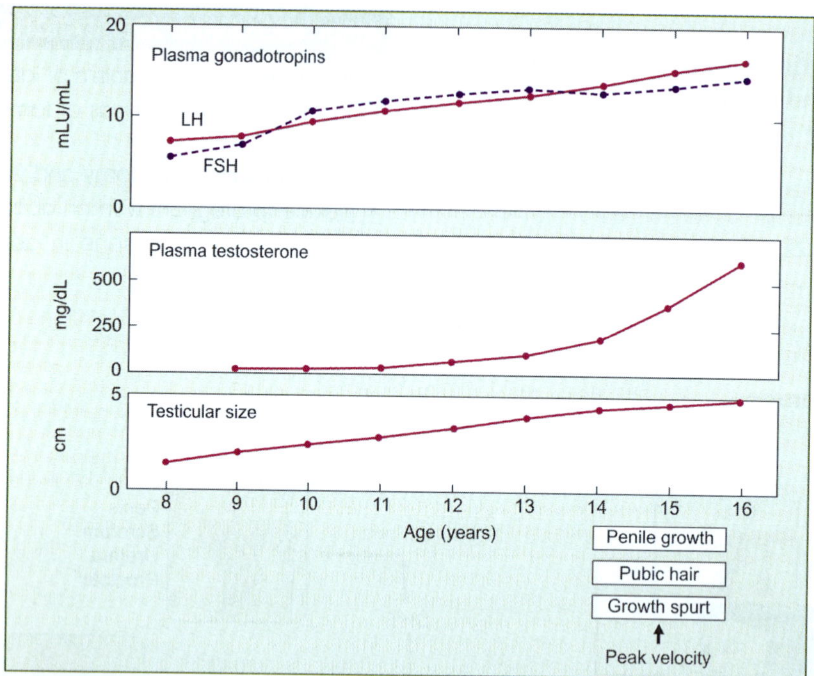

Fig. 10.21: Gonadotropins and testosterone secretion at puberty with functions

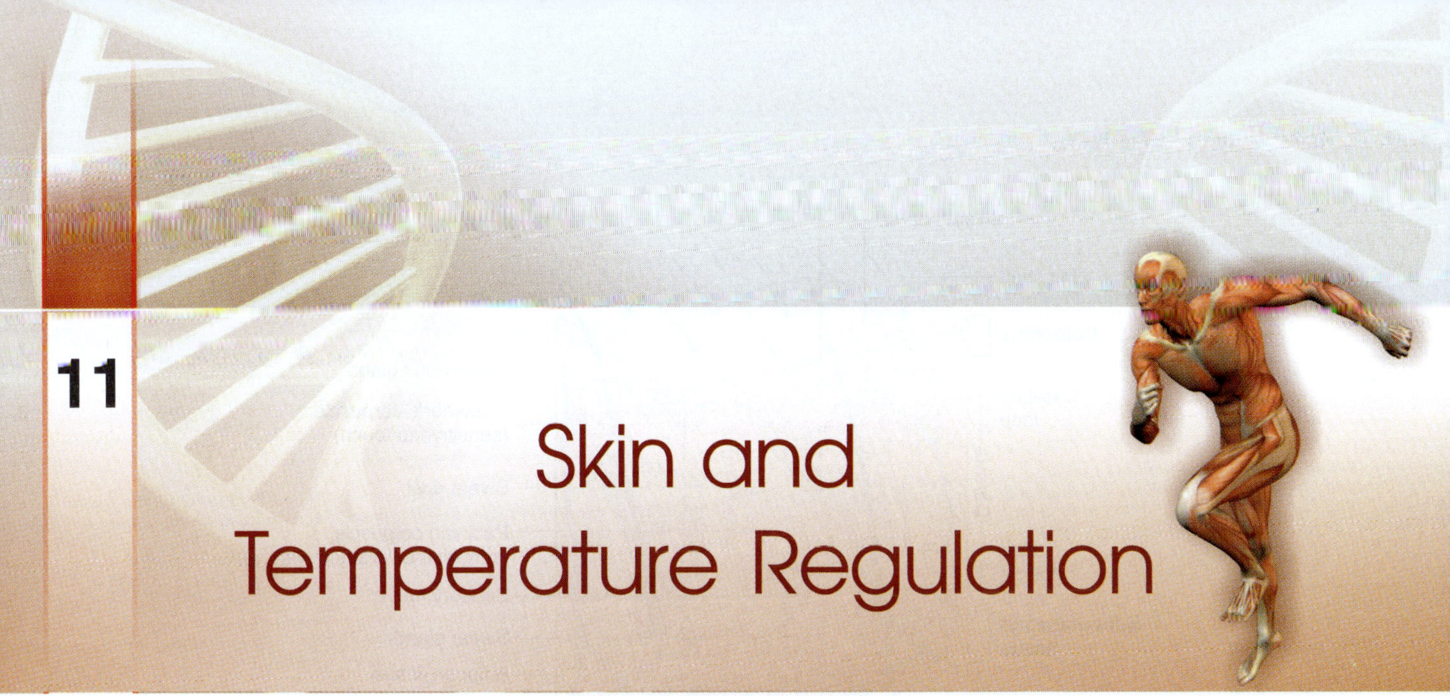

11 Skin and Temperature Regulation

The skin covers the out surface of the body and becomes continuous with the mucous membranes that line the body openings.

It contains sensory nerve endings of touch, temperature and pain, which monitor body's surroundings and produce protective reflex responses.

There are *two layers* (Fig. 11.1) in the skin:

1. Epidermis
2. Dermis.

EPIDERMIS

This is the superficial layer of the skin and is composed of stratified (many layered) squamous (upper layers are flat) epithelium that is keratinized (cells produce keratin). The thickness of this layer varies in different parts of the body, being thick over the sole and palm of the hand. There are no blood vessels or nerves in this layer.

The deeper layers are bathed with tissue fluid from dermis from where this layer gets requirements of oxygen and nutrition.

The deepest layer is germinal layer, the **stratum germinativum**. The cells in this layer multiply to give rise to superficial layer. The most superficial layer is thick and horny and is called the **stratum corneum**. The cells on the surface are flat, nonnucleated, dead cells where the cytoplasm has been replaced by fibrous protein, the keratin. These cells are constantly being shed off and replaced by cells that originate from germinal layer that gradually pass through the layers during which the cells die and fill with keratin which is tough waterproof protein, which also forms hair and nails, and reach and replace the superficial cells that are shed off by friction and washing. Complete replacement of epidermis takes place in 40 days.

There are melanocytes in the epithelium that secrete melanin. Color of the skin is due to melanin which is a dark brown pigment, formed from amino acid tyrosine in the deep germinal layer; this is absorbed by the surrounding epithelial cells. People of all races have the same number of melanin producing cells in the epidermis but due to genetic differences the amount of melanin produced varies. Sunlight also causes more melanin to be produced to protect the skin from the damaging effects of ultraviolet rays of sunlight. Albinos have no melanin because they lack an enzyme for its production.

Smooth skin is present on the palms of the hand and soles of feet but there are projections on the surface of epidermis, with alternating ridges and grooves forming distinct prints, the fingerprints peculiar to each individual (Fig. 11.2).

The pattern of ridges is different in every individual and forms the basis for finger printing.

Hair and secretions of sebaceous glands and ducts of sweat glands pass through the epidermis to reach the surface.

Blisters form when trauma causes separation of the dermis from epidermis and serous fluid collects between the layers.

DERMIS

This layer is tough and elastic; it is formed of connective tissue and has fibers of protein collagen and elastin which give support to the skin. Rupture of elastic fibers when skin is overstretched, results in

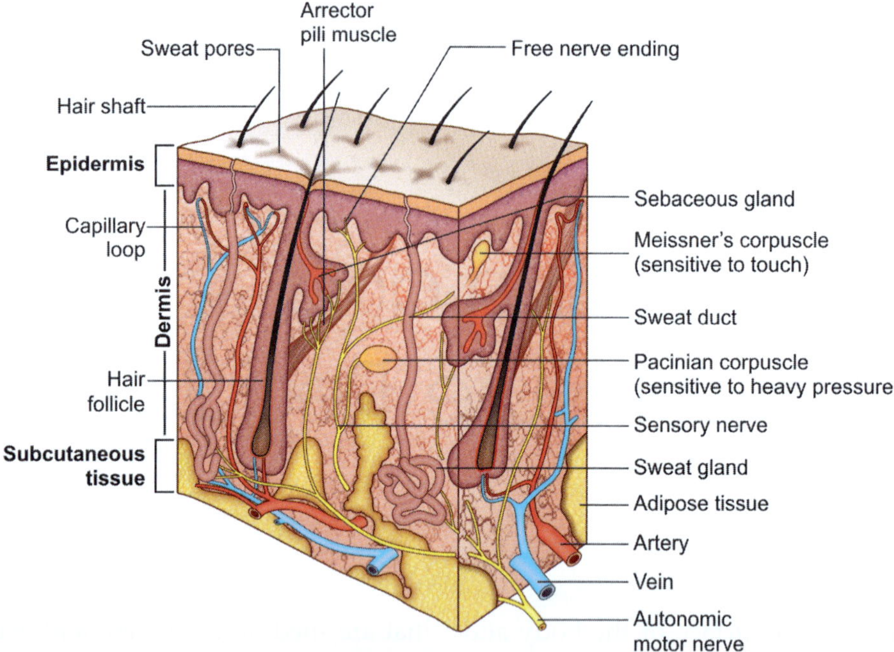

Fig. 11.1: Histological structure of skin

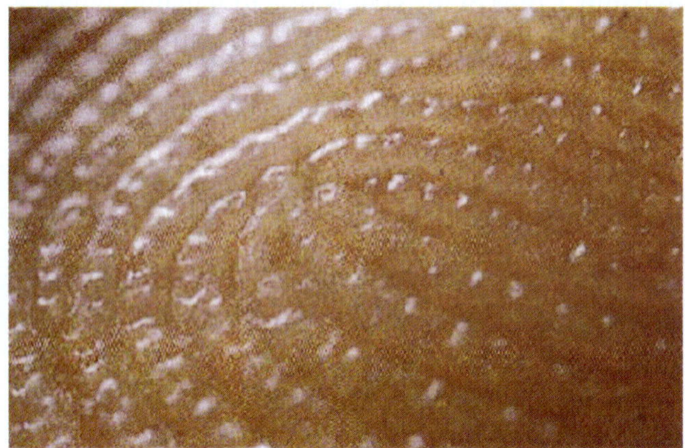

Fig. 11.2: Close-up of a finger tip showing characteristic ridges that form fingerprint, a pattern unique for every individiual

permanent stretchmarks that are found in pregnancy or obesity. Collagen fibers accumulate water and give the skin its tensile strength but this ability declines with age and wrinkles appear. Fibroblasts, macrophages and mast cells are the main cells found in dermis. Beneath the dermis there is areolar tissue and varying amount of adipose tissue (fat). The dermis contains:

- **Small blood vessels:** The arterioles form a fine network with capillary branches that supply sweat glands, sebaceous glands, hair follicles and the dermis.
- **Lymphatic vessels:** These form network throughout the dermis.
- **Nerves and nerve endings** for pain, touch, pressure and temperature. Sensory receptors sensitive to touch, pressure, temperature and pain are widely distributed in the dermis. Individuals receive information about the environment from these receptors. They also produce protective reflex responses.
- **Appendages** of skin.

Appendages of skin are sweat glands of two types eccrine and apocrine; hair to which are attached pilomotor muscles and sebaceous glands.

Sweat Glands

They are composed of epithelial cells. Bodies of the gland lie in subcutaneous tissue. Ducts open on the skin at pores (Fig. 11.1).

Eccrine sweat glands: Distributed all over the body surface and secrete a dilute solution containing sodium chloride, urea and lactic acid. Gland density is most over the palms, soles, and next dense over head, much less dense over trunk and extremities. These sweat glands are stimulated by sympathetic nerves in response to raised body temperature and fear; but, the sympathetic nerves release acetylcholine at the terminals instead of norepinephrine. Atropine inhibits their secretion.

Normal sweat is limited to palms, soles and axilla; but, can be more generalized. It is produced by direct or reflex stimulation of regions in spinal cord, medulla, hypothalamus or cerebral cortex. The secretion is increased when the external body temperature is high. The rise in temperature affects the hypothalamus with the circulating warm blood or from warm endings from skin. In emotional states, sweating is limited to palms, soles and axilla; but, may be generalized and this is due to stimulation of higher centers.

Apocrine sweat glands found mainly in the axilla (eccrine glands are also found here) are also found around nipples and in the females around labia majora and mons pubis.

Not innervated but are stimulated by circulating hormone epinephrine. In the axilla, they secrete an odorless milky fluid which if decomposed by surface microbes causes an unpleasant odor.

The most important function of the *sweat secreted on the surface of the skin is the regulation of body temperature.* Evaporation of the sweat from the body causes loss of heat, and the sweat secretion is regulated for that function. If sweat does not evaporate, it is useless for temperature regulation. *Excessive sweating causes loss of water and salt from the body.* The salt loss decreases if the sweat secretion continues for some days, but water loss has to be made-up.

Hair

Hair is produced by the hair follicles which are tubes within the dermis or subcutaneous tissue. At the base of the hair, follicle is a cluster of cells called the hair matrix (or bulb). Hair is dead cells full of protein keratin.

Hair is formed by multiplication of the cells of the bulb and as they are pushed upwards away from nutrition, the cells die and become keratinized. The part of the hair above the skin is the shaft and the remainder is root. The color of the hair is genetically determined and depends upon the pigment melanin. White hair is due to replacement of melanin by tiny air bubbles. Hair follicle is attached to a small muscle that can contract to raise the hair upright the muscle is called **pilomotor muscle.** These are small smooth muscle fibers attached to the hair follicles. Contraction of the fibers occurs in response to sympathetic stimulation that causes hair to stand, and the skin around is raised described as "goose skin". It occurs in response to fear and cold. This forms a warming mechanism in response to cold though the mechanism is not important in humans.

Sebaceous Glands

These consist of secretory epithelial cells derived from the same tissue as hair follicles. They secrete an oily substance *sebum* into the hair follicles and are therefore present in the skin of all parts of the body except in palm and sole. Sebum oils the hair and keeps the hair soft and pliable and gives it shiny appearance. The glands are most numerous in the skin of the scalp, face, axilla and groin. In the region of the transition from one type of epithelium into another, such as lip, eyelid, nipple, labia minora and glans penis; there are sebaceous glands that are independent of hair follicles, secreting sebum directly on to the surface.

On the skin, the secretion provides some water proofing and acts as a bactericidal and fungicidal agent. It also prevents drying and cracking of skin that may especially occur with exposure to heat and sunshine. The activity of these glands increase at puberty and is less at the extremes of age, making infants and elderly more prone to effects of excessive moisture, e.g. nappy rash.

Nails

Nails are derived from same cells as epidermis and hair and consist of a hard horny keratin plate. They have a protective role. The root of the nail is embedded in the skin covered by cuticle (Fig. 11.3) and forms the hemispherical pale area called the lunula. The nail plate of the nail is the exposed part grown out from the germinal zone of the epidermis called the nail bed. The nail except in lunula is transparent and pink in color, reflects that of the nail bed.

The oxygenation of the hemoglobin and the blood circulating in the dermis gives pink color to the skin. If bile pigments are in excess in the blood or carotene in the subcutaneous tissue, that gives yellowish color to the skin.

Functions of the Skin

1. *Protection:* The skin protects the body by providing a barrier, relatively waterproof that protects the deeper structures.
   - It provides nonspecific defense against invasion by bacteria.

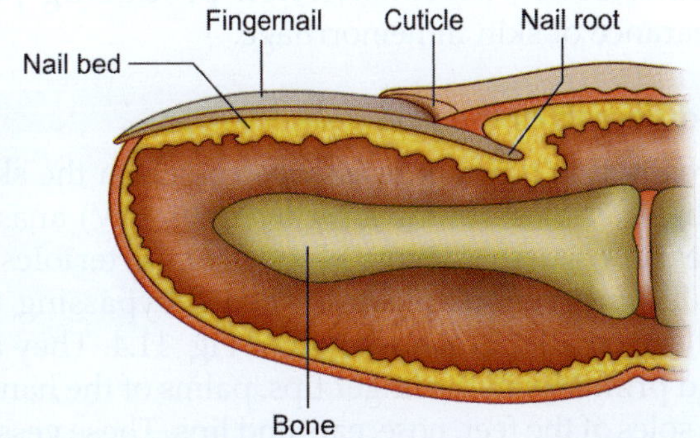

Fig. 11.3: Cross-section of a finger, showing nail structure

- Protection is provided from injury by any chemical and physical agent unless the agent is strong.
- Protection is provided to deeper structures against harm and dehydration by ultraviolet light. Melanocytes have protective role against ultraviolet light.
- In the dermis, they are present specialized immune cells, the *Langerhans cells;* the cells engulf (by phagocytosis) antigens and migrate to lymphoid tissue where they present antigen to "T" lymphocytes; thus, they participate in immune responses.
- The nerve endings present in the skin provide for protective reflex responses when a painful stimulus strikes the skin.

2. *Regulation of body temperature:* Sweat helps to maintain body temperature. The blood flow through the skin is regulated to maintain body temperature. Thermoregulatory adjustments include local responses as well as more generalized responses. Temperature receptors in the skin provide afferent impulses to hypothalamus for temperature regulation. The skin blood vessels when cooled become more sensitive to catecholamines and arterioles and venules constrict.
3. *Formation of vitamin D:* 7-dehydrocholesterol is present in the skin and ultraviolet light from the sun converts it to vitamin D_3.
4. *Absorption:* Skin has limited capacity of absorption. The drugs which can be absorbed from the skin are applied in the form of patches on the skin from where gradual absorption takes place.
5. *Excretion:* Skin has a minor role in excretion of sodium in the sweat; and urea especially when kidney function is impaired.

The vascular bed of the skin is a major blood reservoir in humans. Blood loss evokes profound subcutaneous vasoconstriction producing pale appearance of skin in hemorrhage.

Blood Vessels of the Skin

There are two types of resistance vessels in the skin: (1) the arterioles; (2) the arteriovenous (AV) anastomoses. AV vessels shunt blood from arterioles to venules and venous plexuses; hence bypassing the capillary circulation are shown in Fig. 11.4. They are found primarily in the finger tips, palms of the hands, toes, soles of the feet, nose, ears and lips. These vessels are under control of sympathetic impulses; increase

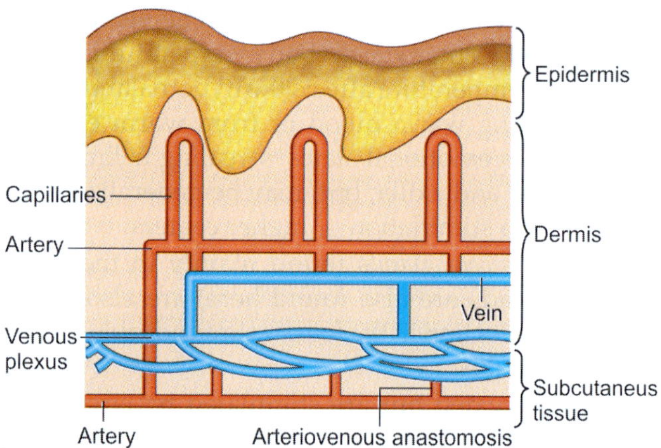

Fig. 11.4: Schematic representation of skin blood vessels

in the number of impulses produces constriction which can reach up to complete obstruction of the lumen. The response is reflex due to activation of temperature receptors in the skin and to the temperature of the blood circulating in the hypothalamus. It is a mechanism to regulate the body temperature. Blood flow in response to thermoregulatory stimuli can vary from 1 to as much as 150 mL/100 g of skin/min, these variations are possible because blood can be shunted through the anastomoses.

The arterioles are similar to those found elsewhere in the body. Arterioles as well as capacitance skin vessels are affected by external temperature. Responses are produced as a result of **direct action** on the blood vessels as well as **reflex action** produced by stimulation of temperature receptors. Hypothalamus regulates the responses to maintain body temperature. It receives afferents from temperature receptors and is affected by the temperature of the blood circulating through it.

When the skin blood vessels are cooled they become more sensitive to catecholamines and the arterioles and venules constrict, the blood is directed away from the skin. The vessels are affected not only in the part exposed but also in the rest of the body.

DISORDER OF SKIN

INFECTIONS

Many harmless organisms naturally live on the skin. The skin is one of the body's defenses against infections, but in some circumstances it can be invaded by infectious organisms, such as viruses, bacteria, fungi and parasites.

Viral Infections

Human Papilloma Virus (HPV)

It causes warts that are spread by direct contact. There is proliferation of epidermis and development of a small firm growth. Common sites are hands, soles of the feet and face.

Herpes Viruses

Chickenpox and shingles are caused by herpes-zoster virus. Other viruses cause cold sores and genital herpes.

Bacterial Infections

Impetigo

It is highly infectious condition commonly caused by *Staphlococcus aureus*. Superficial pustules develop, usually around the nose and mouth. It spreads by direct contact; affects mainly children and immunosuppressed individuals. When caused by *Streptococcus pyogenes* the infection may become complicated, a few weeks later by immune reaction causing glomerulonephritis.

Cellulitis

This is spreading infection caused by some microbes. The spread is facilitated by the formation of enzymes that breakdown the connective tissue that normally isolates an area of inflammation. The microbes enter through break in the skin. If left untreated, infection can enter bloodstream.

Fungal Infections

Ringworm and Dermatitis

These are superficial infections of the skin. In ring worm, there is an outward spreading ring of inflammation. The fungus lives on skin or scalp producing circular bald patches or rings covered with grayish scales. It may be carried in comb or brushes, or headscarfs. It can also be contacted from animals, it most commonly affects the scalp.

When it affects smooth skin, it usually appears as round area with a spreading edge. The fungus can also affect the nails; transmitted from animals; found in cattle from which infection can be spread.

Tina pedis (athlete's foot) affects the between the toes. Both infections are spread by direct contact.

NONINFECTIVE CONDITIONS

Eczema and Dermatitis

Inflammatory conditions which can be acute or chronic. In acute dermatitis, there is redness, swelling and exudation of serous fluid usually accompanied by itching. This is often followed by crusting and scaling. If the condition becomes chronic, the skin thickens and may become leathery due to long-term scratching.

Nappy Rash

In infants, nappy rash is common form of dermatitis and it can spread to involve the rest of the body. It may be a reaction to: ammonia formed by the urine; to drugs or a result of other disease.

Atopic Dermatitis

It is caused by allergens and commonly affects atopic individuals. Children who suffer from hay fever or asthma are often affected.

Contact Dermatitis

It is caused by direct contact with irritants like cosmetic soap or due to hypersensitivity reaction to synthetic rubber or dyes or chemicals.

Psoriasis

This condition is genetically determined. There are exacerbations and periods of remission of varying duration. It is a common in all ages. There is proliferation of the cells of the basal layers of epidermis and the more rapid upward progress of these cells through the epidermis resulting in incomplete maturation of the upper layer. Bleeding may occur when scales are scratched or rubbed off. The elbow, knee and scalp are common sites but other parts can be affected. Sometimes, psoriasis is associated with arthritis.

Acne Vulgaris

It is common condition in adolescents. Sebaceous glands in hair follicles become blocked and infected leading to inflammation and pimple formation.

Pressure Sores

Occur over pressure points where skin is compressed resulting in impaired blood flow.

ALBINISM

The child is born without any melanin pigment in the skin. It is usually inherited.

BURNS

It can be as a result of excessive heat, excessive cold, by electricity, ionizing radiation or chemicals. Infection is common complication as barrier formed by skin is lost.

Classified according to the depth:

- Partial thickness when only skin is involved full thickness when dermis and epidermis are destroyed.
- The burns are painless when dermis is involved as nerves are destroyed.
- The extent of the burn is classified using the rule of nine (Fig. 11.5). In adults hypovolemic shock usually develops when 15% of surface area is affected.

TUMORS

Tumors can be benign or malignant. **Benign growths** take many forms, although few of them give rise to malignant tumors, most are harmless.

Malignant Tumors

Basal Cell Carcinoma

This is least malignant and most common type of skin cancer. It is associated with long-term exposure to sunlight; hence most common sites are head and neck. It appears as a tiny nodule and then forms an ulcer. It is locally invasive but rarely metastasize.

Malignant Melanoma

It is a malignant multiplication of melanocytes, usually originating in a mole which has an irregular outline. It may bleed. Most commonly affects young and middle-aged. Predisposing factors are fair skin and repeated exposure to sunlight. Metastases develop early and common sites of spread are liver, brain, lungs, bowl and bone marrow.

REGULATION OF BODY TEMPERATURE

Normal Body Temperature

The temperature of the body is maintained constant at about 37°C or 98.6°F (range 36.3–37.1°C or 97.3–98.8° F). The extremities are usually cooler than rest of the body. The rectal temperature represents the core body temperature and varies least with environmental temperatures; the oral temperature is normally 0.5°C lower than rectal temperature (Fig. 11.6). The core temperature undergoes a regular circadian (daily) fluctuation of 0.5–0.7°C with rise in the evening and lowest at 6 A.M. Core temperature remains almost constant everyday except when there is fever. In women there is rise of about 0.5°C after ovulation in secretory phase of the cycle. The temperature of the scrotum is regulated at 32°C.

Temperature regulation is less precise in children and may remain 0.5°C above that of adults.

The skin temperature in contrast to the core temperature rises and falls with the temperature of the surroundings. This is the ability of the skin to lose heat to the surroundings.

The core body temperature varies somewhat with exercise and with extremes of the surrounding temperature. With strenuous exercise, the rectal temperature can rise to as high as 100–104° F. On the other hand, if exposed to cold rectal temperature can even fall to below 97°F.

Mechanisms of Temperature Regulation

Body temperature is controlled by balancing heat loss against heat production.

Mechanisms are regulated to maintain body temperature constant as required when the metabolic rate of the body rises or falls.

Heat loss is also regulated with change of environmental temperature. Thermoregulatory responses include local as well as general reflex responses.

Hypothalamus regulates the heat loss and heat conservation mechanisms. Anterior hypothalamus controls heat loss responses and posterior hypothalamus heat conservation responses. It (hypothalamus) receives information from sensory receptors in the skin, deep tissues, spinal cord, hypothalamus itself and other parts of the brain. It acts as an integrating center that on receiving afferents activates appropriate reflex responses to maintain the temperature constant; functioning like a **thermostat** that regulates temperature at the normal body temperature.

Most of the heat produced in the body is in the deep organs especially during exercise. This heat is transferred from deeper organs and tissues to the skin where it is lost to the air and surroundings. Hence, the rate at which it is lost depends on two factors: (1) conduction from the core to the surface and (2) transfer from the skin to the environment.

Heat Production

The body metabolism produces heat (Table 11.1). There is ***basal metabolism*** and ***metabolism due to activity***. The main organs that produce heat are the muscles. The ***ingestion of food increases*** the heat production by small amount. The ***hormones*** can vary the heat production independent of these two mechanisms. *Epinephrine* and *norepinephrine* produce short-lived increase in heat production; *thyroid hormones* produce a slowly developing but prolonged

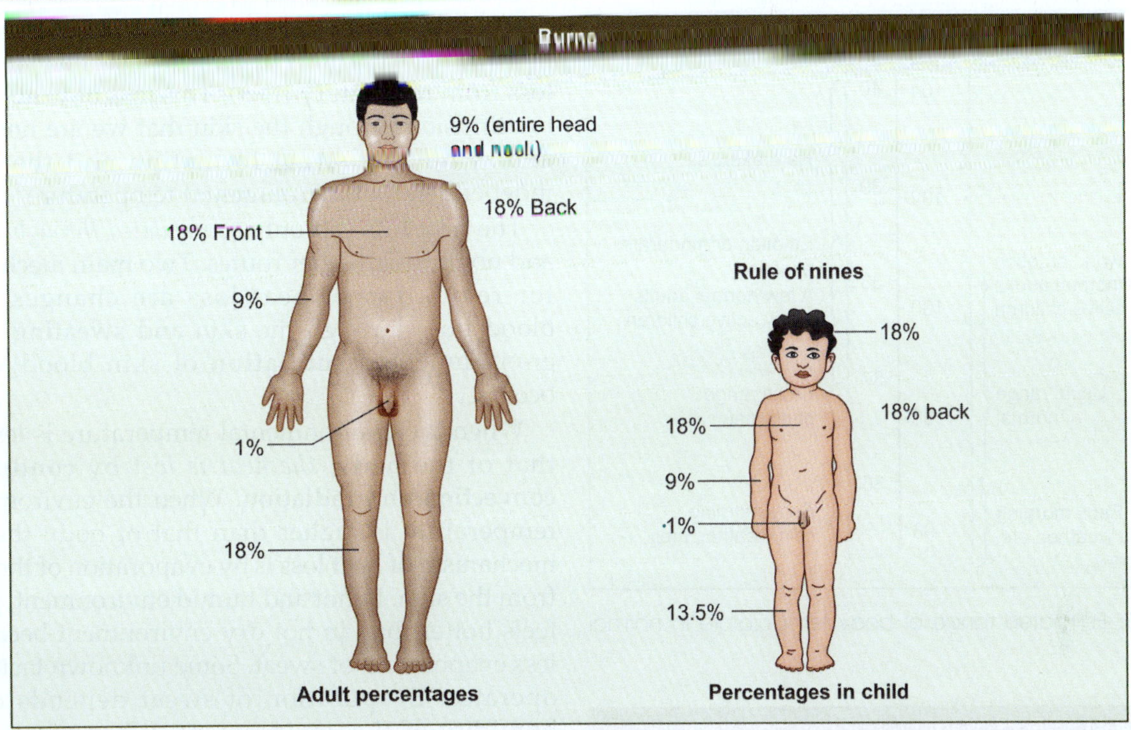

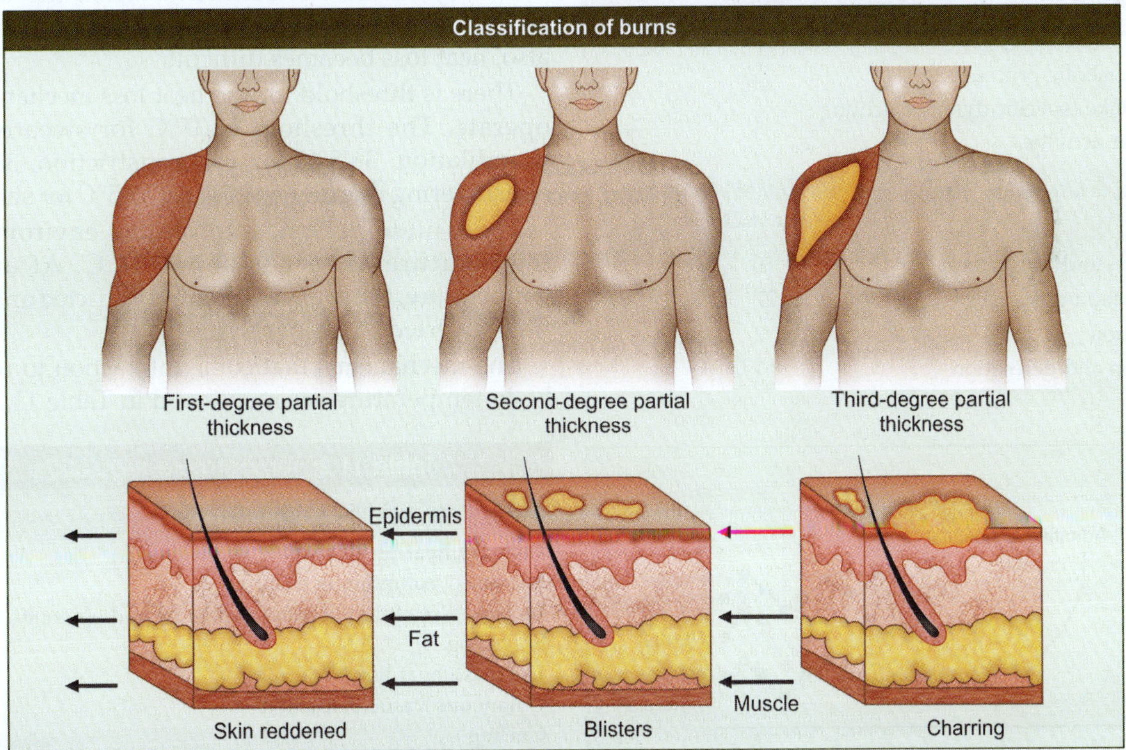

Fig. 11.5: Classification of burns

increase; in hyperthyroidism body temperature is higher than average normal (Fig 11.7). When there is danger of body temperature to fall, is *shivering* produced (activity of skeletal muscles) to produce more heat.

Heat Loss

Most of the heat loss occurs through the *skin*. Small amounts are lost from the *lungs*, in the *urine* and in the *feces*.

At all environmental temperatures, some heat is constantly lost from the skin by evaporation of water

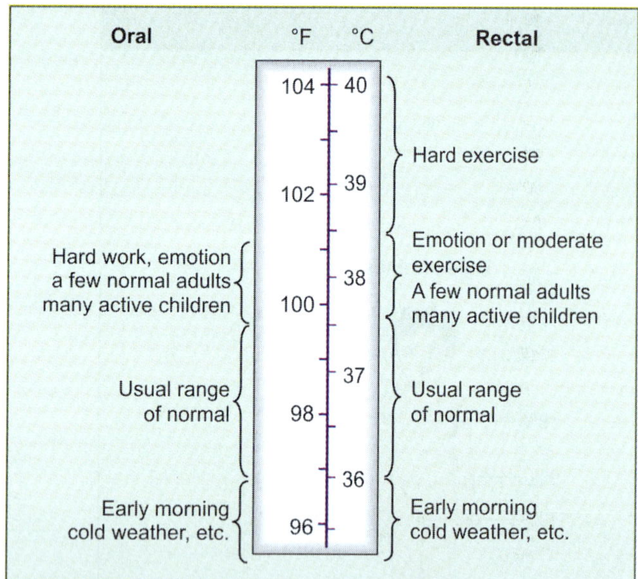

Fig. 11.6: Estimated range of body temperature in normal persons

Table 11.1: Body heat production and heat loss

Body heat is produced by	
Basic metabolic processes	
Food intake (specific dynamic action)	
Muscular activity	
Body heat is lost by	*Percentage of heat lost at 21°C*
Radiation and conduction	70
Vaporization of sweat	27
Respiration	2
Urination and defecation	1

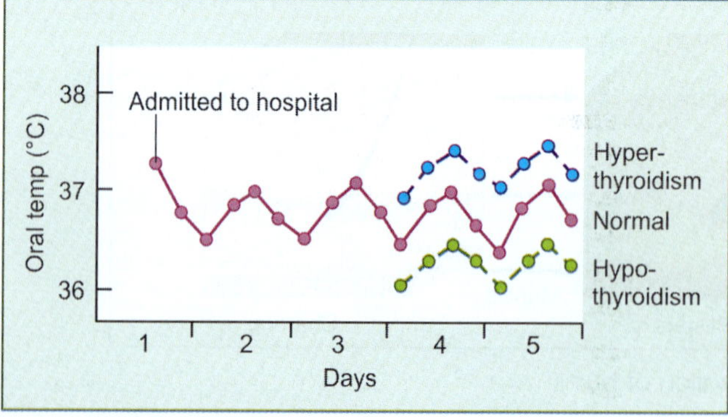

Fig. 11.7: Typical temperature chart of a hospitalized patient who does not have a febrile disease. Slight rise in temperature, due to excitement and apprehension, at the time of admission to the hospital; note regular circadian temperature rhythm. Also temperature record in hypothyroidism and hyperthyroidism

that is called **insensible water loss** that causes a loss of water from the body of about 500 mL/day (includes loss from respiratory tract). This loss of water occurs by diffusion through the skin that we are not aware and is not the sweat formation and the loss is independent of environmental temperature.

The heat loss can only *be regulated through the skin* and not through other routes. Two main mechanisms for regulation of heat loss are changes in the blood flow through the skin and **sweating**. In hot environment **vasodilation** of skin blood vessels occurs.

When the environmental temperature is less than that of the body, *the heat is lost* by **conduction**, **convection** and **radiation.** When the environmental temperature is higher than that of body the main mechanism of heat loss is by evaporation of the sweat from the skin. In hot and humid environment, person feels hotter than in hot dry environment because of less evaporation of sweat. Some unknown factor also operates. Evaporation of sweat depends on the humidity of the environment. When the external environment is above body temperature and is humid also, heat loss becomes difficult.

There is threshold for the heat loss mechanisms to operate. The threshold is 37°C for sweating and vasodilation, 36.8°C for vasoconstriction, 36°C for nonshivering thermogenesis and 35.5°C for shivering.

For a nude person, comfortable environmental temperature at rest is about 27°C. At a lower temperature, the skin vessels are constricted and blood flow diverted to deeper tissues.

The mechanisms that come into action to regulate body temperature are mentioned in Table 11.2.

Table 11.2: Temperature regulation

Mechanisms activated by cold
Increase heat production
Increased voluntary activity
Increased secretion of norepinephrine and epinephrine
Shivering
Decrease heat loss
Cutaneous vasoconstriction
Curling up
Mechanisms activated by heat
Increase heat loss
Cutaneous vasodilation
Sweating
Increased respiration
Decrease heat production
Inertia

Clothes in Temperature Control

Air is poor conductor of heat, and when layers of air are trapped in clothing; between the skin and the clothing, they act as insulators against heat loss.

HYPOTHERMIA

When skin or blood is cooled ***enough*** to lower body temperature, the metabolic and physiological processes in the body slow down. Respiration, heart rate and blood pressure are low and consciousness is lost. At rectal temperatures of about 28°C, the ability to spontaneously return to normal temperature is lost but individual continues to survive and if warmed with external heat returns to normal state.

Humans tolerate body temperature of 21–24°C (70–75°F) without permanent ill effects and induced hypothermia has been used for surgery. Accidental hypothermia due to prolonged exposure to cold air or cold water is a serious problem and requires careful monitoring and prompt reversing.

FEVER

It usually is produced by infections due the pyrogens released from the tissues affected. It is a feature of disease. The regulatory mechanisms behave as if the hypothalamic thermostat is adjusted at higher level to a temperature above 37°C and mechanisms come into action to raise body temperature; as the normal temperature is sensed as low. There is chilly sensation due to vasoconstriction of skin vessels and occasionally shivering also.

Toxins from bacteria act on monocytes, macrophages and Kupffer cells to produce cytokines that act as endogenous pyrogens (EPs). The fever produced due to pyrogens is due to local release of prostaglandins in the hypothalamus. *Prostaglandin 2*, (PGE_2) is one of the prostaglandins that produces fever (Fig. 11.8).

The hypothalamic thermostat is reset to higher temperature, activating heat producing mechanisms, vasoconstriction and shivering until new temperature is reached. When the hypothalamic thermostat is reset to normal temperature with removal of effects of pyrogens heat loss mechanisms are activated, sweating and vasodilation; till normal temperature is reached.

When it is over 41°C (106°F) for *prolonged periods*, some permanent brain damage usually results. When it is above 43°C heat stroke develops and death is common (Fig. 11.9).

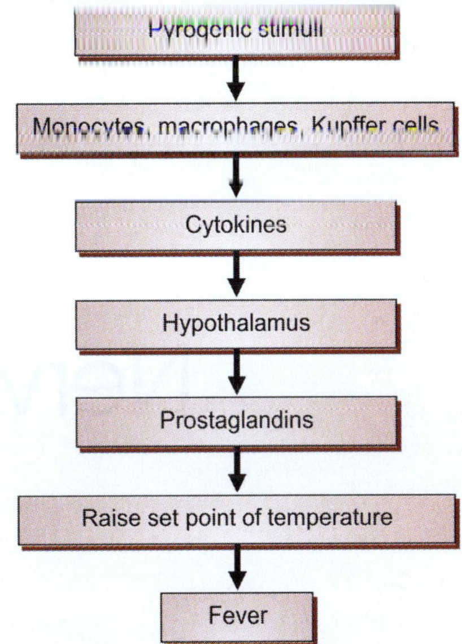

Fig. 11.8: Pathogenesis of fever

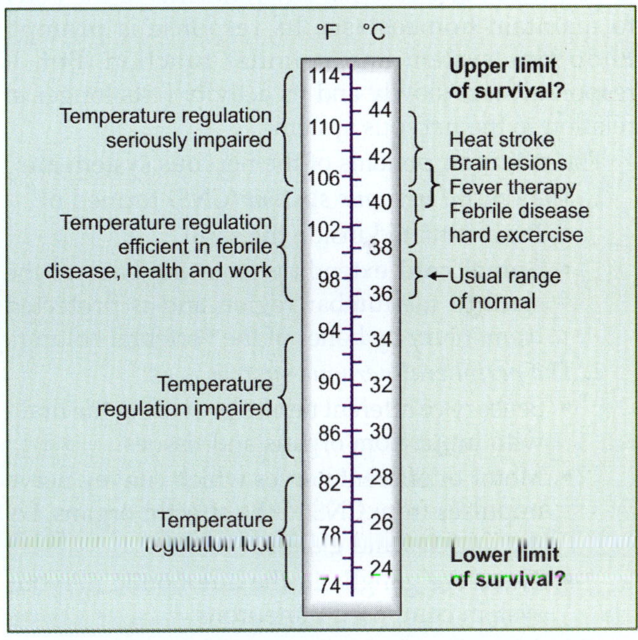

Fig. 11.9: Temperatures under different conditions

IMPLICATIONS AND APPLICATIONS

The student should be able to:

- Recognise normal colour of skin; identify if it is pale due to anaemia or yellowish in colour due to jaundice.
- Give intradermal injection for testing of allergy to the injectable drug.
- Give intradermal injection for mantoux test to check tubercular infection.
- Test any dye on the skin before using it externally.

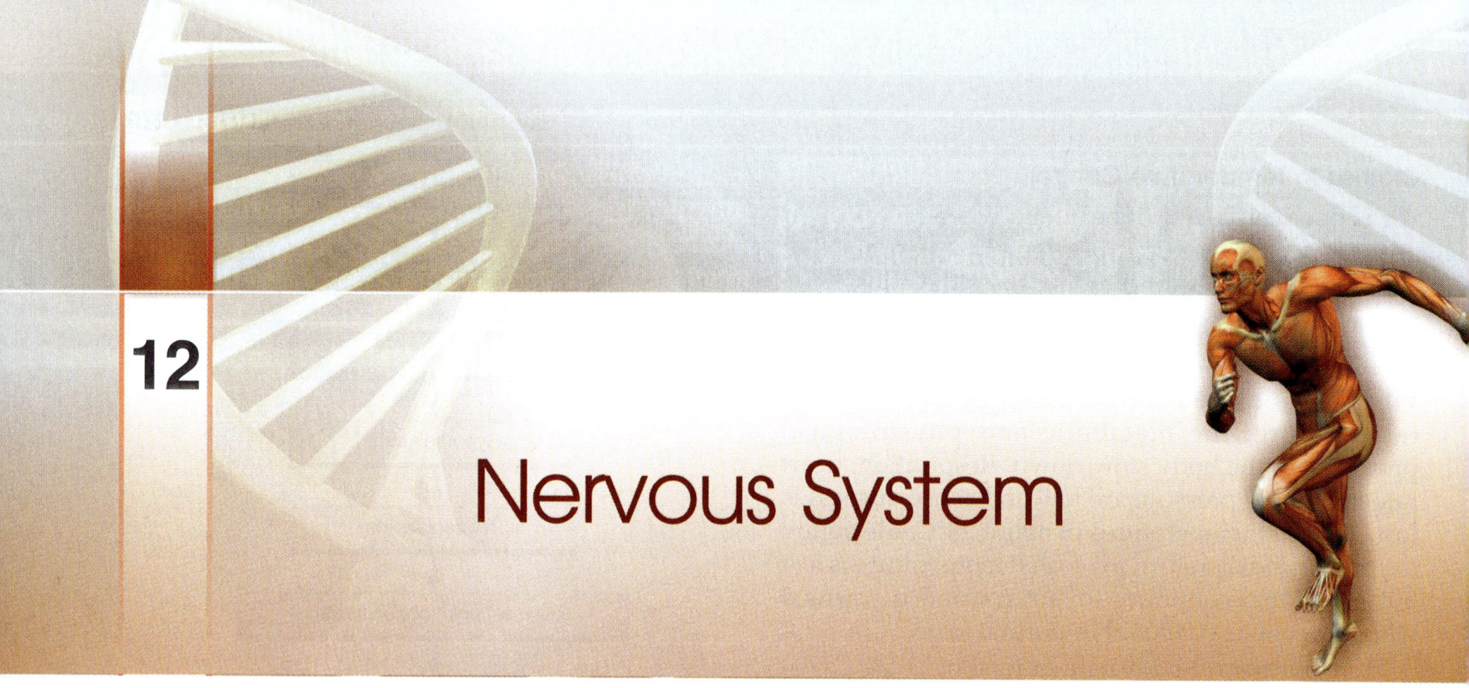

12 Nervous System

Nervous system is a network that responds to the internal and external environments of the body to maintain homeostasis. Its response is prompt. Endocrine system has a similar function. But, it responds more slowly and its activity lasts longer in relation to the nervous system.

The main components of the nervous system are:

1. *The central nervous system (CNS)* formed of:
   - **Brain** situated inside the skull
   - **Spinal cord** extending from the base of the skull to the lumbar region and is protected from injury by bones of the vertebral column.
2. *The peripheral nervous system* is as:
   - Sensory or afferent nerves providing the brain with input from organs and tissues.
   - Motor or efferent nerves which convey nerve impulses from CNS to the effector organs, i.e. the muscles and glands.
   - There are ganglia in the autonomic nervous system composed of neurons.

Functions of Nervous System

Broadly can be grouped as: Sensory detection, information processing and behavior. Learning and memory are specific forms of information processing which permit behavior to change in response to environmental challenges. Other systems the endocrine and the immune systems also share these functions but nervous system is specialized.

Sensory Detection

Sensory detection is the process by which neurons transduce environmental energy into neural signals. Sensory detection is achieved by special neurons with sensory receptors. Various forms of energy can be sensed, mechanical forces, light, sound, chemicals, temperature.

Excitability is a property of neurons. The property involves electrical signals that enable the neurons to receive and transmit information. Excitability appears as electrical events, such as receptor potentials, action potentials and synaptic potentials. Chemical events accompany the electrical events.

Information Processing

- Transmission of information in neuronal networks.
- Integration of information between signals from different sources, i.e. neural integration.
- Storage of information in memory and retrieval of memory.
- Sensory perception with use of sensory information.
- Thought processes.
- Learning.
- Planning and implementation of motor commands.
- Emotions.

Information processing including **learning** and **memory** depends on intercellular communications in neuronal circuits both by electrical and chemical events (to be described in subsequent chapters).

Behavior is organism's responses to its environment. Behavior may be in **cognition** but often is a motor act, such as **movement** or an **autonomic response. Language** is an important set of behaviors in humans.

TRANSMISSION OF IMPULSE ALONG THE NERVRES

All messages are transmitted along the nerves in the form of electrical impulses, the action potentials.

While the impulses are transmitted along the nervous system, they are also *transmitted from one neuron to another neuron* at *junction called* ***Synapse,*** e.g. from sensory to effector neuron and similarly a number of neurons may be involved along with a pathway inside the central nervous system. During communication there is no anatomical continuity between neurons but there is a small gap between them, called synaptic cleft where a chemical transmitter is involved in the conduction of impulse from one neuron to another.

THE SENSORY SYSTEM

The somatic or general sensations are of **touch, pain, heat** and **cold;** are perceived by specialized sensory receptors that are the endings of the sensory nerves; all over the skin. There are other receptors situated in the muscles and joints that respond to changes in position and orientation of the body; that provide **awareness** of **movement** and **position**. There are receptors for special senses also. A list of different receptors in the body is tabulated (Table 12.1).

Nerve impulses travel at a great speed along with nerve fibers and lead to responses, i.e. the perception of sensations or adjustments of body posture.

THE MOTOR SYSTEM

The motor nerves transmit impulses from the central nervous system to the effector regions; which may be the **skeletal muscles** in somatic nervous system or **autonomic nerves** to the viscera.

The autonomic nervous system is not under the voluntary control and is composed of two parts, i.e. parasympathetic system and sympathetic system. The viscera receive fibers from both divisions of autonomic nervous system with activity of one system opposite to the other. This applies to most viscera as they are supplied by both systems.

THE NERVE CELLS AND THE NEUROGLIAL CELLS

Nerve cells are called **neurons**. There are large numbers of these cells in the CNS and some are also present outside the CNS in ganglia. The neurons are surrounded by supporting cells called **neuroglia.** The neuroglial cells are much more numerous than the neurons. They provide support to the neurons and have other functions; one of these is that they form myelin sheath around the nerves.

Parts of Neuron

Each neuron consists of a cell body, containing a nucleus and the processes which are called axon and dendrites (Fig. 12.1). Usually, there is one axon and a number of dendrites. The axon conducts impulses *from* the neurons, and dendrites conduct *to* the neuron.

Table 12.1: Principal sensory modalities

Sensory modality	*Receptor*	*Sense organ*
Vision	Rods and cones	Eye
Hearing	Hair cells	Ear (organ of corti)
Smell	Olfactory neurons	Olfactory mucous membrane
Taste	Taste receptor cells	Taste bud
Rotational acceleration	Hair cells	Ear (semicircular canals)
Linear acceleration	Hair cells	Ear (utricle and saccule)
Touch-pressure	Nerve endings	Various
Warmth	Nerve endings	Various
Cold	Nerve endings	
Pain	Naked nerve endings	
Joint position and movement	Nerve endings	Various
Muscle length	Nerve endings	Muscle spindle
Muscle tension	Nerve endings	Golgi tendon organ
Arterial blood presure	Nerve endings	Stretch receptors in carotid sinus and aortic arch
Central venous pressure	Nerve endings	Stretch receptors in walls of great veins, atria
Inflation of lung	Nerve endings	Stretch receptors in lung parenchyma
Temperature of blood in head	Neurons in hypothalamus	
Arterial PO_2	Glomus cells	Carotid and aortic bodies

The first 11 are conscious sensations.

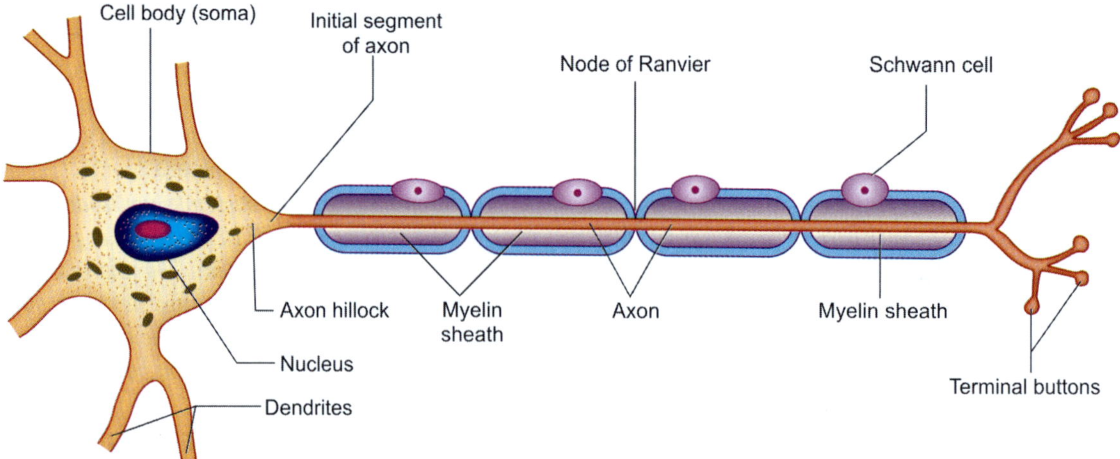

Fig. 12.1: Motor neuron with myelinated axon

Cell Bodies

Nerve cells cannot be seen with naked eye. They can be examined under the microscope and they have various sizes and shapes. The cell bodies form the grey matter of the nervous system which forms the outer surface of the brain but central region in the spinal cord. In the peripheral, nervous system groups of cell bodies are called ganglia.

Axons and Dendrites

Axons and dendrites form the white matter of the nervous system.

Axons are found under the grey matter in the brain and in the spinal cord form groups called tracts that surround the grey matter. The white matter in the spinal cord exists as ventral (anterior), dorsal (posterior) and lateral columns surrounding the grey matter which is in the form of letter H, with a central canal (Fig. 12.2).

Dendrites

Dendrites are short processes and usually branching processes and mostly receive impulses.

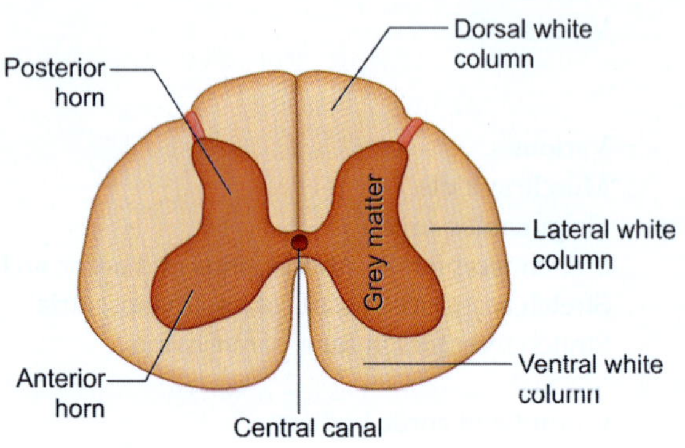

Fig. 12.2: Section of spinal cord

Nerve Fibers-Myelinated or Unmyelinated

The axon of many neurons is myelinated (Fig. 12.1), i.e. acquires a sheath of myelin, a protein-lipid complex that is wrapped around the axon. Outside the CNS the myelin is produced by ***Schwann cells*** which are neuroglial cells found along the axon. Myelin is formed by Schwann cell as its membrane wraps around the axon, number of times (Fig. 12.3A). The myelin sheath envelops the axons except at regular, repeating intervals of about 1 mm, called the nodes of Ranvier (Fig. 12.1). All neurons are not myelinated, some are unmyelinated, and they are surrounded by Schwann cell *without wrapping* of the Schwann cell membrane around the axon that produces myelin (Fig. 12.3A).

Inside the CNS most of the neurons are myelinated but another type of neuroglial cells called the ***oligodendrocytes*** form the myelin sheath rather than Schwann cells. Unlike the Schwann cells which form the myelin between two nodes of Ranvier on a single neuron; oligodendrocytes give rise to number of processes that form myelin around many adjoining axons (Fig. 12.3B).

> **Diseases Involving Myelin**
>
> ***Mutation of the Gene for the Component of Myelin*** causes peripheral neuropathies. Many different mutations occur that cause symptoms ranging from mild to severe.
>
> **Multiple sclerosis** is an autoimmune crippling disease. There is patchy destruction of myelin in CNS. It results in delayed or blocked conduction in these axons.

PERIPHERAL NERVES

Membrane Potentials

Electrical potentials exist across the membranes of essentially all cells of the body. In addition, nerve and muscle cells are "excitable". The following discussion

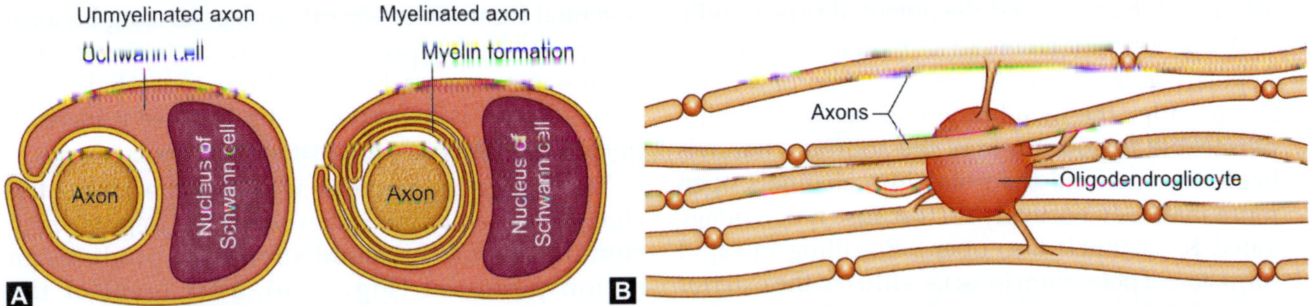

Figs 12.3A and B: Relation of Schwann cells to axons in nerves. (A) The left is an unmyelinated axon, and on the right is a myelinated axon. Cell membrane of the Schwann cell has wrapped around the axon making myelin sheath, (B) myelination of axons in the central nervous system by oligodendrogliocytes. One oligodendrogliocyte sends processes to a number of axons

is concerned with membrane potentials that are generated both at rest and during action potentials in nerve. It is also applicable to skeletal muscle cells.

Resting Membrane Potential

In the resting state the nerve cell membrane is polarized, i.e. there is charge difference ***across*** the membrane, the inside of the membrane is negatively charged in relation to the outside of the membrane. This potential difference across the membrane is called the ***resting membrane potential*** (Fig. 12.4).

Ionic Basis of Resting Membrane Potential

Inside the cell, the main positive ion is potassium with higher concentration then on the outside in the extracellular fluid (ECF) where the main positive ion with higher concentration is sodium. The resting membrane is *not very* permeable to sodium but is relatively more permeable to potassium, hence K^+ tend to ***diffuse out*** from inside of the membrane due to this difference in concentration (**concentration gradient**). But, along with them the negatively charged ions the protein and phosphates from inside the cell cannot diffuse out (being large in size). This results in *more negative charges* to spread along the *inner side of the membrane*, and more positive charges along the outside of it; that produce the potential difference across the membrane, called the **resting membrane potential (RMP)** which is negative potential (inside negative), the magnitude is about –70 mV in the neuron. The sodium potassium pump present in the membrane maintains this state as it pumps out sodium and pumps in potassium across the membrane, using energy from ATP. But, for each molecule of ATP used, it pumps out 3 Na^+ and pumps in 2 K^+. Hence, it keeps the concentration of sodium low inside the cell; and as it *moves out more positive* charges than it moves in, it contributes to the magnitude of RMP.

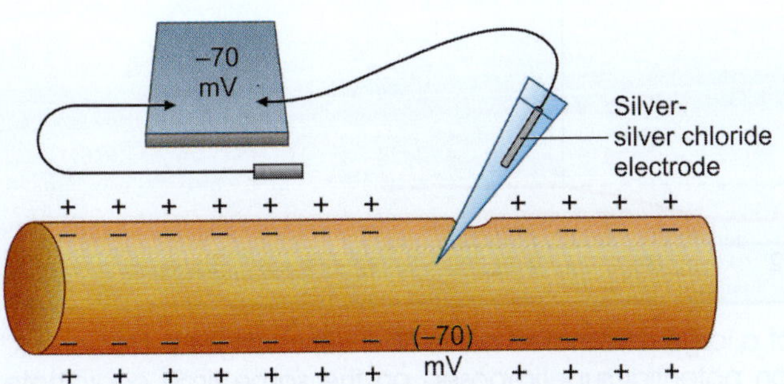

Fig. 12. 4: Recording of RMP in a nerve

RMP is written with negative sign as it expresses the charge on the inside of the membrane.

The number of ions contributing to the RMP is small and inside the cell the number of positive ions and negative ions balance each other.

RMP is present in almost all cells in the body but magnitude differs in different cells. In excitable tissues, i.e. muscle and nerve, it is essential for their activity. Magnitude in skeletal muscle and cardiac muscle is about –90 mV. In inexcitable cells the value of RMP is low.

Nerve Action Potential and Ionic Basis

Nerve signals are transmitted by action potentials which are rapid changes in the membrane potential. Each action potential begins with a sudden change from the normal resting negative potential to a positive membrane potential and then with an equally rapidity changes back to negative potential.

The successive stages of the action potential are as follows:

- Resting membrane potential before the action potential
- *Depolarization stage:* At this time, the membrane suddenly becomes permeable to sodium ions, (due to opening of Na^+ channels) allowing large numbers of positively charged sodium ions to flow to the

interior of the axon, and the potential rises rapidly in the positive direction, recorded as upstroke.

- Repolarization stage: Within a fraction of a millisecond after the membrane had becomes highly permeable to sodium ions the sodium channels begin to close and the potassium channels open more than they normally do (because now voltage gated K^+ channels also open). Resulting in rapid diffusion of potassium ions; i.e. efflux to the exterior reestablishes the normal negative resting membrane potential recorded as downstroke (Figs 12.5A and B).

When an external electrical stumulus is given to an of excitable tissue the characteristics of action potential (AP) and the ionic events producing AP can be studied.

Electronic Potentials, Local Response and Firing Level

Current pulses of electrical stimulus can be depolarizing or hyperpolarizing. A change in membrane potential from –70 to –55 mV is depolarizing because it decreases the potential difference across the membrane; conversely a membrane potential from–70 to –90 mV is hyperpolarizing because it increase potential difference across th membrane.

The larger the current stimulus the larger the change in membrane potential. If the depolarizing stimulus is of a **threshold** strength it produces an action potential (Fig. 12.6). This level of the membrane potential that initiates an AP is called firing level. But when the current strength (stimulus) applied on membrane produces less depolarization than the firing level the stimuli are subthreshold. Fig. 12.6 shows the changes in potential when *subthreshold* stimuli have been given. The potential changes are observed mainly near the site of passage of current (stimulus). The changes are not propogated (as are action potentials) they are called local responses.

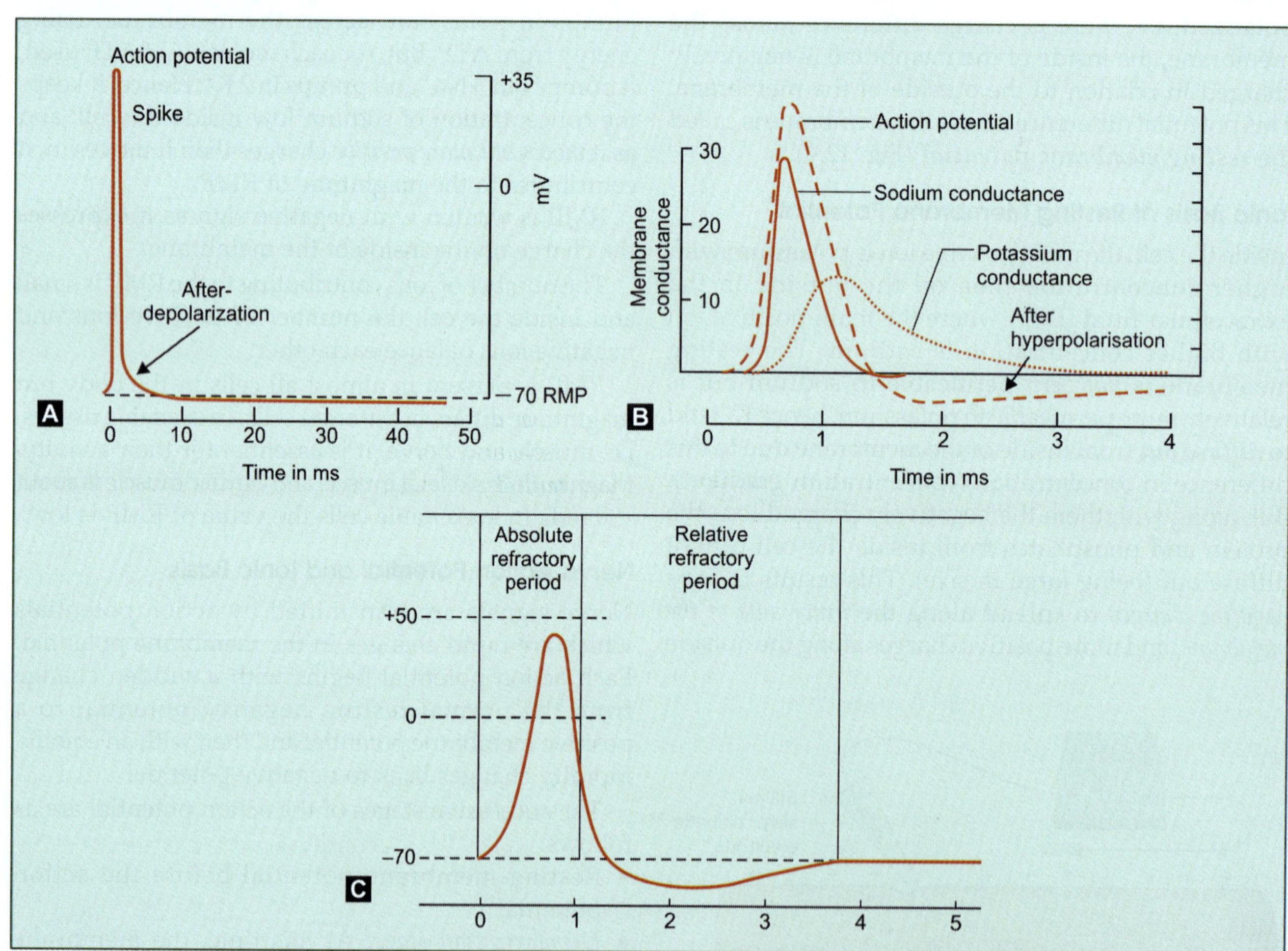

Figs 12.5A to C: (A) Diagram of the complete action potential of a large myelinated nerve fiber; (B) changes in Na^+ and K^+ membrane permeability during the action potential. The action potential superimposed on the same time coordinate; (C) refractory peroids during action potential

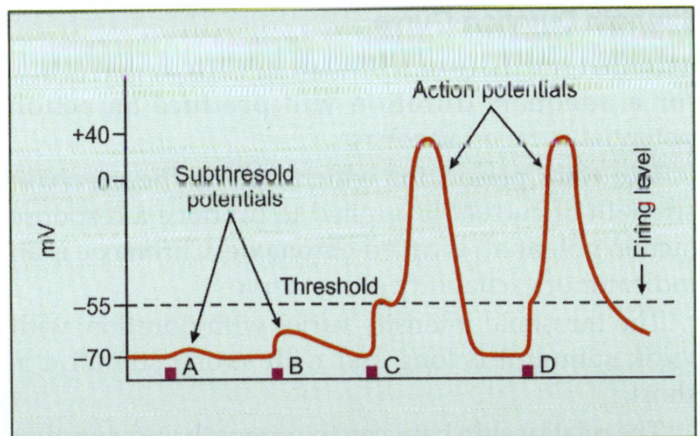

Fig. 12.6: Subthreshold stimuli at A and B fail to produce action potentials. Depolarization to threshold level produces action potential as in C and D

When larger depolarizing current is applied to membrane a threshold membrane potential can be reached at which a response different, from local responses, i.e. an action potential occurs. The action potential differs from local response in two ways (1) it is a larger response in which the polarity of the membrane is reversed (interior becomes positive), (2) action potential is conducted without decrement down the length of the nerve or muscle fiber, i.e. the size and shape of the action potential remains the same as it travels. The size does not decrease with distance as in the local response (Fig. 12.6). Also when a stimulus larger then threshold, suprathreshold stimulus is applied the size and shape of the action potential does not change but remains the same. A stimulus either fails to produce an action potential (subthreshold stimulus) or it produces a full sized action potential (AP). Action potential is **all-or-none response.**

Voltage-Gated Sodium and Potassium Channels are Activated and Inactivated during the Course of an Action Potential

The factor for both depolarization and repolarization of the nerve membrane during the action potential is the *voltage-gated sodium channel*. The voltage-gated potassium channel also plays an important role in increasing the rapidity of repolarization of the membrane.

The events that cause the action potential can be summarized as follows:

- *RMP:* Before the action potential begins, the conductance for potassium ioins is 50–100 times as great as the conductance for sodium ions. This is causes much greater leakage of potassium ions (efflux) than sodium ions (influx) through the **leak channels.**
- *At the onset of the action potential:* When a stimulus causes depolarization up to firing level the sodium channels sudenly become activated and allow great increase in sodium conductance and influx of Na^+ (due to concentration and electrical gradient) produce rapid depolarization. Then the inactivation process within a few fractions of a millisecond closes the sodium channels. Hence, rapid depolarization is terminated and repolarization occurs. The onset of the action potential also causes voltage-gated potassium channels to begin opening but more slowly. Hence, they contribute in repolarization.
- *At the end of the action potential:* The return of the membrane potential to the negative state causes the potassium channels back to their original status i.e. the resting state where K^+ channels remain open but, the voltage-gated K^+ channels that opened during repolarization close again, only after a delay, which results in after hyperpolarization before reaching RMP level (Fig. 12.5B).

An Action Potential does not Occur Until the Threshold has been Reached

A sudden decrease in the membrane potential in a large nerve fiber from –70 millivolts to about –55 millivolts usually causes explosive development of the action potential due to opening of voltage-gated Na^+ channels. This level of –55 millivolts then is said to be the threshold for stimulation (Firing level).

Refactoring Period

A new action potential cannot occur so long as the membrane is still depolarized from the preceding action potential: After the action potential is initiated, the sodium channels soon then become inactivated and any amount of excitatory signal applied to these channels does not open the inactivation gates. The only condition that can reopen them is when the membrane potential returns either to, or almost to the original resting membrane potential level. Then, inactivation gates of the channels open and a new action potential can then be initiated.

- *Absolute refractory period:* An action potential cannot be elicited during the absolute refractory period even with a strong stimulus. This period for large myelinated nerve fibers is from depolarization till the repolarization is one-third complete (Fig. 12.5C).
- *Relative refractory period:* This period follows the absolute refractory period. During this time, stronger than normal stimuli can excite the fiber and an action potential can be initiated.

Conduction of an Impulse

The nerve impulse is conducted because of electrotonic depolarization of membrane ahead of action potentials and and when threshold depolarization is reached AP is produced.

The impulse travels along the nerve (or muscle membrane). Positive charges from the membrane ahead of the action potential flow into the area of negativity due to action potential (current sink). By drawing positive charges this flow decreases the polarity of the membrane ahead of the action potential. Such electrotonic depolarization intiates a local response, and when the firing level is reached, a propagated response occurs that in turn electronically depolarizes the membrane in front of it.

The impulse travels in the *forward direction* because for *sometime after* passage of an action potential that region of the nerve remains in **refractory state**, i.e. it cannot transmit another action potential for a short period after an action potential and hence the impulse travels ahead and not backwards.

Impulses are conducted at a faster rate in myelinated fibers as the impulse, jumps from one node to the next one; as in between two nodes, the myelin acts as an insulator. This type of conduction is called **saltatory conduction**. It results in ***faster conduction*** of the impulse. In unmyelinated fibers, the impulse is conducted slowly by successive depolarization of the neighboring regions (Figs 12.7A and B).

Even amongst the myelinated fibers, *speed of conduction* varies with the *diameter of the axon*. The larger diameter fibers conduct at faster rates (Table 12.2).

Transmission of impulse in all nerves involves similar mechanism, i.e. nerve signals are transmitted by action potentials.

Strength Duration Curve

Minimal intensity of stimulating current that acting for a adequate duration will produce an action potential is called **rheobase.**

The **time period** for which double the rheobase strength of current is applied to produce a response (action potential) is called **chronaxie**. Chronaxie is an indicator of excitability of the nerve.

The threshold intensity varies with duration; with weak stimuli it is long and with strong stimuli it is short.

The relationship between the **strength** and **duration of a stimulus** is called **strength-duration curve.**

Accomodation in Nerve

When a nerve or muscle cell is depolarized slowly it may not respond with an action potential. This property is called accomodation. It is because during the slow depolarization some sodium channels become inactivated and normal threshold may be passed without an action potential. Hence, if depolarization is slow the critical number of open Na^+ channels required to trigger an action potential may not be reached.

Compound Action Potential

The action potential described is as recorded from a single nerve fiber with one electrode inserted into the fiber (Fig. 12.4) while the other is on the outer surface of the membrane of the fiber (intracellular recording). If a recording is made from a mixed nerve which has many types of fibers, by placing electrodes on the whole nerve; on the outside of the nerve, the two electrodes stimulating and recording being separated by a distance, a compound action potential (Fig. 12.8) is recorded which has ***multiple peaks***. Peripheral nerves are made-up of a number of axons bound together in a fibrous envelope called epineurium.

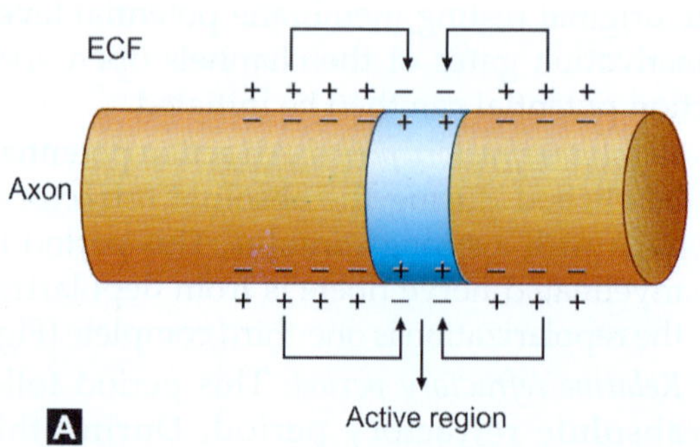

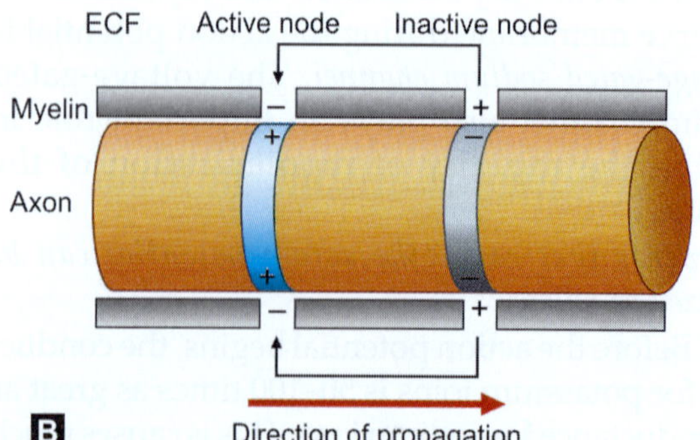

Figs 12.7A and B: Local current flow (movement of positive charges) for an impulse in an axon. (A) Unmyelinated axon; (B) Myelinated axon

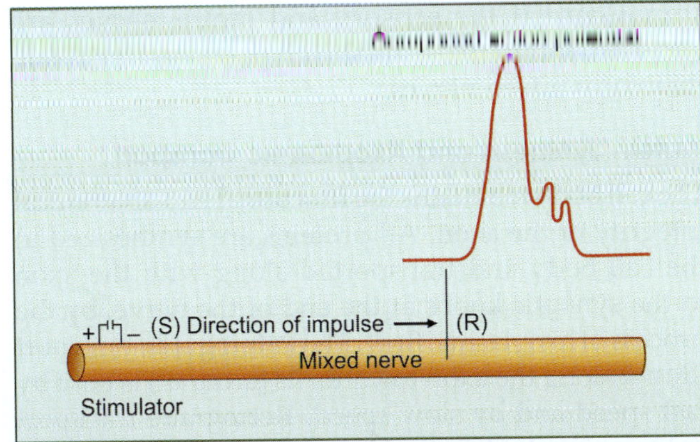

Fig. 12.8: Compound action potential. The drawing shows the record obtained with recording electrodes (R) at a distances from the stimulating electrodes; (S) along a mixed nerve

Potential changes recorded extracellularly from such nerves represent algebraic summation of the all-or-none action potentials of many of the axons; this is a **compound action potential**.

The *threshold* for stimulation (i.e. production of action potential), for the individual axons in the nerve vary. When stimuli are subthreshold none of the axons are stimulated and no response occurs. When the stimuli are of threshold intensity, axons with low threshold get stimulated; as intensity of stimulation is increased axons with higher threshold also get stimulated. The maximal stimulus excites all the axons and supramaximal stimulus does not increase the response.

Types of Nerve Fibers

The peripheral nerve fibers are classified (Erlanger and Gasser) according to their diameter into A, B, C types, with further sub-classification of A type to alpha, beta, gamma and delta (Aα, Aβ, Aγ, Aδ).

A and B type of fibers are myelinated, C type are unmyelinated. Table 12.2 shows the classification that includes both, motor and sensory peripheral nerve fibers and the functions served.

Another numerical classification is for sensory fiber (Table 12.3).

Table 12.3 shows type of classification used only for sensory nerve fibers.

The various types of fibers in peripheral nerves differ in their sensitivity to hypoxia and anesthetics (Table 12.4). This fact has clinical significance. Local anesthetics depress transmission in group C (pain) fibers before they affect the touch fibers in the group A. On the other hand, pressure on the nerve can cause loss of conduction in large diameter motor and touch-pressure fibers while pain sensation remains intact. Sometimes, when people sleep with their arm under their head for long periods, resulting compression of the nerves produces numbness.

Table 12.3: Numerical classification sometimes used for sensory nerve fibers

Number	*Origin*	*Fiber type*
Ia	Muscle spindle, annulospiral ending	Aα
Ib	Golgi tendon organ	Aα
II	Muscle spindle, flower-spray ending, touch, pressure	Aβ
III	Pain and cold receptors, some touch receptors	Aδ
IV	Pain, temperature and other receptors	Dorsal root C

Table 12.4: Relative susceptibility of A, B and C nerve fibers to conduction block by various agents

Suceptibility to:	*Most susceptible*	*Intermediate*	*Least susceptible*
Hypoxia	B	A	C
Pressure	A	B	C
Local anesthetics	C	B	A

Table 12.2: Nerve fiber types

Fiber type		*Function*	*Fiber diameter (μm)*	*Conduction velocity (m/s)*
A	α	Proprioception, somatic motor	12–20	70–120
	β	Touch, pressure	5–12	30–70
	γ	Motor to muscle spindle	3–6	15–30
	δ	Pain, cold, touch	2–5	12–30
B		Preganglionic autonomic	<3	3–15
C	Dorsal root	Pain, temperature, some mechanoreception	0.4–1.2	0.5–2
	Sympathetic	Postganglionic sympathetic	0.3–1.3	0.7–2.3

m/s—Meters per second

Sensory or Afferent Nerves

The *endings of the nerves* serve as receptors which receive the different stimuli external or internal. An appropriate stimulus for the endings (e.g. pain stimulus for pain endings) produces depolarization of the endings (a local response) and if depolarization produced reaches the firing level an action potential is initiated in the nerve (Fig. 12.6) that travels as an impulse. At the receptor, the nerve fiber loses myelin sheath if it is a myelinated nerve. The ending (receptor) may be encapsulated with covering of fibrous tissue or may be naked nerve ending (Figs 12.9A to F). Pain receptors are naked nerve endings.

Motor or Efferent Nerves

Motor nerves originate in the brain, spinal cord and autonomic ganglia. They transmit impulses to the effecter organs, muscles or glands. The two groups are:

- **Somatic nerves** involved in *voluntary* and *reflex* skeletal muscle *contractions*
- **Autonomic nerves** (sympathetic and parasympathetic) involved in *cardiac and smooth muscle* contraction and *glandular secretion*.

Mixed Nerves

In the spinal cord, sensory and motor fibers are arranged in separate groups or tracts. Outside the spinal cord if the sensory and motor nerves are enclosed within the same sheath of connective tissue they form mixed nerves.

Protein Synthesis and Axoplasmic Transport

The cell body maintains the functional and anatomical integrity of the axon. All proteins are synthesized in the cell body and transported along with the axon to the synaptic knobs at the end of the nerve, by the process of axoplasmic flow. The **anterograde** transport (down along the axon towards its terminal) is both by fast speed and by slow speed. **Retrograde** transport in the opposite directions also occurs (up along with the axon towards the cell body). Some substances are taken up at the nerve endings by endocytosis, e.g. nerve growth factor and various viruses and are transported back to the cell body. The transport (Figs 12.10A and B) along the axon takes place along the microtubules.

Wallerian Degeneration

If the axon is cut, the part distal to it degenerates. Repair may take place with the growth from the central end of the fiber provided the gap between two cut ends can be bridged (Figs 12.11A to C).

With a cut of axon, there are harmful effects on the cell body for several weeks after the injury. The Nissl

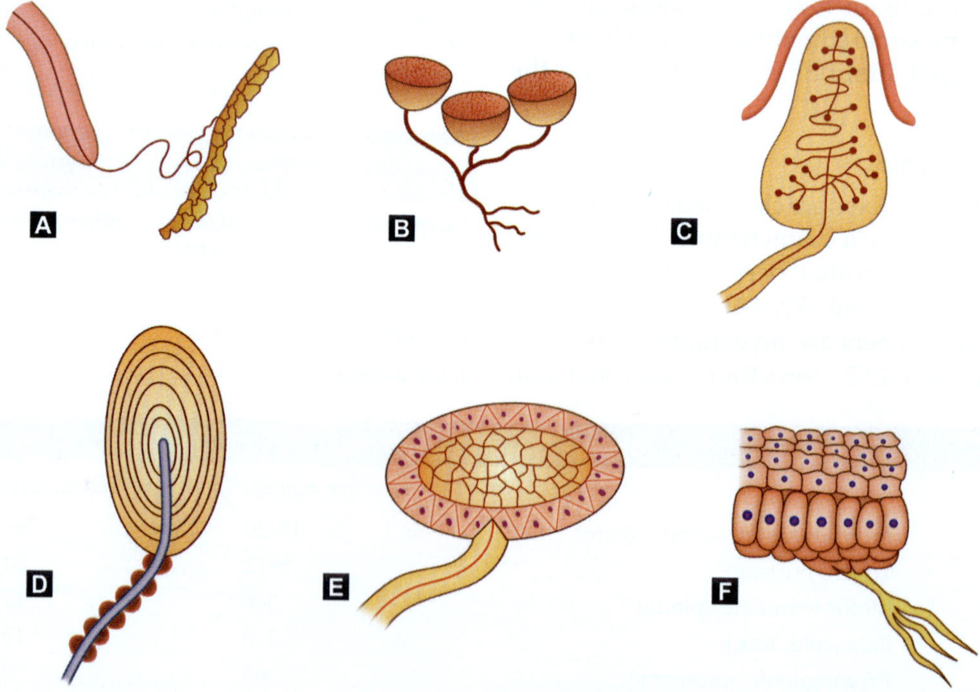

Figs 12.9A to F: Sensory receptors in the skin. (A) Ruffini endings and (B) Merkel's disks are expanded ends of sensory nerve fibers. (C) Meissner's corpuscles; (D) Pacinian corpuscles; (E) Krause's end-bulbs; (F) Naked nerve endings between cells in tissue. Except (F) all are encapsulated endings

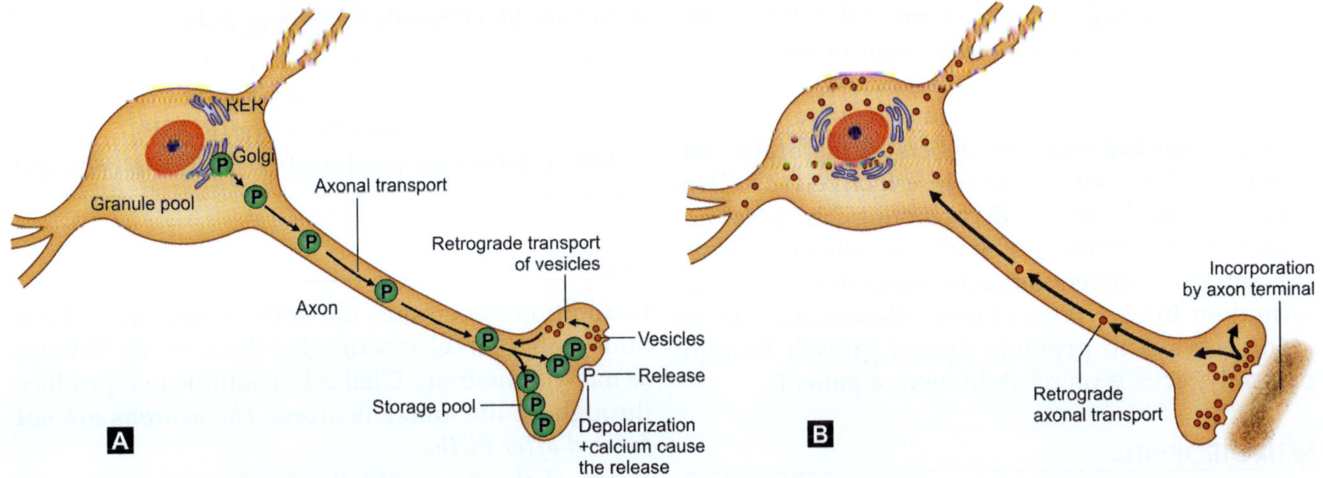

Figs 12.10A and B: (A) Anterograde axonal transport (B) Retrograde axonal transport

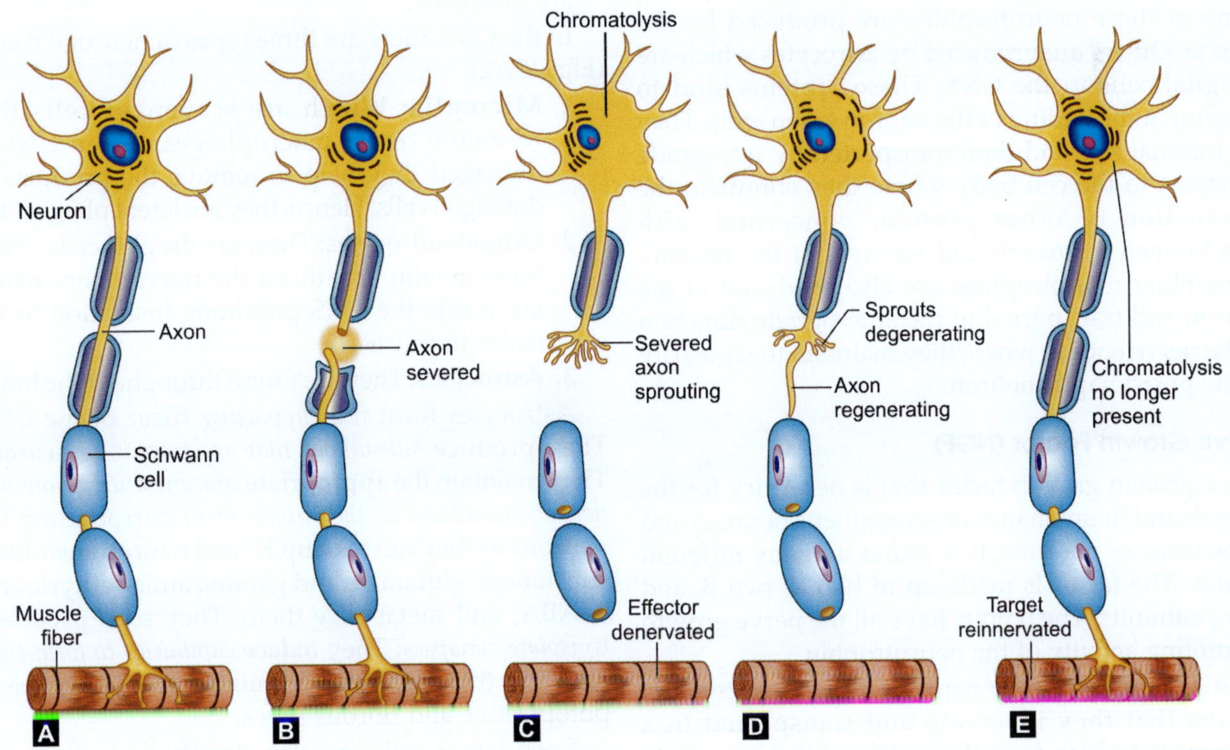

Figs 12.11A to E: (A) Normal motoneuron innervating a skeletal muscle fiber; (B) Motor axon has been severed, and the cell body is undergoing chromatolysis; (C) This is associated with sprouting of axon terminal; (D) with regeneration of the axon the excess sprouts degenerate; (E) when the target cell is reinnervated, chromatolysis is no longer present

bodies in the cell undergo chromatolysis (i.e. the RNA of ribosomes of the endoplasmic reticulum lose their staining characteristics); the cell may die or recover with restoration of Nissl substance in the cell body. A completely severed peripheral nerve has some capacity to repair itself. Schwann cells proliferate to bridge the gap. The axon of the central end divides and these endings begin to sprout out of the end of the nerve. Some of the sprouting ends cross the gap and enter the neural tubes of the peripheral ends (Figs 12.11D and E). This results from growth promoting factors secreted by Schwann cells that attract axons towards distal stump. Adhesion molecules of immunoglobulin super family promote axonal growth along cell membranes and extracellular tissues. Inhibitory molecules in the perineurium direct the neuronal growth. Denervated distal stumps upgrade production of neutrophins to promote growth. The growth rate is 1–2 mm per day. If suitably matched connections are made with terminals, i.e. sensory terminals for sensory nerves and with motor end plate for motor nerves, functions are restored although not full recovery. Fibers of the brain and spinal cord do not regenerate effectively as CNS neurons do not have growth promoting chemicals and CNS myelin is inhibitor of axonal growth and events like astrocyte proliferation, activities of microglia, scar formation hinder regeneration. Research is on to identify ways to promote axonal growth though presently focus is on rehabilitation of patients.

NEUROTROPHINS

A number of proteins are necessary for the ***survival*** and ***growth of neurons*** and are called ***neurotrophins***. Some of these neurotrophins are produced by the muscle. Others are produced by astrocytes which are the glial cells in the CNS. These proteins bind to receptor at the ending of the neuron (axon end). They are internalized and then transported by retrograde transport to the cell body where they stimulate the production of other proteins concerned with developments, growth and survival of the neuron. Some other neurotrophins are also produced in the neuron and transported in the anterograde direction to the nerve ending where they maintain the integrity of the postsynaptic neuron.

Nerve Growth Factor (NGF)

It is a protein growth factor that is necessary for the growth and maintenance of sympathetic neurons and some sensory neurons. It is found in many different tissues. The factor is made-up of two α, two β, and two γ subunits. The β units have all the nerve growth promoting activity of the neurotrophin.

NGF is picked up by neurons in the extracerebral organs that they innervate and transported in a retrograde fashion from the ending of the neurons to their cell bodies. It is also present in the brain and is likely responsible for growth and maintenance of cholinergic neurons in the basal forebrain and striatum. Possibly NGF produces reduction in apoptosis. Brain-derived neurotrophic factor (BDNF) is another **Neurotrophin**.

Other Factors Affecting Neuronal Growth

- Ciliary Neurotrophic Factor (CNTF)
- Glial Cell Line-derived Neurotrophic Factor (GDNF)
- Leukemia Inhibitory Factor (LIF)
- Insulin-like Growth Factor I (IGF-I)
- Transforming Growth Factor (TGF)
- Fibroblast Growth Factor (FGF) and
- Platelet-Derived Growth Factor (PDGF)

The first two are produced by Schwann cells and astrocytes.

NEUROGLIA

In addition to neurons, the nervous system contains numerous glial cells (neuroglia) these are 10–50 times as many as neurons. Glial cells continue to reproduce throughout life unlike neurons. ***The neurons are not formed after birth.***

The glial cells are of following types:

Schwann cells in the *peripheral nervous system* are glial cells.

In the CNS, there are three types of neuroglial cells (Fig. 12.12).

1. **Microglia:** Which are scavenger cells that resemble tissue macrophages. When CNS is damaged they help to remove the products of damaged cells. Hence, they are latent phagocytes.
2. **Oligodendrocytes:** These are the glial cells which form myelin sheath on the nerve fibers which are inside the CNS providing insulation to the nerve impulses.
3. **Astrocytes:** They are found throughout the brain.

Astrocytes form the *supporting tissue* of the CNS. They produce *substances that are trophic to neurons*. They maintain the **appropriate** *concentration of ions and neurotransmitters in the environment* surrounding the neurons as they can take up K^+ and neurotransmitters substances, glutamate and gamma aminobutyric acid (GABA) and metabolize them. They send processes to *isolate synapses*. They *induce capillaries to form tight junctions* that form blood brain barrier. They are of potoplasmic and fibrous types.

Ependymal cells are also classified as glial cells. These cells form the epithelial lining of the ventricles of the brain and the central canal of the spinal cord.

THE SYNAPSE AND NEUROTRANSMITTER SUBSTANCES

There is always more than one neuron in the pathway for the transmission of nerve impulses from their origin to the destination whether it is a sensory or motor sensation. At these points, there is no continuity of the *nervous tissues* between the two neurons. The region at which the nerve impulse passes from one to another neuron is called a **synapse**. At its free end the axon of the presynaptic neuron breaks up into minute

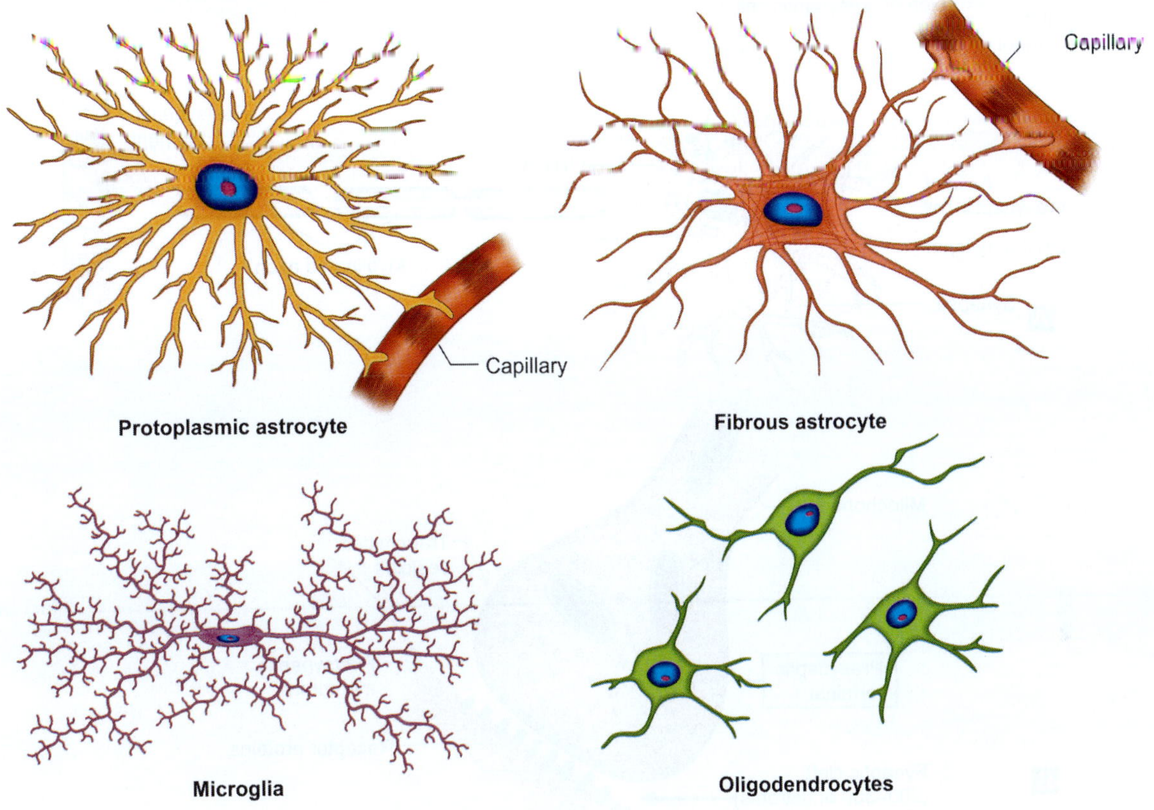

Fig. 12.12: Glial cells in the brain

branches, each of which terminates in small swelling called synaptic knobs or terminal button. These are in close proximity to either the dendrites or the cell body of the postsynaptic neuron or postsynaptic motor end plate in muscle. (Fig. 12.13A). A narrow space between them is called the synaptic cleft (Fig 12.13B). In the synaptic knob there are synaptic vesicles containing neurotransmitter substance.

There are a number of neurotransmitter substances, and *usually* it is one type of neurotransmitter which is present at anyone nerve terminal. The arrival of an impulse at the presynaptic knob causes opening of voltage gated Ca^{2+} channels and influx of calcium ions from the ECF into the synaptic knob then releases neurotransmitter (Fig. 12.13B) in the synaptic cleft. Neurotransmitter is released by exocytosis and diffuses across the synaptic cleft to the postsynaptic cell membrane to bind with ***specific receptors*** for that transmitter. The binding with the receptors results in changes in the ionic permeability of the postsynaptic membrane; producing **diffusion of ions** across the membrane that results in change in the membrane polarity, resulting in either increase or decrease in the excitability of the postsynaptic neuron due to depolarization (EPSP) or hyperpolarization (IPSP) in the postsynaptic membrane. The action of the neurotransmitter is short lived and is terminated by its inactivation by enzymes present at the synapse or by reuptake of the neurotransmitter into the synaptic knob. The neurotransmitters either have an excitatory or inhibitory effect on the excitability of the postsynaptic neuron, i.e. result in the production of either excitatory postsynaptic potential (EPSP) or inhibitory postsynaptic potential (IPSP) (Figs 12.14A to C). 'EPSP' and 'IPSP' are local changes in the membrane.

If the binding of the neurotransmitter with its receptors results in opening of sodium ion channels, diffusion of sodium (influx) across the cell membrane produces EPSP that increases excitability of the neuron. If the binding of a transmitter (which is now a different transmitter substance) with its receptors results in increase of permeability to chloride ions which are negatively charged, the diffusion (influx) across the cell membrane produces IPSP, similarly if it produces increased efflux of K^+ it results in decrease of excitability of the neuron. A neuron is subjected to a number of impulses at anyone time at its different synapses (Fig. 12.13A) if the sum total effect of these impulses arriving at one time is

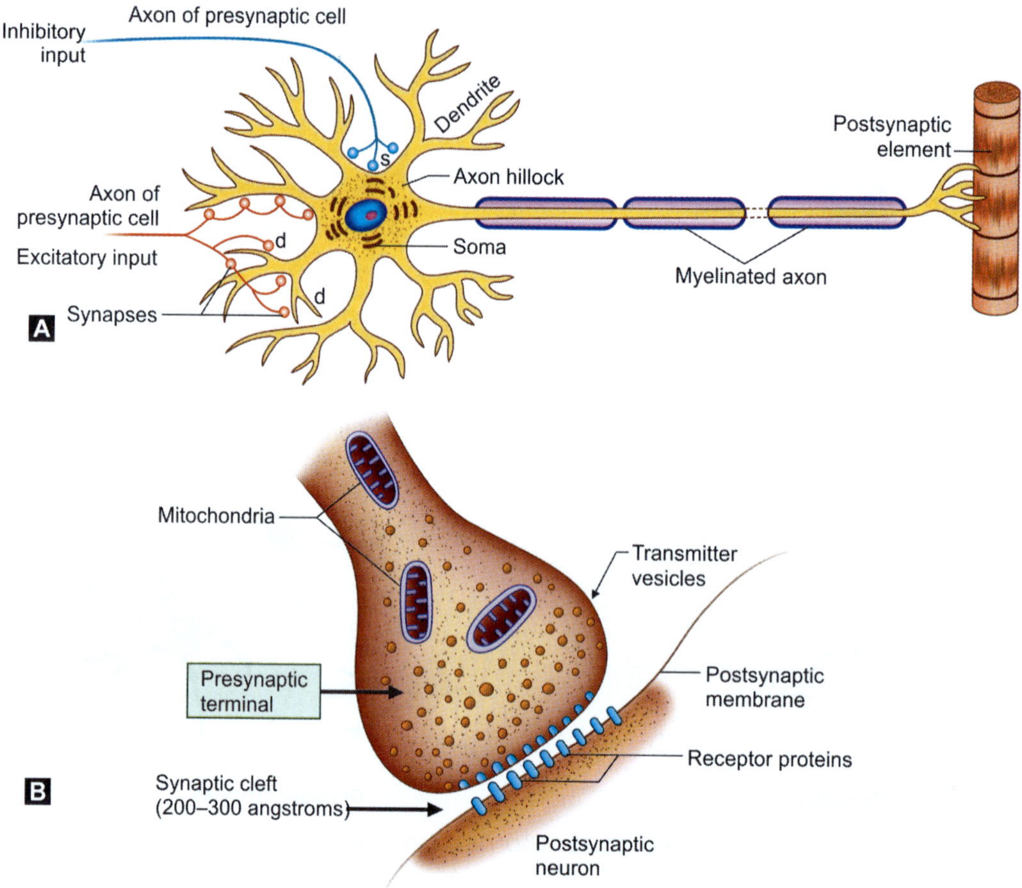

Figs 12.13A and B: (A) Schematic diagram of an idealized neuron and its major components. Most afferent input from axons to cells terminates in synapses on the dendrites (d), although some may terminate on the soma (S). Excitatory terminals tend to terminate more distally on dendrites than do inhibitory ones, which often terminate on the soma. (B) Physiological anatomy of the synapse

increase in the excitability of the postsynaptic neuron, up to a threshold level it results in an action potential (Fig. 12.14D); that travels along axon of postsynaptic cell to its destination. If no action potential is initiated local changes in the membrane regress with time.

There are various neurotransmitter substances known which act at different synapses in the CNS. Neurotransmitters are also involved in autonomic nervous system. The neurotransmitter substances are **acetylcholine**, **epinephrine**, **norepinephrine**, **serotonin, histamine, glutamate, aspartate, glycine, GABA, dopamine, β endorphin, enkephalins, substance P** and also many other substances are as neurotransmitters (Table 12.5).

Glycine and GABA are inhibitory neurotransmitters whereas glutamate and aspartate have excitatory action.

The endings of **autonomic nerves** on smooth muscle and glands, branch near the effector organ and release a neurotransmitter, either **acetylcholine** or **norepinephrine** which may have excitatory or inhibitory action (described in relevant sections).

Inhibition and Facilitation at Synapses

Inhibition in the CNS can be **postsynaptic** or **presynaptic.** Postsynaptic inhibition is direct inhibition caused by release of inhibitory neurotransmitter by the presynaptic terminal on the postsynaptic neuron producing IPSP. The presynaptic inhibition is due to inhibitory transmitter released at the excitatory presynaptic terminal of an axon so that the excitatory neurotransmitter release is decreased at its synapse with postsynaptic neuron (Fig. 12.15A).

There is still another type of inhibition in CNS called **Renshaw cell inhibition** where a motor neuron axon gives a branch to an inhibitory neuron called Renshaw cell this cell inhibits motor neuron from which impulse arises. This is called feedback inhibition (Fig. 12.15B).

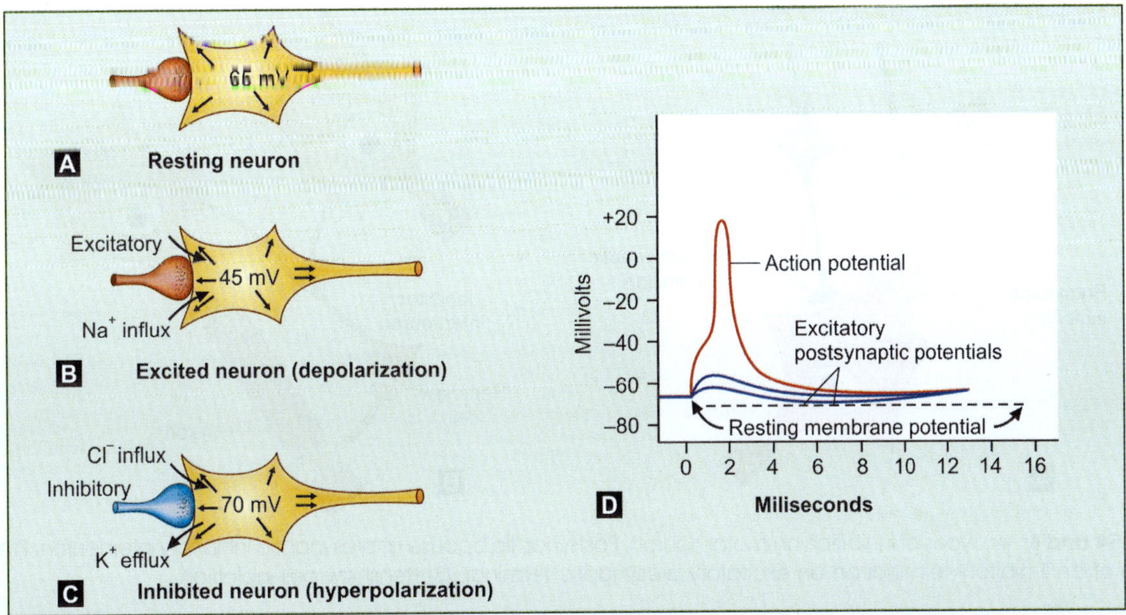

Figs 12.14A to D: (A) Resting neuron; (B) EPSP in the neuron, membrane polarization has decreased, depolarization. If many excitatory endings are active at one time depolarization reaches firing level and action potential is initiated in its axon, (C) The membrane is hyperpolarized (more negative) excitability is decreased with IPSP; (D) When depolarized is to the firing level action potential is produced, depolarization less than that only produces EPSP

Table 12.5: Neurotransmitter substances

Small Molecule Rapidly Acting Transmitters	
Class I:	Acetylcholine
Class II:	The amines:
	Norepinephrine
	Epinephrine
	Dopamine
	Serotonin
	Histamine
Class III :	Amino acids:
	γ-aminobutyric acid (GABA)
	Glycine
	Glutamate
Neuropeptide Slowly Acting Transmitters	
Hypothalamic releasing hormones (refer to text)	
Pituitary peptides	
β-Endorphin	
α-Melanocyte-stimulating hormone	
Peptides that act on gut and brain	
Leucine enkephalin	
Methionine enkephalin	
Substance P	
Gastrin	
Cholecystokinin	
Vasoactive intestinal polypeptide (VIP)	

SOMATIC AND VISCERAL SENSATIONS

The somatosensory system transmits information from sensory receptor organs in the skin, muscle, joint and viscera. The sensory information that is transmitted includes touch, pressure, vibration, proprioception (position sense and joint movement), thermal sense (warmth or cold), pain and visceral distension. The information from sensory receptor organs reaches CNS by way of **first order neurons** which are primary afferent neurons with their cell bodies in the dorsal root ganglia of the spinal cord (or ganglia for cranial nerves). The impulses travel in the central processes of the neurons and pass through the dorsal root of the spinal cord, to reach the **grey matter** in the spinal cord (or enter the brainstem from a cranial nerve). These processes make synaptic connections at various levels in the spinal cord or in the brainstem (as described later in this section) to finally relay information to the cerebral cortex. They also make polysynaptic connections in the spinal cord with motor neurons for reflex responses (Fig. 12.16).

1. Cutaneous Sensations

They originate in the skin. The sensations are touch (fine touch, crude touch) and pressure, vibration, pain, warmth and cold. Pressure sense is maintained touch. Endings of the sensory nerves are the receptors (Fig. 12.9) and are without myelin sheath. The

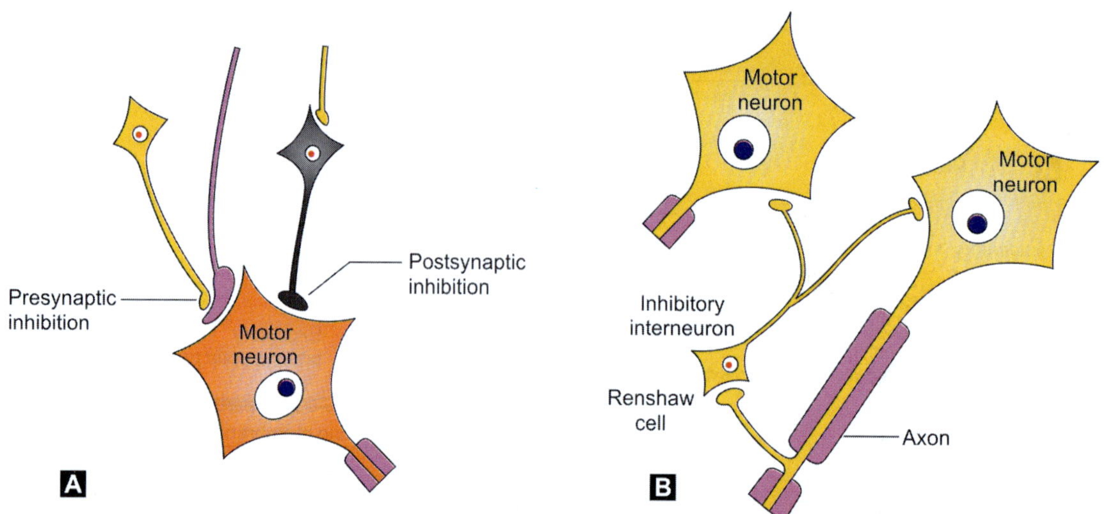

Figs 12.15A and B: (A) Types of inhibition on motor neuron, Postsynaptic bcause of presynaptic inhibitory interneuron. Presynaptic because of an inhibitory terminal on an excitatory presynaptic terminal, (B) Renshaw cell inbibition

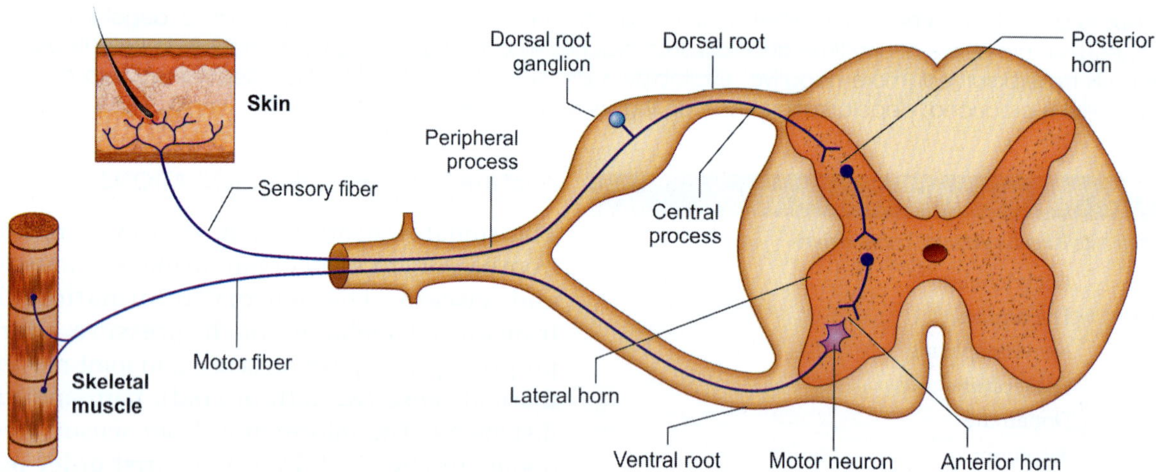

Fig. 12.16: A diagram of the spinal cord, spinal roots and spinal nerve. A primary afferent neuron is with its cell body in the dorsal root ganglion and its central and peripheral processes distributing, respectively, to the spinal cord grey matter and to a sensory receptor in the skin. A motor neuron is shown to have its cell body in the anterior horn of spinal cord grey matter and to project its axon out of the ventral root to innervate a skeletal muscle fiber forming a circuit for reflex action

appropriate stimulus for the endings generates an impulse in the nerve (Fig. 12.17).

The **pain sensations** are carried by **small diameter** axons of both myelinated and unmyelinated nerves (Tables 12.2 and 12.3). The receptors are naked nerve endings.

The **touch sensation** is carried by **myelinated nerve** fibers which have large diameter (Tables 12.2 and 12.3). The endings which are receptors are encapsulated with fibrous tissue coverings (Fig. 12.9).

Cold and warmth sensations are carried by the myelinated nerves of smaller diameter than those for touch sensation and also by unmyelinated nerves (Tables 12.2 and 12.3).

Since pain sensation is carried by both myelinated and unmyelinated nerve fibers, there are two types of pain felt: one is fast pain, the impulses travel via myelinated fibers and the other is slow pain that is transmitted by unmyelinated fibers. A pain stimulus may give both types of sensations, i.e. two pain sensations that are called fast (or first) and slow (or second) pain. The fast pain is sharp, bright localized sensation; the slow pain is dull, intense, diffuse and unpleasant sensation.

2. Muscle, Joint, and Visceral Sensations

Skeletal muscle contains mechanoreceptors (mainly) but also nociceptors (pain receptors). The most

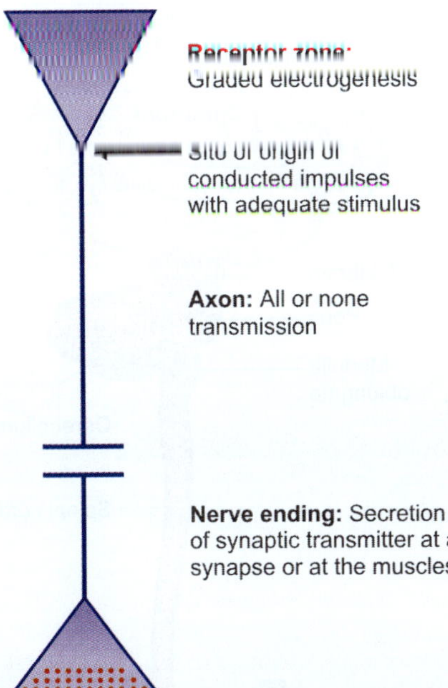

Fig. 12.17: Functional organization of neurons. Nonconducted local potentials are integrated in the receptor zone, and action potentials are initiated at a site close to the receptor zone. The action potentials are conducted along the axon to nerve endings where they release neurotransmitter

important functionally are stretch receptors which include muscle spindles (Fig. 12.18A) and Golgi tendon organs (Fig. 12.18B). They are important in proprioception and also in motor control. Nociceptors in muscle respond to pressure applied to the muscle and to release of metabolites (pain producing metabolites).

Joints are associated with mechanoreceptors and nociceptors.

Viscera are *sparsely* supplied with sensory receptors which are mainly involved in reflexes and have *minor* role in sensory experience. But, they are sensitive to sensation of distension; though visceral nociceptors also signal visceral pain. Being sparsely innervated, visceral pain is poorly localized.

CENTRAL NERVOUS SYSTEM

BRAIN

The parts of brain are (Figs 12.19A and B):

- Cerebrum
- Cerebellum
- Midbrain
- Pons
- Medulla oblongata.

  The last three together are called brainstem.

Cerebrum

The superficial parts of cerebrum are composed of cell bodies of neurons that form the grey matter of the cerebral cortex and the deeper parts consist of nerve fibers or white matter. The surface of the cortex is

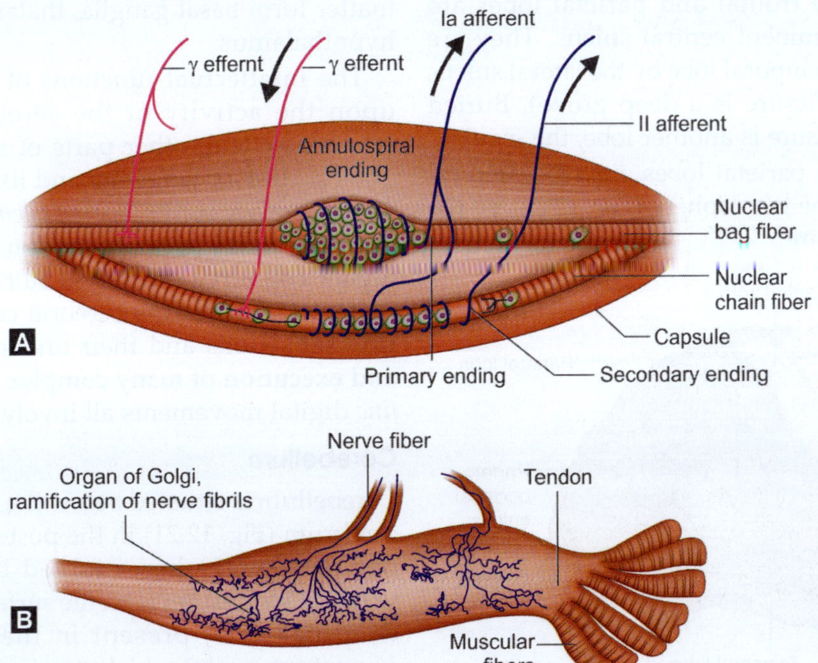

Figs 12.18A and B: (A) Diagrammatic representation of the main components of muscle spindle. Each spindle has a capsule and usually contains two nuclear bag fibers and four or more nuclear chain fibers; (B) Golgi tendon organ

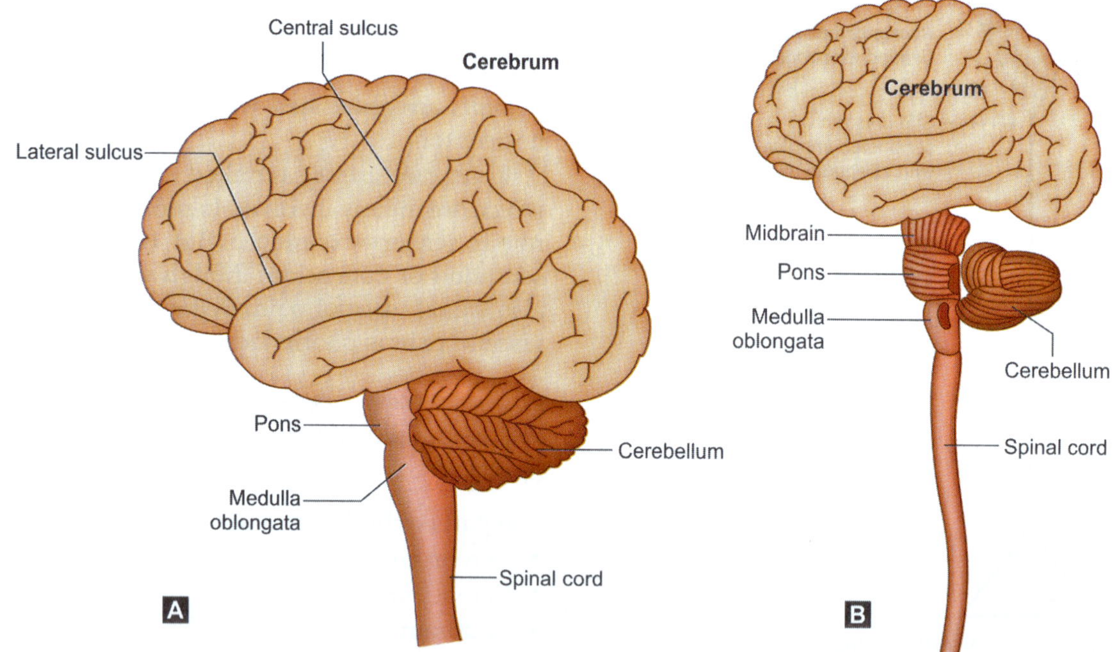

Figs 12.19A and B: (A) Parts of the brain with spinal cord, midbrain is not seen here; (B) View of the major parts of the CNS. Midbrain has been pulled down to show it

highly folded into ridges called gyri, separated by grooves called sulci. The gyri greatly increase the surface area of the cerebrum. The cerebral cortex is subdivided into number of lobes for descriptive purposes; frontal, parietal, temporal and occipital lobes (Fig. 12.20) which are names of the bones under which they lie. The frontal and parietal lobes are separated by a prominent central sulcus. They are separated from the temporal lobe by the lateral sulcus (or lateral fissure; fissure is a deep grove). Buried within the lateral fissure is another lobe, the insula.

The occipital and parietal lobes are separated on the medial side of the hemisphere (Fig. 12.21) by the parietooccipital fissure.

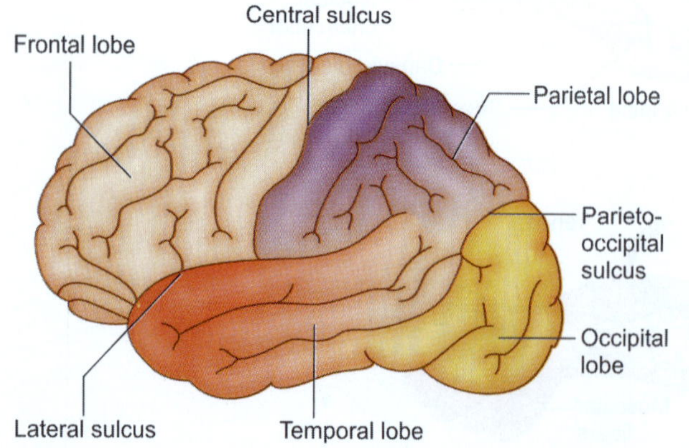

Fig. 12.20: Lateral surface of cerebral cortex showing different lobes

The limbic lobe is formed on the medial side of the hemisphere by the limbic cortex, the cingulate gyrus (Fig. 12.21). The hippocampal formation which is a part of the limbic lobe is enclosed in the temporal lobe on the base of the brain (Fig. 12.43).

Other collections of grey matter deep in the white matter form basal ganglia, thalamus (Fig. 12.22) and hypothalamus.

The **intellectual** functions of the human depend upon the activity of the cerebral cortex and its interaction with other parts of the nervous system. The function of **language** and its grasp is dependent on the cerebral cortex. *Special talents* like **mathematical** or **musical abilities** depend on it. It is involved in higher **cognitive** functions. Storage of **memory** and its recall involves the cerebral cortex. **Perception of fine sensations** and their understanding; **planning and execution** of many complex **motor activities** the *fine* digital movements all involve the *cerebral cortex*.

Cerebellum

Cerebellum is situated below the posterior part of the cerebrum (Fig. 12.21) in the posterior cranial fossa. It has two hemispheres joined by narrow median vermis. Grey matter is on the surface and white matter deep below it; present in the white matter are ***important nuclei*** which receive afferents and give efferent fibers that have important role in ***motor functions***.

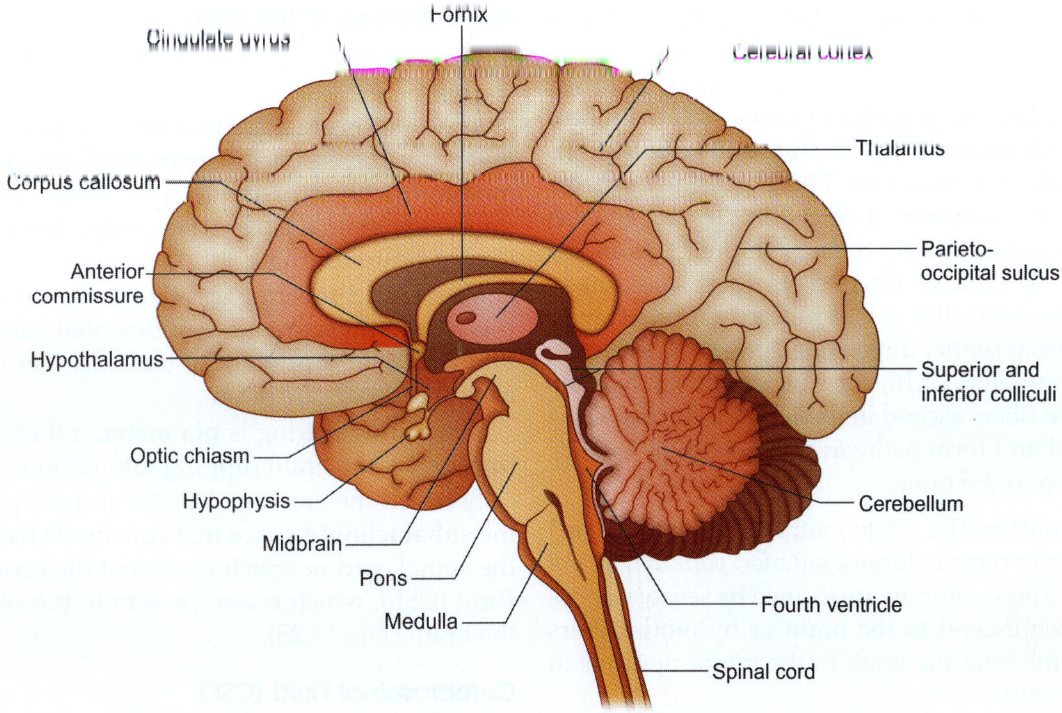

Fig. 12.21: Section showing medial surface of the right hemisphere of the brain

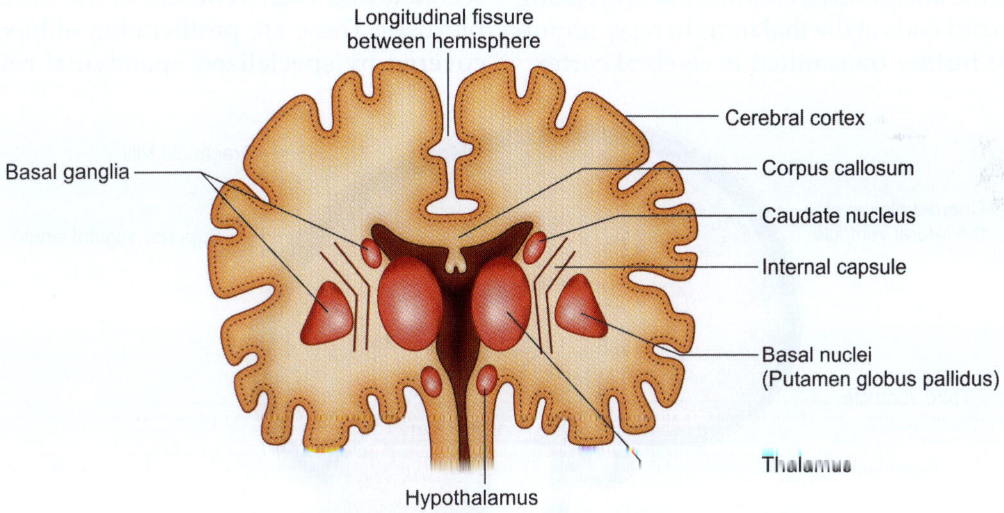

Fig. 12.22: A section of the cerebrum

Midbrain

It is the area of the brain around the cerebral aqueduct between the cerebrum above and the pons below.

Pons

It is situated **in front of the cerebellum,** below the midbrain and above the medulla.

Medulla Oblongata

It extends from the pons above to the spinal cord below.

Midbrain, Pons and Medulla oblongata are grouped as brainstem.

Spinal Cord

The grey matter is in the center in the form of letter H and white matter surrounds the grey matter. The nerve roots arise from the spinal cord (Fig. 12.16).

Grey matter: It forms *two anterior horns, two posterior horns* and at places *small lateral horn.* The two sides are connected and here it is pierced by the central canal, an extension from the fourth ventricle containing cerebrospinal fluid. The anterior (or ventral) horn is composed of cell bodies of lower **motor neurons; alpha motor neurons, gamma motor neurons** and interneurons (which are connector neurons linking different neurons). The posterior horn (or dorsal horn) is composed of cell bodies of neurons which are stimulated by sensory impulses from the periphery. The nerve fibers from these cells make connections with: the spinal motor neurons (lower motor neurons) either directly or through intervening interneurons (Fig. 12.16) for reflex action while the other nerve fibers ascend in the white columns of the spinal cord and form pathways that conduct sensory information to the brain.

White matter: The white matter of the spinal cord is arranged in three columns: *anterior; posterior; lateral* (Fig. 12.2). These columns are formed by sensory nerve fibers which ascend to the brain or by motor fibers that descend from the brain to the motor neurons in the spinal cord.

The nerve fiber tracts are named according to the point of origin to the destination, e.g. lateral spinothalamic tract is in the lateral white column and originating in the spinal cord ends at the thalamus to relay impulses which are further transmitted to cerebral cortex.

The Coverings of the Brain

There are three membranes, the meninges which cover the brain.

The outermost called **dura mater**, is made-up of **two layers**; two layers enclose **cranial venous sinuses**. The meningeal layer or inner layer forms folds which divide the cranial cavity into compartments that are intercommunicating.

The second covering is called the arachnoid mater. It is a thin transparent membrane that surrounds the brain without dipping into the sulci, but bridges all irregularities in the brain.

The third covering is **pia mater,** a thin membrane that covers the brain dipping into various sulci.

Between the arachnoid mater and the pia mater is the **subarachnoid space** that surrounds the brain and the spinal cord in which is present the **cerebrospinal fluid** (CSF), which is also present in the ventricles of the brain (Fig. 12.23).

Cerebrospinal Fluid (CSF)

Within the substance of the brain is the ventricular systems a series of spaces filled with CSF. CSF is secreted into each ventricle of the brain by choroid plexuses. These are proliferation of blood capillaries covered by specialized ependymal cells lining the

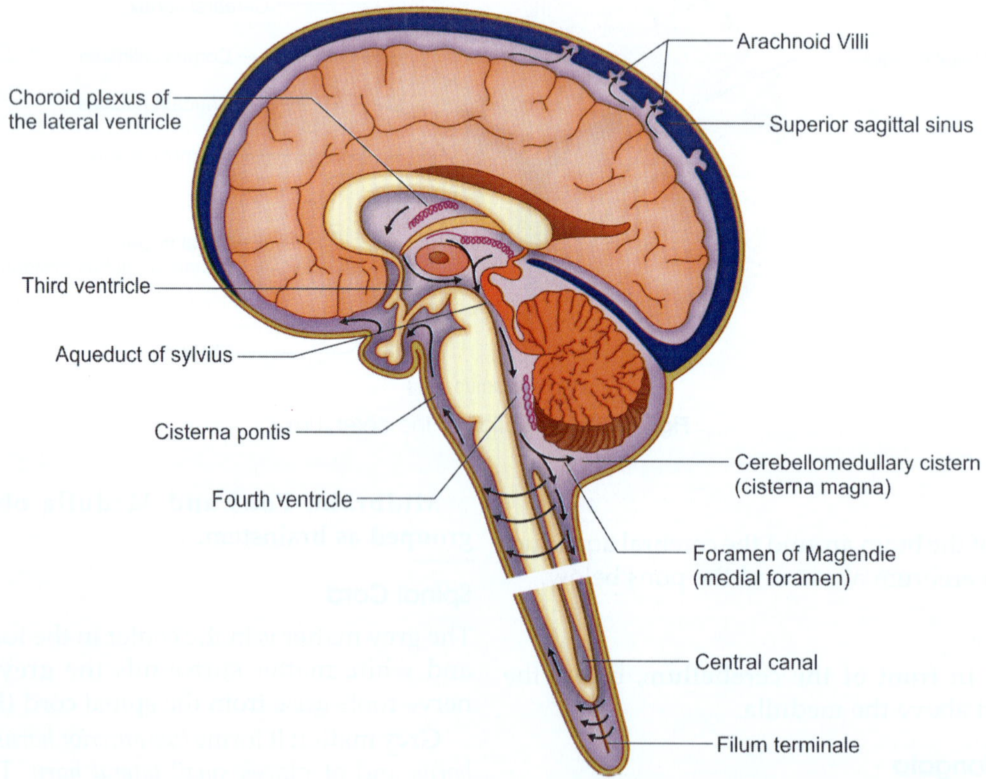

Fig. 12.23: A section of the cerebrum and spinal cord to show circulation of CSF

ventricle walls (Fig. 12.23). CSF is secreted continuously and absorbed at the same rate to maintain its volume. *It fills the ventricles and subarachnoid space*, the volume is about 150 mL. CSF is absorbed mainly (bulk flow) through the **arachnoid villi** into the *dural venous sinuses* (Fig. 12.23). Bulk flow is about 500 mL/day and additional amounts of CSF are absorbed by diffusion into cerebral blood vessels (the CSF is turned over approximately 4 times a day).

The *choroid plexuses are located in the lateral, third and fourth ventricles* (Fig. 12.23). The lateral ventricles are located within the two cerebral hemispheres connect with the third ventricle through the *interventricular foramen* (of Monro). The third ventricle lies in the midline between the diencephalon on the two sides. The cerebral aqueduct of sylvius traverses the midbrain and connects third ventricle with fourth ventricle. The fourth ventricle is interposed between the pons and medulla below and cerebellum above. From the fourth ventricle, the central canal of spinal cord continues cadually (in adults it is generally not patent).

The CSF *escapes from the ventricular system to the subarachnoid space* through three apertures in the roof of the fourth ventricle, *one medial aperture* (Fig. 12.23), and *two lateral apertures* (foramens of Luschka). After leaving the ventricular system, the CSF circulates through the subarachnoid space that surrounds the brain and the spinal cord. Regions where spaces are distended are called *subarachnoid cisterns*. The *lumbar cistern* which surrounds the lumbar and sacral spinal roots below the level of termination of the spinal cord is the largest cistern.

CSF pressure is measured using a vertical tube to a lumbar puncture needle in the lumbar cisterna (below the level where spinal cord ends with subject lying in the horizontal position and on the side) and the pressure is normally *70–180 mm CSF*. At the pressure of 112 mm CSF, which is average normal CSF pressure, filtration and absorption are equal. Below a pressure of 68 mm CSF, absorption stops.

The composition of the CSF (Table 12.6) is almost the same as that of brain ECF. *CSF is clear, alkaline fluid with specific gravity of 1.005*, consists of:

- Water
- Na^+ and others. K^+ concentration less than that in blood
- Glucose concentration less than that of blood
- Plasma proteins: Only small amounts of albumin and globulin
- Urea
- A few leucocytes

Table 12.6: Concentration of various substances in human CSF and plasma

	Substance	*CSF*	*Plasma*
Na^+	(meq/kg H_2O)	147.0	150.0
K^+	(meq/kg H_2O)	2.9	4.6
Ca^{2+}	(meq/kg H_2O)	2.3	4.7
Cl^-	(meq/kg H_2O)	113.0	99.0
HCO^-	(meq/L)	25.1	24.8
pH		7.33	7.40
Osmolality	(mosm/kg H_2O)	289.0	289.0
Protein	(mg/dL)	20.0	6000.0
Glucose	(mg/dL)	64.0	100.0
Urea	(mg/dL)	12.0	15.0

The ECF within CNS communicates with CSF. Thus, the composition of the CSF is an indication of the composition of ECF environment of neuron in the brain and spinal cord.

Functions

CSF cushions the brain and regulates the extracelluler environment of neurons. CSF *supports* and *protects* the brain and the spinal cord, acts as *shock absorber* between brain and cranial bones. The meninges of the brain assist in this function. The dura mater is attached firmly to the bone. There is normally no "subdural space"; the arachnoid is held to the dura by the surface tension of the thin layer of fluid between two membranes. The brain itself is supported within the arachnoid by the blood vessels and nerve roots and numerous fine fibrous arachnoid trabeculae. Brain weighs about 1,400 gm but in CSF ("water bath") it has net weight of 50 gm. The *buoyancy* and *attachments* suspend it efficiently. When the head receives a blow, the arachnoid slides on the dura and brain moves. But, its motion is checked by CSF cushion and by arachnoid trabeculae.

Removal of *excess* CSF during lumbar puncture can cause *severe headache* after fluid is removed because the brain hangs on vessels and nerve roots and traction on them stimulates pain fibers. The pain can be relieved by treatment.

Exchange across CSF and extracellular fluid around the nerve cells for the *nutrients* and *waste products* may also be a function.

If the brain is enlarged by, e.g. hemorrhage or tumor, some compensation is made by a reduction in the amount of CSF. This helps as the brain is inside a closed space. When the volume of brain tissue is reduced, as in degeneration or atrophy, the volume of CSF is increased to fill the space.

Hydrocephalus

Obstruction of the circulation of CSF leads to increase CSF pressure and hydrocephalus, abnormal accumulation of the fluid in cranium.

When foramens of Luschka (lateral opertures) and Magendie (medial foramen) are blocked or if there is obstruction within the ventricular system, the fluid is accumulated proximal to the block and distends the ventricles. This is ***internal hydrocephalus***, or ***non communicating hydrocephalus***. If the pressure increase is sustained, brain substance may be damaged and lost.

Large amounts of fluid accumulate when absorption in villi is decreased this is called ***external hydrocephalus*** also called ***communicating hydrocephalus***.

Special Features of Cerebral Circulation

Blood reaches the brain through the internal carotid arteries and vertebral arteries. The latter join to form the basilar artery, which with branches of internal carotid arteries forms circle of Willis. The rate of blood flow to the brain remains fairly constant within a narrow range. The average adult brain weighs about 1,400 gm and the **flow for whole brain is about 756 mL/min.** The volume of blood flow and extracellular fluid must remains constant; change in either of these volumes must be accompanied by reciprocal change in the other.

Regulation of Cerebral Blood Flow

The cerebral circulation lies within a rigid cranium, and as the intracranial contents cannot be compressed, any increase in arterial flow as with arteriolar dilatation must be accompanied by comparable increase in venous outflow.

The brain is least tolerant to ischemia of all other tissues in the body. *Interruption of cerebral blood flow for as little as 5 seconds results in loss of consciousness, and ischemia lasting just a few minutes results in irreversible brain damage.*

Local regulatory mechanisms and reflexes originating in the brain tend to maintain cerebral circulation **constant.**

An elevation of intracranial pressure as in a growing intracranial tumor produces *increase in systemic blood pressure* that regulates the blood flow to the brain as it tends to decrease because of compression to blood. This response is called **Cushing's reflex,** is due to ischemic stimulation of vasomotor region in the medulla and there is also *bradycardia* due to stimulation of cardiac center.

Local factors: Generally, **total cerebral blood** flow remains **constant.** Though regional cortical blood flow is affected with regional neural activity. Glucose uptake also corresponds with regional cortical activity. Cerebral blood vessels are very sensitive to **carbon dioxide tension**. Increased arterial CO_2 tension produces marked cerebral **vasodilation.**

Cerebral vessels show **autoregulation** between blood pressures of 60 mmHg and 160 mmHg. Hence, blood flow remains regulated during changes in systemic blood pressure within this range. Mean arterial pressures below 60 mmHg result in reduced cerebral blood flow and fainting; pressures above 160 mmHg may lead to increased permeability of the blood–brain barrier and cerebral edema. Autoregulation of cerebral blood flow is abolished by hypercapnia or with strong vasodilator.

The Blood–Brain Barrier

There are tight junctions between endothelial cells in the vessels of the brain and between epithelial cells in the choroid plexuses. It is because of these barriers that proteins are prevented from entering into the brain in the adults and that the penetration of smaller molecules, e.g. those of urea is slow. This limits exchange between blood and brain ECF and blood and CSF, is called blood–brain barrier. But, there are numerous carrier-mediated and active transport systems in the cerebral capillaries. These move substances out of as well as into the brain. The movement out of the brain is freer than movement into it because of bulk flow of CSF into venous blood via arachnoid villi.

ASCENDING PATHWAYS IN THE CNS

The *general pattern* of transmission of impulses is as follows:

The fibers of the first-order neurons; the cell bodies of which lie in the *dorsal root ganglia* of the spinal cord, make synaptic connections with neurons either in the spinal cord *or* in the medulla which are the *second-order neurons*, the fibers of which cross over to the **other side of midline (opposite side),** and these travel up to make synaptic connections in the thalamus with specific relay nuclei [ventral basal group of nuclei/ ventral posterior (VP)] for relay of impulses. Fibers from face area form medial part of VP (VPM) thalamic nucleus. The thalamic neurons are *third-order neurons.* All the sensations from the right side of the body reach left thalamus and vice versa; the third order neurons conduct impulses to the cerebral cortex to the **postcentral gyrus** (the same side as the thalamus) for **perception** (Fig. 12.24).

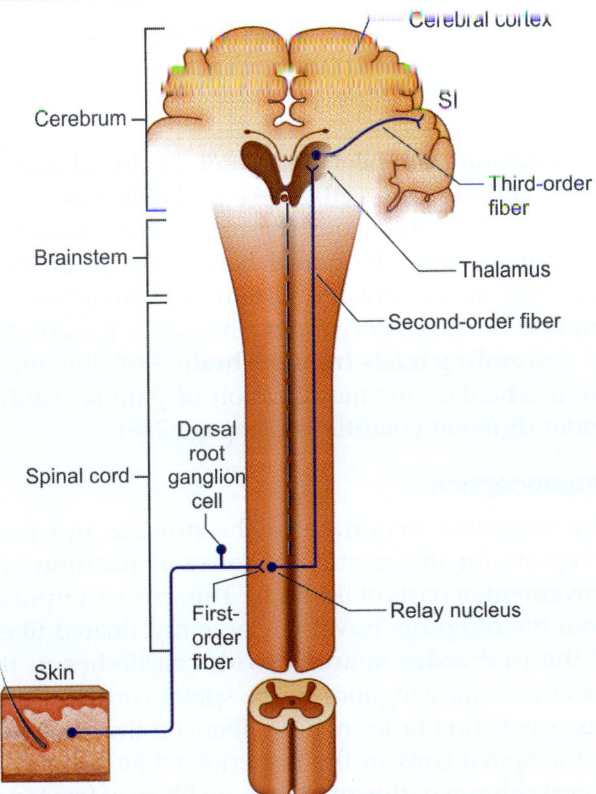

Fig. 12.24: General arrangement of sensory pathways. First, second, and third-order neurons are shown. Note that the axon of the second-order neuron crosses the midline, so that sensory information from one side of the body is transmitted to the opposite side of the brain

The pathways in the spinal cord differ for different somatic sensations though they all project to the postcentral gyrus of the opposite side for perception after relay in the ventral basal group of nuclei (VP) in the thalamus.

The pathways for different sensations to thalamus are as follows:

Pain and Temperature Sensations

The fibers of first order neurons for pain sensations with cell bodies in posterior root ganglion, relay in the neurons in the dorsal horn of the spinal cord as they enter; the fibers of these second-order neurons crossover to the opposite side in the spinal cord and travel up as lateral spinothalamic tract in the lateral white column of spinal cord. The fibers for cold and warmth sensations have similar course, i.e. the fibers of first-order relay in the spinal cord in the dorsal horn cells and fibers of these second-order neurons crossover to the other side and travel up with the fibers for pain sensation. The fibers of both sensations together form the **lateral spinothalamic tract** responsible for transmission of pain and temperature sensation from the opposite side of the body (Fig. 12.25).

Touch sensation. The fibers for touch sensations take two different paths in the spinal cord, one type of touch sensation travels on the same side in the spinal cord; the other type crosses over and travels on the opposite side.

For **fine touch**, the first-order fibers travel up in the **dorsal columns** of the spinal cord on the *same side*, and make synaptic connections with neurons in the medulla in the **nucleus gracilis and nucleus cuneatus;** fibers of the second-order from these nuclei crossover to the opposite side and travel up in the brain as **medial lemniscus** to end in the thalamus. Sensation for **vibration, two point discrimination** and **stereognosis** is carried by these fibers.

The fibers that carry **crude touch** sensation relay in the spinal cord as they enter, in dorsal horn and the fibers of second-order from dorsal horn neurons *crossover* to the other side in the spinal cord; travel up as anterior (or ventral) spinothalamic tract to reach thalamus. The anterior (ventral) spinothalamic tract,

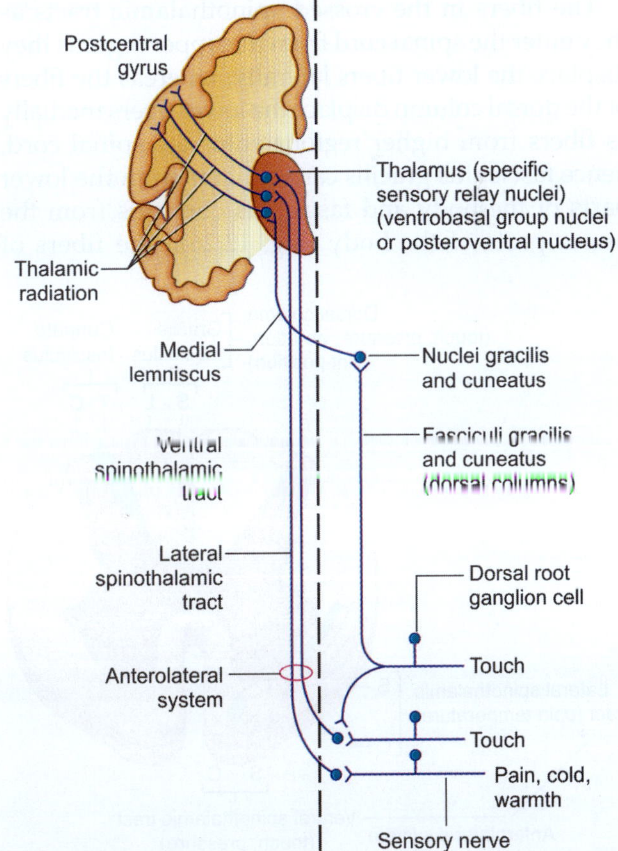

Fig. 12.25: Touch, pain, and temperature pathways. The anterolateral system includes ventral and lateral spinothalamic ascending tracts

and the lateral spinothalamic tract together are often called anterolateral system in the spinal cord; fibers in these tracts are crossed fibers, carry sensations from the opposite side of the body, (unlike the fibers of dorsal column which are uncrossed in spinal cord carry sensations from the same side till they reach the medullary nuclei of gracilis and cuneatus).

The sensory fibres of spinothalamic tracts (anterolateral system) relay in the specific sensory nuclei of the thalamus, the ventral posterior group also called ventrobasal group. Those from head region relay in the medial part of the nucleus (VPM nuclei) and those from the rest of the body in the lateral part (VPL nuclei). These nuclei are the specific sensory nuclei of the thalamus which relay information to the primary sensory cortex for perception of sensations.

Anterolateral system of sensory pathway also relays in the reticular formation of the brainstem and in nonspecific relay nuclei of the thalamus which project diffusely and nonspecifically to all areas of cerebral cortex and this pathway is responsible for the alert state of the cerebral cortex which makes perception of sensations possible.

The fibers in the crossed spinothalamic tracts as they enter the spinal cord from the upper regions they displace the lower fibers laterally, whereas the fibers of the dorsal column displace the lower fibers medially as fibers from higher regions enter the spinal cord, hence fasciculus gracilis carries fibers from the lower parts of the body and fasciculus cuneatus from the upper parts of the body (Fig. 12.26). The fibers of

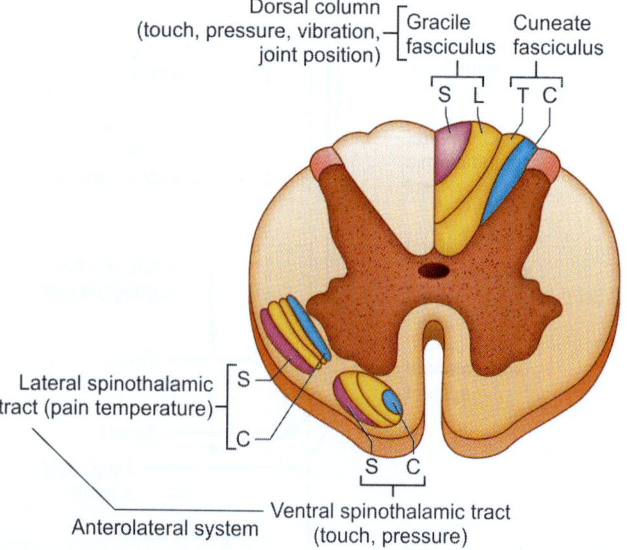

Fig. 12.26: Section of spinal cord showing location of ascending sensory pathways from one side of the body. C-Cervical; T-Thoracic; L-Lumbar; S-Sacral

the third-order neurons in the thalamus transmit all touch sensations from contralateral (opposite) side of the body to its own side postcentral gyrus for sensory perception.

Collateral from fibers that enter the dorsal column pass to **dorsal horn cells**; these probably modify the input of other cutaneous sensory systems including the pain system. The **dorsal horn** is the **gate** where impulses in the sensory system are converted into impulses in the sensory tracts. The **gate** is also affected by **descending tracts from the brain**. Probably this is the mechanism for modification of pain sensibility under different conditions (*See* page 276).

Proprioception

The impulses originate in the muscle and joint receptors for information of **sense of position** and **movement** of parts of the body. The sensory impulses from the receptors travel via large myelinated fibers of the first order neurons (with cell bodies in the posterior root ganglion) to the spinal cord and then pass up as first order neuron fibers on the same side in the spinal cord in the posterior white column as **dorsal column pathway** along with fibers of fine touch (Fig. 12.25) and reach medulla to make synaptic connection with second-order neurons in nuclei of gracilis and cuneatus; the fibers of these crossover to the opposite side and travel up in medial lemniscus to reach thalamus and make synaptic connections with neurons in the thalamus, VP group (ventrobasal group) from where the third-order neurons *project to* the postcentral gyrus (sensory cortex) like all other somatic sensory sensations from the opposite side of the body. The sense of position and movement is perceived in the postcentral gyrus as are other somatic sensations.

Summary of Ascending Sensory Pathways

The fibers for fine touch, vibration and proprioception ascend in spinal cord in the dorsal columns as fasciculus gracilis and fasciculus cuneatus. This ascending system in the spinal cord is called dorsal column or lemniscal system. Gracilis fibers from lower parts of the body, cuneatus from upper parts; and synapse in nuclei of gracilis and cuneatus in medulla; the second-order neuron fibers cross to opposite side travel up in the medial lemniscus. The medial lemniscus ends in the thalamus in the ventrobasal group of nuclei (ventral posterior nucleus and related specific sensory relay nuclei, i.e. ventrobasal group) which relay the information to its own side somatosensory area, S1 in postcentral gyrus.

The other fibers touch (for crude touch) along with and those carrying temperature and pain, synapse with neurons in dorsal horn, the axons of these cross the midline and ascend as anterolateral system of ascending fibers (in general touch is associated with ventral spinothalamic tract and pain and temperature with the lateral spinothalamic tract though there is no rigid localization of function). The fibers reach thalamus and relay in ventral posterior nucleus (VP); fibers of these relay nuclei connect with its own side somatosensory cortex S1 for perception of sensations.

There is also a major input from the anterolateral system into the mesencephalic (midbrain) reticular formation. It activates the reticular activating system that maintains the cortex in alert state.

The fibers of the lemniscal and anterolateral columns are joined by impulses from head region in the brainstem. All sensory fibers relay in the same groups of nuclei of the thalamus from head area in VPM and for rest of the body in VPL nuclei which relay information to its own side sensory cortex (postcentral gyrus of the opposite side from that of the origin of sensations).

Cerebral Cortex and Higher Functions of the Nervous System

Activity of the cerebral cortex in the two hemispheres is coordinated by interconnections through the cerebral commissures, the largest of which is the corpus callosum (Fig. 12.21).

Main Functions of Cerebrum

Figure 12.27A shows the areas for the functions of the cerebral cortex. Areas are also known by the numerical figures given by Brodmann (Fig. 12.27B).

Sensory Functions of Cerebrum

The perception of sensations is by the sensory cortex, the area known as somatic sensory area 1 (also called S1). The area is in the whole of postcentral gyrus

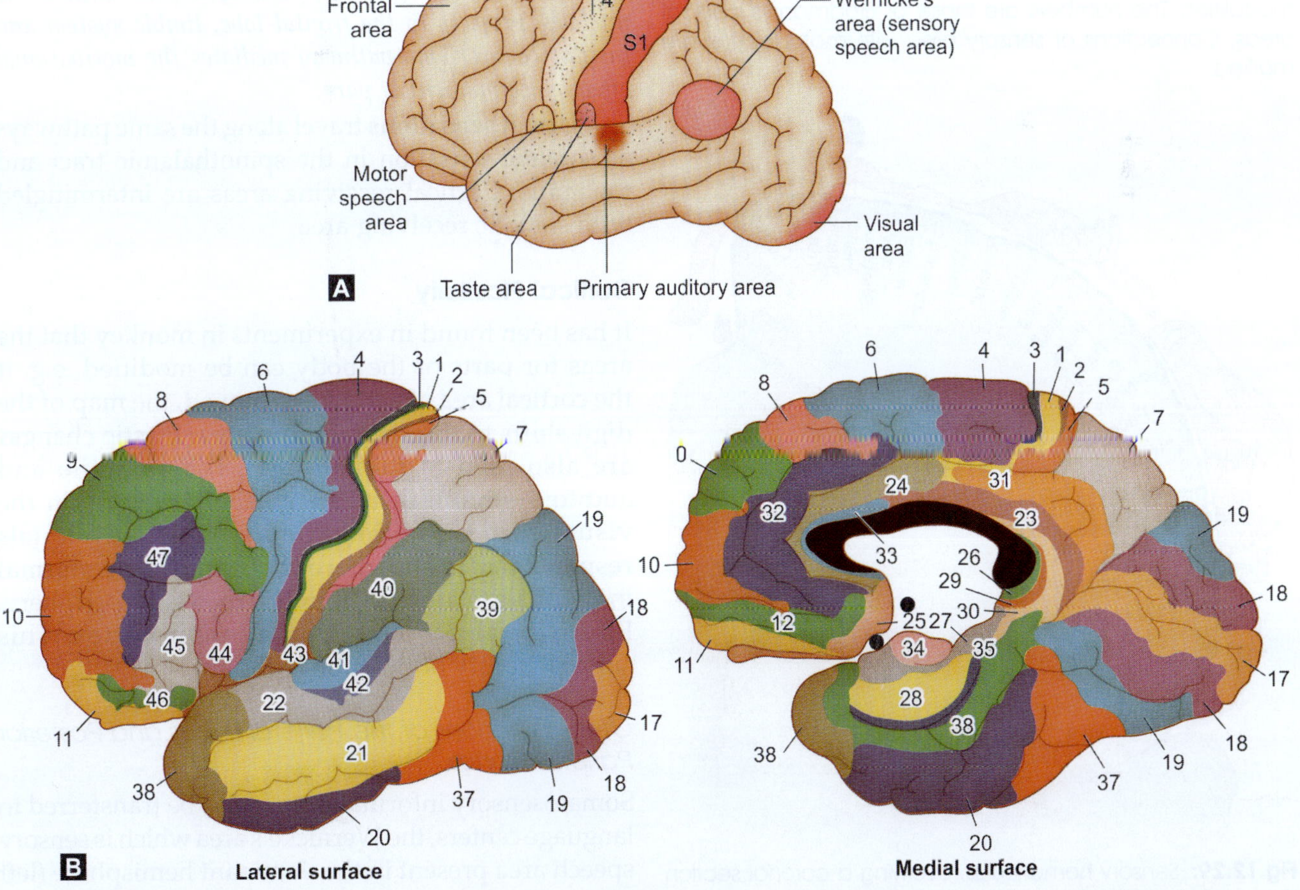

Figs 12.27A and B: (A) The cerebrum showing the functional areas, (B) Brodmann numerical classification of areas

(Fig. 12.27). The area is also referred as 3, 1, 2 in Brodmann's classification. Here, sensations of pain, temperature, pressure, touch, vibration, muscular movement and position sense are perceived. The sensory area of the right hemisphere receives impulses from the left side of the body and vice versa. The area has somatotopic organization, i.e. parts of the body are represented in order (Figs 12.28 and 12.29) along the postcentral gyrus with legs at the upper part and head at the lower end of the gyrus (upside down representation of the body but face upside). The areas of the body where receptors for sensation are more numerous have larger representation in the cortical area. Therefore, hand area and face area are larger than the area for the back of the body.

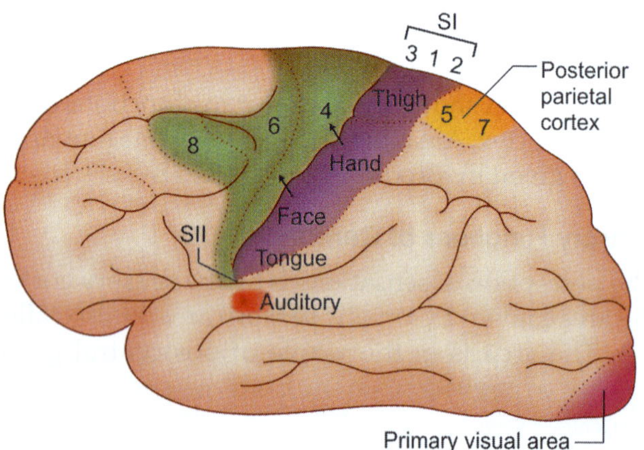

Fig. 12.28: Brain areas concerned with somatic sensation, and some of the cortical receiving areas for other sensory modalities. The numbers are those of Brodmann's cortical areas. Connections of sensory area with motor cortex are marked

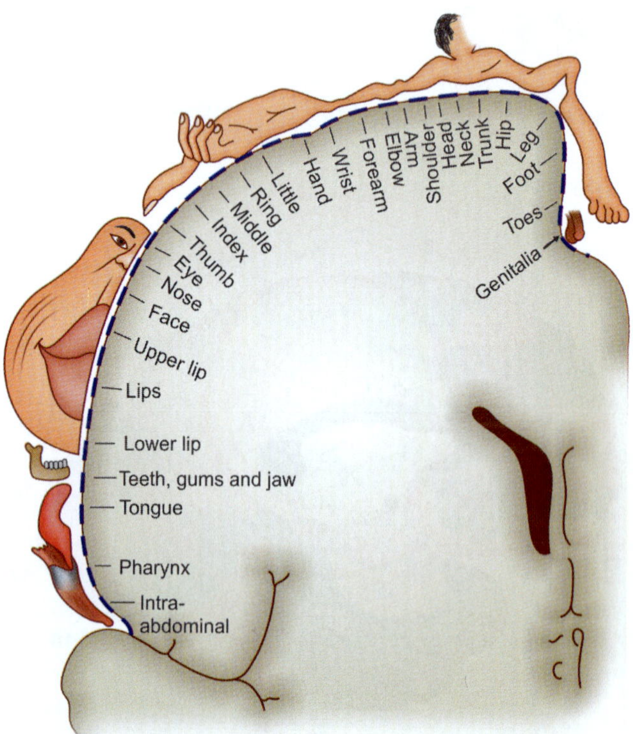

Fig.12.29: Sensory homunculus, overlying a coronal section through the postcentral gyrus

Connections of the sensory area with the frontal lobe (Fig. 12.28) allow somatosensory information to guide voluntary motor activity.

There is another somatosensory area called S11, present in the sylvian fissure (Fig. 12.28). Here, the representation of the body is not as complete as in area S1. It receives connections from S1 area.

Positron emission tomographic (PET) and functional magnetic resonance imaging (fMRI) in humans indicate that pain activates the primary and secondary somatosensory cortex and cingulate gyrus on the side opposite to the stimuls. Also the amygdala, frontal lobe and insular cortex are activated. This indicates two components of **pain pathway.** The pathway to the ***primary somatosensory cortex*** is responsible for the *discriminative aspect of pain.* The other pathway that includes *synapses in the brainstem reticular formation and centrolateral thalamic nucleus, projects to the frontal lobe, limbic system and insular cortex. This pathway mediates the motivational affective component of pain.*

Visceral sensations travel along the same pathways as somatic sensation in the spinothalamic tract and thalamus. Cortical receiving areas are intermingled with somatic receiving area.

Cortical Plasticity

It has been found in experiments in monkey that the areas for parts of the body can be modified, e.g. if the cortical area of a digit is removed, the map of the digit shifts to the surrounding area. Plastic changes are also seen in human beings, e.g. tactile and auditory stimuli increase metabolic activity in the visual cortex of blind people. Deaf individuals respond faster and more accurately than normal individuals to moving stimuli in the visual periphery. Plasticity also occurs in the motor cortex. This suggest ability of the brain to adapt.

Other Functions of the Parietal Lobes and Posterior Parietal Cortex

Somatosensory information can also be transferred to language centers, the Wernicke's area which is sensory speech area present in the dominant hemisphere (left hemisphere in right handed individuals).

Stereognosis

The ability to identify objects by handling them without looking at them is called **stereognosis**. Normal persons can identify objects, such as coins of different denominations by their weight, size and texture with eyes closed. This sensation depends upon intact touch and pressure sensation, and it has a cortical component involving the parietal lobe posterior to the postcentral gyrus; impaired stereognosis (astereognosis) is an early sign of damage to the cerebral cortex and occurs in the absence of any defect in touch or pressure sensation when there is lesion in the *parietal lobe posterior to the postcentral gyrus*.

Two Point Discrimination

The minimal distance by which two points must be separated to be perceived as separate is called the two point threshold. It depends upon touch sensation and cortical component. Its magnitude varies in different parts of the body and is smallest where touch receptors are most numerous. Back of the body is least sensitive for two point discrimination.

The **parietal lobe** in the **nondominant hemisphere** is involved **spatial analysis**. Patients with right parietal lobe lesions have difficulty in recognizing or drawing three dimension objects and recognizing spatial relationships. Similar problems on the left side are masked by language.

Clinical Significance

A lesion on the S1 cortex in humans causes sensory loss that depends upon the area affected. A lesion of the thalamus in the somatosensory region also produces somatosensory loss on the opposite side of the body. However, cortical lesions affect fine touch, discriminatory touch, proprioception but pain and crude sensations of temperature may still be appreciated, possibly at the level of thalamus.

MOTOR AREAS OF THE CEREBRUM

The **precentral gyrus** immediately anterior to the central sulcus **(Broadmann's area 4)** (Fig. 12.30) is the **primary motor cortex (M1)**. Here, the cell bodies of neurons (Betz's cells) are pyramidal shaped and they are classified as **upper motor neurons** and are involved in the production of voluntary movements in the corresponding parts on the opposite side of the body.

The movements are controlled on the opposite side of the body, i.e. the right hemisphere controls the movements of the left side and left hemisphere controls the movements on the right side. The area for controlling the movement for any part is localized. The figure (Fig. 12.31) shows the representation of the body in the primary motor area. Face is represented in the lowermost part of the gyrus and legs on the uppermost part and on to the medial side of the hemisphere. **The body except the face is represented**

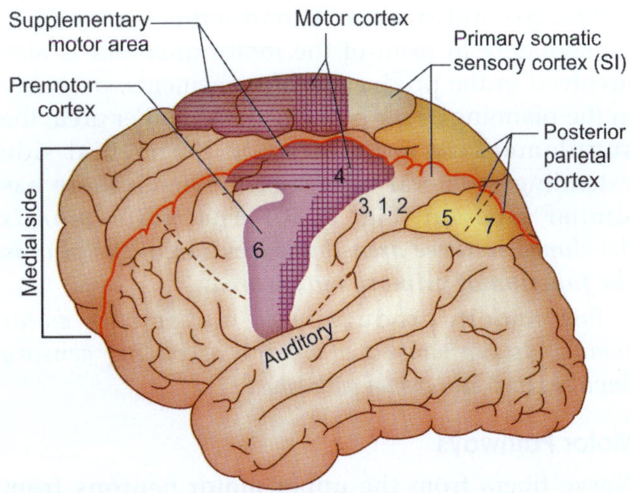

Fig. 12.30: Medial (above) and lateral (below) views of the cerebral cortex, showing the motor cortex (Brodmann's area 4) and other areas concerned with control of voluntary movement along with the numbers assigned by Brodmann

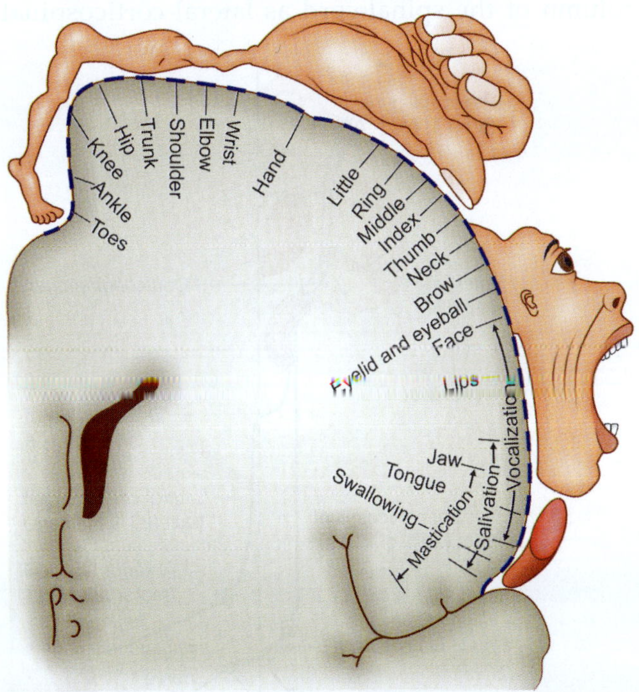

Fig. 12.31: Motor homunculus. The figure represents on a coronal section the precentral gyrus, the location of the cortical representation of the various parts. The size of the various parts is proportionate to the cortical area devoted to them

upside down in each hemisphere. The size of the areas of the primary motor cortex for different parts of the body vary with the type of movement produced by the part. The part responsible for production of **fine**, voluntary **movements** has much **larger representation.** The areas involved in **speech** and **hand movements are large** in the cortex.

The **premotor area (Broadmann's area 6)** is immediately in front of the motor area and is also involved in the production of movements, probably in the planning of the movements. Another area, the **supplementary motor area** on the medial side extending to lateral surface of the hemisphere has similar function (Fig. 12.30). The ***motor plan is developed in these areas but execution of the plan is the function of primary motor area.***

For smooth production of movements *motor commands are monitored* by the *ascending sensory impulses* and the *visual pathways*.

Motor Pathways

Nerve fibers from **the upper motor neurons from cerebral motor area** pass downwards through the internal capsule to the medulla oblongata forming pyramids of medulla and then 80% of the fibers cross over to the opposite side to descend in the lateral white column of the spinal cord as lateral corticospinal pathway (Fig. 12.32A). These fibers make synaptic connections with the motor neurons, and terminate at these **lower motor neurons** in the grey matter in ventral horn (in the corresponding segment of the spinal cord). Some of the fibers first make connections with interneurons in the segment and via these with motor neurons; others make direct connections with motor neurons and these are fibers for skilled motor activity. Twenty percent of the fibers after passing through medulla do not cross at the level of medulla and descend in the anterior (or ventral) white column of the spinal cord as anterior (or ventral) corticospinal tract; these fibers cross the midline at the level of the muscles it controls. At this point, the fibers end on interneurons which makes contact with motor neurons on both sides of spinal cord in medial region of ventral horn, i.e. with the medial group of motor neurons (Figs 12.32A and B). These neurons control axial musculature and thereby contribute to balance and postural support. They also contribute to proximal limb muscles and gross movements. The nerve fibers from the motor cortex to the lower motor neurons (nuclei) of cranial nerves are called corticobulbar fibers.

The lateral corticospinal pathway is concerned with the control of muscles in the distal portions of limbs, the muscles which mediate fine, skilled

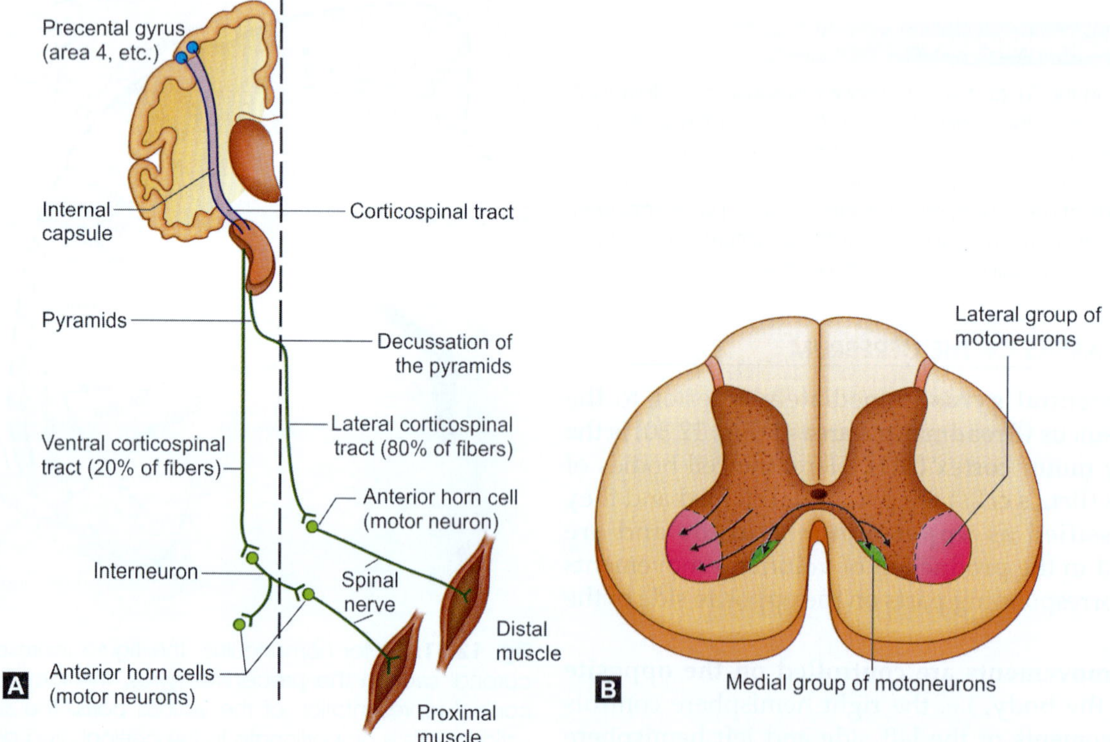

Figs 12.32A and B: (A) The corticospinal tracts, (B) Note that medial group of motor neurons have bilateral connections

movements and the supporting musculature in the proximal limb. The ventral corticospinal pathway as mentioned is for postural adjustments and gross movements.

The Lower Motor Neurons

The axon of the lower motor neuron leave the spinal cord via its ventral (anterior) spinal root and form the motor nerve for the muscle, to end at the motor end plate of the muscle fibers (Fig. 12.33).

Hence, the **upper motor neurons** in the cerebral motor areas send impulses via the descending fibers to the lower motor neurons. The motor neurons in the spinal cord (or its cranial equivalent) which receive these impulses and send impulses to the skeletal muscle are called the **lower motor neurons**. They are the final pathways to muscles.

Motor Speech Area (Broca's Area)

The area in the inferior frontal gyrus (i.e. area inferior to the premotor area just above the lateral sulcus) has a group of neurons that constitute motor speech (Broca's) area (Fig. 12.34), which plans the movements necessary for speech. It is dominant in the left hemisphere in the right handed persons and also for most proportion of left handed persons. New terminology for dominant hemisphere is **categorical hemisphere.**

Clinical Significance

The lower motor neuron is the final and only pathway to the skeletal muscle and hence its lesion produces paralysis of the muscles, innervated by it. The muscles lose tone (hypotonic), as *no impulses* including even for any reflex activity are transmitted to the muscles. Since there is no activity in the muscle, atrophy of the muscle takes place. On the other hand, if there is lesion of the **upper motor neuron**, the lower motor neuron, is cut off from impulses from the upper motor neuron, it is *unable to execute voluntary contraction* but because of presence of reflex activity due to its connections with afferent spinal neurons (Figs 12.33 and 12.35) the tone of the muscles innervated by the lower motor neurons is not lost rather the tone is exaggerated due to activity of brainstem reticular formation (Fig. 12.36) that becomes imbalanced because of decrease of inhibitory impulses that makes the facilitatory areas of the descending reticular formation dominant. Normally the activity of the excitatory and inhibitory areas of reticular formation on lower motor neurons is kept in balance. But in lesions of upper motor neurons, there is decrease in the inhibitory control resulting in increased tone of muscles affected; and exaggeration of deep muscle reflexes.

Therefore a *lesion in the upper motor neuron* produces the syndrome of spastic paralysis and hyperactive stretch reflexes and there is absence of muscular atrophy as the muscles are active in maintenance of tone. *If the lesion is in the right hemispheres the affected side is the left side of the body and vice versa.*

In lower motor neuron lesions, paralysis is flaccid, hypotonia of muscles and absent deep reflexes on the same side.

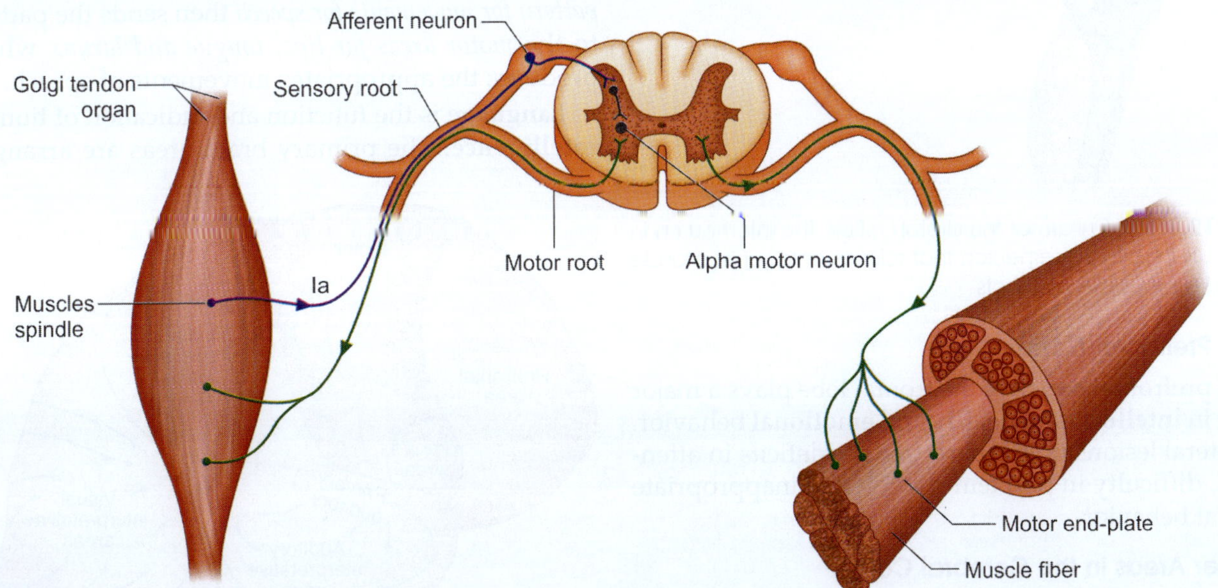

Fig. 12.33: Simple reflex arc consisting of an afferent neuron arising from muscle spindle and an efferent lower motor neuron (alpha) whose cell body is in anterior horn within the spinal cord. Note that the efferent neuron terminates on muscle fibres at motor end plates

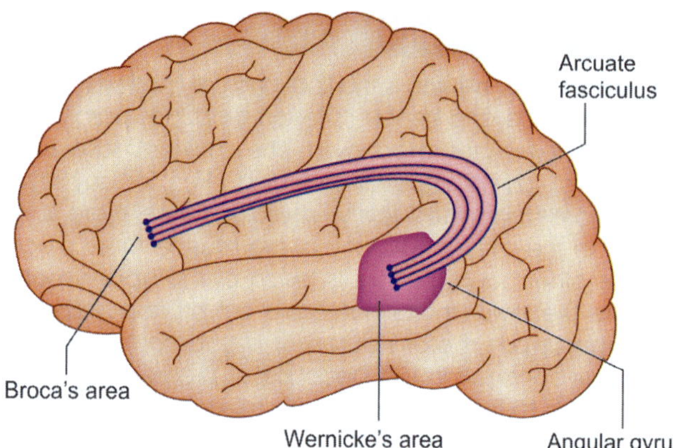

Fig. 12.34: Location of some of the areas that in the categorical hemisphere are concerned with language functions

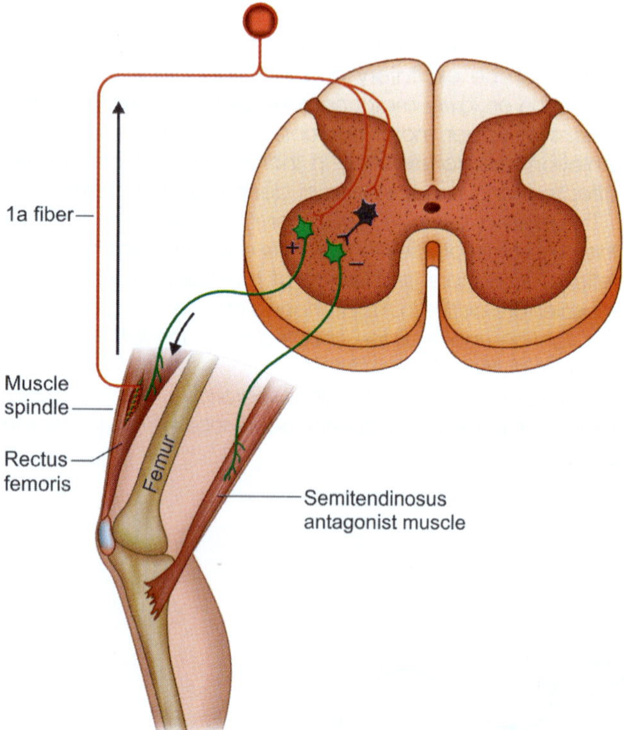

Fig. 12.35: Refex arc of the stretch reflex. The interneuron in black is inhibitory interneuron that relaxes antagonist muscle when protagonist contracts

The Prefrontal Cortex

The prefrontal cortex of the frontal lobe plays a major role in **intellect, personality** and **emotional** behavior. Bilateral lesions in this part produce deficits in attention, difficulty in problem-solving and inappropriate social behavior.

Other Areas in the Cerebral Cortex

The Auditory (Hearing) Area

The area lies below the lateral sulcus in the temporal lobe in the superior temporal gyrus (Fig. 12.37). The

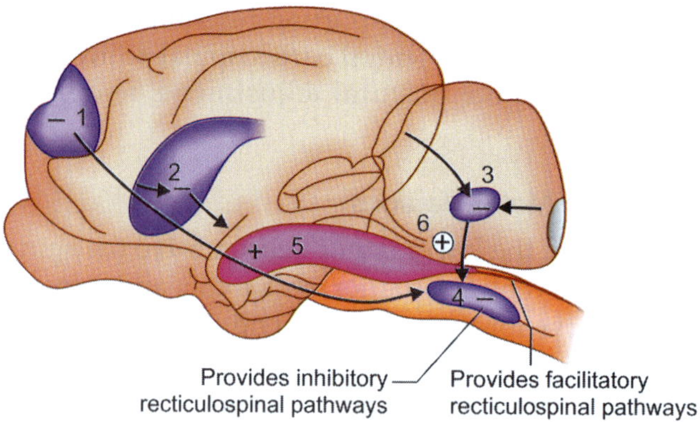

Fig. 12.36: Areas in the animal brain where stimulation produces facilitation (plus signs) or inhibition (minus signs) of stretch reflexes: 1. Motor cortex; 2. Basal ganglia. 3. Cerebellum; 4. Reticular inhibitory area; 5. Reticular facilitatory area; 6. Vestibular nuclei

area receives auditory impulses transmitted by the cochlear part of the vestibulocochlear nerves (VIIIth cranial nerve). The temporal lobe *interprets* the auditory impulses (Fig. 12.37). Each side receives from both ears.

The Sensory Speech Area (Wernicke's Area)

Posterior to the auditory area is the Wernicke's area (Fig. 12.37) which is sensory speech area and it is concerned with interpretation of auditory and visual information for speech. It sends the information to Broca's area which is motor speech area in the frontal lobe immediately in front of the inferior end of motor cortex (Fig. 12.37). Broca's area processes the information received from Wernicke's area to make a *pattern for movements for speech* then sends the pattern to the *motor areas for lips, tongue and larynx* which produces the appropriates movements of speech.

Language is the function and indication of human **intelligence.** The primary brain areas are arranged

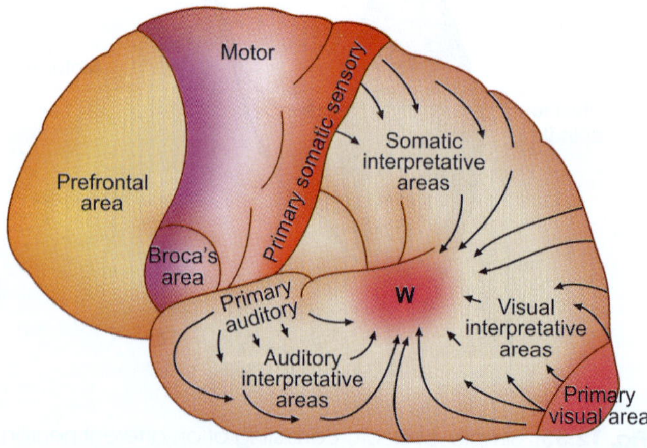

Fig. 12.37: The cerebral cortex showing areas for different functions. W=Wernicke's area

along with the lateral cerebral sulcus of the categorical hemisphere.

The Taste Area

It lies in the sensory area for the face. The impulses from nerve endings in the taste buds, carried by VIIth, IXth and Xth cranial nerves on the tongue and the adjoining regions are perceived after the impulses have passed through and relayed in the thalamus.

The Visual Area

The primary visual area (Brodmann's area 17) is located mainly on the sides of calcarine fissure. The greater part of the occipital lobe is involved in receiving and interpreting the visual impulses (Fig. 12.37).

The Olfactory Area

Prepyriform cortex, amygdaloid nucleus and part of the cortex of basal forebrain are involved in the interpretation of olfactory sensation.

Other Areas of the Cerebrum

Deep within the cerebral hemispheres, there are groups of cell bodies called nuclei where impulses are passed from one neuron to another. They have important role in physiological functions.

Important masses of grey matter include:

- Basal ganglia
- Thalamus
- Hypothalamus.

BASAL GANGLIA

These are a group of nuclei on each side forming grey matter which lies deep in the cerebral hemisphers. The main actions of basal ganglia are with the motor areas of the cerebral cortex by way of thalamus. Hence, they have a role in motor functions and are generally known as ***extra pyramidal system***.

Lesions of basal ganglia produce **abnormal movements** and **posture.**

The basal ganglia include **caudate nucleus, putamen,** and the **globus pallidus** (Fig. 12.38) caudate and putamen are also referred to as striatum. Putamen and globus pallidus combined is referred to as lentiform nucleus. Associated with basal ganglia are **subthalamic nucleus** of diencephalon and **substantia nigra** of midbrain. Which are grouped under basal ganglia.

The caudate nucleus and putamen collectively form the **striatum;** the putamen and globus pallidus form the **lenticular nucleus**, as mentioned.

The globus pallidus is divided into external and internal segments (GPe and GPi); both contain inhibitory GABAergic neurons. The substantia nigra is divided into a **pars compacta** which uses dopainine as a neurotransmitter and a **pars reticulata** which uses GABA as a neurotransmitter. The striatal neurons are neurons that use GABA as a neurotransmitter and interneurons that form acetylcholine.

Figure 12.38B shows the major connection to and from and within the basal ganglia along with the neurotransmitters within these pathways. There are two main inputs to the basal ganglia: they are both excitatory (glutamate), and they both terminate in the striatum. They are from a wide region of the cerebral cortex (corticostriate pathway) and from intralaminar nuclei of the thalamus (thalamostriatal pathway). The two major outputs of the basal ganglia are from GPi and substantia nigra pars reticulata, both inhibitory (GABAergic) and both project to the thalamus. From the thalamus, there is an excitatory (presumably glutamate) projection to the prefrontal and premotor cortex. This forms full cortical basal ganglia-thalamic-cortical loop.

The connections within the basal ganglia include a ***dopaminergic* nigrostriatal projection** from the substantia nigra pars compacta to the striatum and a GABAergic projection from the striatum to substantia nigra pars reticulata. There is an inhibitory projection from the striatum to both GPe and GPi. The subthalamic nucleus receives an inhibitory input from GPe, and in turn the subthalamic nucleus has an excitatory (glutamate) projection to both GPe and GPi.

Functions of the Basal Ganglia

Functions of the basal ganglia are in the **planning** and **programming of movements.** Basal ganglia (the caudate nuclei) also play a role in some cognitive processes

Parkinson's disease (Paralysis Agitans) is a common disorder especially in the elderly. It is characterized by ***tremor; rigidity*** (excessive muscles tone of the skeletal muscles); paucity and slowness of movements, i.e. ***bradykinesia.*** There is difficulty in *initiating movements* and *decreased spontaneous movements* like swaying of arms during walking and emotional expressions of face while talking. The **walk** may become difficult to start and **shuffling** (short steps). There is also difficulty in **delicate movements** such as in ***handwriting.***

The **face becomes mask** like as the muscles become rigid. Later, there may be difficulty in eating. Body **posture becomes flexed.**

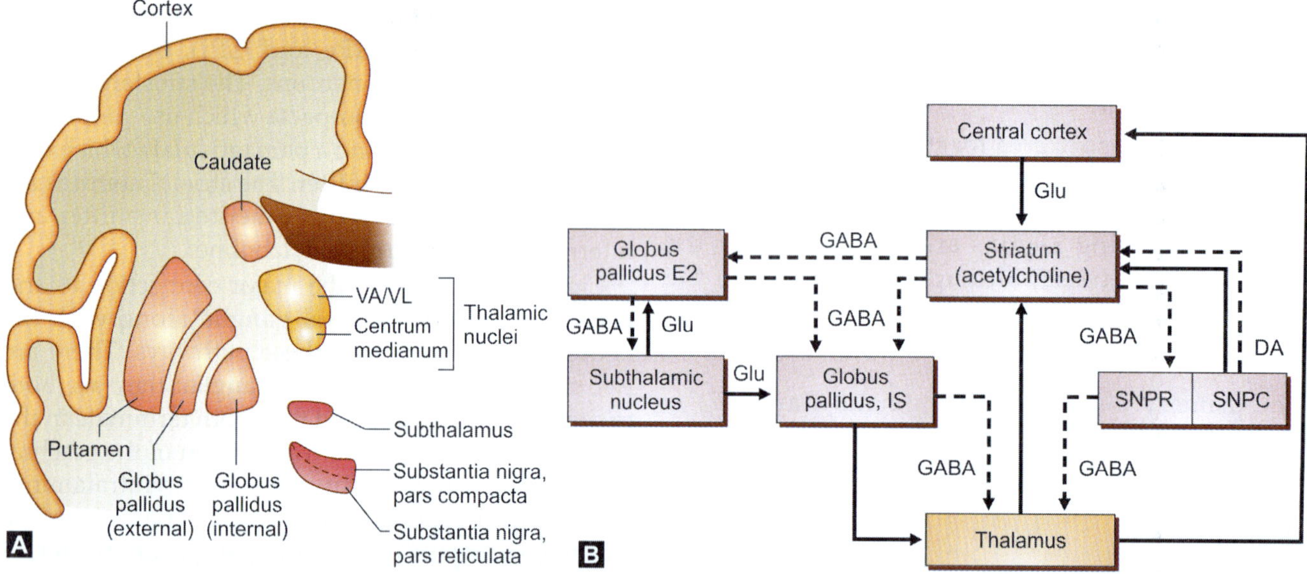

Figs 12.38A and B: (A) Basal ganglia and associated nuclei. VA/VL, ventral anterior and ventral lateral thalamic nuclei (B) Diagrammatic representation of the principal connections of the basal ganglia. Solid lines indicate excitatory pathway, dashed lines inhibitory pathways. The transmitters are indicated in the pathways, where they are known DA, dopamine to; Glu, glutamate. Acetylcholine is the transmitter produced by interneurons in the striatum. ES, external segment; IS, internal segment; SNPC, substant nigra, pars compacta; SNPR, substantia nigra, pars reticulata. The subthalamic nucleus also projects to the pars compacta of the substantia nigra; pathway has been omitted.

The **tremor** is present at **rest**, disappears with activity. It often begins in one hand and gradually spreads to other limbs.

The main pathology in this disease **is loss of neurons in the substantia nigra** in the midbrain. The axons of these neurons project to the **striatum** of basal ganglia and release neurotransmitter, **dopamine** at that site. The loss of dopamine at the striatum (due to degeneration of neurons at the midbrain) is responsible for the symptoms of the disease (Parkinsonism). It is a degenerative disease.

Before the dopaminergic neurons are completely lost, administration for L-dopa can relieve some of the motor deficits in Parkinson's disease. L-Dopa is a precursor of dopamine and it can cross the blood brain barrier. The possibility is being explored of transplanting dopamine synthesizing neurons into the striantum with focus on the potential for human embryonic stem cells to play such a role.

The deficits which occur in some other diseases of basal ganglia are ***abnormal involuntary movements*** like **tremors, athetosis, chorea, dystonia** and **ballism.**

The tremor of the basal ganglion disease is a "**pill rolling**" tremor that occurs when the limb is at rest. It increases during excitement and decreases during sleep.

- *Athetosis* is continuous slow involuntary movement of the extremities and facial muscles.
- *Chorea* is rapid dancing movements which are involuntary usually involving extremities.
- *Dystonic movements* are slow movements of the trunk that result in distorted body positions.
- *Hemiballismus* is violent, flailing and intense movement due to partial lesion of the subthalamic nucleus.

Another basal ganglion disturbance is **Huntington's disease.** This results from genetic defect that involves an autosomal dominant gene. This defect leads to loss of GABAergic and cholinergic neurons of the striatum producing choreiform movements.

In all of these basal ganglia disorders, the motor dysfunction is contralateral to the diseased component. This is because the main final output of the basal ganglia is mediated by the corticospinal tract.

Cerebellum

Cerebellum connected to the brainstem. It has two hemispheres joined by narrow median vermis (Figs 12.39A). Grey matter is on the surface and white matter deep below it where important nuclei are present.

Anatomical Features of the Cerebellum

The cerebellum consists of a three-layered cortex surrounding four pairs (four on each side), of centrally located nuclei in the white matter (called the dentate, globose, emboliform and fastigial nuclei). The surface cortex has numerous folds called folia that are similar to the gyri of the cerebral cortex. The cerebellar cortex is divided into three major subdivision: *anterior, posterior and flocculonodular lobes.* The anterior and posterior lobes are futher divided in the plane into a midline portion, the *vermis;* a slightly more lateral portion with ill-difined borders, the *intermediate zone;* and most laterally, the large *lateral hemisheres.*

The vermis and the intermediate zone contain a somatotopic map of the body surface that reflects peripheral sensory input from muscles, tendons, joint capsules and some cutaneous receptors.

The sensory information is transmitted to the cerebellum by fiber tracts known as spinocerebellar; dorsal and ventral spinocerebellar tracts. These pathways do not reach the conscious level but have role in the coordination of movements.

The lateral hemispheres receive input primarily from the cerebral cortex via the pontine nuclei.

Subdivisions of the cerebellum. Phylogenetically, the cerebellum can be subdivided into the archicerebellum, paleocerebellum, and neocerebellum. These subdivisions correspond to regions of the cerebellum that are dominated by vestibular input (the **vestibulocerebellum)** by spinal cord input (the **spinocerebellum**), and by indirect input from the cerebrum by way of the pontine nuclei (the **corticocerebellum** or called **cerebrocerebellum**). The vestibulocerebellum consists chiefly of the floculonodular lobe. However, it also includes a small part of the vermis and intermediate cortex of the posterior lobe. The spinocerebellum is composed of most of the vermis and intermediate region. The corticocerebellum consists of the hemispheres (Fig. 12.39B).

Functional Neuronal Circuits of the Cerebellum

There are three layers in the cerebellar cortex. The *molecular layer*, the *Purkinje cell layer* and the *granular layer* (Fig. 12.39C). The principal cell type is the Purkinje cell (which are amongs the largest neurons) which receives input to its fan-shaped dendritic tree located in the molecular layer. This input comes from two main sources: (1) *climbing fibers* that originate from cells of the inferior olivary complex and (2) *parallel fibres* that represent the axons of granule cells. The granule cells receive synaptic input from *mossy fibres* which are formed by all the other cerebellar afferent systems. Recently, however, another class of afferent fibers apparently form synaptic contact with Purkinje cells, *multilayered fibers*, originating from biogenic amine cell groups, such as the locus ceruleus, and other nuclei including portions of the hypothalamus.

The fundamental cerebellar circuit is completed by the axon of the Purkinje cells which form synaptic contact with one of the cerebellar nuclei, (although a few Purkinje axons extend directly into the vestibular nuclei in the brainstem). The transmission of signals through the fundamental circuit is influenced by three additional considerations.

1. Purkinje cells and cerebellar nuclear cells exhibit a high level of background activity, which can be modulated upward or downward.
2. The cells of the central nuclei receive direct excitatory input from climbing fibers and most mossy fiber systems whereas the output from Purkinje cells is inhibitory.
3. Three other inhibitory interneurons (basket cells, stellate cells, Golgi cells) in the cerebellar cortex also influence the transmission of signals through the fundamental circuit.

The cerebellar nuclei send efferents as mentioned below.

Physiological Anatomy of Cerebellum

Vestibulocerebellum (or flocculonodular lobe) is the oldest part of the cerebellum has *vestibular connections* and is concerned with ***equilibrium and eye movements***. The rest of the vermis and adjacent medial portions of the hemisphere the **spinocerebellum** receives *proprioceptive input from the body as well as motor plan from motor cortex.* By comparison it ***coordinates and smoothes on going movements***. The *vermis projects to the brainstem area* concerned with control of axial and proximal limb ***muscles whereas hemispheres of spinocerebellum*** project to the *brainstem areas for distal limb muscles* and *also contralateral thalamus*. The lateral portions of the cerebellar hemispheres are called **cerebrocerebellum** and they interact with motor cortex in *planning and programming* movements (Fig. 12.39B).

Most of the vestibulocerebellar output passes directly to the brainstem lateral vestibular nucleus but rest of the cerebellar cortex projects to deep nuclei, which in turn project to brainstem. The deep nuclei provide the only output for the spinocerebellum and cerebrocerebellum. The medial portion of the spinocerebellum projects to the **fastigial nuclei** from these to the brainstem. The adjacent hemispheric portions of the spinocerebellum project to **emboliform** and **globose** nuclei from thereto the brainstem.

The cerebrocerebellum projects to **dentate nucleus** and from thereto the contralateral ventrolateral nucleus of the thalamus. The thalamic neurons project to premotor and primary motor complex.

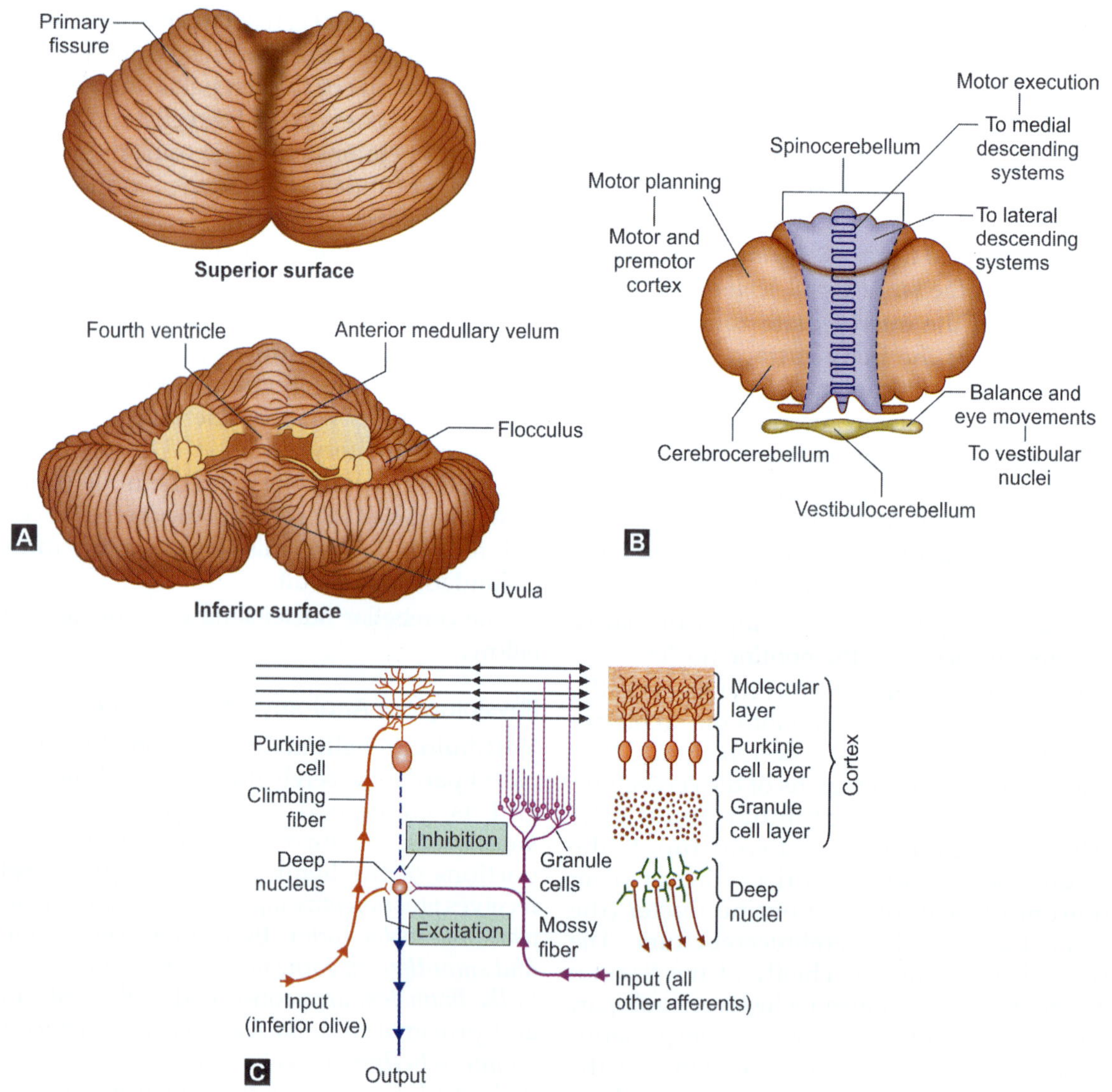

Figs 12.39A to C: (A) Anatomy of cerebellum, (B) Functional divisions, (C) Basal neuronal circuits

Functions

Cerebellum has *no role in production of voluntary* movements but has important role in **coordination of voluntary movements** and in **maintaining posture and balance of the body.** ***Cerebellum coordinates the movements so that they are smooth and accurate*** (it controls the rate, range, force and direction of movements). It receives sensory input from muscles, joints, skin receptors, eyes and ears and with this information it functions in coordination of muscular movements and in the maintenance of balance and posture of the body.

Cerebellum and Role in Learning

Cerebellum in concerned with **motor learning** that makes coordination easier when task is performed over and over again.

Lesions in the cerebellum results in **unsteady movements.** As a result, the gait becomes wide-based, unsteady (***drunken gait***), ***speech*** may ***become slurred*** or **scanning.** Dysarthria in which some syllables are held others dropped too quickly. There is no paralysis or sensory deficit. The person if asked to touch his nose with a finger, the hand moves beyond the point (this is described as ***dysmetria or past-pointing***, it initiates a gross correction, but the correction overshoots to the other side; then with movements back and forth it touches the nose. This is ***intention tremor***, i.e. the **tremor is during movements but absent at rest,** unlike the resting tremor in Parkinsonism. The tremor in cerebellum disease appears when the patient attempts to perform some voluntary action. Another test to detect cerebellar lesion is that the patient is unable to perform rapidly alternating opposite movements, such as repeated pronation and supination of the hands, i.e. patients show *adiodochokinesia*.

Tone in affected muscles is decreased (**hypotonnia**). In unilateral lesions the ***same side of the body*** is affected.

Cerebellar nystagmus: Tremor of the eyes when attempting to fix on a point in the periphery of visual field.

THALAMUS

Thalamus consists of large masses of nerve cells and fibers situated within the cerebral hemispheres below the corpus callosum (Fig. 12.22) one on each side of the third ventricle. Internal medullary lamina divides it into 3 nuclear masses (Fig. 12.40A) medial, lateral and anterior. ***Thalamus participates in sensory, motor and limbic functions.*** Almost all information to the cortex is processed before, in the thalmus. All sensosry impulses with the exception of olfaction relay in the thalamus. Thalamus is a **great relay station.** Fibers make synaptic connections with the **specific sensory relay** nuclei situated in the thalamus; nucleus **ventral posterior** (VP) for somatic sensory pathways (VPM-for head and VPL for rest of body); lateral geniculate body for **visual pathway**; medial geniculate body for **auditory pathway.** Fibers from these neurons project to the cerebral cortex to the specific regions where sensations are perceived. **Motor fibers** from **basal ganglia** and **cerebellum** relay in the thalamus in the ventral anterior and ventral lateral nuclei and from thalamic nuclei protect to the motor cortex in the cerebrum.

There are other nuclei, the intralaminar and the medial, in the thalamus called ***nonspecific projection nuclei*** which receive impulses from the **reticular activating system** in the brainstem and their fibers project diffusely and nonspecifically to all areas of the neocortex (Fig. 12.40B). The impulses are responsible for ***attention*** and ***arousal***. Thalamus also has a role in **sleep wakeful cycles** and in the production of the waves recorded in the **electroencephalogram** (EEG).

A **memory** pathway relays in the anterior nucleus of thalamus, thalamus is said to be related to memory.

Destruction of the VPL or VPM nuclei diminishes sensations on the contralateral side of the body or face respectively. The sensory qualities lost are those that are transmitted mainly by the dorsal column medial lemniscus pathway and its trigeminal equivalent. The discriminative component of pain sensation is lost.

The motivational-affective component of pain is still present if the medial thalamus is intact. Perhaps it persists because of the spinothalamic and spinoreticulothalamic projections to this part of the thalamus. A lesion of the somatosensory thalamus sometimes results in a central pain state, known as **thalamic pain**. Pain indistinguishable from thalamic pain can also be produced by lesions in the brainstem or cortex.

HYPOTHALAMUS

It is a part of diencephalon. It has a number of nuclei (group of neurons) associated with different functions. Some important nuclei include supraoptic, paraventricular, tuberal and mammillary nuclei. Continuing anteriorly from hypothalamus are telencephalic structures the preoptic region and septum, which help regulate autonomic functions.

Functions of Hypothalamus

- It *produces* **posterior pituitary hormones** in the neurons in supraoptic and paraventricular nuclei; the axons of these neurons pass through the pituitary stalk to the posterior pituitary; and the hormones, oxytocin and antidiuretic hormone (ADH, vasopressin) travel down by axoplasmic flow and are stored at the endings. The hormones are secreted when there is appropriate stimulus from hypothalamus to posterior pituitary and from there enter capillary blood. The stimulus travels as action potential along these axons.
- Hypothalamus ***controls*** **anterior pituitary secretions** because it forms and secretes local hormones called releasing factors which travel via portal circulation along the pituitary stalk to anterior pituitary where they stimulate or inhibit its different secretions (Fig. 14.41). These are:
  1. Growth Hormone Releasing Hormone (GRH)
  2. Growth Hormone Inhibiting Hormone (GIH)
  3. Prolactin Inhibiting Hormone (PIH) (Dopamine)
  4. Prolactin Releasing Hormone (PRH) (Not established)
  5. Corticotropin Releasing Hormone (CRH)
  6. Thyrotropin Releasing Hormone (TRH)
  7. Gonadotropin Releasing Hormone (GnRH)

  (Refer to anterior pituitry for influence on the different hormones of anterior pituitary).
- **Body temperature** is regulated; *maintained* at *normal level* by *controlling appropriate regulatory mechanisms;* whenever, it deviates from normal set point at the hypothalamus. The mechanisms are discussed with temperature regulation in the chapter with skin. Hypothalamus acts as a **thermostat**.

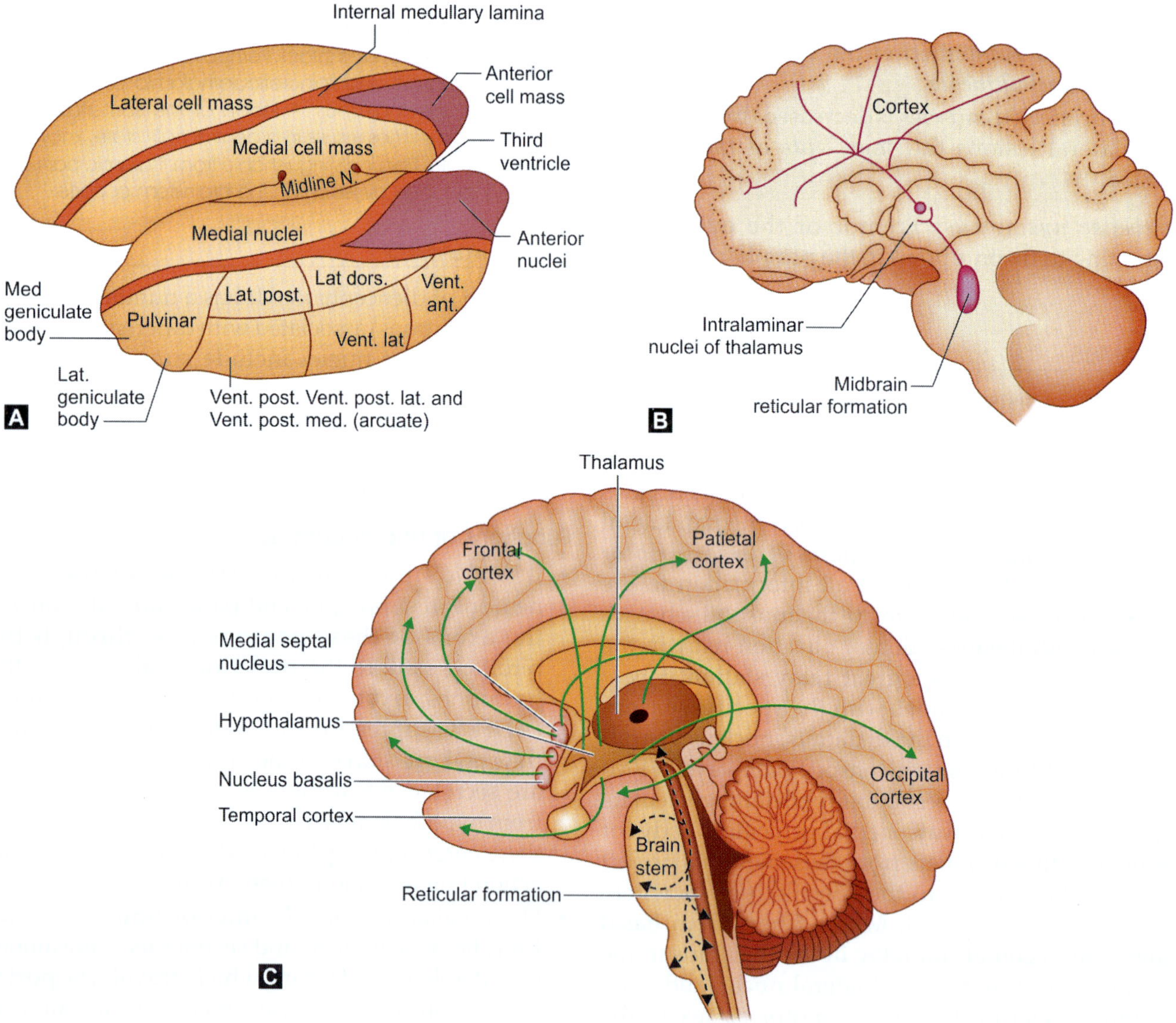

Figs 12.40A to C: (A) Schematic representation bilaterally of the thalamus, location of the thalamic nuclei, (B) Shows ascending reticular system in the midbrain, its projection into the intralaminar nuclei from thereto many parts of cerebral cortex, (C) Other pathways of RAS

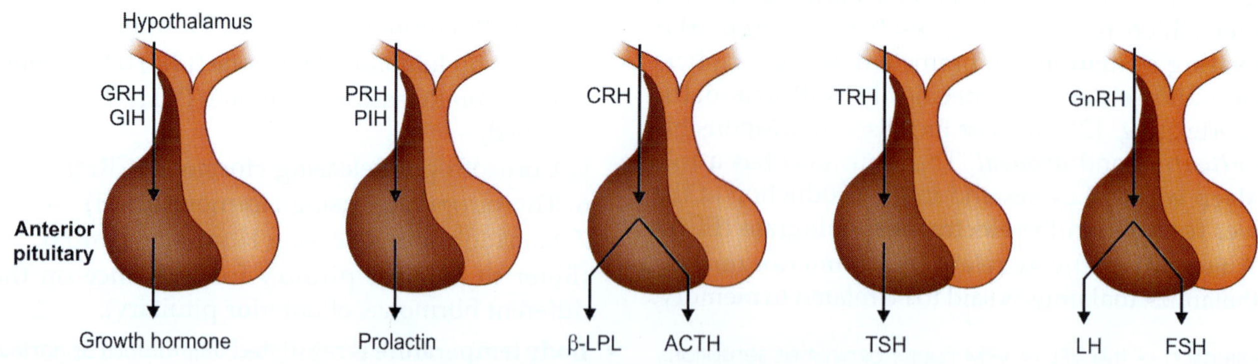

Fig. 12.41: Hypothalamic control of anterior pituitary

- **Feeding behavior:** There is a **satiety center** and a ***feeding center***, the activity of these centers regulates feeding behavior.
- **Leptin and Ghrelin:** ***Leptin*** is a satiety producing hormone secreted by fat cells (adipose tissue) acts at hypothalamic receptors in producing its effects

(anorexigenic). *Ghrelin* is a fast-acting hormone that stimulates food intake. It is produced by stomach, levels increase before food and decrease after a meal. Believed to be involved in meal initiation. The effects (orexigenic) are produced at hypothalmic level.

- **Thirst and water balance:** There is a thirst center which is activated with increase of osmolality of ECF or decrease of ECF volume (Fig. 12.42) and by psychological factors; produces thirst sensation that activates drinking behavior. The osmoreceptors which sense ECF osmolality are also situated in the hypothalamus.
- **Autonomic nervous system:** It functions as a higher control over autonomic nervous system.
- **Emotional reactions** of ***pleasure, fear and rage***: It has a role in these emotions along with limbic system.
- **Circadian rhythms** are produced because of biological clock located in the suprachiasmatic nuclei (SCN) of hypothalamus. There are rhythmic fluctuations in some functions of the body, the cycles have duration of 24 hours, i.e. they are circadian. The efferents from SCN initiate *neural* and *hormonal signals that produce circadian rhythms*. There is circadian rhythm for *sleep wakeful cycles, body temperature* and for *secretions of some hormones.*
- **Sexual behavior, *maternal behavior***: It has a role in these functions.
- **Memory:** Hypothalamus has role in memory as mamillary bodies in the hypothalamus have extensive connections with hippocampus (Fig. 12.43) via fornix. The mamillary bodies project to anterior thalamus from where fibers for memory project to prefrontal cortex. Memory is discussed later.

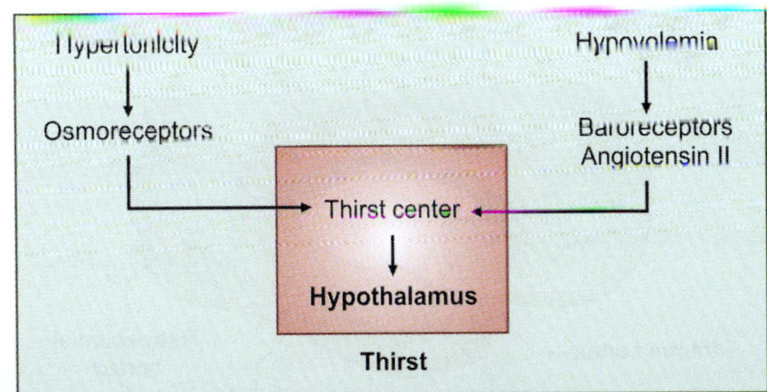

Fig. 12.42: Diagrammatic representation of the way in which changes in plasma osmolality and changes in ECF volume affect thirst

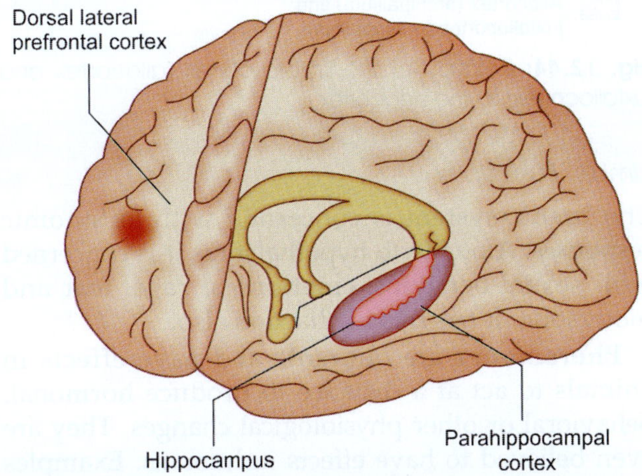

Fig. 12.43: Areas concerned with explicit memories

Neural Influences on Immune System

Environmental stress can cause immunosuppression in which the number of helper T cells and the activity of natural killer cells is reduced. One mechanism for the effect involves the release of CRF from hypothalmus.

EMOTIONS

The **hypothalamus** and **limbic lobe** are concerned with **genesis** of emotions and **expression** of emotions.

Emotions have both **mental** and **physical** components. The mental component consists of cognition, affect and conation. The example are: I hear a loud sound which I recognize that of a firing by gun (cognition), I feel frightened (affect), I want to go away from here (conation). The physical side of emotions consists of changes in the viscera and skeletal muscles. These are widespread and involve coordinated activity of both the autonomic and somatic nervous systems. The changes include hypertension, tachycardia, respiratory affects and sweating.

The limbic lobe or limbic system is applied to the part of the brain that consists of a rim of cortical tissue around the hilum of cerebral hemisphere and the associated deep structures, the hypothalamus, the hippocampus (Fig. 12.43), the amygdala, septal nuclei and anterior thalamic nucleus.

The **limbic cortex** is phylogenetically the oldest part of the cerebral cortex that is called the **allocortex,** (made-up of three layers of cells in histological sections) and another layer of transitional cortex called **juxtallocortex** next to it (Fig. 12.44) in the cingulated gyrus (composed of 3–6 layers of cells).

The rest of the cerebral cortex (nonlimbic portions) is the **neocortex** which has six layers of cells and is most highly developed type and reaches its greatest development in human beings.

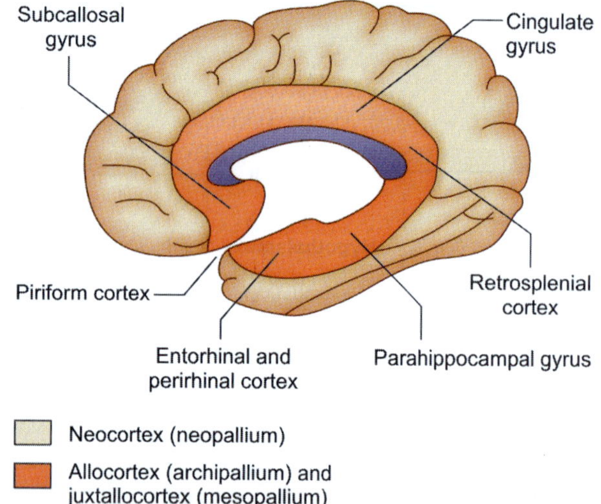

Fig. 12.44: Relation of the limbic cortex (allocortex and juxtallocortex) to the neocortex

Limbic Functions

The limbic system is concerned with autonomic responses. Along with hypothalamus it is concerned with sexual behavior, emotions of rage, fear and motivation. It has role in olfaction also.

Pheromones are odorants and have effects in animals to act at a distance to produce hormonal, behavioral or other physiological changes. They are even believed to have effects in humans. Examples are that women who are room mates often have their menstrual cycles that are synthronized.

BRAINSTEM

Midbrain

It is situated between the cerebrum above and the pons below (Fig. 12.19B). It formed of neurons and nerve fibers. Fibers connect the cerebrum with lower parts of the brain and with spinal cord. The nerve cells and the fibers are also a part of **reticular formation**. Reticular formation has an important role in the **alert state of the cerebral cortex** which makes perception of sensations possible. This system is called the reticular activating system (RAS). Any injury in the reticular formation in this part of the brain is likely to result in coma. Descending fibers of nuerons via reticulospinal pathways influence gamma motor neurons which produce effects on the tone of muscles.

Pons

Situated in front of the cerebellum, below midbrain and above medulla (Fig. 12.19). Consists mainly of nerve fibers between the two hemispheres of cerebellum and fibers which pass between the higher centers and the spinal cord.

Pons has centers for controlling the rate and depth of respiration (refers to respiratory system).

Medulla Oblongata

Situated between pons above and the spinal cord below. Its outer surface is formed of white matter; of fibers that pass between the brain and the spinal cord; grey matter is present centrally. Some cells are relay stations; but other cells are forming the vital centers for the control of respiration, heart rate and blood pressure. These centers are:

- Respiratory centre
- Cardiac centre
- Vasomotor centre
- Swallowing centre
- Vomiting centre

Control of Respiration, Heart Rate and Blood Pressure

The medullary areas for the reflex control of the circulation, heart and lungs are called the *vital centers* because damage to them is fatal.

The respiratory centre is responsible for the respiratory movements (refer to respiratory system).

The *vasomotor centre* controls the blood pressure, via *sympathetic impulses* to the *heart* and *blood vessels*. Increase in the frequency of impulses increases blood pressure.

Cardiac centre sends impulses by *vagal nerves* to the heart. Increase in the frequency of impulses lowers the heart rate.

The vasomotor centre and cardiac centre regulate the blood pressure as they are constantly receiving impulses form the baroreceptors situated in the carotid sinus and arch of the aorta. The regulation maintains the blood pressure at the normal level. These centers also receive impulses from the higher areas of brain, i.e. cerebral cortex and hypothalamus; emotions affect the heart rate and blood pressure via these impulses. Anger raises the heart rate and blood pressure whereas depression has the opposite effect. Pain impulses also affect the vasomotor centre and raise the blood pressure but severe pain may cause fall in the blood pressure.

Vomiting Centre

The "vomiting centre" is in the reticular formation of the medulla; consists of scattered groups of neurons that control different components of vomiting reflex.

Vomiting starts with salivation and sensation of nausea. Reverse peristalsis empties material from the upper part of small intestine into stomach. The glottis closes, preventing aspiration into trachea. The breath is held in mid-inspiration. The muscle of the abdominal wall contract and raise intra-abdominal pressure. The esophagus and the lower esophageal sphincter relax and gastric contents are pushed out.

The afferents for stimulation of the center are:

- Afferent impulses (via visceral afferents in the sympathetic and vagal nerves) from the upper part of gastrointestinal tract as a result of irritation of the mucosa.
- Afferents from vestibular nuclei mediate the nausea and vomiting of motion sickness.
- Emotional stimuli may result in vomiting because of impulses from the diencephalon and limbic system, e.g. when there is unpleasant smell.
- Vomiting is also initiated if the chemoreceptor cells present in the chemoreceptor trigger zone in the medulla get stimulated by chemical agents present in the blood, e.g. vomiting that occurs in uremia or by injection of apomorphine or by a number of other emetic drugs. The chemoreceptor zone is situated in the lateral walls of the 4th ventricle. (Refer to section on GIT for afferent and efferents to vomiting centre).

Swallowing

Swallowing is controlled by a central program generator in the medulla. It is ***initiated by voluntary act*** of propelling bolus from the mouth towards the back of the pharynx and *beyond that are the involuntary activities* that *involve carefully timed responses of the respiratory as well as gastrointestinal system, coordinated by swallowing center.*

The Reticular Formation

It is phylogenetically old reticular core of the brain; is present in midventral portion of the midbrain and medulla. It contains centers for respiration, heart rate and blood pressure as described above (also refer to relevant sections).

The lower brainstem in the medulla contains reticular inhibitory area. Projections from here inhibit the spinal motor neurons to antigravity muscles.

Reticular excitatiory area is located in the reticular formation of the Pons and Midbrain. The area projects to spinal cord and exerts an excitatory influence on motor neurons that innervate antigravity muscles. This area also sends fibers to thalamus that form RAS (Fig. 12.40B).

The descending pathways from the facilitatory and inhibitory areas (Fig. 12.36) to motor neurons (Fig. 12.15) are concerned with adjustment of stretch reflexes and are responsible for the normal tone of the skeletal muscles and balance of the body.

The gamma motor neurons innervate the intrafusal muscle fibers of the muscle spindles (Fig. 12.18A) present in the muscle (Fig. 12.45). The contraction of these fibers stretches the central region of the intrafusal fibers from where the 1a afferents (Fig. 12.46A) arise which get stimulated and impulses impinge on the alpha motor neurons of the same muscle (Fig. 12.46A) and increase their excitability. This is **stretch reflex** (Fig. 12.35) also called **tendon reflex.**

In upper motor neuron lesions, there is spasticity of muscles as the inhibitory area in the reticular formation is cut off from higher areas which normally activate it. Its activity decreases whereas the facilitatory area in the reticular formation remains active (does not require stimulation from higher areas) and the balance shifts towards facilitation that increases the excitability of gamma motor neurons which reflexly increase the excitability of alpha motor neurons (Figs 12.46A and B), that results in increased tone of the muscles.

This is the function of the ***descending path of the reticular system***. In addition, the reticular formation has **ascending connections** with the cerebral cortex responsible for the alert state of the cerebral cortex as described above. The neurons of reticular formation form clusters and a polysynaptic network which receives nerve impulses from all the *ascending spinal sensory pathways;* from *Vth cranial* nerve; *auditory, visual* and olfactory systems. Due to complexity of network it losses specificity and the system is activated equally

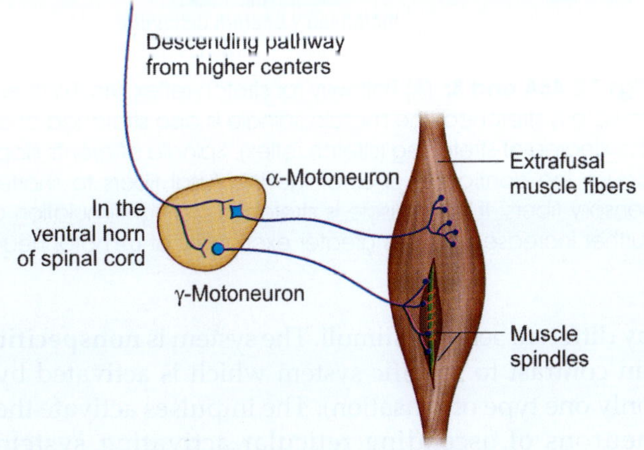

Fig. 12.45: Coactivation of an α- and a γ-motoneuron by a descending motor pathway

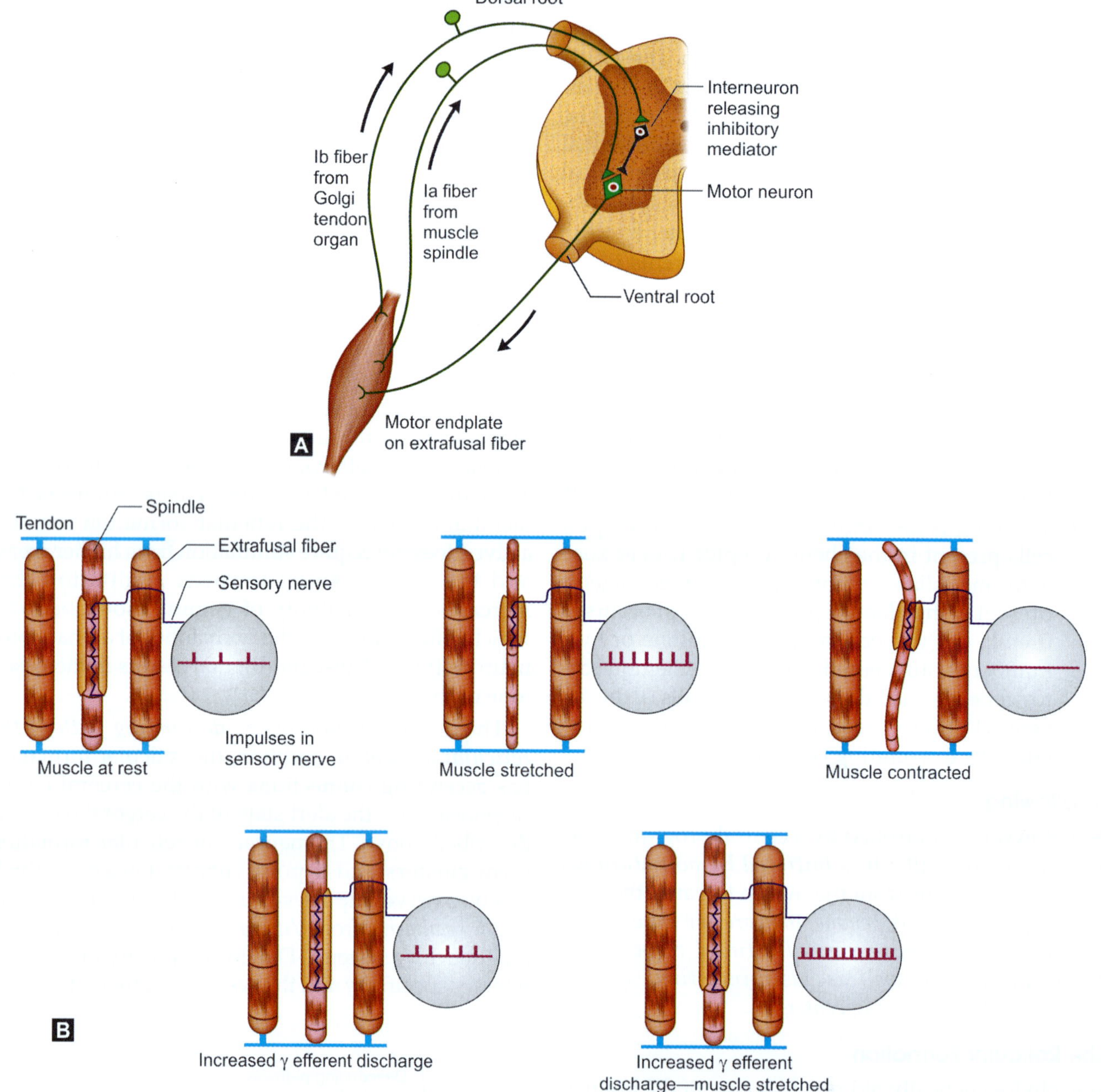

Figs 12.46A and B: (A) Pathway for stretch reflex (via 1a fiber) and inverse stretch reflex (via Golgi ending); (B) When the whole muscle is stretched, the muscle spindle is also stretched and its sensory endings are activated at a frequency proportional to the degree of stretching (stretch reflex). Spindle afferents stop firing when the muscle contracts. Stimulation of γ-motor neurons cause the contractile ends of the intrafusal fibers to shorten. This stretches the nuclear bag region, increases impulses in sensory fibers. If the muscle is stretched during stimulation of the γ-motor neurons, the rate of discharge in sensory fibers is further increased causes greater excitability of α-motor neuron.

by different sensory stimuli. The system is **nonspecific** (in contrast to specific system which is activated by only one type of sensation). The impulses activate the neurons of ascending reticular activating system (**ARAS or RAS**). The axons of which project to all parts of cerebrum (Fig. 12.40B and C). Part of it passes through thalamus in the intralaminar and midline nuclei, i.e. nonspecific relay nuclei; the rest passes without relay in the thalamus to the cortex; the activity is described as Reticular Activating System is responsible for the alert state of the brain that enable the perception of sensations.

The Electroencephalogram

The background activity of the brain was first analysed by German psychiatrist Hans Berger; hence, these waves are also known as Berger waves. The EEG can be recorded with scalp electrodes and unopened skull or by electrodes on the brain. Electrocorticogram (ECG) is a record with electrodes on the surface of piameter.

The recordings may be with bipolar electrodes or unipolar electrodes.

The following rhythms are described:

Alpha Rhythm: When the person is awake but at rest with mind wandering (not concentrating) and eyes closed. The most prominent component is fairly regular pattern of waves at a frequency of 8–12 Hz and amplitude of 50–100 µV. This pattern is alpha rhythm (Fig. 12.47A). It is most marked in parieto-occipital region. When attention is focused on something alpha rhythm is replaced by irregular low voltage fast activity. This is called alpha block. It is also called arousal or alerting response or desynchronization (Figs 12.47B).

Other rhythms: 18–30 Hz with lower amplitude is called **beta rhythm** sometimes seen over frontal regions. Gamma oscillations at 30–80 Hz are often seen when an individual focuses attention on something. This is replaced by irregular fast activity with initiation of motor activity in response to stimulus.

A pattern of large amplitude, regular 4–7 Hz waves is called **theta rhythm** (Fig. 12.48). Large slow waves with a frequency of less than 4 Hz is called **delta waves** present in deep sleep (Fig. 12.48).

During coma the EEG is dominated by delta activity. Brain death is defined by flat EEG.

Sleep Patterns

There are two different types of sleep: (1) rapid eye movement sleep called **REM sleep** and (2) **slow wave sleep** also called **non-REM sleep.**

REM sleep is so called because there are rapid roving eyes movements during this sleep. The EEG activity is rapid low voltage activity (Fig. 12.48) (this is like the activity seen in awake state) but on the other hand the threshold for arousal by sensory stimuli is increased, hence it is called *paradoxical sleep*. Muscle tone is hypotonic in neck muscles. REM sleep is associated with dreams. Another characteristic of this type of sleep is pontogeniculo-occipital (PGO) spikes, phasic potentials that originate in pons pass to lateral geniculate then to occipital cortex.

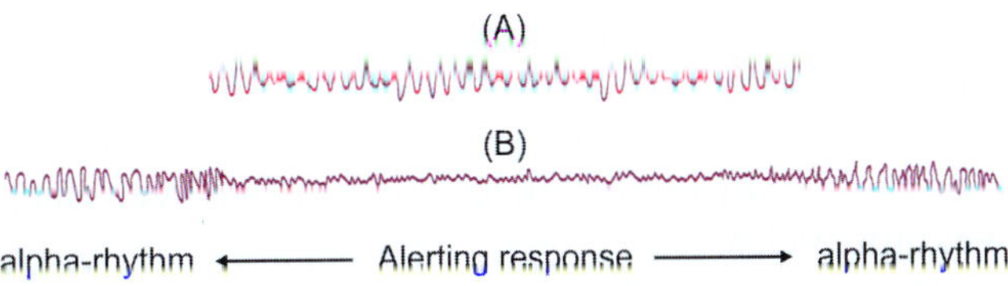

Figs 12.47A and B: (A) EEG showing alpha rhythm, (B) alerting response produced by a stimulus blocking alpha rhythm

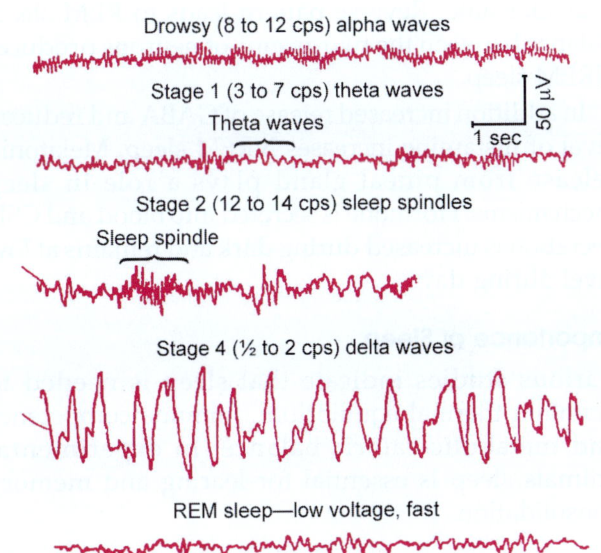

Fig. 12.48: ECG different waves in drowsiness and stages 1, 2 and 4 of slow wave (non-REM) sleep and in REM sleep

PET studies in humans in REM sleep show increased activity in pontine area, amygdala, anterior cingulate gyrus and decreased activity in prefrontal and parietal cortex. Activity in visual areas is increased but decreased in primary visual cortex, could explains the role of emotions in production of dreams.

Slow wave sleep: It is divided into four stages during which the EEG waves become slower, the maximum slowing occurring in stage 4 (Fig. 12.48). Dreams do not occur during non-REM sleep.

Both types of sleep normally occur during whole night sleep with cycles repeating during the night.

A circuit connecting cortex and thalamus is important in sleep-wakeful states. Transition between sleep and wakefulness is a circadian rhythm consisting of 6–8 hr sleep and 16–18 hr of wakefulness. Nuclei in brainstem and hypothalamus are involved. Electrical stimulation of hypothalamus or RAS produces arousal and stimulation of anterior hypothalamus and adjacent basal forebrain region induces sleep. Damage to midbrain reticular formation produces coma. Brainstem RAS is composed of several group of neurons that release norepinephrine, secrotonin or acetylcholine. Preoptic neurons (hypothalamus) release GABA and posterior hypothalamic neurons release histamine. Orexin produced by hypothalamus is believed to be important in switching between sleep wakeful cycles.

When activity of norepinephrine and serotonin containing neurons is dominant there is reduced level of acetylcholine neurons in reticular formation. This is awake state. Reverse pattern leads to REM sleep. Balance between the two groups of neurons produces NREM sleep.

In addition increased release of GABA and reduced level of histamine increases NREM sleep. Melatonin release from pineal gland plays a role in sleep mechanisms. Hormone is secreted into blood and CSF. Secretion is increased during dark and remains at low level during day.

Importance of Sleep

Various studies indicate that sleep is needed to maintain thermal equilibrium, immune competence and metabolic-caloric balance. In experimental animals sleep is essential for learing and memory consolidation.

HIGHER FUNCTIONS OF THE BRAIN

Learning, memory, judgment, and language are grouped as higher functions of the brain.

Humans have the ability to alter behavior on the basis of experience. ***Learning*** is ***acquisition*** of the information that makes it possible and ***memory*** is the ***retention and storage*** of that information.

Memory is divided into ***explicit memory*** that is associated with consciousness or awareness and is dependent for its retention on hippocampus and other parts of the medial temporal lobes of the brain. ***Implicit memory*** does not involve awareness and is called reflex memory. Its retention does not involve processing in the hippocampus and in most instances involves skills, habits, and conditioned reflexes that once acquired become automatic.

Explicit memory involve: (1) **short-term memory** which lasts seconds to hours during which processing in the hippocampus and elsewhere lays down long-term changes and (2) **long-term memory** (remote memory) which stores memories for years and sometimes for life. *During short-term memory the memory is subject to disruption by trauma and various drugs but long-term memory is resistant to disruption.* Working memory is a form of short-term memory that keeps information available usually for short periods while the person plans action based on it, e.g. dailing telephone number.

According to current views during working memory, information is stored in areas of prefrontal cortex, and also transmitted into medial temporal lobe and specifically to ***parahippocampal gyrus*** from where it is passed to ***hippocampus*** and processed there. During this stage, it is vulnerable, subsequent output from here strengthens circuits in many different neocortical areas forming stable memories that can be triggered by various different clues.

In humans, bilateral destruction of the **ventral hippocampus or Alzheimer's disease** causes effects in short-term memory but with intact working memory and remote memory, and the implicit memory processes remain intact. Subjects perform in terms of conscious memory so long they concentrate on what they are doing; but, if distracted even for a short time, all memory of what they were doing is lost. They are capable of new learning and retain old pre-lesion memories ***but cannot form new long-term memories.***

The amygdala is closely associated with hippocampus and is concerned with encoding emotions related to memories. Amygdaloid lesions make animals less fearful. In normal humans, events associated with strong emotions are remembered better than events without emotions. In Japan, amygdaloid lesions had been produced in subjects for relief of excessive tension to give relief.

Long-term memories are stored in various parts of the neocortex and they can be accessed by a number of different associations. The memory of a scene can be revived by that scene or the sound or smell associated with it.

Conditioned Reflexes (Associative Learning)

A conditioned reflex is a reflex response to a stimulus that previously did not produce that response. But it is acquired by repeatedly pairing the stimulus with that which normally does produce that response. Classically, it has been shown by experiments of scientist Pavlov. Salivation was produced in dogs when bell was rung after the bell had previously been paired a number of times with presentation of meat. The meat is unconditioned stimulus (US) the bell was the conditioned stimulus (CS).

If the CS is presented many times without the US, the response dies down (extinction).

A number of somatic, visceral and other neural changes can be made to occur as conditioned reflex responses. Conditioning of visceral reflexes is called **Biofeedback**. The changes that can be produced include alterations in heart rate, and conditioned decrease in blood pressure. But, the effects are mild only.

Biofeedback has also been called an educational process for learning of specialized mind or body skills (it is also called by many as trial and error learning), is also known as "Operant conditioning". It is used to establish learned control of specific physiological responses. The technique has been used recently in upper neuron paralyzed patients in an attempt to recruit active and intact neurons for the damaged ones by possibility of forming new neuronal connections.

New Brain Cells

Traditional view that neurons are not formed after birth is being doubted as it is now being considered that neurons form from stem cells throughout life in two areas: (1) the hippocampus and (2) olfactory bulb.

Complementary Specialization of Hemispheres

Activity in the two hemispheres of the cerebral cortex is coordinated by interconnections through the cerebral commissures. *Most of the neocortex on the two sides is connected through the* ***corpus callosum****. Parts of the temporal lobes* connect through the *anterior commissure*, and the *hippocampal formations on the two sides communicate through the hippocampal commissure* formed between the formices on the two sides, as they pass under the corpus callosum.

The function of Language is believed to be that of the neocortex only. ***Language*** functions are more or less localized to one hemisphere. That has been called the **dominant hemisphere**. But, it has been realized that the other hemisphere is not less developed but developed for other functions like spatiotemporal relations. It is concerned with identification of objects by their form; recognition of musical themes and has role in recognition of faces. Hence, this hemisphere has been called the **representational hemisphere** and the other as **categorical** (instead of dominant) hemisphere.

Lesions of the categorical hemisphere produce language disorders, the lesion of representational hemisphere do not. Instead lesions of representational hemisphere produce astereognosis and other agnosias. Agnosia is general term for *inability* to recognize objects by a particular sensory modality even though the sensory modality itself is intact. Lesions producing these defects are in the parietal lobe, especially when they are in the representational hemisphere.

Hemisphere specialization is related to handedness which is probably genetically determined. About 91% of people are right handed, in majority of these people (about 96% of them) left hemisphere is categorical hemisphere and in remaining 4% the right hemisphere is dominant.

In most of the left-handed individuals (in about 70%) the left hemisphere is the dominant hemisphere, but in about 15% the right hemisphere is dominant, in about remaining 15% there no definite lateralization. Learning disabilities, such as dyslexia are found to be more common in left-handed people; but many talented artists, musicians and mathematicians are left-handed individuals.

Language Disorders

Aphasias are dysfunctions of language that are not due to defects in vision or hearing or due to motor paralysis. They are caused by lesions in the categorical hemisphere. Commonly are produced by obstruction to the blood supply. They are classified as *fluent*, *non-fluent* and *anomic* aphasias. In nonfluent aphasia, the lesion is in the Broca's area. Speech is slow and words are difficult to come. In fluent type, the lesion may be in the Wernicke's area when speech is normal and patient may talk excessively but what they talk does not make sense. The patient is not able to comprehend the meaning of spoken or written words. When there is damage to the angular gyrus without affecting Broca's area or Wenicke's area there is no difficulty with speech or understanding of auditory information. But, there is trouble in understanding of written language or of pictures as there is problem with processing of visual information to be transmitted to the Wernicke's area. This is called anomic aphasia.

Frequently aphasia is general (global) speech is scant and nonfluent.

SPINAL REFLEXES AND POSTURE

White matter: The white matter of the spinal cord is arranged in three columns; anterior, posterior or lateral.

The lower motor neurons (alpha motor neurons) which have cell bodies in the anterior horn of the spinal cord; the axons (myelinated) leave by anterior root which joins the posterior root to form mixed nerve which passes through the intervertebral foramen. Near its termination in the muscle the axon branches into a number of fibers which end at the motor end plate making a synaptic junction the neuromuscular junction (already described). The **lower motor neuron** has been called the final common pathway for transmission of impulses to the skeletal muscle. The cell bodies of the *neurons are influenced by upper motor neurons, and some neurons in the dorsal horn of the spinal cord which are involved in reflexes*. These impulses regulate the activity of lower motor neurons.

In the ventral horns are also present smaller motor neurons gamma motor neurons which send nerve impulses by their fibers to muscle spindles, to their intrafusal fibers. The *muscle spindles* are present in the voluntary muscles, the impulses *do not cause voluntary contraction of the muscle but regulate the tone in the muscle*. The gamma-motor neurons receive impulses from the descending reticular formation in the brainstem which regulate the tone of the muscles and posture of the body (explained already).

Spinal Reflexes

A reflex action is an immediate motor response to a stimulus, e.g. when a hot object is touched the hand is immediately withdrawn before the conscious perception of the sensation. There may be two or three or more neurons involved in the reflex arc; they function as:

- **Sensory neuron** to perceive the stimulus
- **Connector neuron** in the spinal cord that acts as center to receive sensory input and sends impulses to motor neuron
- **Lower motor neuron** to produce a response.

When there are only two neurons one sensory and one motor in the reflex it is monosynaptic reflex, e.g. stretch reflex. When connector neurons are involved in between it is a polysynaptic reflex (Fig. 12.49).

The connector neurons, may be many in number, e.g. when a hot object is touched, the hand, arm and the upper arm may move which involves many connector neurons and lower motor neurons supplying all these muscles.

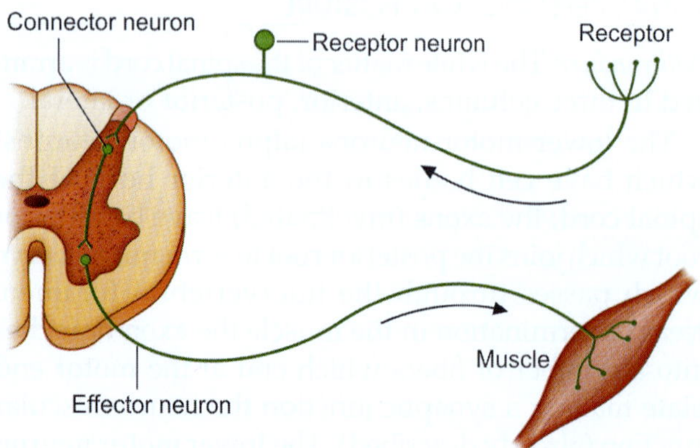

Fig. 12.49: Bisynaptic reflex pathway

Other similar reflexes may involve one or more inter neurons in the spinal cord, between the afferent and efferent neurons (Fig. 12.49 and 12.50).

Monosynaptic Reflex

A reflex action is **monosynaptic**, if it involves only two neurons, one sensory and the other motor, e.g. when we tap the patellar tendon it results in contraction of the quadriceps muscle on the same side and the foot kicks forward. The sensory impulses (from muscle spindles) on tapping enter the spinal cord and relay on the lower motor neurons of the same quadriceps muscle. This is **stretch reflex** (Fig. 12.46A).

Polysynaptic Spinal Reflexes

In a polysynaptic reflex pathway afferent nerves may branch in a complex fashion (Fig. 12.50). The number of synapses in each of their branches varies, conseqently a **prolonged response** occurs. Because of the **synaptic delay at each synapse**, activity in the branches with fewer synapses reaches the motor neurons earlier. More the interneurons involved in reflex action more the reaction time. Some of the branch pathways turn back (Fig. 12.50) permitting activity to reverberate until it becomes unable to cause a prolonged response and dies out. Such **reverberating circuits** are common in the brain and spinal cord.

The **withdrawal reflex** is a **polysynaptic reflex** that occurs in response to a noxious stimulus to the skin or subcutaneous tissues and muscle. The response is flexor muscle contraction and inhibition of extensor muscles, so that the body part is withdrawn from the stimulus. When a strong stimulus is applied to a limb, the response includes not only flexion and withdrawal of that limb but also extension of the opposite limb. This **crossed extensor response** is a part of the withdrawal reflex. Strong stimuli can generate activity in the interneuron pool that spreads to all four extremities. This spread of excitatory impulses up and

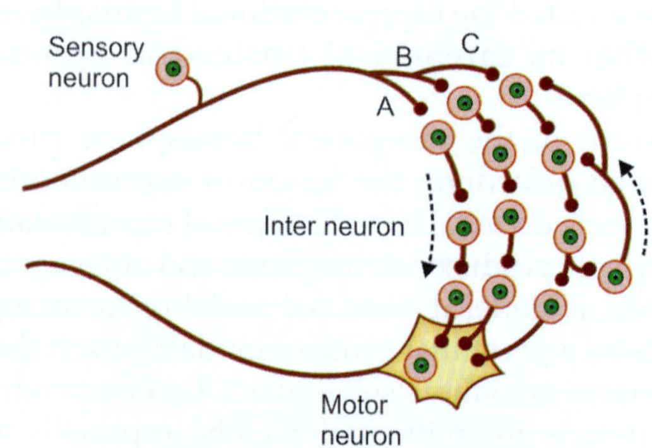

Fig. 12.50: Polysynaptic reflex pathway

down the spinal cord to more motor neurons is called **irradiation of the stimulus**, and the increase in the number of active motor units is called **recruitment of motor units**.

Importance of the Withdrawal Reflex

Flexor responses can be produced by **innocuous** stimulation of the skin or by stretch of the muscle, but strong flexor responses with withdrawal are initiated only by stimuli that are **noxious.**

The reaction time for withdrawal reflex is shortened if the strength of the noxious stimulus is increased. Spatial and temporal facilitation in the polysynaptic pathways occurs.

Stronger simuli produce more action potentials per second in the active branches of sensory nerves **(temporal facilitation)** and cause more sensory branches to become active **(spatial facilitation)**; hence in motor neurons EPSP for threshold level for action potential occurs more rapidly.

FUNCTIONS OF MUSCLE SPINDLES AND CENTRAL CONNECTIONS OF AFFERENT FIBERS

When the muscle is passively stretched, the spindles are also stretched. Its sensory endings are distorted and receptor potentials are generated. These in turn sets up action potentials in the sensory 1a fibers at a frequency proportional to the degree of stretching. These nerves end directly on motor neurons supplying the extrafusal fibers of the same muscle (Fig. 12.46A). This initiates **reflex** contraction of the extrafusal fibers in the muscle. This is monosynatic stretch reflex.

The time between the application of the stimulus and the response is called the **reaction time.** In humans, the reaction time for a stretch reflex, such as the knee jerk is 19–24 ms.

Effects of γ-Motor Neuron Discharge

Stimulation of γ-motor neurons produces different picture from that produced by stimulation of the α-motor neurons. Stimulation of γ-motor neurons does not lead directly to contraction of the muscles because the intrafusal fibers of the spindles, are not strong enough to cause shortening. But, stimulation does cause the contractile ends of the intrafusal fibers to shorten and hence stretch the nuclear bag portion deforming the nerve endings and initiating impulses in the 1a fibers (Fig. 12.46A). This in turn leads to reflex contraction of the muscle. Thus, muscles can be made to contract via stimulation of the α-motor neurons that innervate the extrafusal fibers or the γ-motor neurons that initiate contraction via the stretch reflex.

If the whole muscle is stretched during stimulation of the γ-motor neurons, the rate of discharge in the 1a fibers is further increased (Fig. 12.46B). Increased γ-motor neuron activity increases **spindle sensitivity** during stretch.

In response to descending excitatory input to spinal motor system both α- and γ-motor neurons (Fig. 12.45) are activated. Because of this "α–γ coactivation", intrafusal and extrafusal fibers shorten together and spindle afferent activity can occur throughout the period of muscle contraction. In this way, the spindle remains capable of responding to stretch and reflexly adjusting α-motor neuron discharge.

Control of γ-Motor Neuron Discharge

The γ-motor neurons are regulated by descending tracts from a number of areas in the brain via **reticulospinal pathways** and **pathways to α-motor neurons** (Fig. 12.36 and 45). Via these pathways, the sensitivity of the muscle spindles and hence, the threshold of the stretch reflexes in various parts of the body can be adjusted and shifted to meet the needs of postural control.

Other factors also influence γ-motor neuron. Anxiety causes an increased discharge, the hyperactive tendon reflexes in anxious patients. Stimulation of the skin, especially by noxious agents, increases γ-motor neuron discharge to ipsilateral flexor muscle spindles. Trying to pull the hands apart when the flexed fingers are hooked together facilitates the knee jerk reflex **(Jendrassik's maneuver)**, and it may be due to increased γ-motor neuron discharge initiated by afferent impulses from the hands.

Reciprocal Innervation

When a stretch reflex occurs, the muscles that antagonize the action of the muscle, the antagonists relax. This is due to **reciprocal innervation**. Impulses in the 1a fibers from the muscle spindles of the muscle cause via postsynaptic pathway inhibition of the motor neurons of the antagonists beacause of a collateral from 1a fiber to an inhibitory interneuron that synapses on a motor neuron supplying the antagonist muscles. The pathway mediating this effect is bisynaptic (Fig. 12.35).

INVERSE STRETCH REFLEX

Up to a point, the harder a muscle is stretched, the stronger is the reflex contraction. When the tension becomes great enough, contraction suddenly ceases and the muscle relaxes. This relaxation in response to strong stretch is called the **inverse stretch reflex.** The receptor for the inverse stretch reflex is in the **Golgi tendon organ** (Fig. 12.33 and 46A). This organ consists of collection of knobby nerve ending in the tendon (Fig. 12.18B). The fibers from the Golgi tendon organs make-up the 1b group of myelinated, rapidly conducting nerve fibers. Stimulation of these 1b fibers leads to the production of IPSPs on the motor neurons that supply the same muscle from which the fibers arise because the 1b fibers end in the spinal cord on inhibitory interneurons that in turn terminate directly on the motor neurons, to produce IPSP.

Because the Golgi tendon organs, unlike the spindles, are in series with the muscle fibers, they are stimulated by both passive stretch and active contraction of the muscle. The degree of stimulation by passive stretch is not great because the elastic muscle fibers take up much of the stretch and this is why it takes a strong stretch to produce relaxation. But, discharge is regularly produced by contraction of the muscle and the Golgi tendon organ thus functions in a feedback circuit that regulates muscle **force** in a fashion the spindle feedback circuit regulates muscle length.

MUSCLE TONE

The resistance of a muscle to stretch is often referred to as its **tone** or **tonus.** If the motor nerve to a muscle is severed, the muscle offers very little resistance and is said to be **flaccid**. A **hypertonic (spastic)** muscle is one in which the resistance to stretch is high because of hyperactive stretch reflexes. Between the states of flaccidity and spasticity is the area of normal tone. The muscles are generally **hypotonic** when the rate of γ-motor neuron discharge is low and hypertonic when it is high.

When the muscles are hypertonic, the sequence of moderate stretch → muscle contraction, strong stretch → muscle relaxation is clearly seen. Passive flexion of the elbow, for example, meets resistance as a result of the stretch reflex in the triceps muscle. Further stretch activates the inverse stretch reflex. The resistance to flexion suddenly collapses and the arm flexes. This sequence of resistance followed by give in when a limb is moved passively is known as the **clasp-knife effect** because of its resemblance to the closing of a pocket knife. It is also know as the **lengthening reaction.**

Posture Regulating Systems

This involves a number of **nuclei** in the **spinal cord, brainstem** and **cerebral cortex**. They are concerned with **static posture,** also along with corticospinal and corticobulbar systems with **initiation and control of movement**. At the **spinal cord level afferent impulses produce simple reflex responses.** At higher levels in the nervous system increasingly complicated responses occur (Table 12.7). Postural reflexes maintain the body in upright position and provide a stable background for movements. These are integrated at various levels of the CNS (Table 12.7) and affected through various motor pathways. An important factor is the ***variation in the threshold of stretch reflexes due to affect of gamma efferent discharge on muscle spindle*** that reflexly affects excitability of motor neurons in the spinal cord. In the **upper motor neuron** lesion such increase in excitability is responsible for the increase in **muscle tone and exaggerated deep reflexes.**

Babinski's sign: Damage to the lateral corticospnial tract in humans produces the Babinski's sign, i.e. dorsflexion of the great toe and fanning of **other toes** when lateral aspect of sole of foot is scratched. Normal response is plantar flexion of all toes. In **an infant Babinski's sign may be present normally.**

Locomotion generator: There are two ***pattern generators*** **for locomotion** in the spinal cord; one is in the **cervical region** and the other is in the **lumbar region.** But spinal humans (when spinal cord is cut off from higher centers) cannot walk by themselves; because the ***pattern generator has to be turned on by tonic discharge of an area in the midbrain, the mesencephalic locomotor region.*** This can be possible with incomplete transection when some connecting fibers to spinal cord with higher centers remain.

Trail in experimental animals shows that generator can be turned on with the drug levodopa after complete transaction of spinal cord.

Spinal Cord Injury

In all vertebrates, transection of the spinal cord is followed by a period of **spinal shock** during which all spinal reflex responses are profoundly depressed. Subsequently, reflex responses return and become hyperactive. The **duration** of spinal shock is proportional to the degree of encephalization of motor function in the species. In frogs, it lasts for minutes; in dogs and cats, it lasts for 1–2 hours; in monkeys, it lasts for days; and in ***humans, it usually lasts for about 2 weeks.***

Absence of tonic influence on spinal motor neurons by excitatory impulses in descending pathways has a role in development of spinal shock. In addition, spinal inhibitory interneurons normally themselves inhibited may be released from descending inhibition to become disinhibited. This would inhibit motor

Table 12.7: Principal postural reflexes

Reflex	*Stimulus*	*Response*	*Receptor*	*Integrated*
Stretch reflexes	Stretch	Contraction of muscle	Muscle spindles	Spinal cord, medulla
Positive supporting (magnet) reaction	Contact with sole or palm	Foot extended to support body	Proprioceptors in distal flexors	Spinal cord
Negative supporting reaction	Stretch	Release of positive supporting reaction	Proprioceptors in extensors	Spinal cord
Tonic labyrinthine reflexes	Gravity	Contraction of limb extensor muscles	Otolithic organs	Medulla
Tonic neck reflexes	Head turned:	Change in pattern of extensor contraction	Neck proprioceptors	Medulla
	• To side	• Extension of limbs on side to which head is turned		
	• Up	• Hind legs flex		
	• Down	• Fore legs flex		
Labyrinthine righting reflexes	Gravity	Head kept level	Otolithic organs	Midbrain
Neck righting reflexes	Stretch of neck muscles	Righting of thorax and shoulders, then pelvis	Muscle spindles	Midbrain
Body on head righting reflexes	Pressure on side of body	Righting of head	Exteroceptors	Midbrain
Body on body righting reflexes	Presure on side of body	Righting of body even when head held sideways	Exteroceptors	Midbrain
Optical righting	Visual cues	Righting of head	Eyes	Cerebral cortex
Placing reaction	Various visual, exteroceptive, and proprioceptive cues	Foot placed on supporting surface in position to support body	Various	Cerebral cortex

neurons. The later recovery of reflex excitability may be due to the development of denervation hypersensitivity to the mediators released by the remaining spinal excitatory endings; and sprouting of collaterals from existing neurons with the formation of additional excitatory endings on interneurons and motor neurons.

The **first reflex response to appear** *as spinal shock wears off in humans is often a slight contraction of the leg flexors and adductors in response to a noxious stimulus,* the withdrawal reflex. In some patients, the knee jerk reflex recovers first. The interval for return of reflex activity is about 2 weeks but if complications are present it is much longer. When the spinal reflexes begin to reappear after spinal shock, their threshold steadily drops.

In quadriplegic humans, the threshold of the withdrawal reflex is very low; even minor noxious stimuli may cause prolonged withdrawal of one extremity or marked flexion-extension patterns in the other three limbs. Stretch reflexes are also hyperactive. Afferent stimuli irradiate from one reflex center to another. When a relatively minor noxious stimulus is applied to the skin, it may activate autonomic neurons and produce evacuation of the bladder and rectum, sweating, pallor, and blood pressure swings. This distressing **mass reflex** can be used to give paraplegic patients a degree of bladder and bowel control. They can be trained to initiate urination and defecation by stroking or pinching their thighs. If the cord section is incomplete, the flexor spasms initiated by noxious stimuli can be associated with bursts of pain.

Summary of Voluntary Movement

The ***contraction of the muscles*** which move the joint are under voluntary control, and the stimulus to contract originates at **conscious level in the cerebrum.** But, some nerve impulses which control ***tone and posture*** in the muscles are initiated in the **brainstem and cerebellum.** This involuntary activity is associated with coordination of muscle activity, e.g. when very fine movement is required and in the maintenance of posture and balance (Table 12.8).

The motor pathways from the brain to the muscles are made-up **at least two neurons.** The tracts are **pyramidal** (corticospinal) or **extrapyramidal.** The motor fibers of the ***pyramidal tract*** originate in the cerebral cortex and after crossing over in the medulla descend

Table 12.8: Summary of functions of different components of CNS

Region	*Function*
Spinal cord	Sensory input; reflex organization; somatic and autonomic motor output
Medulla	Cardiovascular control; respiratory control; brainstem reflexes
Pons	Respiratory and urinary bladder control; vestibular control of eye movements
Cerebellum	Motor control; motor learning
Midbrain	Acoustic relay; control of eye movements; motor control
Thalamus	Sensory and motor relay to cerebral cortex. Role in arousal and selective attention; EEG waves
Hypothalamus	Autonomic and endocrine control
Basal ganglia	Motor control
Cerebral cortex	Sensory perception; cognition; learning and memory; motor planning and voluntary movement.

down to the spinal **motor neurons in the ventral horn of the spinal cord,** the latter neuron is called **lower motor neuron.** In the case of *extrapyramidal pathways* that maintain posture the neurons involved **have many relays in the brainstem.** Any neuron above the lower motor neuron in the spinal cord (or equivalent motor neuron of cranial nerve in the brainstem) is called **upper motor neuron.**

Table 12.8 gives the summary of functions of different components of CNS.

AUTONOMIC NERVOUS SYSTEM

Autonomic nervous system is involuntary and not under the control of will. It is divided into two divisions.

1. Sympathetic
2. Parasympathetic

   The organs where they produce their effects are:
   - Cardiac muscle
   - Smooth muscles
   - Glands in the gastrointestinal system

The effects produced by autonomic nervous system are rapid. The two divisions produce opposite effects in an organ. Most of the structures receive both divisions. The smooth muscle in the wall of hollow viscera is generally innervated by both noradrenergic (sympathetic fibers) and cholinergic fibers (parasympathetic fibers) and activity of one system increases the intrinsic activity of the smooth muscle whereas activity in other decreases it, there is no uniform rule about which system stimulates and which inhibits.

In a general way, the functions promoted by activity of **parasympathetic division** of the autonomic nervous system are those concerned with **day-to-day living,** e.g. promoting *digestion* and *absorption* of food by increasing the activity of *gastric glands, stimulating mobility* of the intestinal musculature and relaxing the pyloric sphincter; and hence this division of the autonomic nervous system is **anabolic** against the **sympathetic nervous system which is called catabolic.**

The **sympathetic nervous system** has role in maintaining homeostasis and in emergency situations it discharges as a unit. The effects produced help an individual to cope with emergency, e.g. there is dilatation of the pupil, and relaxation of accommodation in the eye, acceleration of the heart beat and rise of blood pressure (providing better profusion to vital organs and muscles) and constriction of the blood vessels of skin to reduce bleeding if any. It also alerts the individual by *activating reticular formation* and raises the blood glucose and fatty acid levels making *more energy available* for *fight or flight* reactions that have been described by Cannon.

The autonomic nervous system is organized on the basis of the reflex action, similar to the functioning of somatic nervous system.

The *afferent nerves carry the sensations* from visceral receptors and the impulses are *integrated* at *various levels of CNS* and transmitted by efferent autonomic pathways to the viscera.

The efferent pathways are as follows. There are *two efferent neurons* in each of the divisions of autonomic system:

- Preganglionic neuron
- Postganglionic neuron.

General Features

The cell body of the preganglionic neuron is the brain or spinal cord. Its axon terminals synapse with the cell bodies of the postganglionic neurons which are situated outside the CNS in the autonomic ganglia or in the organ itself. Postganglionic neurons release the neurotransmitter in the organ where the effects are produced.

Preganglionic neurons of both the systems release acetylcholine at the synapse with postganglionic neurons (Fig. 12.51). The postganglionic neurons of the parasympathetic system at the nerve endings

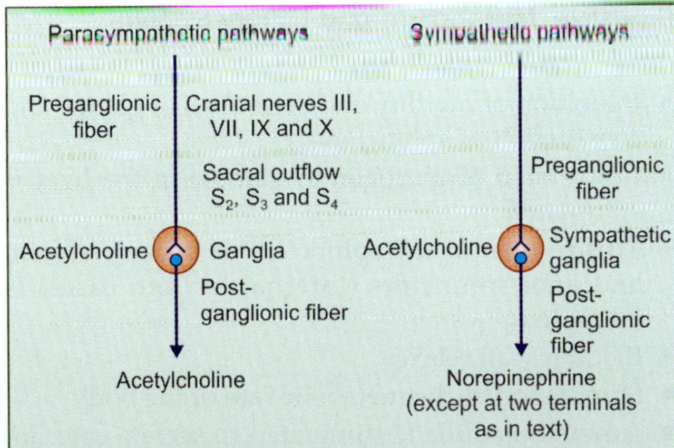

Fig. 12.51: Neurotransmitters at the terminals of preganglionic and postganglionic fibers of the parasympathetic and sympathetic pathways

release acetylcholine which produce the effects in the organ. The postganglionic neurons of sympathetic system release norepinephrine (noradrenaline) at all terminals except at two regions, i.e. at sweat glands and at some blood vessels in skeletal muscles where they release again acetylcholine.

Norepinephrine, epinephrine, and dopamine are all found in plasma. The epinephrine and some of the dopamine come from the adrenal medulla, but norepinephrine diffuses into the bloodstream from sympathetic nerve endings. The norepinephrine released from sympathetic postganglionic fibers binds to adrenoceptors. These are several types: α_1, α_2, β_1, β_2, and β_3.

Adrenal Medulla: The main secretions of the epinephrine, norepinephrine, and dopamine. The adrenal medulla is in effect a sympathetic ganglion in which the postganglionic neurons have lost their exons to become secretory cells. The cells secrete when stimulated by preganglionic nerve fibers that reach the gland via splanchnic nerves. Adrenal medullary hormones prepare the body for emergencies and that are called **fight and flight** responses.

Sympathetic Nervous System

The Preganglionic Neurons

These have cell bodies in the lateral column of grey matter in the spinal cord extending from the 1st thoracic to the 3rd or 4th lumbar segments. The fiber pathways have been described in anatomy section. The fibers make the synaptic junction with the post-synaptic neurons where the presynaptic neurons release acetylcholine at the synapse.

The postganglionic neuron has a cell body in a ganglion and its terminals are in the organ (or tissue) supplied. The postganglionic neuron releases transmitter norepinephrine (noradrenaline) at all the endings except at two regions, e.g. sweat glands and some skeletal muscle blood vessels (forming sympathetic vasodilator pathway where at endings the transmitter released is acetylcholine.

Parasympathetic System

The Preganglionic Neurons

Preganglionic neurons have the cell body in the brain or spinal cord and the fibers come out as:

- Cranial outflow
- Sacral outflow.

Cranial outflow: Preganglionic neurons are situated in the brain and their axons travel in III, VII, IX and Xth cranial nerves (the fibers originate in the nuclei situated in the brainstem).

Sacral outflow: Cell bodies of the sacral outflow are in the lateral horn of grey matter in the sacral segment of the spinal cord. The fibers come out of the spinal cord in the anterior roots of 2nd to 4th sacral segments.

The postganglionic neurons for the parasympathetic system are situated either in the ganglia or in the organ itself.

In the case of parasympathetic system, the chemical transmitter at the synapse of presynaptic with postsynaptic neurons and also at the endings of postsynaptic neurons, i.e. at both the sites is acetylcholine.

Higher Centers Controlling Autonomic Nervous System

The hypothalamic and other centers in the brainstem control the functions of the autonomic nervous system by producing effects on the preganglionic neurons. The levels of the autonomic integration within the CNS are arranged like the somatic nervous system. Simple reflexes, such as **contraction of the full bladder** are integrated in the spinal cord (in the sacral portion). A collection of urine in the bladder can initiate reflex contraction of the bladder wall, but the spinal reflex is facilitated and inhibited by higher brain centers (is subjected to voluntary facilitation and inhibition). The complex reflexes that regulate respiration and blood pressure are integrated in the medulla oblongata. Swallowing, coughing, sneezing and vomiting are also reflex responses integrated in the medulla oblongata. The reflexes controlling pupillary responses to light and accommodation are integrated in the midbrain. The autonomic mechanisms of maintenance of temperature of the internal environment are integrated in the hypothalamus.

Coughing is initiated by irritation of the lining of trachea and extrapulmonary bronchi.

Vomiting is another example of the way visceral reflexes are integrated in the medulla and these are coordinated and timed with somatic as well as visceral components.

Control of Respiration, Heart Rate and Blood Pressure

There are areas for the autonomic reflex control of the circulation, heart and respiration that have been described already. The motor responses are graded and delicately adjusted.

The effects of stimulation of the autonomic nervous system on each of the body systems are as follows:

Cardiovascular System

Sympathetic Stimulation

- Increase in the heart rate and force of contraction of the ventricles as a result increase in cardiac output is produced.
- Dilatation of blood vessels supplying skeletal muscles during exercise increasing supply of oxygen and nutrition for increased muscular activity.
- Constriction of arterioles to maintain blood pressure and regulation of arterial pressure via feedback mechanisms from the carotid and aortic baroreceptors.
- Constriction of blood vessels in skin and splanchnic regions to divert more blood supply to the vital regions in some situations like hemorrhage in effort to maintain their needs at the expense of supply to nonvital regions.

Parasympathetic Stimulation

Decrease the rate and force of heart beat. The parasympathetic nervous system exerts little if any direct effect on blood vessel musculature except in the case of sexual functions.

Respiratory System

Sympathetic Stimulation

Produce dilation of the airways, especially bronchioles.

Parasympathetic Stimulation

Produce constriction of bronchioles

Digestive, Metabolism and Urinary System

Sympathetic Stimulation

- Inhibition of motility and secretions of glands and constriction of sphincters
- Conversion of glycogen to glucose in the liver is stimulated
- Muscle tone of the sphincters of urinary system and anal sphincters (internal in both cases) is increased
- Bladder wall relaxes
- Stimulation of the metabolic rate of the body
- Adrenal medulla is stimulated to secrete catecholamines (epinephrine and norepinephrine) hormones into the blood which potentiate and sustain the effects generalized sympathetic stimulation during stressful conditions.

Parasympathetic Stimulation

- Digestion in the stomach and digestion and absorption in the intestine stimulated; pancreatic juice secretion is stimulated.
- Contraction of the muscle of bladder and relaxation of internal sphincter responsible for micturition (when external sphincter is relaxed voluntarily).
- Relaxation of internal anal sphincter and contraction of rectal muscles that is responsible for defecation (when external sphincter is voluntarily relaxed).

EYE

Sympathetic Stimulation

Dilatation of pupil due to contraction of the radial muscle fibers of the iris.

Parasympathetic

- Miosis (contraction) of pupil by contraction of circular muscle fibers of iris.
- Contraction of ciliary muscle for near vision (accommodation reflex).

SKIN

Sympathetic Stimulation

- Increased secretion of sweat by postganglionic cholinergic fibers
- Constriction of blood vessels to prevent heat loss
- Contractions of the muscle of the hair follicles of the skin giving appearance of goose flesh.

There is no parasympathetic supply to skin blood vessels.

Summary of the Functions of the Autonomic Nervous System

Autonomic nervous system is involved in reflex activities depending on the sensory input to the spinal cord or brain. The response of the systems is rapid, involving contraction or inhibition of contraction of smooth or cardiac muscle or secretion of glands. The reflexes are coordinated at the subconscious level in the brain. Sensory information for some reflexes like micturition reflex does reach the conscious level in the cerebrum and the reflex can be inhibited by voluntary activity though only temporarily. Similarly the respiration can be held voluntarily but only for a brief period.

The parasympathetic and sympathetic system having opposing action in the organs regulate the functioning in an optimum manner.

Sympathetic system prepares the body to deal with stressful situations. The adrenal medulla is stimulated in such situations and the hormones epinephrine and norepinephrine liberated are released into the blood stream and the hormones reinforce the effects of sympathetic stimulation. It is said that the sympathetic system stimulation prepares the body for fight or flight. The sympathetic system discharges as a unit in emergency situations. But, the sympathetic system also subserves other functions, e.g. tonic noradrenergic discharge to the arterioles maintains arterial blood pressure and variations in this discharge is the mechanisms by which carotid feedback regulation of blood pressure is affected. Sympathetic discharge is decreased in fasting animals and increased when fasting animals are fed again. These changes may explain the decrease in blood pressure and metabolic rate produced by fasting and opposite changes produced by feeding. **Hence, there is role of sympathetic system in maintaining homeostasis besides the mass discharge in emergency situations.**

The effects of **parasympathetic stimulation** are promotion of functions which are concerned with **vegetative aspects of day-to-day living,** e.g. digestive and absorptive activities of the gastrointestinal tract.

Afferents from Viscera

Sensory fibers from viscera travel along with the autonomic fibers, the nerves from the viscera and are referred as autonomic afferents. They are responsible for reflex actions involving the autonomic nervous system and are responsible for following effects.

- Visceral reflexes mostly at subconscious level, e.g. coughing, blood pressure maintenance
- Sensation of hunger, nausea, rectal, or bladder distention.

Visceral Pain

Viscera are generally insensitive to cutting, burning and crushing. But visceral pain can be felt as dull, poorly localized and may be associated with nausea and autonomic symptoms. Visceral pain often radiates or is referred to other areas. Pain is experienced when:

- Visceral nerves are stretched
- Ischemia and local accumulation of metabolities
- During inflammation as the sensitivity of nerve endings is increased
- Distention of the intestines
- Large number of fibers are stimulated.

If the cause of the pain is with inflammation of parietal layer of serous membrane (pleura, peritoneum) the pain is acute and localized over the site because the somatic nerve branches supply these structures and transmit information to the cerebral cortex.

Referred Pain

In some cases the visceral pain is perceived in a superficial tissue (it is referred pain) away from the site of viscera. This occurs when the somatic fibers and sensory fibers from the viscera are entering the same segment of the spinal cord (Fig. 12.52) and the pain is perceived in the superficial area of the somatic structure. The pain is referred to a structure that developed from the same embryonic segment or dermatome as the structure in which pain originates. The cardiac pain is referred to the inner side of left arm.

Pain on the top of shoulder is caused by irritation of central part of diaphragm.

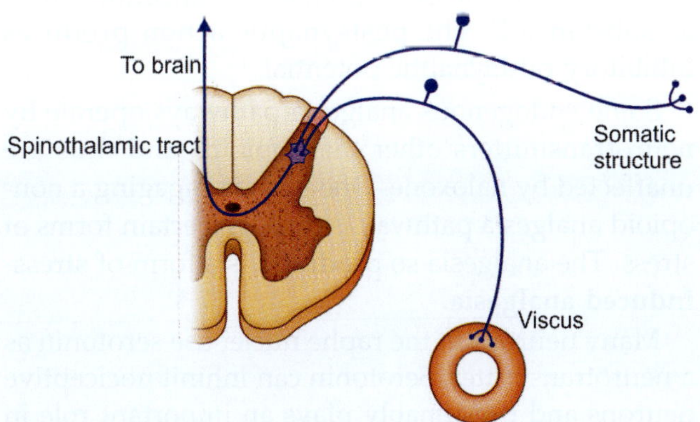

Fig. 12.52: Diagram of the way in which convergence in the dorsal horn cell may cause referred pain

Modulation of Pain Transmission

Interest is in the descending control system that regulates the transmission of nociceptive information. This system suppresses excessive pain under certain circumstances. It is well known that soldiers on the battlefield, accident victims, and athletes in competition often feel little or no pain at the time a wound occurs. At a later time, pain may develop and become severe. The pain control system is important medically it is distinguished as a special system called the **endogenous analgesia system.**

Several centers in the brainstem and descending pathways from these contribute to the endogenous analgesia system. Stimulation in the periaqueductal grey, the locus ceruleus, or the medullary raphe nuclei (Fig. 12.53A) inhibits nociceptive neurons at spinal cord and brainstem levels, including spinothalamic tract and trigeminothalamic tract cells. Pathways also originate in sensorimotor cortex, hypothalamus and reticular formation.

The endogenous analgesia system can be subdivided into two components: one component uses one of the endogenous **opioid peptides** as neurotransmitters or modulators and the other does not. The endogenous opioids are neuropeptides that activate one of several types of opiate receptors (Fig. 12.53B). Some of the endogenous opioids include enkephalin, dynorphin, and β-endorphin. Opiate analgesia can generally be prevented or reversed by the narcotic antagonist naloxone.

The opioid-mediated endogenous analgesia system can be activated by exogenous administration of morphine or other opiate drugs. Opiates typically inhibit neural activity in nociceptive pathways. Two sites of action for opiate inhibition, presynaptic and postsynaptic (Fig. 12.53B). The presynaptic action of opiates on nociceptive afferent terminals is thought to prevent the release of excitatory transmitter, such as substance P. The postsynaptic action produces inhibitory postsynaptic potential.

Some endogenous analgesia pathways operate by neurotransmitters other than opioids and thus are unaffected by naloxone. One way of engaging a non-opioid analgesia pathway is through certain forms of stress. The analgesia so produced is a form of **stress-induced analgesia.**

Many neurons in the raphe nuclei use serotonin as a neurotransmitter. Serotonin can inhinit nociceptive neurons and presumably plays an important role in the endogenous analgesia system. Other brainstem neurons release catecholamines, such as norepinephrine

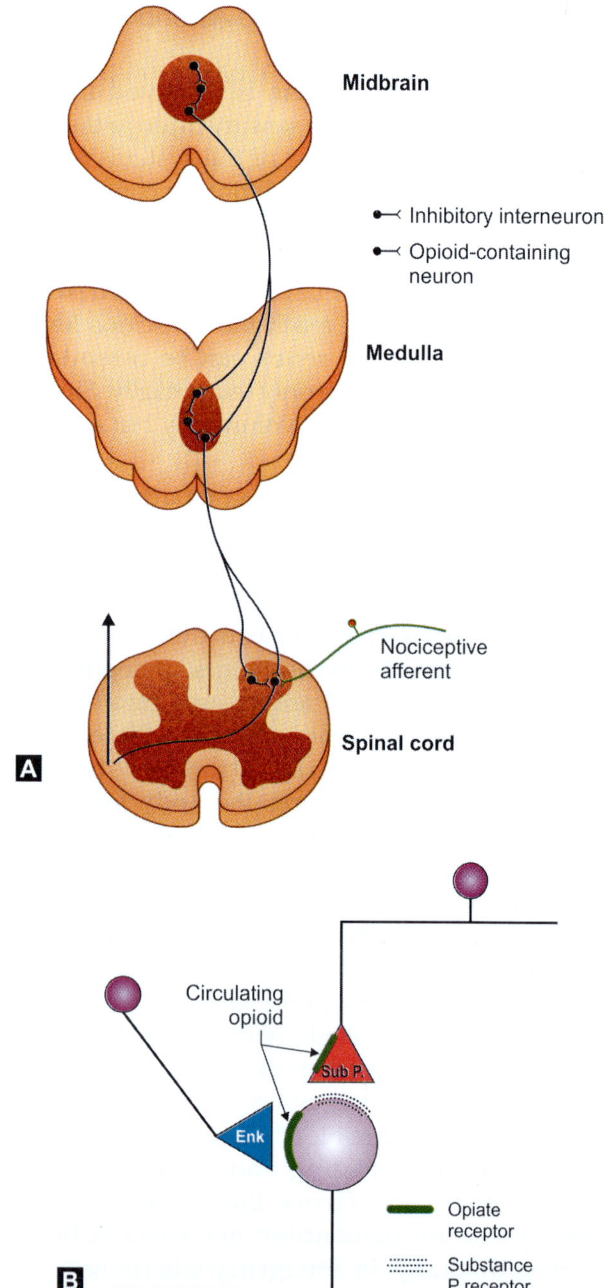

Figs 12.53A and B: (A) Some of the neurons may have a role in the endogenous analgesia system. Neurons in the midbrain periaqueductal grey activate the raphe-spinal tract, which in turn inhibits nociceptive spinal neurons, such as those of the spinothalamic tract. Interneurons containing opioid substances are involved in the system at each level, (B) Possible presynaptic and postsynaptic sites of action of enkephalin (*Enk*). The presynaptic action might prevent the release of substance P. from nociceptors

and epinephrine, in the spinal cord. These catecholamines also inhibit nociceptive neurons; therefore, catecholaminergic neurons may contribute to the endogenous analgesia system. Furthermore, these monoamine neurotransmitters interact with endogenous opioids. Many other substances are likely involved in the analgesia system.

The analgesic effect of acupunture may involve release of opioids.

Rubbing an injured area for pain relief is belived to be due to collaterals of mechanoreceptors fibers inhibiting pain transmission in dorsal horn.

Cranial Nerves

Refer to Anatomy for pathways.

Ist cranial nerve is olfactory nerve which carries sensory afferents from olfactory receptors from the upper part of nasal cavity.

IInd cranial nerve is optic nerve which carries sensory impulses from ganglion cells of retina in the eye to the brain.

IIIrd, IVth and VIth, cranial nerves are called oculomotor, trochlear and abducent nerves respectively, are motor nerves to the eye muscles. IVth supplies the superior oblique muscle of the eyeball, VIth supplies external rectus, and IIIrd all the other eye muscles and levator palpebrae superioris and has parasympathetic component for ciliary muscle and pupil and responsible for accommodation reflex and pupillary constriction. Paralysis leads to ptosis (dropping of upper eyelid) due to paralysis of levator palpebrae superioris.

Vth nerve is trigeminal nerve has both motor and sensory components. It is motor for muscles of mastication and sensory for the face by its three divisions and sensory for the anterior two-thirds of the tongue.

VIIth cranial nerve is facial nerve and it supplies all the muscles of the face and scalp except the levator palpebrae superioris. Hence, it is responsible for facial expressions. It has a sensory component that brings taste impulses from anterior two-thirds of the tongue. Its parasympathetic fibers supply lacrimal gland; and submandibular and sublingual salivary glands. When there is paralysis of the nerve, patient is unable to whistle, food tends to collect in between the teeth and the fluids escape from the affected angle of the mouth.

VIIIth cranial nerve carries sensory impulses from hearing apparatus and vestibular apparatus to the brain.

IXth, Xth and XIth cranial nerves are glossopharygeal, vagus and accessory nerves respectively. Glossopharygeal nerve gives secretory parasympathetic fibers to the parotid salivary gland, also carries sensory impules from the posterior third of the tongue (including taste impulses from the same region), palate, pharynx and tonsils. Lesions produce difficulty in swallowing, impairement of taste over posterior third of tongue. Vagus gives parasympathetic fibers to stomach, small intestine and part of large intestine. Vagus also has sensory fibers, which carry impulses from the same parts. Lesion produce pharyngeal paralysis, laryngeal paralysis and abnormality of motility of esophagus and motility and secretion of GIT. IXth nerve is motor to sternocleidomastoid and trapezius muscles.

XIIth cranial nerve is motor to tongue muscles. If the nerve is paralyzed and the person is asked to protrude the tongue, the tongue is pushed to the paralyzed side due to the action of the genioglossus muscle of the normal side.

DISORDERS OR DISEASE OF NERVOUS SYSTEM

Headache

It is a very common symptom with many different possible causes most of them minor and self-limiting. One type is severe and recurrent headache, known as migraine.

Migraine is accompanied by symptoms, such as disturbance of vision, nausea and sometimes vomiting and diarrhea. The attack may last several hours with person unable to carry out normal activities and so must rest. Bright light and noise is disturbing during the attack and may prolong it. It has some genetic component. The possible triggers for the attack are stress like that of anxiety, tiredness, excitement, travel, hunger, noise, menstruation, and other factors like intake of alcohol, certain foods and bright light.

It cannot be cured but can be treated with drugs. Action taken at the earliest sign of the onset, splashing cold water on face, taking bedrest in a dark and quiet room helps. Meditation helps as it reduces stress.

For the other types of headache, a number of different parts of head and neck may be responsible for causing pain of the headache and the types of pain produced differ. The brain itself cannot feel pain, but the surrounding meninges and arteries passing through the brain may be source of pain if they become inflamed or overstretched. The bones of the skull cannot feel pain but the covering periosteum is sensitive to pain if stretched or inflamed.

Sleep Disorders

Insomnia

It is defined as a subjective problem of insufficient or nonrestorative sleep despite an adequate opportunity to sleep. Difficulty in going to sleep or of maintained sleep.

Sleep walking (somnambulism), **bedwetting** (nocturnal enuresis), and night terrors occur during slow wave sleep or more specifically during arousal from slow wave sleep. **Somnambulist** walk with their eyes open and avoid obstacles, but when awakened cannot recall the episodes.

Narcolepsy

It is a disease when there is sudden loss of tone in muscles and irresistible urge to sleep during day time activities. In some cases, it starts with sudden onset of REM sleep.

Obstructive sleep apnea (OSA) is the most common cause of daytime sleepiness due to fragmented sleep at nighty. Breathing ceases for more than 10 s during episodes of obstruction of the upper airway (especially the pharynx) due to reduction in muscle tone. The apnea causes brief arousals from sleep in order to reestablish upper airway tone, individual begins to snore soon after falling asleep. The snoring gets louder then is interrupted by an episode of apnea, which is then followed by a loud snort and gasp, as individual tries to breathe. OSA is not associated with a reduction in total sleep time, but individuals with OSA experience a much greater time in stage 1 NREM sleep and a marked reduction in slow-wave-sleep (stages 3 and 4 NREM sleep). The pathophysiology of OSA includes a reduction in neuromuscular tone at the onset of sleep and a change in the central respiratory drive.

Congenital Malformations

Spina Bifida

Developing spinal cord fails to develope properly. Vertebral defect.

Mental Handicap

A child may be born with severe mental handicap. The severe forms are due to an abnormality of brain structure, the condition may be hereditary or congenital caused by infection during pregnancy such as German measles. The birth process is also important for the brain which should not suffer from oxygen lack or later from excess of bile pigment.

The causes for mild handicap are not well understood but the finding is of delayed milestones.

Circulatory Disturbances Affecting the Brain

Cerebral Hypoxia

If severe hypoxia is persistent for more than a few minutes (over 5 minutes), irreversible brain damage takes place. The neurons are most sensitive and are affected first, then the neuroglial cells.

Conditions leading to severe hypoxia are:

- Cardiorespiratory arrest
- Sudden severe hypotension. If the blood pressure falls below 60 mmHg, the mechanisms that autoregulate the blood supply to the brain fail.
- Carbon monoxide poisoning

Conditions affecting cerebral blood vessels that may lead to hypoxia are: Occlusion of cerebral artery by atheroma or degenerative changes in elderly.

If the individual survives the initial episode of ischemia, infarction, necrosis and loss of function may result.

Stroke

It is common cause of death and disability especially in the elderly. Predisposing factors include:

- Hypertension
- Diabetes mellitus
- Cigarette smoking
- Atheroma.

It is caused by a disturbance in the brain activity due to interference with its blood supply. If the **blockage** occurs in one of the arteries supplying oxygenated blood to a part of the brain, that part of brain will stop functioning and the cells concerned may die if the stoppage continues for more than a few minutes. The blockage may be due to **clot** forming in the artery itself (**thrombosis**) or from clot elsewhere in the blood circulation and traveling to the brain (**embolism**). There are also several types of **hemorrhages** which may cause stroke.

A person who suffers a major stroke on the right side of the brain and survives will be left with a left hemiplegia, i.e. paralysis of the left arm and left leg and lower half of the face. Sensations on the same areas may be diminished and loss of awareness of objects in the left half of the field of vision. A stroke in the left side of the brain will cause similar disturbances but on the right side of the body and in addition interference with speech function varying from total loss (aphasia) to difficulty in finding correct words (dysphagia).

Recovery from stroke is usually slow, and encouragement of the patient from medical staff, and others is important to restore bodily functions.

A temporary condition that resembles a mild stroke called ***transient ischemic attack*** is caused by temporary blockage of a small artery in the brain but clears shortly and symptoms fade after a few hours, the patient should consult a doctor as there is increased risk of stroke in future.

Cerebral Hemorrhage

It is most serious condition. It occurs in elderly people who have had high blood pressure for long periods or an aneurysm. The artery ruptures deep in the brain and the tissue is damaged by flow of blood under high pressure and the patient loses consciousness within a few minutes of the onset of attack which can be fatal.

The escaped blood may cause arterial spasm, leading to ischemia, infarction or fibrosis and hypoxic brain damage.

A severe hemorrhage may be instantly fatal.

Small repeated hemorrhages have a cumulative effect in brain damage.

If the patient survives the initial stroke a clot of blood forms in the brain and increased pressure inside the skull stops the bleeding. The increase in pressure may lead to interference with the brains control of respiration so that breathing may becomes more labored and may stop unless helped artificially. Such cases surgical treatment may be effective because if clot is removed, life is saved. Disability usually follows.

Cerebral Thrombosis

Cerebral thrombosis is found in older people whose cerebral arteries are the site of atherosclerosis. It is often less dramatic event than cerebral hemorrhage. Consciousness may be preserved and it is not unusual for the patient to find that one arm and leg are weak and mouth distorted by the pull of unopposed face muscles on the nonparalysed side. If the left side of the brain is involved, there is difficulty in speaking. In such cases, recovery may be expected in a few weeks or months.

Intracerebral Hemorrhage

Prolonged hypertension leads to formation of microaneurysms in the wall of very small arteries in the brain. Rupture of one or more of these due to continuing rise in blood pressure is usually the cause of intracerebral hemorrhage. The most common sites are the branches of the middle cerebral artery in the region of the internal capsule and the basal ganglia.

Subarachnoid Hemorrhage

This is mostly due to rupture of an aneurysm in one of the major cerebral arteries or bleeding from a congenital malformed blood vessel. The blood may remain localized but usually spreads to the subarachnoid space around the brain and spinal cord causing generalized increase in ICP without distortion of the brain. The irritant effect of the blood may cause arterial spasm, leading to ischemia, infarction, and the effects of localized brain damage. It occurs most commonly in middle life but occasionally in younger people due to rupture of a malformed blood vessel. This condition may be fatal or results in permanent disability.

Degenerative Diseases

Selective degeneration with ageing can occur in three different types of cells in the CNS, causing three different progressive, crippling and eventually fatal diseases. Degeneration of ***hippocampal neurons*** is associated with ***Alzheimer's disease***. ***Parkinson's disease*** is due to degeneration in ***substantia nigra***. Degeneration of cholinergic motor neurons in the brainstem and spinal cord is associated with one form of ***amyotrophic lateral sclerosis (ALS** or **Lou Gehrig's disease).***

Cytoplasmic form of superoxide dimutase (SOD) is found in many parts of the body. It is defective as a result of genetic mutation in the familial form of amyotrophic lateral sclerosis (ALS). Therefore, it may be that O_2^- (free radical) accumulates in motor neurons and kills them.

Dementia

It is caused by progressive degeneration and atrophy of the cerebral cortex which is irreversible change and results in mental deterioration and progresses over years. There is gradual impairment of memory, especially the short-term memory, intellect and reasoning. Emotional lability and personality changes may occur.

Alzheimer's Disease

This is a dementia of unknown etiology although there is genetic component and occurs after the age of 60 years. Females are more commonly involved. The severity of the disease increases with age. There is progressive atrophy of the cerebral cortex accompanied by deteriorating mental functioning. Death usually occurs in short span of some years after onset.

Huntington's Disease

Usually manifests itself ages of 30 and 50 years, lesion in the neurons in the caudate and putamen caused by genetic abnormality (autosomal dominant disorder) associated with deficient production of GABA from these neurons projecting to pallidum. Rapid uncoordinated jerky movements of the limbs and involuntary twitching of facial muscles occurs.

Demyelinating Diseases

These diseases are caused either by injury to axons or by disorders of cells that secrete myelin, i.e. oligodendrocytes or Schwann cells.

Multiple (Disseminated) Sclerosis

This disease involves loss of part of myelin covering the nerve fibers. Any part of the brain, spinal cord or optic nerves may be affected. The demyelinated white matter, called plaques are irregularly distributed throughout the brain and spinal cord. In early stages, there may be little damage to axons. Most commonly it arises between the ages of 30 years and 45 years.

Some cases start with **episode of partial** or **complete loss of vision in one eye.** Other common early symptoms include double vision, tingling or numbness in one limb, unsteadiness when walking or paralysis of the legs (paraplegia). The cycles of recovery and relapse can go on for many years but there is tendency towards partial or total invalidity. No cure is known at present through certain drugs may help. In some cases, there may be chronic progression without remission or acute disease rapidly leading to death.

Genetically, abnormal myelin is present in many patients and may be antigenic, causing development of autoimmunity. Viral infection by slow-growing viruses that attack myelin has been suggested but no virus has been identified.

Infections of the Central Nervous System

The brain and the spinal cord are fairly well protected from microbial infection by the blood brain barrier. When infection does occur microbes may be:

- Blood-borne from infection elsewhere in the body, e.g. lung abscess
- Introduced through the skull fracture
- Spread through the skull bones from, e.g. ear infection, mastoiditis, skull bone infection
- Introduced during surgical procedure, e.g. lumbar puncture.

The microbes usually involved are bacteria and viruses occasionally protozoa and fungi. The infection may originate in the meninges (meningitis) or in the brain (encephalitis).

The brain, spinal cord and the peripheral nerves may all become infected or inflamed. When the brain is involved it is called encephalitis, or meningitis when meninges are involved. Infection of the spinal cord is myelitis and infection of the nerves is neuritis.

Encephalitis

It is usually caused by virus infection and may cause headache, fever, nausea, drowsiness or coma. Paralysis, numbness, blindness and deafness may also result. Although full recovery may be made, some infections can be fatal or lead to permanent disability.

Meningitis

Meningitis is the inflammation of the membranes that cover the brain and spinal cord. The symptoms of meningitis include headache which may be severe in front of the head or all over.

There is often pain in the back and limbs. The fever may be accompanied by vomiting or in children by fits. Bright light hurts the eye. Patient lie still and want to be left alone, if untreated mental state gradually deteriorates leading to confusion, drowsiness and coma. Viruses are common cause of meningitis. The meningitis may be the only sign of infection or may be complication of mumps, measles glandular fever, hepatitis or other viral infections though this is rare. Meningitis may also be caused by bacteria either spreading from tuberculosis, pneumonia, osteomyelitis or may be only sign of infection. One form is meningococcal meningitis, the result of infection with bacteria.

In all cases of suspected meningitis, a lumbar puncture is performed and CSF examined. There is usually an increase in CSF pressure, pus in the fluid is evidence of bacterial infection, appropriate antibiotic is required. If viral infection is present patient is rested and nursed, complications are watched for to be treated if they arise. Most patients recover.

Rabies

All warm blood animals are susceptible to the rabies virus. The main reservoirs of virus are wild animals some of which may be carriers. There may infect domestic pets which then become the main source of human infection.

The viruses multiply in the salivary glands and are present in large numbers in saliva. They enter the body through skin abrasions and travel to the brain along with the nerves. The incubation period varies about 2 weeks to may be several months. Extensive damage to the basal nuclei, midbrain, medulla oblongata and the posterior root ganglia of the peripheral nerves causes meningeal irritation, extreme hyperesthesia, muscle spasm and convulsions.

Hydrophobia and overflow of saliva from the month are due to painful spasm of the throat muscles that inhibit swallowing. In the advanced stage, muscle spasm may alternate with flaccid paralysis and death may occur due to respiratory muscle spasm or paralysis.

Not all people exposed to virus contact rabies but in those who do, the motality rate is high.

Human Immunodeficiency Virus (HIV)

- Brain is often infected in individuals with AIDS
- Opportunistic infections occur, i.e. minor infections which normally do not produce symptoms of disease affect the individual, as immune system is damaged by the virus. The virus attacks the 'T' helper lymphocytes resulting in their destruction and weak cellular and humoral immunity.
- Infective condition is caused by slow virus and the symptoms of disease may appear after a number of years after the infection with virus.
- The transmission of virus is through blood or body fluids. Hence, infection spreads through sexual intercourse, blood transfusion or by contaminated syringes and needles. It can also spread from mother to child during pregnancy or breastfeeding.

There may be progressive form of dementia for which there is no treatment and hence is fatal.

Neuritis

It is a term for large group of disorders affecting the peripheral nerves anywhere in the body. It is not necessarily due to inflammation, pressure over a nerve or nerve root is a common cause. Occasionally other nerves are involved, and in addition to pain, there is widespread muscular weakness and sometimes paralysis. This condition is called polyneuritis which can have many causes. Polyneuritis may be caused by infections; diphtheria and leprosy are typical examples, or it may be due to untreated diabetes or vitamin B_{12} deficiency. A common form occurs in alcoholics who may experience severe cramp like pains particularly at night, the milder form may be in the form of experience of needles and numbness.

Ophthalmic division of Vth cranial nerve causes trigeminal neuralgia or vesicles form in the cornea when affected, leads to ulceration, virus pass along the sensory nerve to the surface tissue supplied, e.g. skin, cornea. Recovery is slow infection is usually unilateral.

Herpes Zoster Neuritis (Shingles)

Herpes zoster viruses cause chickenpox (varicella) mainly in children and shingles (zoster) in adults. Susceptible children may contact chickenpox from a patient with shingles. Adults infected with viruses may show no immediate signs of disease. The viruses may remain dormant in posterior root ganglia and become active after years causes shingles. Reactivation may be either spontaneous or associated with following factors:

- Local trauma involving dermatome
- Exposure of dermatome to irradiation, e.g. sun, X-ray.
- Depression of immunological system, e.g. drugs, old age, AIDS.

Herpes zoster is a virus infection of a group of nerves. Pain and irritation followed by blister formation in the skin along the course of the nerve. The pain may be severe and last for weeks, and discomfort may last for months.

Acute Disseminating Encephalomyelitis

It is rare but serious condition that may occur during or soon after viral infection, e.g. measles, chickenpox, mumps, respiratory infection. It may develop following primary immunization against viral diseases, mainly in older children or adults.

Guillain-Barré Syndrome

It is a rare condition in which immune system attacks nerves leading to muscle weakness even paralysis. Often occurs after viral or bacterial infection. There is sudden, acute, progressive, bilateral ascending paralysis, beginning with lower limbs and spreading to the arms, trunk and cranial nerves. It usually occurs 1–3 weeks after upper respiratory tract infection. There is widespread inflammation accompanied by some demyelination of spinal, peripheral and cranial nerves and spinal ganglia. Paralysis may affect all the limbs and the respiratory muscles. Patients who survive acute phase usually recover completely in weeks or months.

Motor Neuron Disease

This is progressive degeneration of the motor neurons, occurring mainly in men between 60 and 70 years of age. The cause is unknown. Motor neurons in the cerebral cortex, brainstem and anterior horn of the spinal cord are destroyed and replaced by gliosis. Early affects are usually weakness and twitching of the small muscles of the hand and muscle of the arm and shoulder girdle. The legs are affected later. Death is usually due to involvement of respiratory center in the medulla oblongata.

Sensory Neurons

The sensory functions are lost as a result of disease or injury depending on which neurons have been damaged and their position in the brain or spinal cord or the peripheral nerve involved.

Mixed Motor and Sensory Conditions

Subacute combined degeneration of the spinal cord: This condition most commonly occurs as a complication of pernicious anemia. Vitamin B_{12} is associated with formation and maintenance of myelin sheath by Schwann cells and oligodendrocytes. Although degeneration of the spinal cord may be apparent before anemia, it is arrested by treatment with vitamin B_{12}. This type of degeneration occasionally complicates chronic conditions, such as diabetes mellitus, leukemia and carcinoma. The degeneration of myelin of nerve fiber occurs in the posterior and lateral columns of white matter in the spinal cord, especially the upper thoracic and lower cervical regions. Less frequently in the posterior root ganglia and peripheral nerves are involved. Demyelination of proprioceptive fibers leads to ataxia; and involvement of upper motor neurons leads to increased muscle tone and spastic paralysis.

Diseases of the Peripheral Nerves

Neuropathies

This is a group of diseases of peripheral nerves not associated with inflammation. They are classified as:

Parenchymal (polyneuropathy): When several neurons are affected.

Interstitial (mononeuropathy): A single neuron is usually affected

Parenchymal Neuropathy

Damage to a number of neurons and their myelin sheaths occurs in metabolic or toxic disorders, e.g.

- Nutritional deficiency of folic acid or vitamin B_1, or B_2, or B_6, or B_{12}.
- Metabolic disorders, e.g. diabetes mellitus
- Chronic diseases, e.g. renal failure, hepatic failure, carcinoma
- Toxic reactions, e.g. lead, arsenic, mercury, carbon tetrachloride, aniline dyes and some drugs, such as phenytoin or chloroquine
- Infections, e.g. influenza, measles, typhoid fever, diphtheria, leprosy.

The long neurons are usually affected first, e.g. those supplying the feet and legs. The outcome depends upon the cause of neuropathy and extent of damage.

Interstitial Neuropathy

Usually one neuron is damaged (mononeuropathy) and most common cause is ischemia due to pressure, e.g.

- Pressure applied to cranial nerves in cranial bone foramina due to distortion of the brain by increased BP.
- Compression of the nerve in a confined space caused by surrounding inflammation and edema, e.g. median nerve in carpal tunnel.
- External pressure on a nerve, e.g. an unconsciousness person lying with arm hanging over the side of a bed or trolley.
- Compression of axillary (circumflex) nerve by ill/fitting crutches.
- Trapping of a nerve between broken ends of bones.
- Ischemia due to thrombosis of blood vessel suppling a nerve.

The resultant dysfunction depends on the site are extent of injury.

Bells' Palsy

Compression of facial nerve in temporal bone foramen causes paralysis of facial muscles with dropping and loss of facial expression on the affected side. The immediate cause is inflammation and edema of the nerve but underlying cause is unknown. The onset may be sudden or develop over several hours. Distortion of the features is due to loss of muscle tone and the affected side being expression less. Recovery is usually complete in few months.

Sciatica

The pain is felt in buttock, thigh or leg produced by pressure on the sciatic nerve or on its roots as they emerge from the spinal cord. The most common cause is an intervertebral disc protruding and lying in contract with one or more nerve roots; other causes are disorders within the spinal cord, such as collapse of a vertebra, tumors affecting nerve roots and meninges and disorders within the nerve canal.

The pain of sciatica begins in the back and shoots down the back of the leg to the sole or over to the top of the foot. There may be spasms of the muscles of the back and some movements may become difficult. The treatment includes bedrest and physiotherapy. Use of surgical corset may give relief if required.

Metabolic Disorders

Phenylketonuria

This is a genetic disorder in which the gene needed for synthesizing the enzyme phenylalanine hydroxylase is absent. The enzyme converts phenylalanine to tyrosine in the liver. Phenylalanine is the intermediate metabolite that accumulates in the liver cells and overflows into the blood. In high quantities, it is toxic to the nervous system and if untreated this condition results in brain damage and mental retardation within a few months. Tyrosine is a constituent of the skin pigment melanin and depigmentation occurs: affected children are fair skinned and blonde.

Neuronal Damage

Damage to the nerve cells or their processor can lead rapid necrosis with sudden functional failure or to slow atrophy with gradually increasing dysfunction. These changes are associated with:

- Hypoxia
- Nutritional deficiencies
- Hypoglycemia
- Trauma
- Ageing
- Infections
- Poisons, e.g. organic lead.

Neuronal Regeneration

Neurons of the brain, spinal cord and ganglia reach maturity a few months after birth and are not replaced when they are damaged or die.

The axons of the peripheral nerves may regenerate if the cell body remains intact. Distal to the damage the axon and myelin sheath disintegrate and are removed by macrophages but Schwann cells survive and proliferate within the neurilemma. The live proximal part of the axon grows along with the original tract (about 3 mm per day), provided the two parts of neurolemma are correctly positioned and in close opposition. Restoration of function depends on the reestablishment of satisfactory connections with the end organ. When neurolemma is out of position or destroyed, the sprouting axons and Schwann cells form a tumor; traumatic neuroma that produces severe pain, e.g. following some fractures, and in amputation of limb.

NEUROGLIA DAMAGE

Astrocytes

When severely damaged undergo necrosis and disintegrate. In less severe cases and chronic conditions, there is proliferation of astrocyte processes and later cells atrophy (gliosis). The process occurs in many diseases and is like fibrosis in other tissues.

Oligodendrocytes

They increase in number around degenerating neurons and are destroyed in demyelinating diseases, such as multiple sclerosis.

Microglia

Microglia are derived from monocytes that migrate from blood; found mainly around blood vessels. When there is inflammation and cell destruction microglia increase in size and become phagocytic.

EFFECTS OF POISON ON THE CNS

Many chemical substances either drugs or in the environment may damage nervous system. Neuron metabolism may be disturbed directly or result of damage to other organs, e.g. liver, kidney. The outcome depends upon the toxicity of the substance, the dose, and duration of exposure ranging from short-term neurological disturbance to encephalopathy which may cause coma and death.

EPILEPSY

The epilepsies are a group of disorders characterized by chronic, recurrent paroxysmal changes in neurological function caused by abnormalities in the electrical activity of the brain. Each episode of neurological dysfunction is called a seizure. Isolated nonrecurrent seizures may occur in otherwise healthy individuals for a variety of reasons, and under these circumstances the individual is not said to have epilepsy.

The **seizure** is defined as a paroxysmal involuntary disturbance of brain function that may manifest as an impairment or loss of consciousness, abnormal motor activity, behavioral abnormalities, sensory disturbances or autonomic dysfunction. Some seizures are characterized by abnormal movements without loss or impairment of consciousness. EEG for evidence of generalized or focal abnormality is recorded.

Computed tomography (CT), magnetic resonance imaging (MRI) is done for evidence of structural lesion or idiopathic epilepsy or metabolic abnormality.

Tumors of Nervous System

Tumors involve neuroglial cells as neurons do not multiply. Metastases of these tumors are rare. The growth of the tumor has a space occupying effect that may lead to increased intracranial pressure. Slow growing tumors are called benign and rapidly growing malignant. Signs of raised intracranial pressure appear as the limit of compensatory mechanisms are reached. Hemorrhage in the tumor may suddenly raise the ICP. The compensatory mechanismss involve reduction in the volume of CSF and circulating blood.

Metastases in the brain: Metastases from the tumor cells from breast or lungs are common. May occur in leukemias.

IMPLICATIONS AND APPLICATIONS

- To test various reflexes like biceps, triceps and patellar reflexes.
- To test babinski sign.
- To assist in "Lumbar Puncture".
- To read EEG
- To be able to identify developmental defects like meningocele or meningomyelocele.
- To be able to test all the 12 cranial nerves.
- To be able to test most of the 31 spinal nerves.
- Identify Parkinson's disease (Fig. 12.54).

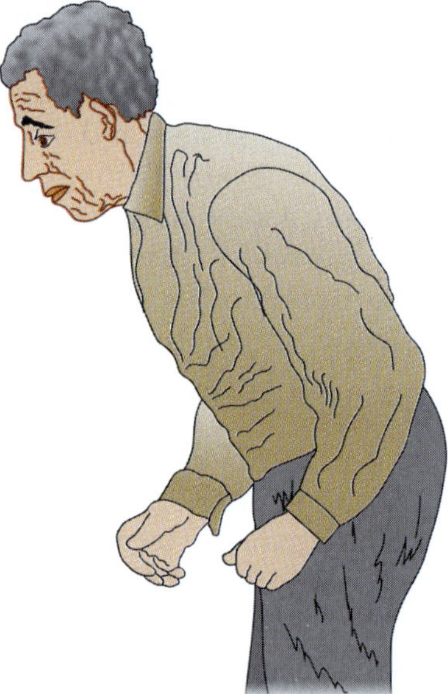

Fig. 12.54: Parkinson's disease

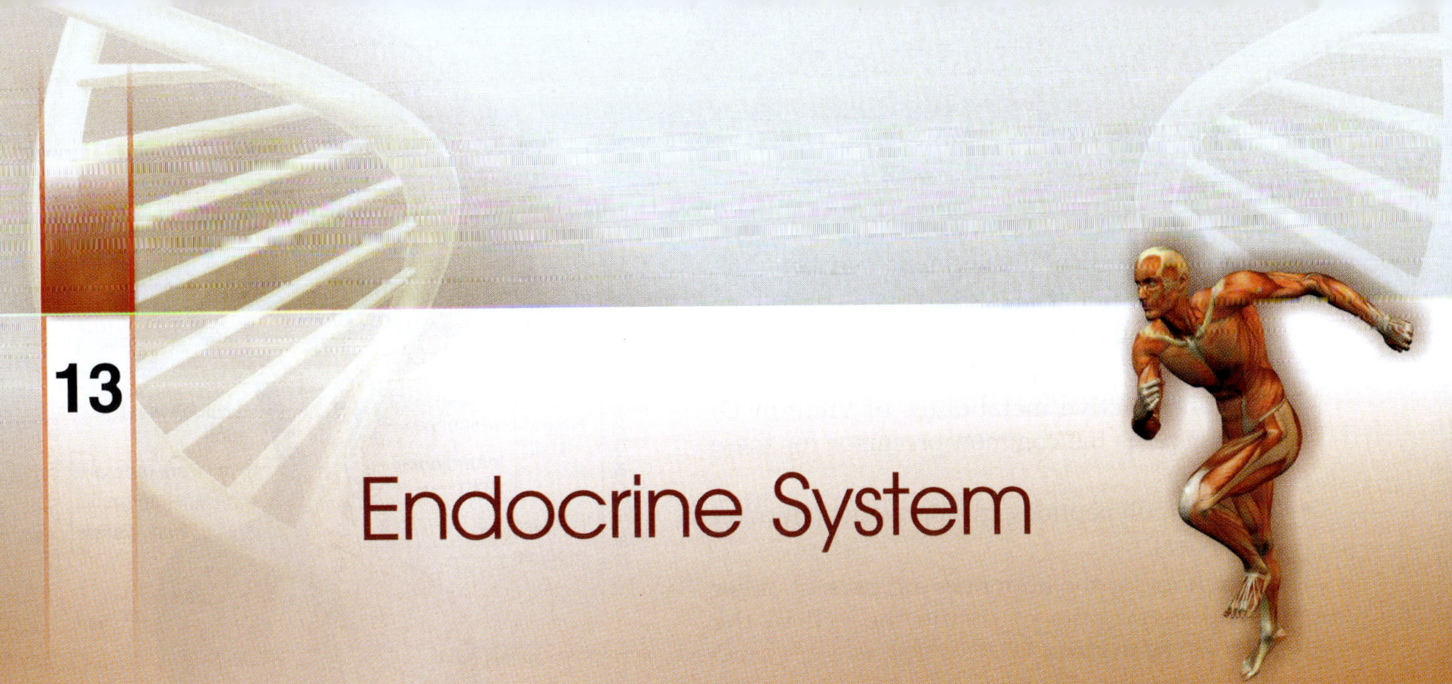

13 Endocrine System

TRANSMISSION OF SIGNALS FROM CELL TO CELL

Involves the following functions:

Endocrine function: Transmission of a chemical signal from an endocrine cell *through bloodstream* to a distant target cell.

Neurocrine function: Transmission of a signal from a neuron *down its axon to release a chemical into blood stream for action* to a distant target cell (as the hormones of posterior pituitary gland).

Synaptic transmission is also chemical transmission, occurs at synaptic cleft from presynaptic neuron to postsynaptic neuron or to muscle end plate.

Paracrine function: Transmission of a chemical signal from one cell type to a neighboring different cell type by *diffusion through intercellular fluid (somatostatin in the islets of pancreas).*

Autocrine function: Transmission of a signal released into the extracellular fluid *back to the cell of origin* or to neighboring identical cells.

Gap junction: Transmission of signal from cell to cell directly without passing through ECF as in cardiac and smooth muscle.

ENDOCRINE GLANDS

The endocrine glands are the glands which pour their secretions (i.e. hormones) directly into the blood to act at a distant site. Hence, these glands are also called ductless glands. The **hormones act** on the cell of the target organ by combining with their **receptors** on these cells.

The combination with the receptors leads to events responsible for the action of the hormone.

The **hypothalamus is the highest center** for the control of hormonal secretions of anterior pituitary, which in turn controls most of the endocrine glands.

The **external environment** influences the functions of some of the endocrine glands and mechanism is by the neural impulses reaching the hypothalamus. Therefore, the nervous system and endocrine system together integrate incoming stimuli to produce changes in responses to the external and internal environment.

The control of the secretions is also under the **negative feedback** effect of hormones; the effect limits the output of each hormone, e.g. when a hormone A stimulates the secretion of hormone B; when the concentration of B hormone is in excess it inhibits the secretion of A, which in turn would reduce the secretion of B: if the concentration of the hormone B is reduced the negative feedback effect on A is reduced, the secretion of A increases and it stimulates the secretion of B. This is the most significant mechanism of regulation of hormone concentration.

Hormones are secreted in the body by:

- Pituitary gland (anterior lobe is also called adenohypophysis and posterior lobe is also called neurohypophysis)
- Thyroid gland
- Parathyroid glands
- Suprarenal glands (adrenal cortex and adrenal medulla)
- Pancreas (Islets of Langerhans)
- Ovaries (Graafian follicles and corpus luteum)
- Testes (Leydig's cells)
- Pineal gland

- Thymus gland
- *Kidneys* and *heart*.

The chemical nature of the hormone may be:

- Amines the catecholamines and iodine containing amino acids the thyroid hormones.
- Steroids (e.g. adrenal cortical hormones, sex hormones, active metabolites of vitamin D) Cholesterol is the common precursor for these hormones.
- Proteins, polypeptides, glycoproteins (all other hormones).

The receptors for the hormones are present either on the cell membrane or inside the cell in the cytoplasm or the nucleus.

THE PITUITARY GLAND

INTRODUCTION

The pituitary gland lies in the hypophyseal fossa of the sphenoid bone below the hypothalamus to which it is attached by a stalk (Fig. 13.1). The fosa is roofed by the diaphragma sellae. The stalk (Fig. 13.2) of the hypophysis cerebri pierces the diaphragma sallae and is attached above to the floor of third ventricle. The gland is of the size of a pea and decreases with age and consists of three parts that originate from two separate structures, the posterior lobe is a downgrowth of neural tissue below the third ventricle, the anterior lobe arises from the Rathke's pouch, an evagination of the roof of the pharynx (Fig. 13.3) but it is closely adherent to the posterior lobe in the adult with the intermediate lobe in between the two; intermediate lobe is rudimentary in humans.

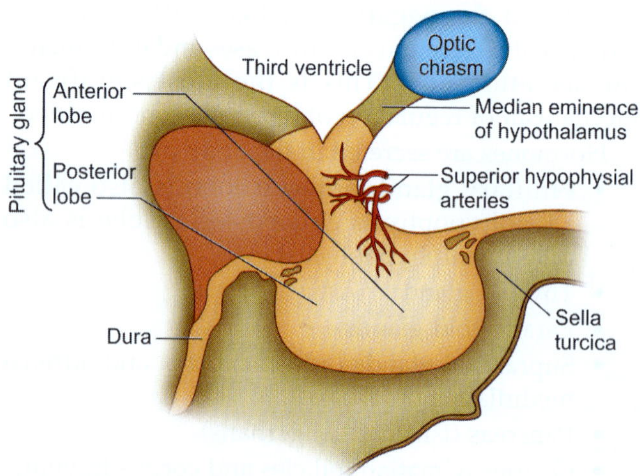

Fig. 13.1: Anatomy of the sella turcica and surrounding structures sagittal view

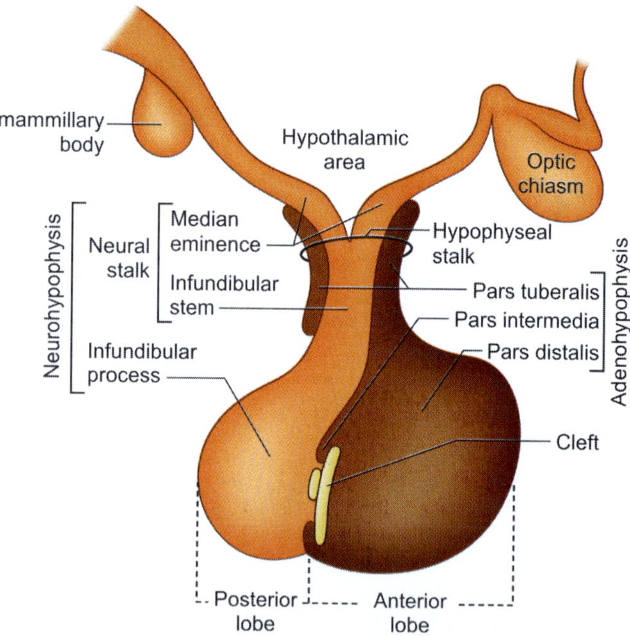

Fig. 13.2: Pituitary stalk and two lobes of pituitary gland

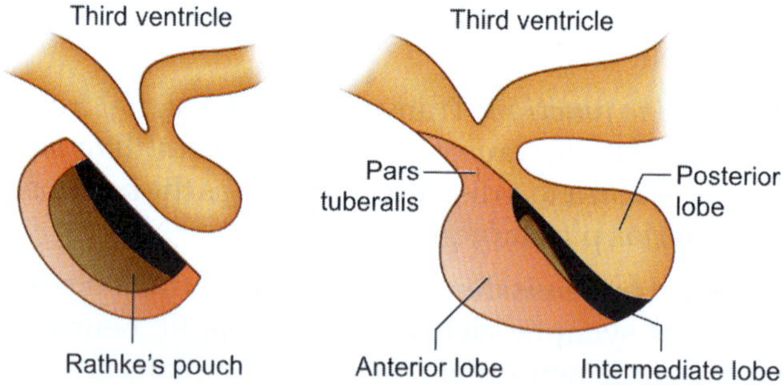

Fig. 13.3: Diagrammatic outline of the formation of the pituitary and the parts of the organ in the adult

Hypothalamic Control

Hypothalamic releases factors called releasing and inhibiting factors, now commonly called **hypophysiotropic hormones**, since they are secreted into the bloodstream and act at a distance from their site of origin.

Hypophysiotropic hormones: The hypothalamic releasing and inhibiting hormones are:

- **Corticotropin-releasing hormone (CRH);**
- **Thyrotropin-releasing hormone (TRH);**
- **Growth hormone-releasing hormone (GRH);**
- **Growth hormone inhibiting hormone (GIH),** (generally called **somatostatin);**
- **Luteinizing hormone-releasing hormone (LHRH)** generally known as **gonadotropin-releasing hormone (GnRH);**

- **Prolactin-inhibiting hormone (PIH)**
- **Prolactin-releasing hormone (PRH)**

Portal Blood Vessels to Anterior Pituitary

The ***portal hypophysial vessels*** form a direct vascular link between the hypothalamus and the anterior pituitary. Arterial twigs form a network of capillaries called the primary plexus on the ventral surface of hypothalamus. The capillaries drain into set of long portal vessels that carry the blood downward to anterior pituitary. These portal vessels give rise to secondary capillary plexus (Fig. 13.4) that supplies the endocrine cells of anterior pituitary with majority of their blood. The system begins and ends in capillaries without going through the heart hence, it is a portal system. The median eminence is generally defined as that portion of ventral hypothalamus from which portal vessels arise.

Anterior pituitary gland lies outside the blood brain barrier.

Hypothalamic Control Over Pituitary Secretions

The hypothalamus influences the secretions of pituitary both anterior and the posterior lobes the nature of control is different.

In the posterior lobe, there are **endings** of the axons of the **cells situated in the hypothalamus**. The hormones of the posterior pituitary are ***synthesized in the hypothalamus***, travel via the axons to the posterior pituitary and they are released from these endings (Fig. 13.4) into the blood vessels of posterior pituitary when appropriate stimuli come from the hypothalamus via these axons to the posterior pituitary.

There are two hormones of the posterior pituitary: **oxytocin** and **antidiuretic hormone (ADH)** also called **vasopressin.** Cells of the posterior pituitary are pituicytes cells which are modified astrocytes.

The anterior lobe is made of cells which secrete the hormones of anterior pituitary. The hormones are **growth hormone prolactin** adrenocorticotopic hormone **(ACTH)** thyroid stimulating hormone **(TSH)** follicle stimulating hormone **(FSH)** and luteinizing hormone **(LH)** FSH and LH are called the gonadotropins.

The anterior pituitary seacretion are controlled by the hypothalamic hormones that reach anterior pituitary through portal hypophysial blood vessels. These hypothalamic hormones (Table 13.1) stimulate and some inhibit the secretions of the anterior pituitary hormones. Five of the hormones are stimulatory for secretions and two of them are inhibitory (Table 13.1).

Hypothalamic Role in Endocrine Functions

Hypothalamus plays a key role in regulating pituitary functions. It can be considered as central relay station for collecting and integrating signals from different sources to affect the function of pituitary. As a result,

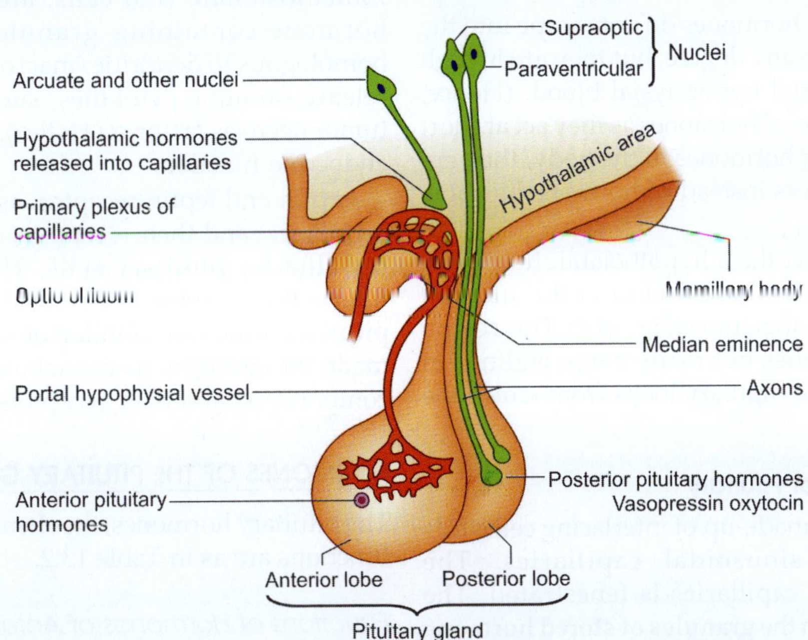

Fig. 13.4: Secretion of hypothalamic hormones. The hormones of the posterior lobe are released into the general circulation from the endings of supraoptic and paraventricular neurons, but hypophysiotropic hormones are secreted into the portal hypophysial circulation from the endings of arcuate and other hypothalamic neurons to reach anterior lobe via portal vessels

Table 13.1: Hypothalamic releasing or inhibitory hormones on target pituitary hormones

Hypothalamic releasing or inhibitory hormones	*Target pituitary hormones*
1. Growth hormone releasing (GRH)	Growth hormone
2. Growth hormone inhibiting hormone (GIH) (somatostatin)	Growth hormone (prolactin, thyrotropin)
3. Prolactin inhibiting hormone (PIH), (dopamine)	Prolactin
4. Prolactin releasing hormone (PRH) (not established)	Prolactin
5. Corticotropin releasing hormone (CRH)	ACTH
6. Thyrotropin releasing hormone (TRH)	TSH (prolactin)
7. Gonadotropin releasing hormone (GnRH)	FSH LH

the pituitary function can be influenced by pain; sleep or wakefulness; emotions; light.

The nervous system receives information about changes in the internal and external environments from the sense organs. It brings about adjustments to these changes through mechanisms which include changes in the rate at which hormones are secreted.

The hypothalamus pituitary axis is also under the influence of blood borne substances from the periphery.

The hypothalamic hormones do not escape into the general circulation to any degree, but they are in high concentration in portal hypophysial blood. (Hence, these are also called local hormones as they act at short distance unlike other hormones in the body; they are also called local factors instead of hormone by some others).

The area from where these hypothalamic hormones are secreted into the bloodstream is the median eminence of the hypothalamus (Fig. 13.4). This region contains few cell bodies but many nerve endings in close proximity to the capillary loops from which the portal vessels arise.

Cell Types in Anterior Pituitary

Anterior pituitary is made-up of interlacing cell cords and network of sinusoidal capillaries. The endothelium of the capillaries is fenestrated. The pituitary cells contain the **granules of stored hormone** that are extruded from the cell by exocytosis, which then enter the capillaries to be conveyed to the target tissues.

Five types of secaretory cells have been identified in the anterior pituitary by immunocytochemistry and electron microscopy. The cell types are somatotropes, which secrete growth hormone; lactotropes (also called mammotropes), which secrete prolactin; corticotropes, which secrete ACTH; thyrotropes, which secrete TSH; and gonadotropes, which secrete FSH and LH. Some cells may contain two or more hormones. The three pituitary glycoprotein hormones, FSH, LH and TSH, while being made-up of two subunits, all share a common α subunit that is the product of a single gene and has the same amino acid composition in each hormone, although their carbohydrate residues vary. The α subunit must be combined with a β subunit characteristic of each hormone for maximal physiologic activity. The β subunits are produced by separate genes. The α subunits are remarkably interchangeable and hybrid molecules can be created. The placental glycoprotein human chorionic gonadotropin (hCG) has α and β subunits.

The anterior pituitary also contains folliculostellate cells that send processes between the granulated secretory cells. Anterior pituitary cells cannot be completely distinguished from each other by conventional histological staining and they are not localized to exclusive areas. Immunohistochemical techniques have permitted each type to be identified.

About 10% of anterior pituitary cells, known as folliculostellate (FS) cells, are devoid of protein hormone-containing granules. These cells are homologous to dendritic/macrophage cells, and they release immune cytokines, such as IL-1, IL-6, and tumor necrosis factor-α (TNF-α), which can modulate endocrine function.

Leptin and leptin receptor, as well as interleukins (cytokines) and their receptors, are also expressed in the anterior pituitary cells. This gives leptin and interleukins a possible role in regulating anterior pituitary function. Similar observations have been made for endogenous cannabinoids (marihuana-like components) and their receptors.

HORMONES OF THE PITUITARY GLAND

The pituitary hormones, the chemical nature and main functions are as in Table 13.2.

Functions of Hormones of Anterior Lobe of Pituitary

Figure 13.5 gives summary of the functions of anterior pituitary hormones, with their sites of action.

Table 13.2: The chemical nature and main functions of the pituitary hormones

Name of the hormone	*Nature of hormone*	*Principal actions*
Anterior Lobe		
1. Growth hormone (GH, somatotropin)	Polypeptide	Accelerates body growth, stimulates secretions of IGF-1 from liver
2. TSH (thyrotropin)	Glycoprotein	• Stimulates growth of thyroid gland • Stimulates thyroid secretions
3. ATCH (corticotropin)	Polypeptide	• Stimulates growth of adrenal cortical zones (zona fasciculata and zona reticularis) • Stimulates the secretions of these zones
4. Prolactin (PRL)	Protein	• Milk production and breast development • Stimulates secretions of milk and maternal behavior
5. FSH	Glycoprotein	• Stimulates ovarian follicle growth in female or spermatogenesis in male
6. LH	Glycoprotein	• Stimulates ovulation and luteinization of ovarian follicles and its secretion in female • Testosterone secretions stimulated in male
Posterior Lobe		
Antidiuretic hormone (ADH), Vasopressin	Peptide	• Promotes water retention
Oxytocin	Peptide	• Causes milk ejection • Contraction of pregnant uterus

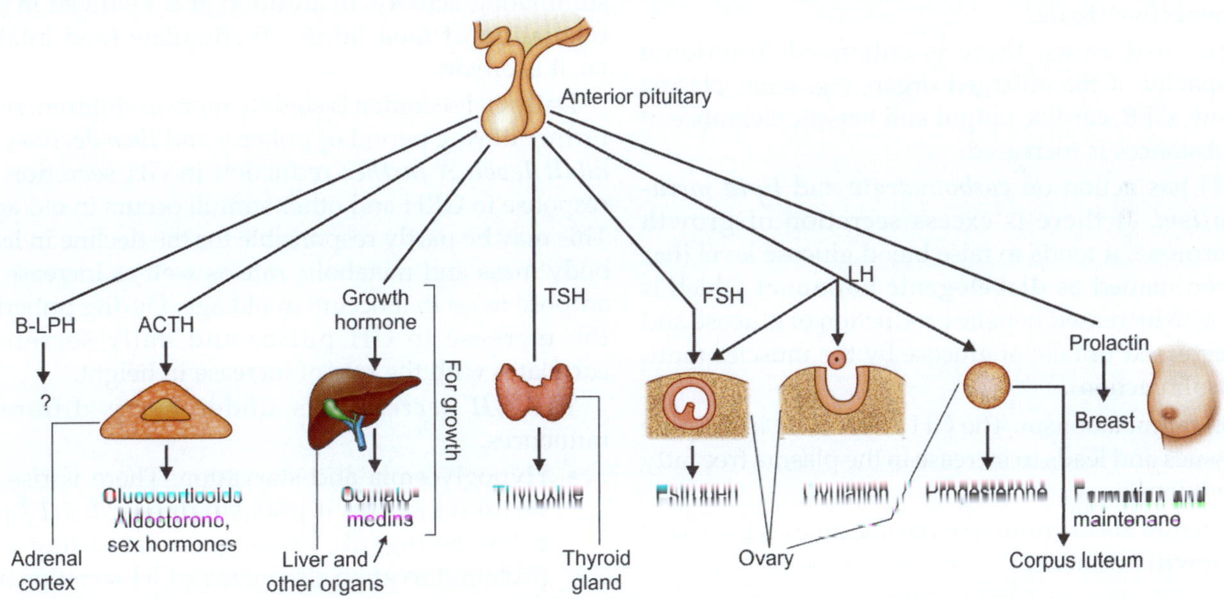

Fig. 13.5: Anterior pituitary hormones. In women, FSH and LH act in sequence. In men, FSH has role in spermatogenesis and LH in secretion of testosterone that has also role in spermatogenesis

Growth Hormone

It stimulates postnatal ***somatic growth*** and development. It helps to maintain normal lean body mass and bone mass in adults. It has numerous actions on ***protein, carbohydrate*** and ***fat metabolism***. It originates in anterior pituitary cells called somatotropes that make-up 40 to 50% of the adult gland. These cells can form tumors that secrete excess growth hormone (GH) that produces disease called acromegaly.

Only primate growth hormone is effective in humans. Until recently, GH deficient individuals were treated with extracts of human pituitary from cadavers. But now, GH is produced by recombinant DNA technology.

Synthesis, Release of GH

The secretion of GH is **increased** by GRH from hypothalamus. Somatostatin from the hypothalamus is powerful **inhibitor** of GH release. Secretion of GH occurs in pulses, that in turn is due to release of pulses of GRH into the portal hypophysial circulation.

Functions of Growth Hormone

- Growth hormone has the most specific effect of stimulating *linear growth of the body* which is as a result of stimulant action on the epiphysial cartilages (or the growth plates), which lay down more bone matrix at the ends of long bones. In its **deficiency,** *growth is stunted.* **Excess secretion** in a child leads to ***gigantism;*** in an adult due to closure of epiphyses linear growth is not possible, but bone and soft tissue deformities occur, the condition is called ***acromegaly.***
- GH stimulates ***uptake of amino acids*** by the cells to increase protein synthesis. Hence, growth hormone has profound **anabolic action**. Visceral organs and endocrine glands share the anabolic response, and also skeletal muscle, heart, skin, connective tissue.

  In most cases, there is enhanced functional capacity of the enlarged organ, e.g. renal plasma flow, GFR, cardiac output and hepatic clearance of substances is increased.
- GH has action on ***carbohydrate*** and ***lipid metabolism.*** If there is excess secretion of growth hormone, it tends to raise blood glucose level (has been named as **diabetogenic hormone**) which is due to increased hepatic production of glucose and decreased uptake of glucose by the muscles (anti-insulin action).
- On fat metabolism. The GH is ***lipolytic*** in adipose tissues and leads to increase in the plasma free fatty acid levels.

Calcium absorption from the intestines is increased by growth hormone.

Mechanism of Action

The growth promoting actions of the GH are believed to be due mostly to the production of **somatomedins** [insulin like growth factors ***IGF***s] produced mainly from ***liver*** and from other tissues due to the action of the growth hormone on these tissues.

Somatomedins are IGFs (i.e. IGF-I and IGF-II). The ***IGF-I*** is believed to promote growth in postnatal life, i.e. after birth, but IGF-II possibly promotes growth in fetal life and not stimulated by GH in postnatal life. When both protein and energy intake is ample, the absorbed amino acids are used for protein synthesis. GH secretion is stimulated by amino acids and with increase in the production of somatomedins, there is increased in the lean body mass. Growth promoting effects of GH are largely by IGF-1. IGFs generated locally by GH in target cells (e.g. osteoblasts) act in an autocrine or paracrine fastion and are more important than plasma IGFs. In hypoglycemia IGF-1 does not increase when GH increase.

Regulation of Secretion of GH

The growth hormone secretion undergoes rapid spontaneous fluctuations in children and young adults and declines in old age. One factor stimulating its secretion is GRH; the factor inhibiting its secretion is somatostatin; both are from hypothalamus; a third factor is probably ghrelin which enhances growth hormone secretion in the presence of stimuli which increase its secretion.

Ghrelin synthesis and secretion occurs mainly in the stomach but it is also produced in the hypothalamus and has a marked growth hormone stimulating activity. In addition, it is involved in the **regulation of *food intake.*** It stimulate food intake, i.e. it is orexin.

Daily GH secretion is slightly more in children, rises further during period of puberty an***d then declines to adult level. A further*** reduction in GH secretion in response to GRH and other stimuli occurs in old age. This may be partly responsible for the decline in lean body mass and metabolic rate as well as increase in adipose mass that occurs in old age. During puberty, the increase in GH pulses and daily secretion correlates with the rate of increase in height.

The GH secretion is under many different influences.

- Hypoglycemia and starvation: There is rise in secretion of GH if ***plasma glucose level falls*** below 50 mg/dL. Prolonged total fasting and protein starvation also increase GH secretion but the somatomedins are not stimulated under such conditions and hence, no growth promoting effects are produced. When protein and energy intake are both ample the absorbed amino acids are used for protein synthesis and to stimulate growth.
- A **high protein meal** or infusion of a mixture of amino acids raises the plasma GH, ***arginine*** is most effective amino acid.
- ***Exercise*** and **stress** of various types increase GH secretion.

- A peak in the growth hormone secretion occurs on going to *sleep* but inhibited during REM sleep.
- GH secretion like other hormones is under the influence of **negative feedback** effects and hence, GH inhibits its own secretion. The mechanism may be via short loop because GH stimulates the synthesis and release of ***somatostatin*** from the hypothalamus.

Somatostatin synthesis and release are also increased by somatomedins which are generated in the periphery mainly from the liver which is now a long loop for inhibition (Fig. 13.6).

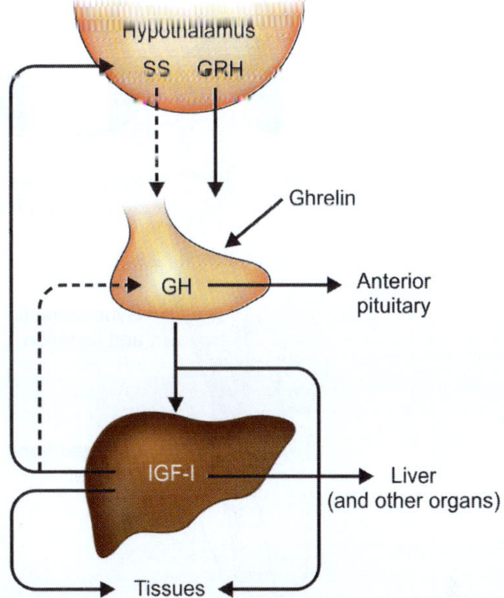

Fig. 13.6: Feedback control of growth hormone secretion. The dashed arrows indicate inhibitory effects and the solid arrows stimulatory effects. GH growth hormone, IGF-1 insulin like growth factor 1, GRH growth hormone stimulating factor, SS somatostatin

Clinical Significance

Clinical Syndromes of GH Dysfunction

Deficiency of GH in children can result from hypothalamic dysfunction; pituitary destruction; a biologically incompetent GH molecule; failure to generate somatomedins normally; or defective receptor of GH or GHRH.

Short stature and delayed bone maturation are the consequences. Puberty is delayed obesity is common.

In adult no obvious signs are evident.

Increased secretion of GH results from pituitary tumors. If hypersecretion of GH begins before puberty is completed, i.e. before fusion of epiphyses of long bones, the individual grows very tall and has long arms and legs condition called **gigantism**.

In adult life, it produces a syndrome of **acromegaly** (Fig. 13.7A and B). In adults, only periosteal bone growth can be increased by GH (as epiphyses are already joined) leading to widened fingers, toes, hands and feet (acro stands for peripheral) prominent bony ridges above the eyes and a prominent lower jaw. Facial features are coarse (Fig. 13.7B). The tongue is enlarged, skin is thick and subcutaneous fat is sparse. All organ sizes are increased. Life span is shortened because of enlargement of heart and atherosclerosis. Glucose intolerance is present and there may be frank diabetes mellitus, damage to the optic chiasm (due to growth of the tumor) causes visual disturbance (Fig. 13.7A).

Prolactin

It is a protein hormone and the main function is **breast development** and **milk production**. Prolactin participates in stimulating the original development of breast tissue and its further hyperplasia during pregnancy. It is the principal hormone responsible for lactogenesis (formation of milk). It influences *reproductive functions.*

The ***cells producing*** this hormone constitute 10–25% of the pituitary cells. They increase in number during pregnancy and lactation and with estrogen treatment. Dopamine inhibits secretion and TRH increases it.

During prepubertal and postpubertal life, prolactin together with estrogen, progesterone, cortisol and growth hormone, stimulates the proliferation and branching of ducts in the female breast.

Prolactin has an important ***role in lactation*** and its ***secretion increases progressively during pregnancy.*** If the new mother does not nurse her child, the plasma level of prolactin declines 3–6 weeks after delivery to normal range of nonpregnant women. With lactation, the suckling maintains elevated level of prolactin secretions.

Normal basal plasma concentration of prolactin is similar in women and men.

Prolactin secretion is tonically inhibited by PIH from hypothalamus; ***PIH*** is possibly ***dopamine*** in nature (unlike other hypothalamic hormones which are peptides in nature).

During pregnancy prolactin along with estrogen and progesterone causes development of lobules of alveoli within which milk production occurs (prolactin action on the milk secretion needs priming by estrogen and progesterone). After parturition prolactin together with insulin and cortisol stimulates milk synthesis and secretion.

However estrogen directly antagonizes the stimulant effects of prolactin on milk production by the breast. Hence, estrogen may be administered to women who do not want to nurse their babies.

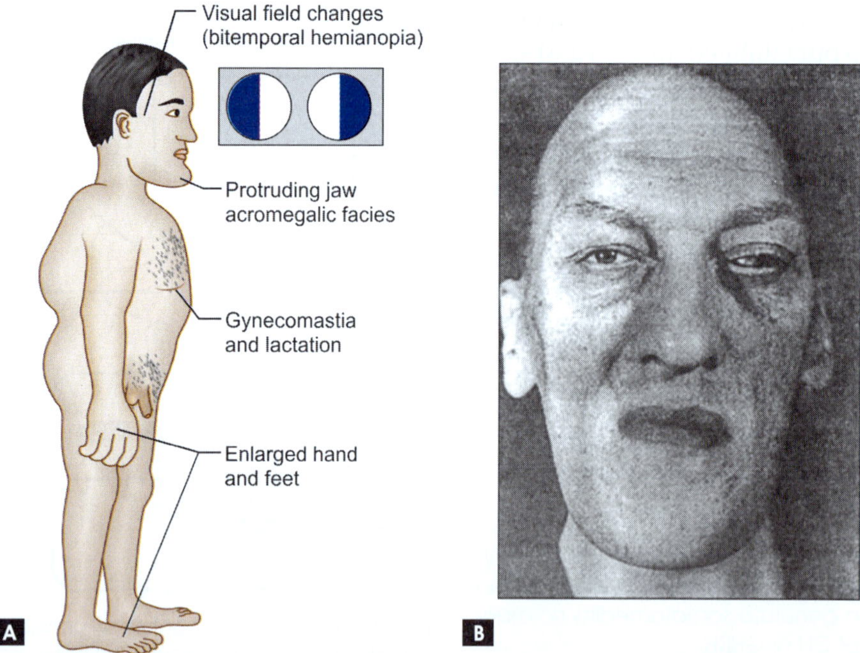

Figs 13.7A and B: (A) Acromegaly (typical findings); (B) Acromegaly in man. Typical facial changes

Prolactin is also present in amniotic fluid; its source is pregnancy modified cells of uterus.

Prolactin has both **stimulating** and **inhibitory** effects on **reproduction**. It possibly is responsible in women who nurse their baby, for not having periods for 25–30 weeks after delivery, against periods after 6 weeks in women who do not nurse. It inhibits ovulation and so only 5–10% women become pregnant again during suckling period. Nursing is known to be important but partly effective method of birth control. Furthermore about 50% of the cycles in the first 6 months after resumption of periods are anovulatory.

Excess prolactin *blocks synthesis and release of GnRH pulses and inhibits its action on pituitary, and antagonizes the action of gonadotropins on the ovaries. It inhibits normal sperm production in males.*

Clinical Significance

Clinical Correlates of Prolactin Dysfunction

Prolactin deficiency in women due to destruction of anterior pituitary results in inability to lactate.

Prolactin excess results from hypothalamic dysfunction or due to tumors of pituitary. In women, this causes complete loss of menses; sometimes lactation unassociated with pregnancy (galactorrhea). In men, decreased testosterone secretion and sperm production results from prolactin excess.

Posterior Lobe of Pituitary

Hormones

The hormones are:

- **ADH or vasopressin**
- **Oxytocin.**

The primary role of **ADH** is to conserve body water and to regulate the **tonicity of body fluids**.

The primary role of the **oxytocin** is to **eject milk** from the lactating breast. It also has a role during **labor.**

Both hormones are synthesized in the cell bodies of the hypothalamic neurons (in the supraoptic and paraventricular nuclei). The hormones travel down the axons in the pituitary stalk; then stored at the endings of axons in the posterior pituitary.

The hormones are released when nerve impulse is transmitted from the cell body in the hypothalamus down the axon. The subsequent passage of the hormone into the bloodstream is by diffusion through pores in the fenestrated capillary endothelium.

Functions of Vasopressin

Its principal effect is retention of water by the kidney and so it is often called **ADH**. It ***increases*** the ***permeability*** of the ***collecting ducts of kidney to water***; allowing it to enter the hypertonic environment of the renal medulla (due to osmotic difference). The receptors on tubular cells with which it combines are called **V_2 receptors.**

The stimulus for ADH secretion is rise in the osmotic pressure of body fluids, **ADH regulates the osmotic pressure of the body fluids.**

As the water is reabsorbed under the action of vasopressin, the urine becomes concentrated and its volume decreases. The overall effect is retention of water in excess of solute and the effective osmotic pressure of body fluids is decreased and regulated.

Hemodynamic control of ADH secretion. A decrease in blood volume or arterial pressure also stimulates ADH secretion. The receptors activated by this response are situated in both the low-pressure (left atrium and large pulmonary vessels) and the high-pressure (aortic arch and carotid sinus) regions.

Both groups of receptors are sensitive to stretch of the wall in which they are located (e.g. cardiac atrial wall, aortic arch and carotid sinus) and are thus called **baroreceptors.** Signals from these receptors are carried in afferent fibers of the vagus and glossopharyngeal nerves to the brainstem. Signals are then relayed from the brainstem to the secretory cells of the supraoptic and paraventricular hypothalamic nuclei. Normally, signals from the baroreceptors inhibit ADH secretion. When blood volume or arterial pressure decreases, this inhibitory input is decreased, ADH secretion is stimulated.

There are three types of stimuli for ADH secretion:

1. Increase in osmotic pressure of ECF
2. Fall in the ECF volume (e.g. hemorrhage)
3. Emotional stimuli, e.g. surgery, exercise, pain, nausea and emotions.

V_1 receptors are present on blood vessels; mediate the vasoconstrictor effect of vasopressin; but relative large amounts of hormone are required to produce vasoconstrictor effect. Hemorrhage is a potent stimulus for ADH secretion. Hence, ADH plays a role in blood pressure homeostasis.

Clinical Significance

In certain clinical conditions, some **nonosmotic stimuli** cause increase in secretion of ADH, e.g. patients who have had surgery may have elevated levels of plasma vasopressin because of pain and hypovolemia. This may cause low plasma osmolality and **low plasma sodium.**

Diabetes insipidus is the syndrome due to vasopressin deficiency or when the kidneys fail to respond to this hormone. Causes of vasopressin deficiency include: disease processes in the region of hypothalamus (supraoptic and paraventricular nuclei), lesion in the hypothalamo-hypophysial tract or in the posterior pituitary gland.

The symptoms of diabetes insipidus are large amounts dilute urine (*polyuria*) that causes thirst that results in drinking of large amounts of fluid (*polydipsia*), provided the thirst mechanism is intact. It is the polydipsia that keeps the patient healthy. If the centre of thirst is depressed for any reason and the intake of fluid decreases, they develop dehydration that can be fatal.

Another cause of diabetes insipidus is inability of the kidney to respond to vasopressin (***nephrogenic diabetes insipidus***) although the secretion of ADH is not affected. In this condition, there is congenital defect in vasopressin receptors (V_2) in the kidney.

Functions of Oxytocin

Oxytocin acts on the breast and uterus. In the lactating breast, it causes contraction of the myoepithelial cells that line the ducts of the breast. This squeezes the milk out of alveoli of the lactating breast into large ducts (sinuses) and hence, out of nipple (*milk ejection*).

Many hormones acting together are responsible for breast growth and secretion of milk into ducts but milk ***ejection requires oxytocin.***

The Milk Ejection Reflex

It is a neuroendocrine reflex. The receptors are touch receptors, which are in the breast especially around the nipple. Impulses are relayed to the hypothalamus, causing secretion of oxytocin; milk is expressed into the sinuses, to flow into the mouth of the infant.

In lactating women, genital stimulation and emotional stimuli also produce oxytocin secretion, sometimes causing milk to spurt from the breast.

Other Actions of Oxytocin

Oxytocin causes contraction of the smooth muscle of the uterus. The sensitivity of the uterine musculature is enhanced by estrogen and inhibited by progesterone. In late pregnancy, the uterus become very sensitive to oxytocin as there is marked increase in oxytocin receptors. Marked increase with oxytocin receptors at this time results in normal levels of oxytocin to initiate contractions. Dilation of the cervix, descend of the fetus down the birth canal initiates impulses that cause increased secretion of oxytocin during labor to enhance labor; setting up a the positive feedback secretion of oxytocin.

THYROID GLAND

The thyroid gland is situated in the neck in front of larynx and trachea weighs about 20 gm. The lobes are about 5 cm long and 3 cm wide. The two lobes of the human thyroid lying on either side of trachea (Fig. 13.8) are connected the thyroid isthmus by a

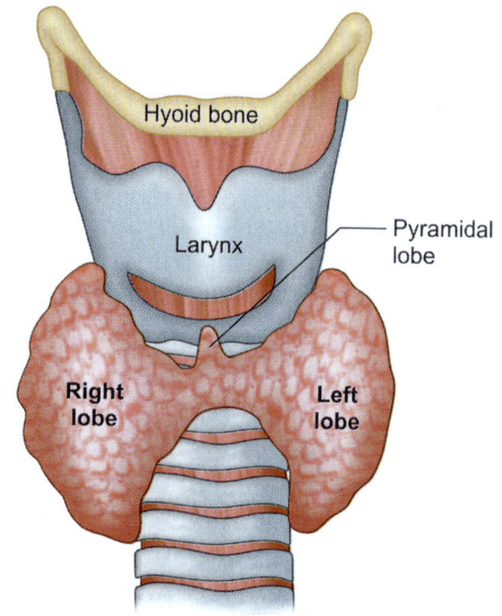

Fig. 13.8: Showing thyroid gland with right, left and pyramidal lobes

bridge of tissue. There is sometimes a pyramidal lobe arising from the isthmus in front of the larynx. The gland receives rich blood supply. The arterial blood supply is through superior and inferior thyroid arteries. The veins from the gland drain into internal jugular veins.

Histological Structure

The thyroid gland is made-up of number of acini (follicles). Each spherical follicle is made-up of single layer of cuboidal epithelial cells and is filled with material called colloid; where newly formed hormone is stored; when the gland is inactive the colloid is abundant, the follicles are large and the cells lining them are flat.

When the gland is active the follicles are small, the cells are cuboidal or columnar and the edges of colloid are scalloped, forming reabsorption "lacunae" (Fig. 13.9). The cell shows droplets of thyroglobulin.

The thyroid cells rest on basal lamina that separates them from adjacent capillaries, the capillaries are fenestrated. Scattered within the gland in close association with the epithelial cells is a separate line of ***parafollicular cells called 'C' cells*** (or clear cells). These are the source of polypeptide hormone, **calcitonin** (Fig. 13.9) which has a role in calcium metabolism.

The hormones of the thyroid gland are:

- Thyroxine (T_4) tetraiodothyronine
- **Triiodothyronine (T_3):** It is also formed in peripheral tissue from T_4.
- Calcitonin.

The T_4 and T_3 are iodine containing amino acids. T_3 is more active than T_4.

Calcitonin is not discussed here but with calcium metabolism. The following description applies to T_4 and T_3.

Synthesis of Hormones

Iodine is raw material for thyroid hormone synthesis. Ingested iodine is converted to iodide and absorbed. The minimum daily iodine intake that maintains normal thyroid function is 150 μg in adults.

Deficiency of iodine intake results in goiter enlargement of thyroid gland due to decreased secretion of its hormones that results in decreased negative

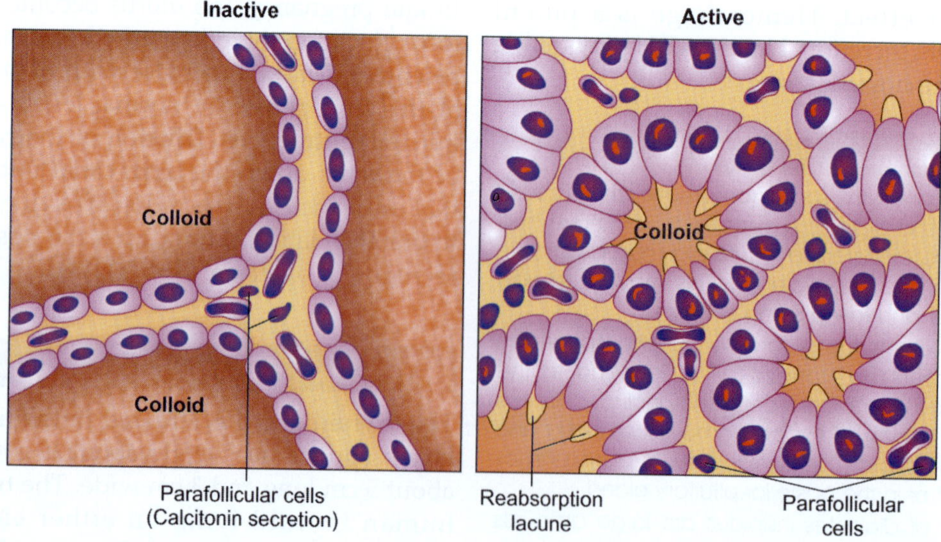

Fig. 13.9: Thyroid histology. "Reabsorption lacunae" in the colloid next to the cells in the active gland

feedback effect on TSH from pituitary, the increased secretion of which enlarges the gland.

The major organs that take-up the iodine are the thyroid which uses it to make thyroid hormones and the kidneys which excrete it in urine.

THE IODIDE PUMP

The thyroid cell membranes facing the capillaries contain a **Na^+/I^- Symporter** (or iodide pump) that transports Na^+ and I^- into the cells against the electrochemical gradient for 1^-.

This pump is capable of producing intracellular 1^- concentrations that are 20–40 times as great as the concentration in plasma. The process is secondary active transport; the I^- enters the cell with sodium that enters due to concentration gradient built up due to transport of Na^+ out of thyroid cells by Na^+ K^+ ATPase, the process that uses energy. The 1^- then diffuses to colloid. The ***Iodide trap*** is essential for normal thyroid function.

Iodide is essential for thyroid function but iodine deficiency and iodine excess both inhibit thyroid function.

Synthesis of Hormone in Thyroid Tissue

In the thyroid gland, iodide is oxidized to iodine and bound to tyrosine residues that are part of thyroglobulin molecule in the colloid.

The thyroid hormones are ***synthesized in the colloid*** (Fig. 13.10), which is then ingested by the thyroid cells; in the cell the hormones T_4 and T_3 are liberated by breaking the bonds with the colloid; and from the cytoplasm of the cell the hormones pas into capillary circulation.

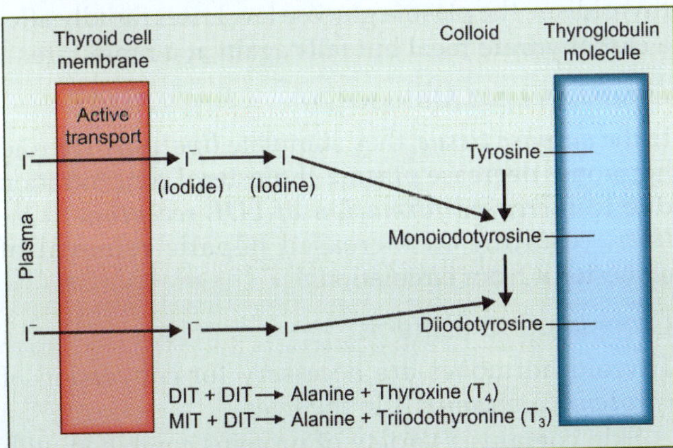

Fig. 13.10: Thyroid hormone synthesis. Iodination of tyrosine takes place at the apical border of the thyroid cells while the molecules are bound in peptide linkage in thyroglobulin

TSH stimulates the process of formation and secretion of the hormones.

Sustained TSH stimulation leads to hypertrophy and hyperplasia of the follicular cells. Thyroid gland blood flow increases.

Plasma Levels of Hormones

Normal total plasma T_4 level in adults is about 8 µg/dL (2 ng/dL is free) and plasma T3 level is approximately 0.15 µg/dL (0.3 ng/dL is free); large amounts of both hormones are bound to plasma proteins. Both hormones are measured by radioimmunoassay. It is the small free level of hormones that are physiologically active; and also inhibit pituitary secretion of TSH in a negative feedback mechanism. The function of the protein binding is for maintenance of readily available part of the hormone.

Physiological Effects of Thyroid Hormones

Calorigenic Action

The most noticeable effect of thyroid hormones is the increase in *basal metabolic rate, oxygen consumption*, and *heat production in all tissues* with the *exception* of adult brain, gonads, spleen and anterior pituitary.

The **resting oxygen consumption** in a normal adult human is about 250 mL/min. In hypothyroid state it may fall to 150 mL/min and in hyperthyroid state increase to about 400 mL/min. In terms of basal metabolic rate (BMR), the BMR may fall up to –40% of normal in hypothyroid state and rise up to +80% of normal in hyperthyroid state. There is a change in the body temperature, a slight rise in body temperature in hyperthyroidism which activates heat dissipating mechanisms. The cardiac output increases to make more oxygen available to tissues in hyperthyroid states, systolic blood pressure is increased and diastolic decreased and there is wide pulse pressure. Decrease in diastolic blood pressure is due to reduction in peripheral resistance because of vasodilatation of skin blood vessels; as the heat loss mechanism are activated. Some of the effects of thyroid hormones in the body are due to stimulation of oxygen consumption.

Effect on Growth and Maturation

Another major effect of thyroid hormones is on **growth** and **maturation** for which it is essential (Fig. 13.11A). In hypothyroid children (Fig. 13.11B), bone growth is slowed and epiphysial closure is delayed An example of role in maturation is their effect on amphibian metamorphosis. Tadpoles treated with T_4

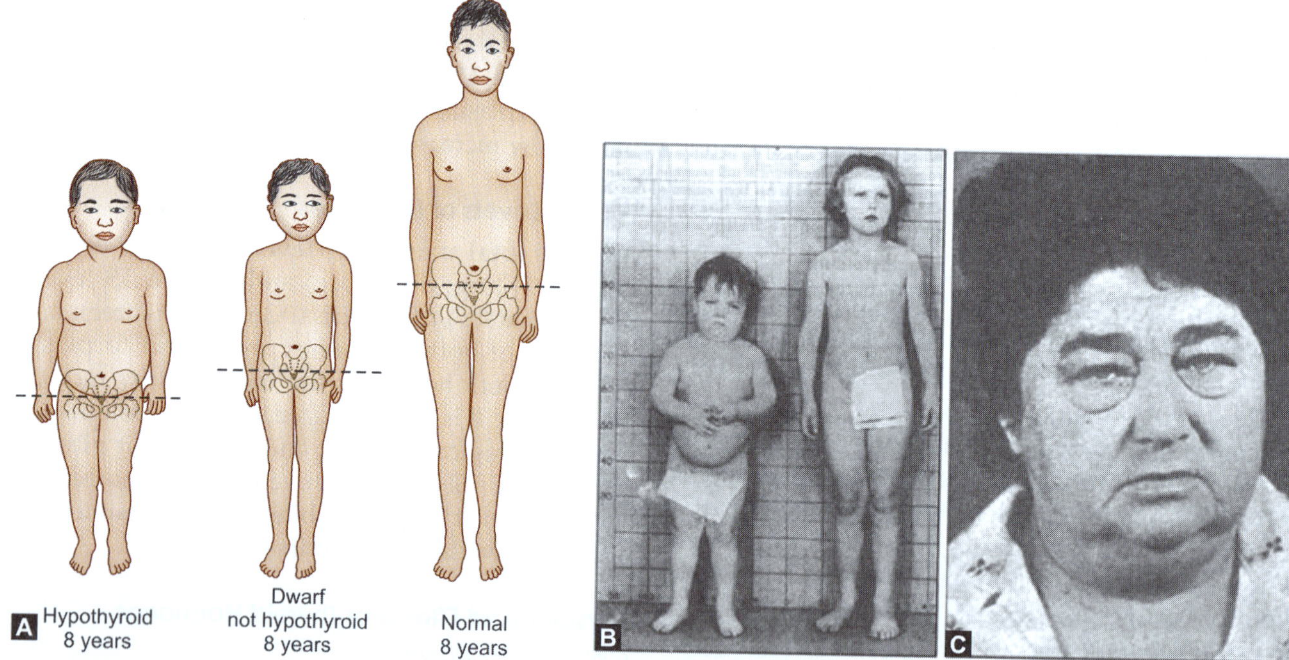

Figs 13.11A to C: (A) Normal and abnormal growth. Hypothyroid dwarfs (cretins) have infantile proportions whereas dwarfs of the constitutional type and of hypopituitary type have proportions characteristic of their chronologic age; (B) Fraternal twins of 8 years age. The boy has congenital hypothyroidism; (C) Hypothyroidism in adult life (myxedema)

and T_3 metamorphose early into dwarf frogs whereas hypothyroid tadpoles never become frogs.

The regular progression of tooth development and eruption is dependent on thyroid hormones; also the normal cycle of growth and maturation of the epidermis and its hair follicles. Excess exposure to T_4 and T_3 also causes desquamation of skin and hair loss.

Clinical Significance

Thyroid hormones have marked effects on **brain development**. The parts of the central nervous system (CNS) most affected are cerebral cortex and the basal ganglia. Cochlea is also affected. Hence, ***deficiency of thyroid hormones during developmental stages causes mental retardation, motor rigidity and deaf-mutism.***

Relation to Catecholamines

The actions of thyroid hormones and catecholamines are related. ***Thyroid hormones increase the number of beta-adrenergic receptors and enhance responses to catecholamines.*** Epinephrine increases the metabolic rate, stimulates the nervous system and produces cardiovascular effects similar to those of thyroid hormones though the duration of action of catecholamines is short.

Although the plasma catecholamine levels are normal in hyperthyroidism, the cardiovascular effects of hyperthyroidism are reduced by drugs which block β-adrenergic receptors responsible for effects by catecholamines.

Effects on Skeletal Muscle

Thyroid hormones increase ***protein breakdown***. Muscle weakness occurs in most patients with hyperthyroidism (***thyrotoxic myopathy***).

Effects on Carbohydrate Metabolism

Thyroid hormones increase the rate of ***absorption of carbohydrates from gastrointestinal tract***. In hyperthyroidism, the plasma glucose level rises rapidly after a carbohydrate meal but falls again at a rapid rate.

Effects on Lipid Metabolism

In the ***adipose tissue,*** they stimulate ***lipolysis***. Thyroid hormones **decrease plasma cholesterol** concentration due to ***increased formation of LDL receptors*** *in the liver*, resulting in increased hepatic removal of cholesterol from circulation.

Other Important Effects

Thyroid hormones are necessary for conversion of ***carotene to vitamin A*** in the liver.

Skin contains a variety of proteins combined with polysaccharides, hyaluronic acid and chondroitin sulphuric acid. In **hypothyroidism,** these complexes accumulate, producing water retention and puffiness of the skin (*myxedema*) (Fig. 13.11C). When thyroid hormones are administered, proteins are metabolized and diuresis clears myxedema.

Regulation of Thyroid Secretion

Thyroid function is regulated primarily by variation in the circulating level of pituitary **TSH. TSH** secretion is increased by ***TRH*** from hypothalamus; and is ***inhibited by negative feedback*** mechanism by circulating free T_4 and T_3 (Fig. 13.12) by the free levels.

TSH secretion is inhibited by **stress** and in experimental **animals it is increased by cold** and decreased by warmth.

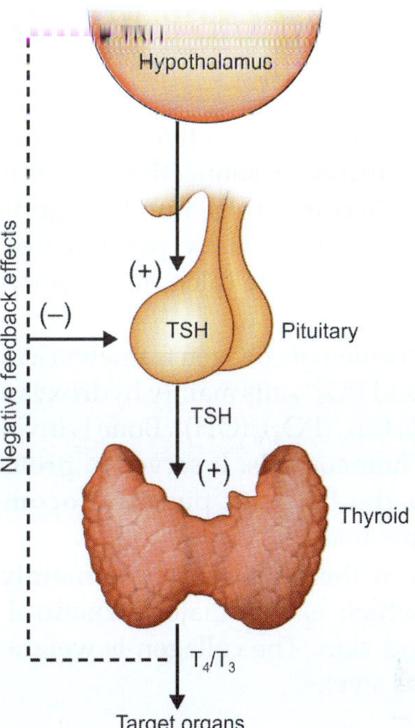

Fig. 13.12: The hypothalamic-pituitary-thyroid axis and negative feedback effects

Clinical Significance

Hypothyroidism

1. **Cretinism:** A child with hypothyroidism from birth or earlier is called a cretin. The child is ***dwarf*** (Fig. 13.11A and B) and ***mentally retarded***. Tongue is enlarged and protruding; potbelly is obvious. If hypothyroidism is present at birth and remains untreated for even 2–4 weeks, the central nervous system will not undergo its normal maturation process in its first year and milestones, such as sitting, standing and walking will be late and severe mental retardation can result in the cretin. Treatment started at birth can result in good prognosis and mental retardation may be avoided.
2. **Myxedema:** Hypothyroidism in adult is called myxedema (Fig. 13.11C).There is **puffiness of the skin**. Hypothyroidism may be a result of disease of thyroid gland, or may be due to pituitary failure or hypothalamic failure. **BMR is low;** ***voice is husky and slow***; hence, myxedema can be diagnosed over telephone. ***Mentation is slow***; memory is poor; plasma cholesterol elevated; hair is coarse; skin is dry and yellowish (carotenemia); ***cold is poorly tolerated***.

Hyperthyroidism

The symptoms are ***nervousness; weight loss***; hyperphagia (increased food intake); ***heat intolerance***; increase in pulse pressure; ***fine tremor*** of stretched fingers; warm soft skin; sweating; a ***high BMR***.

Most common cause is ***Graves' disease*** which is **autoimmune** disease; in which there is formation of antibodies to TSH receptors; these stimulate the receptor rather than blocking them, resulting in marked T_4 and T_3 secretion and enlargement of gland (goiter); ***plasma TSH is low***.

Another feature of Graves disease is the occurrence of swelling of tissues in the orbits, producing protrusion of the eyeballs (**exophthalmos**), in some of the patients (Fig. 13.13).

Causes of hyperthyroidism are enumerated in Table 13.3.

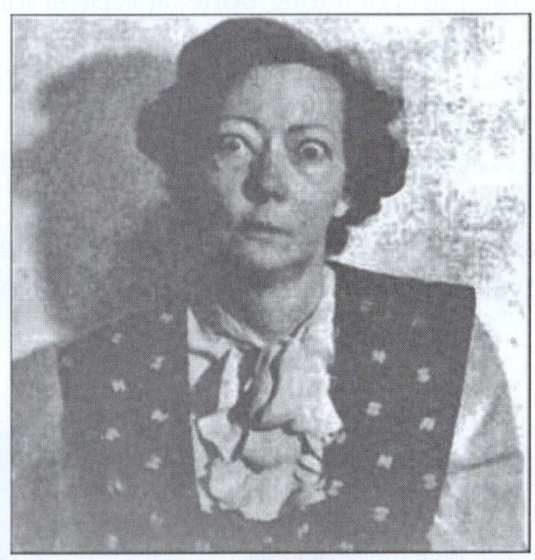

Fig. 13.13: Graves' disease in a woman. Enlargement of thyroid and exophthalmos

Table 13.3: Causes of hyperthyroidism

Causes
Thyroid overactivity
Grave's disease
Mutations causing constitutive activation of TSH receptor
Solitary toxic adenoma
Toxic multinodular goiter
Thyroiditis
TSH-secreting pituitary tumor
Extrathyroidal
Ectopic thyroid tissue
Administration of T_3 or T_4

BONE PHYSIOLOGY

REVIEW OF ANATOMY

Bone is specialized connective tissues having all the common features of connective tissue like ground substance, fibers and cells. But, this rigid supporting tissue is characterized by presence of inorganic mineral salts especially calcium and phosphate in its matrix.

Bone is formed of collagen framework impregnated with Ca^{2+} and PO_4^{3-} salts mainly hydroxyapatites, with the formula $Ca_{10}(PO_4)_6(OH)_2$. Bone is involved in **Ca^{2+} and PO_4^{3-} homeostasis.** It serves to **protect the vital organs** in the body. It permits **locomotion** and **supports** the body.

Protein in the bone matrix is mainly of type 1 collagen which is also major structural protein in tendons and skin. The collagen is weight for weight as strong as steel.

Structure of Bone

The structures of a bone may be analyzed by considering the parts of a long bone. A typical long bone consists of following parts:

1. **Diaphysis** is bone's **shaft,** the long, cylindrical, main portion of the bone.
2. **Epiphyses** are the distal and proximal ends of the bone (Fig. 13.14).
3. **Metaphysis** are regions in mature bone where diaphysis joins the epiphysis. In a growing bone, each metaphysis includes an **epiphyseal plate** (layer of hyaline cartilage that allows diaphysis of bone to grow in length). When bone growth stops in length the resulting bone structure is known as **epiphyseal line.**
4. **Articular cartilage** is a thin layer of hyaline cartilage covering the epiphysis where bone forms a joint with another bone (Fig. 13.14B).
5. **Medullary cavity/marrow cavity** is space within the diaphysis that contains fatty yellow bone marrow in adults.
6. **Periosteum** is tough sheath of dense connective tissue that surrounds the bone surface wherever it is not covered by articular cartilage. Periosteum plays a role in **healing of fractures**. It also serves as an **attachment** point for ligaments and tendons.
7. **Endosteum** is a thin membrane lining the medullary cavity. It contains a **single layer of bone forming cells** and a small amount of connective tissue.

Histology of Bone Tissue

Bone tissue contains an abundant matrix of intercellular material that surrounds the widely separated cells. The matrix contains water (25%), collagen fibres (25%) and crystallized inorganic mineral salts (50%) mainly hydroxyapatite (calcium phsophate and calcium carbonate). These mineral salts are deposited in framework formed by collagen fibres of the matrix. Four types of cells are present in bone tissue.

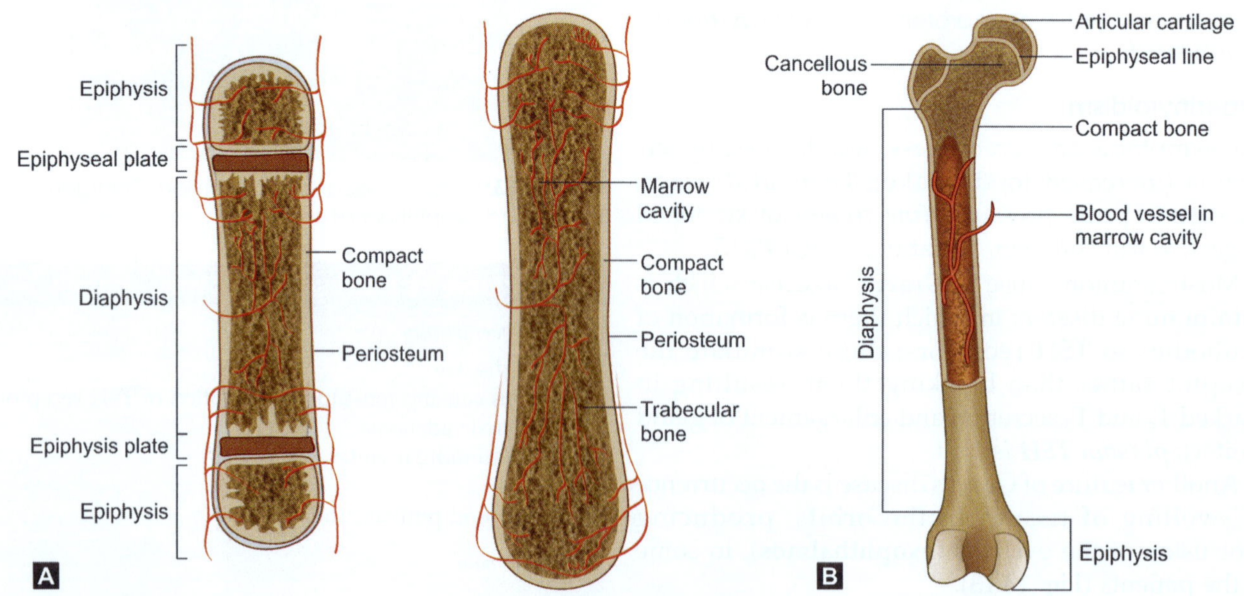

Figs 13.14A and B: (A) Structure of long bone before (left) and after epiphyseal closure (right), (B) Structure of long bone with articular cartilage

1. **Osteogenic cells are stem cells from which bone cells are formed.** They are the only bone cells to undergo cells division, the resulting daughter cells develop into osteoblasts. These are found in periosteum, endosteum and in canals within bone that contain blood vessels.
2. **Osteoblasts** are bone building cells. They *synthesize and secrete collagen fibres* and other organic components needed to build the matrix of bone tissue. They **initiate ossification.** These cells surround themselves within the matrix and become trapped in their secretions and become osteocytes.
3. **Osteocytes** are mature bone cells. They are main cells in bone tissue. They maintain metabolism of bone tissue.
4. **Osteoclasts** are large cells members of monocyte family and are present in endosteum. They cause breakdown of bone matrix, termed **resorption** which is part of normal **development, growth, maintenance** and **repair** of bone.

Bone tissue is classified as either compact or cancellous depending on how its matrix and cells are organized and size and distribution of spaces between its cells and matrix (Fig. 13.15).

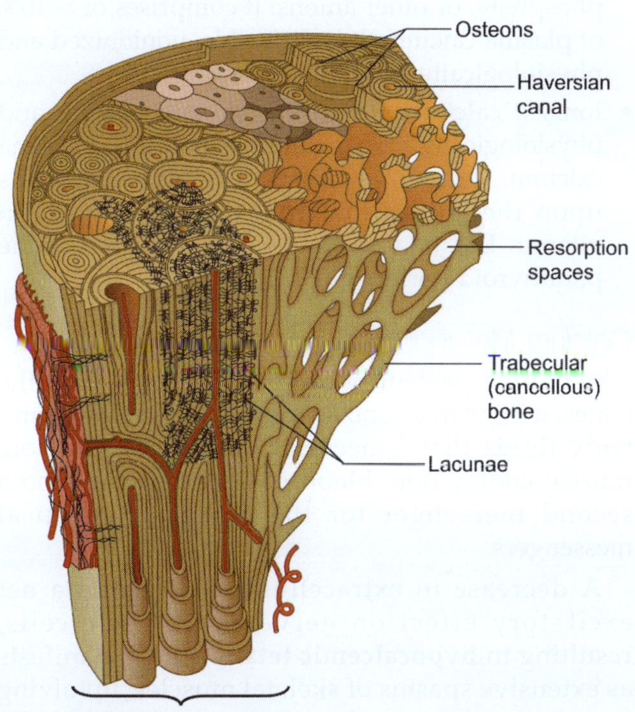

Fig. 13.15: Structure of compact and trabecular bone. The compact bone is shown top and left, cancellous bone on the right

Compact Bone

Compact bone contains few spaces. It forms external layer of all bones and makes up bulk of shaft of long bones. It provides protection and support and resists the stresses produced by weight and movement.

Unit of compact bone is **osteon or Haversian system** (Fig. 13.16).

Blood vessels, lymphatics and nerves from periosteum penetrate the compact bone through transverse **perforating (Volkmann's) canals.** The vessels and nerves of Volkmann's canals connect with those of medullary cavity, periosteum and **central (Haversian canals).** Central canals run longitudinally through the bone.

Around the central canals are **concentric lamellae** (rings of hard, calcified matrix). Between lamellae are small spaces called **lacunae** which contain **osteocytes.** Osteons in compact bone are aligned in same direction along lines of stress. From lacunae, **canaliculi** radiate in all directions. Canaliculi link the lacunae with each other and with Haversian canals. Canaliculi provide route for nutrients and oxygen to reach the osteocytes and for wastes to diffuse away.

The areas between osteons contain **interstitial lamellae** which are fragments of older osteons.

Concellous Bone

The cancellous bone does not contain osteons. It consists of **trabeculae,** an irregular framework of thin columns of bones. Spaces between trabeculae of some bones are filled with **red bone marrow.** Within each trabecula are osteocytes that lie in lacunae. Radiating from the lacunae are canaliculi.

Cancellous or spongy bone is present in short, flat and irregularly shaped bones, epiphyses of long bones and in a narrow rim around the medullary cavity of

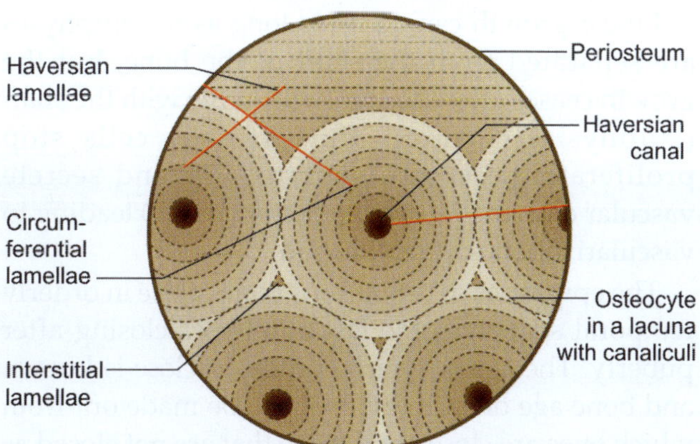

Fig. 13.16: The Haversian system

diaphyses of long bones. Red bone marrow is present in cancellous bone of hip bones, sternum and vertebrae.

In the compact bone the surface to volume ratio is low; **bone cells** lie in the **lacunae.** They receive nutrition by way of canaliculi that ramify throughout the compact bone. **Haversian canals** contain blood vessels. Around each Haversian canal collagen is arranged in concentric rings forming osteons or **Haversian system** (Fig. 13.16). Trabecular bone is made-up of plates which have high surface to volume ratio and there are many cells on the surface of plates. Nutrients diffuse from bone eaxtracellular fluid (ECF) into trabeculae.

Bone Remodeling

Bone is **dynamic** and is constantly being resorbed and new bone formed. This remodeling allows it to respond to stresses and strains. It is living tissue and is well vascularized and has a total blood flow of 200–400 mL/min in adults.

Bone Growth and Development

During fetal life most of the bones are modeled in cartilage and then transformed into bone by ossification (enchondral bone formation). The exceptions are the clavicles, and mandibles and certain bones of the skull in which mesenchymal cells form bone directly (intramembranous bone formation).

During growth areas at the ends of each long bone (epiphyses) are separated from the shaft of the bone by a plate of actively proliferating cartilage the epiphysial plate (Fig. 13.14A). The bone increases in length as this plate lays down new bone at the end of the shaft. The width of the epiphysial plate is proportionate to the rate of growth. The width is affected by a number of hormones most markedly by GH from pituitary and IGF-I.

Linear growth can occur as long as the epiphyses are separated from the shaft of the bone, but the growth ceases after the epiphyses unite with the shaft (epiphysial closure). The cartilage cells stop proliferating, become hypertrophic and secrete vascular endothelial growth factor (VEGF) leading to vascularization and ossification.

The epiphyses of the various bones close in orderly temporal sequence, the last epiphyses closing after puberty. The age at which epiphyses close is known and bone age of an individual can be made out from which ones are closed and those that are not closed as seen on X-ray examination.

Bone Cells

The cells for the formation of bone are osteoblasts and cells responsible for resorption of bone are called osteoclasts.

Throughout life bone is constantly resorbed and new bone is formed. Bone remodeling is mainly a local process carried out in small areas (Fig. 13.17).

Osteoclasts erode and absorb previously formed bone. Bone modeling involves resorption by osteoclasts and then osteoblasts lay down new bone in the same area the process takes about 100 days. Modeling drifts also occur in which shapes of bone change. Osteoclasts tunnel into cortical bone followed by osteoblasts. In trabecular bone remodeling occurs on the surface of trabeculae. With age the periosteum becomes thinner and loses some vasculative. This renders bone to injury and diseases.

Plasma Calcium

Plasma calcium level is 8.5–10.5 mg/dL. It exists in three different forms:

- Protein bound calcium: This form is loosely bound almost entirely to plasma albumin. It is non-diffusible, nonionized calcium comprising of 40–45% of plasma calcium.
- Complexed calcium: It is combined with citrate, phosphate, or other anions. It comprises of 5–10% of plasma calcium. It is diffusible, nonionized and physiologically inactive.
- Ionised calcium. It is diffusible and ionized and physiologically active, comprising of 50% of plasma calcium. The ionized plasma calcium level depends upon the absorption from the gut (hence, on vitamin D_3), and on the level of secretion of the parathyroid hormone (PTH).

Calcium Metabolism

Ninety-nine percent of the body calcium is in the bones. It is the free, ionized calcium in the plasma and body fluids that is necessary for nerve function, muscle contraction, blood coagulation and also a second messenger for the action of chemical messengers.

A decrease in extracellular Ca^{2+} exerts a net excitatory effect on nerve and muscle cells, resulting in **hypocalcemic tetany** which manifests as extensive spasms of skeletal muscles, involving especially the muscles of extremities and the larynx. Laryngospasm may become so severe that the airway is obstructed and fatal asphyxia is produced.

Ca^{2+} plays an important role in clotting, but *in vivo* the level of plasma Ca^{2+} at which fatal tetany occurs is above the level at which clotting defects would occur.

The extent of Ca^{2+} binding by plasma protein is proportionate to the plasma protein level. Plasma ionized calcium can be measured by use of a calcium sensitive electrode. Other **electrolyte and pH affect plasma Ca^{2+}** level. Symptoms of tetany appear at much higher total calcium level if patient hyperventilates as it **increases plasma pH**. Plasma proteins are more ionized when pH is high, providing more protein anion to bind Ca^{2+}.

PARATHYROID GLANDS

There are usually **four parathyroid glands**, two embedded close to the superior poles of thyroid and two in its inferior poles (Fig. 13.18). But, the location and their number can vary. Parathyroid tissue is sometimes found in the mediastinum. The glands contain two types of cells; most plentiful are main cells that synthesize and secrete the parathyroid hormone **(PTH)**; less plentiful are oxyphil cells (Fig. 13.19), the function of which is not known.

PTH is a single chain polypeptide. Synthetic polypeptide has all the action of the hormone. Its

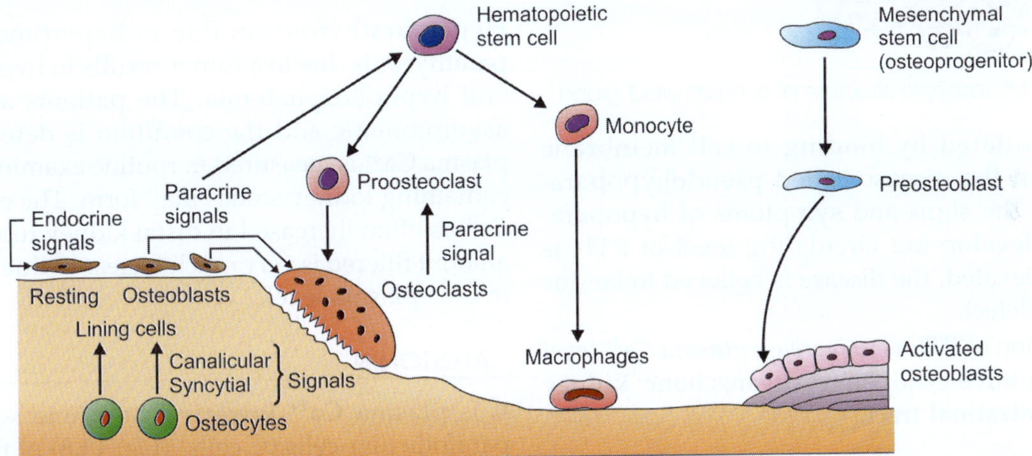

Fig. 13.17: Process of bone remodeling. Signals carried by canalicular and syncytial routes from interior osteocytes, and endocrine signals to resting osteoblasts and lining cells generate local paracrine cytokine signals to nearby osteoclasts and osteoclast precursors. Osteoclasts also recruit their own precursors by paracrine signals. The osteoclasts resorb an area of mineralized bone, and local macrophages complete the clean-up of dissolved elements. The process is then formation as osteoblast precursors recruited to the site and differentiate into active osteoblasts. These lay then new organic matrix and mineralize it. Thus, new bone replaces the previously resorbed mature bone

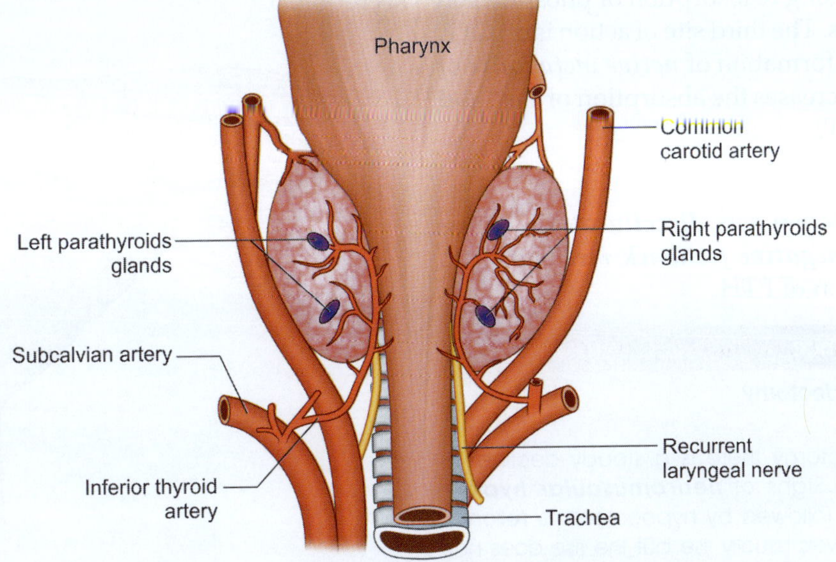

Fig. 13.18: The parathyroid glands, viewed from behind

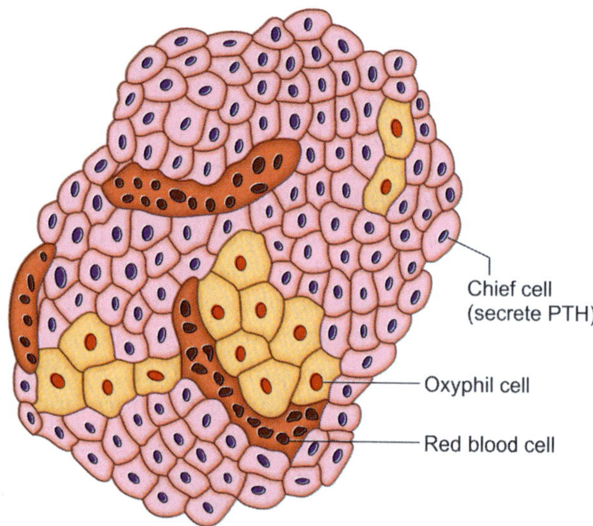

Fig. 13.19: Microscopic structure of a parathyroid gland

action is initiated by binding to cell membrane receptors. In the disease called pseudohypoparathyroidism, the signs and symptoms of hypoparathroidism develop but circulating level of PTH is normal or elevated; the disease is believed to be due to receptor defect.

The function of ***PTH is to increase plasma Ca^{2+} level*** by acting on three major target organs; **bone**; **kidney** and **gastrointestinal tract**.

Functions

PTH acts **directly on bone** to increase bone ***resorption and mobilize Ca^{2+}***. PTH also increases *reabsorption of Ca^{2+} in the distal tubules of* **kidney** and hence, PTH ***increases plasma Ca^{2+} level***; it decreases plasma phosphate level as it increases phosphate excretion in the urine, by decreasing reabsorption of phosphate in the proximal tubules. The third site of action is on **GIT**; PTA stimulates the formation of ***active metabolite of vitamin D*** which increases the absorption of Ca^{2+} and phosphate from GIT.

Regulation of Secretion

Plasma ***ionized calcium*** acts ***directly on the parathyroid glands*** in ***negative feedback mechanism*** to regulate the secretion of PTH.

Clinical Significance

Effects of Parathyroidectomy

PTH is essential for life.

After parathyroidectomy there is a steady decline in plasma Ca^{2+} level. Signs of ***neuromuscular hyperexcitability*** appear, followed by hypocalcemic ***tetany***. Plasma phosphate levels usually rise but the rise does not always occur.

Tetany commonly occurs due to accidental removal of parathyroids during thyroid surgery. Symptoms usually develop 2–3 days after operation but may not appear for several weeks or more.

The sign of tetany in humans include **Chvostek's sign**, a quick contraction of ipsilateral facial muscles on tapping over the facial nerve at the angle of the jaw; and **Trousseau's sign** (Fig. 13.20), a spasm of muscles of the upper extremely that causes flexion of the wrist and thumb and extension of fingers. In individuals with mild tetany in whom spasm is not evident Trousseau's sign could sometimes be produced by occluding the circulation for a few minutes with a blood pressure cuff.

Parathyroid Hormone Excess

Hyperparathyroidism due to hyperfunctioning of parathyroids due to a tumor results in hypercalcemia and hypophosphatemia. The patients are usually asymptomatic and the condition is detected when plasma Ca^{2+} is measured in routine examination. Ca^{2+} containing kidney stones may form. The excretion of Ca^{2+} is often increased in distal kidney tubules as the amount filtered is very much increased due to increase in Ca^{2+} plasma level.

CALCITONIN

It is plasma **Ca^{2+} lowering** hormone secreted by parafollicular cells (C cells) (Fig. 13.8) of the thyroid gland. It lowers both Ca^{2+} and phosphate level in plasma. When plasma Ca^{2+} level rises, the hormone is secreted. It is not secreted until the plasma level Ca^{2+} reaches approximately 9.5 mg/dL; above this level it is secreted in direct proportion to the rise in plasma calcium level. Estrogen also stimulates calcitonin secretion.

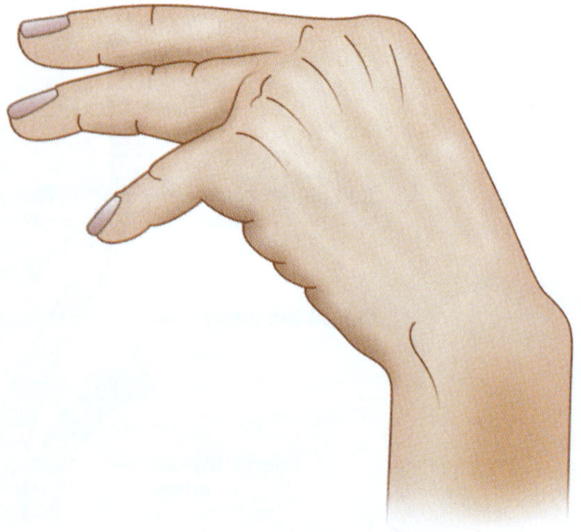

Fig. 13.20: Trousseau's sign in tetany

Functions

Calcitonin lowers the circulating calcium and phosphate levels in the plasma. Its receptors are present in **bone** and **kidney**. In bone, it inhibits bone resorption. It inhibits the activity of osteoclasts. It also increases amount of calcium in the urine as it inhibits calcium reabsorption in the kidney.

Clinical Significance

Calcitonin is useful in treatment of Paget's disease which is due to increased osteoclastic activity resulting in disorganized bone formation.

It is beneficial in severe hypercalcemia, but as the hormone is to be injected the effect wears off.

Estrogens *prevent osteoporosis* by inhibiting the stimulating effect of certain cytokines on osteoclasts.

VITAMIN D

The active absorption of Ca^{2+} and Po_4^{3-} from the intestine is increased by a metabolite of vitamin D. Vitamin D is produced by the action of ultraviolet light on provitamins in the skin. vitamin D_3 also called cholecalciferol, in produced by action of light on the skin.

Vitamin D_3 is also ingested in the diet. In the liver, D_3 is converted to 25-hydroxycholecalciferol (25-OHD$_3$) or calcidiol and this is further converted in the proximal tubules of the kidney to the more active metabolite, 1, 25 dihydroxycholecalciferol, which is also called 1, 25-$(OH)_2D_3$, or calcitriol.

Vitamin D_3 and its derivatives are steroids. 1, 25-$(OH)_2D_3$ is a hormone because it is produced in the body and transported in the bloodstream to produce effects on target cells.

Functions

1, 25-$(OH)_2D_3$ (i.e. active metabolite of vitamin D_3) increases ***Ca^{2+} absorption from intestine***; it facilitates Ca^{2+} reabsorption in the kidneys; increases ***synthetic activity of osteoblasts*** and is necessary for **normal calcification of the bone matrix.**

Recent evidence has shown that it stimulates the **differentiation of immune cells** and keratinocytes in

Clinical Significance

Rickets and Osteomalacia

Vitamin D deficiency causes defective calcification of bone matrix and the disease is called **rickets** in children and **osteomalacia** in adults. The main defect is failure to deliver adequate amounts of Ca^{2+} and Po_4^{3-} to the sites of mineralization. The condition in children is characterized by weakness and bowing of weight bearing bones, dental defects and hypocalcemia.

In adults, the condition is less obvious though if there are repeated pregnancies and the diet is poor in vitamin D_3, the effects may become obvious.

Mutation of the gene for the receptor can cause the disease.

All above three hormones (PTH, calcitonin, and vitamin D_3) operate together to maintain Ca^{2+} levels in the body fluids. Glucucorticoids, growth hormone and estrogen also affect calcium metabolism.

Osteoporosis

It has multiple causes, commonest is involutional osteoporosis. All normal human beings gain bone early in life during growth. After a plateau they begin to lose bone as they grow older. When this loss is accelerated or exaggerated, it leads to osteoporosis. Adult women have less bone mass than adult men, after menopause they lose it more rapidly than men, hence, are prone to develop osteoporosis, the cause of which is primarily estrogen deficiency. Estrogen prevent osteoporosis by inhibiting stimulatory effects of certain cytokines on osteoclasts. Increase intake of calcium and moderate exercise may help to prevent or slow the progress of osteoporosis although their effects are not great. In patients, immobilized for any reason and during space flight bone resorption exceeds bone formation and disuse osteoporosis develops. Large amounts of calcium are lost in urine. Osteoporosis also occurs with excess glucocorticoids secretion.

The diseases produced due to abnormalities of the cells in bone.

In **osteopetrosis**, a rare and usually a severe disease, the osteoclasts are defective and are unable to resorb bone in their normal fashion so the osteoblasts operate unopposed. The result is a steady increas in bone density, neurologic defects due to narrowing and distortion of foramina through which nerves pass, and hematologic abnormalities due to crowding of the marrow cavities.

On the other hand, **osteoporosis** is caused by a relative excess of osteoclastic function. Loss of bone matrix is marked, and the incidence of fractures is increased. Fractures are particularly common in the distal forearm (Colles fracture), vertebral body, and hip. These areas have a high content of trabecular bone, and trabecular bone is more active metabolically, it is lost rapidly. Fractures of the vertebrae with compression cause kyphosis, with the production of a typical "widow's hump" common in elderly women with osteoporosis. Fractures of the hip in elderly individuals are associated with a mortality rate of 12–20%, and half of those who survive require prolonged care.

the skin. There is increased incidence of infections in patients with vitamin D deficiency. The hormone also appears to be involved in the regulation of **growth and production of growth factors.**

ENDOCRINE FUNCTIONS OF PANCREAS

Islets of Langerhans in the pancreas (Fig. 13.21) secrete four hormones; all polypeptide in chemical nature. The islets form the endocrine portion of the pancreas, the rest is exocrine portion which produces pancreatic juice for digestion; the pancreas is both an endocrine and exocrine gland. **Islets of Langerhans** are ovoid collections of cells scattered throughout the pancreas and are more plentiful in the tail of the gland. They make-up about 2% of the volume of the gland, exocrine portion makes up 80% and ducts and blood vessels make-up the rest. Islets have a rich blood supply; blood from islets drains into hepatic portal vein. Following are the hormones secreted by islets:

- **Insulin secreted by "B" cells of the islets**; with role in metabolism of carbohydrates, proteins and fats.
- **Glucagon secreted by "A" cells of the islets**; with role in metabolism of carbohydrates, proteins and fats.
- **Somatostatin secreted by "D" cells of the islets**; has role in secretory activity of islet cells.
- **Pancreatic polypeptide secreted by "F" cells of the islets**; mainly concerned with GIT function.

Glucagon and somatostatin are also secreted by cells in the mucosa of the GIT.

Insulin causes storage of glucose, fatty acids and amino acids and hence, is anabolic in function. *Glucagon mobilizes glucose, fatty acid and amino acids from stores into bloodstream and hence, is catabolic in function.* The two hormones are reciprocal in action and regulate to maintain plasma glucose level in different circumstances.

Somatostatin inhibits insulin and glucagon secretions by the islet cells.

The "B" cells are most common in islets and account for 60–75% of the cells of the islets, the "A" cells make-up 20% of the total, and "D" and "F" cells are less common.

INSULIN

It is a polypeptide hormone having two chains of amino acids linked by disulfide bridges (Fig. 13.22). There are minor differences in the amino acid composition of the molecule from species to species.

These differences make the insulin from other species antigenic and the antibodies formed inhibit the action of injected foreign insulin. Pork insulin differs from human insulin by only one amino acid residue and has low antigenicity. Human insulin produced by recombinant DNA technology in bacteria is being used to avoid antibody formation.

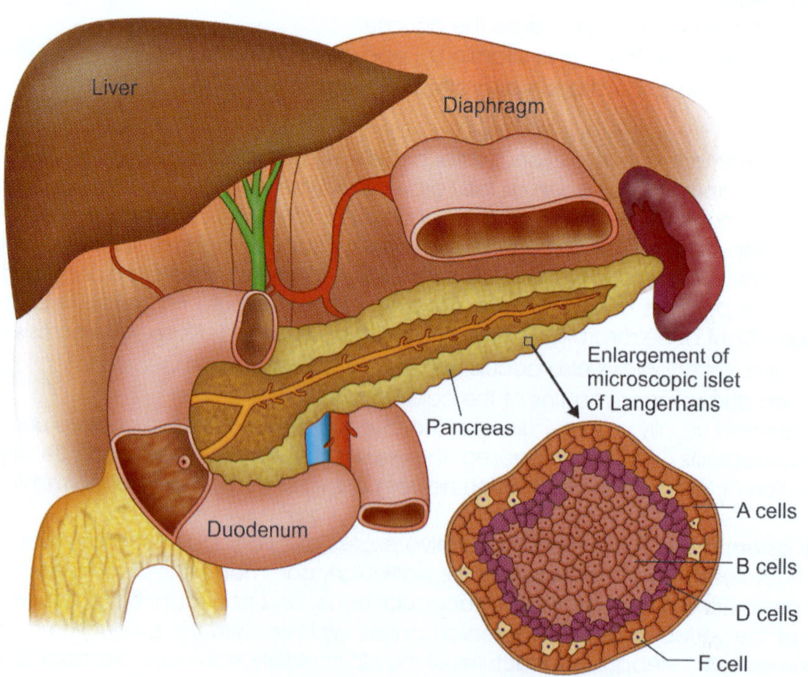

Fig. 13.21: Anatomy of the pancreas. Inset, arrangement of the various cell types in a typical islet of Langerhans

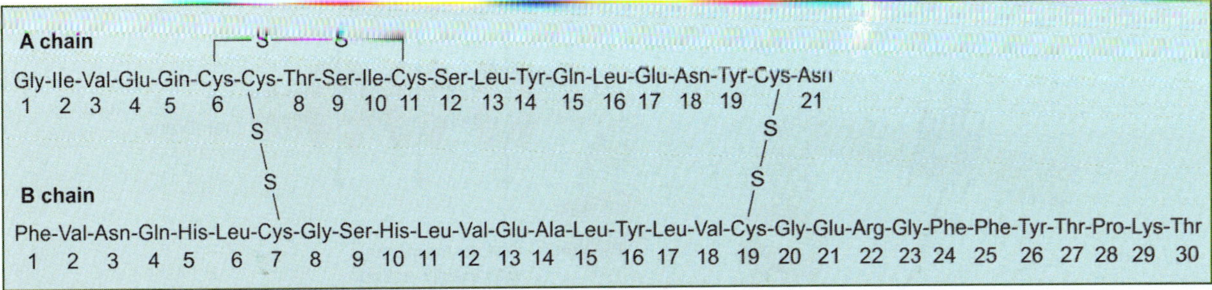

Fig. 13.22: Structure of human insulin (molecular weight 5808)

Insulin and insulin like activity in the blood: Plasma contains a number of substances with insulin like activity in addition to insulin. These substances are mainly IGF–I and IGF–II, which are polypeptide growth factors, small amounts are free in plasma but large amounts are bound to proteins.

But, insulin like activities of IGF-I and IGF-II are weak; as compared to insulin; and are not able to prevent diabetes mellitus in the absence of insulin.

Effects of Insulin

Insulin binds to insulin receptors on the cell membranes. This initiates the actions of insulin.

Glucose Transporters

Glucose enters cells by facilitated diffusion; which requires a transporter in the cell membrane. There are seven different types of glucose transporters (Table 13.4). The intestine and tubules of kidneys contain a transporter which is a cotransporter that transports glucose along with sodium, here mechanism of glucose transfer across the cell membrane is secondary active transport.

GLUT4 is the transporter in the muscle and adipose tissue; which is activated by insulin; when the insulin combines with its receptors on these cells; it results in the transporter molecules present in the cytoplasm to move to the cell membrane to facilitate glucose transport into the cell (Fig. 13.23).

Most of the other glucose transporters are not insulin sensitive and stay in the cell membrane only. Insulin also increases the entry of glucose into liver cells but not by increasing the number of GLUT4 transporters in the cell membrane; it activates enzyme glucokinase and this increases the phosphorylation of glucose in the liver cells; so that intracellular glucose concentration remains low; facilitating the entry of glucose into the cell; due to higher concentration gradient that is so created.

Table 13.4: Glucose transporters

Glucose transporter	*Function*	*Main sites of expression*
Secondary active transport (Na^+ glucose cotransport)		
SGLT 1	Absorption of glucose	Small intestine, renal tubules
SGLT 2	Absorption of glucose	Renal tubules
Facilitated diffusion		
GLUT 1	Basal glucose uptake	Placenta, blood brain barrier, brain, red cells, kidneys, colon, many other organs
GLUT 2	"B" cell glucose sensor; transport out of intestinal and renal epithelial cells	"B" cells of islets, liver, epithelial cells of small intestine, kidneys
GLUT 3	Basal glucose uptake	Brain, placenta, kidneys, many others organs
GLUT 4*	Insulin-stimulated glucose uptake	Skeletal and cardiac muscle, adipose tissue, other tissues
GLUT 5	Fructose transport	Jejunum, sperm
GLUT 6	None	Brain, spleen, leucocyte
GLUT 7	Glucose 6-phosphate transporter in endoplasmic reticulum	Liver, other tissues

*the major insulin responsive glucose transporter.

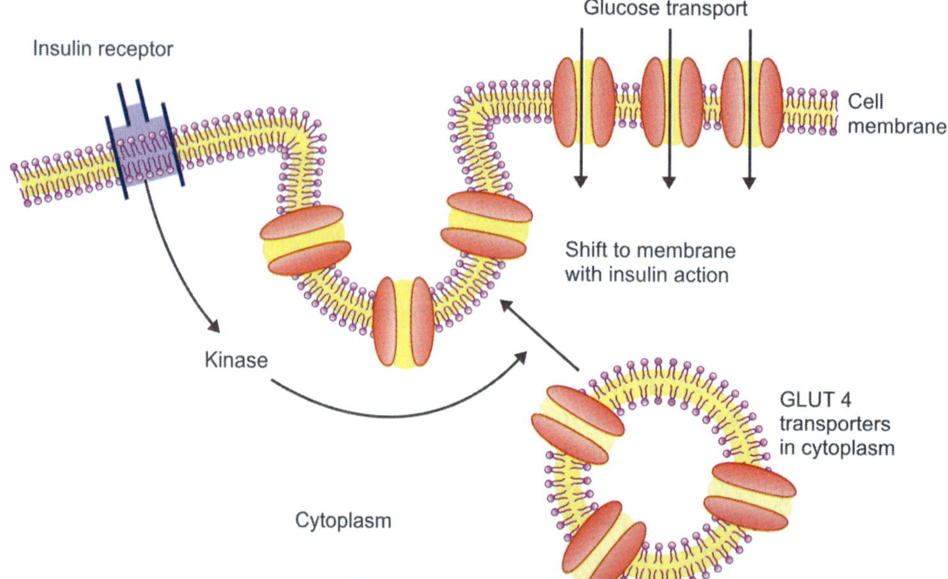

Fig. 13.23: Activation of the insulin receptor causes movement of the GLUT 4—into the cell membrane. The GLUT 4 transporters then mediate glucose transport into the cell

Insulin sensitive tissues also contain a number of GLUT4 vesicles that move into the cell membrane in response to exercise and are independent of the action of insulin. *This is the reason that exercise lowers blood sugar.*

Functions of Insulin

Insulin is the hormone which lowers circulating glucose level and it is secreted to regulate it; *secreted when plasma glucose level rises and it* ***increases peripheral utilization*** *of glucose (Fig. 13.24); in the muscle and adipose tissue, and has action on liver resulting in glycogen synthesis and inhibition of neoglucogenesis* (Table 13.5). *Other actions are:*

- In children failure to grow is a symptom of diabetes; insulin **stimulates growth.** Insulin **increases bone formation** and there is significant bone loss in untreated diabetes.
- **Intestinal absorption of glucose is not affected by insulin; glucose uptake by most of the brain and red cells is unaffected.**

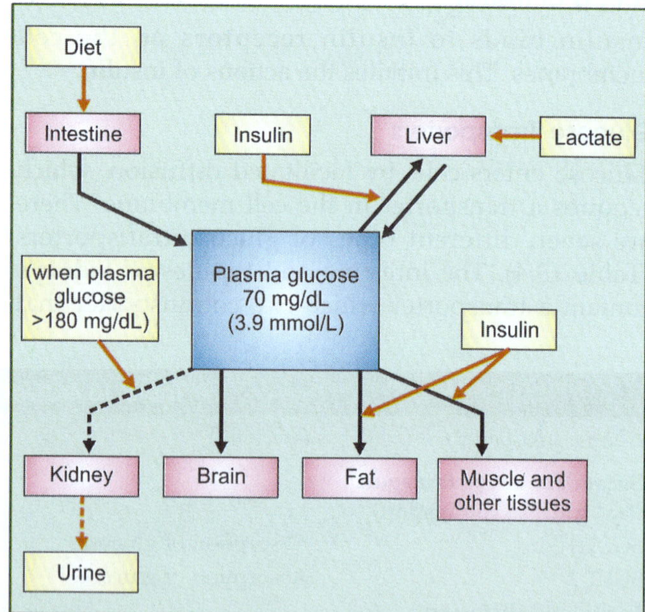

Fig. 13.24: Plasma glucose homeostasis. Liver has glucostatic function. Loss of glucose in the urine when plasma glucose level exceeds the renal threshold (dashed arrows)

Regulation of Insulin Secretion

There is basal level of insulin secretion; the amount of secretion increases after food intake to about 5–10 fold of basal level. The average amount secreted per day is about 40 units in an adult. Regulation of secretion is by direct action of glucose level on "B" cells of pancreas.

Intestinal factors have role in stimulating insulin secretion. Gastric inhibitory peptide (GIP) stimulates insulin secretion. It is produced by 'K' cells in the mucosa of duodenum and jejunum, is stimulated by glucose and fat in the lumen. It is often called **glucose dependent insulinotropic peptide.**

The glucagon derivative GLP-1 (7–36) also stimulates insulin secretion and said to be more potent than GIP. This is believed to be physiological B cell of pancreas stimulating hormone of GIT.

Table 13.5: Action of insulin on some tissues

Muscle	*Adipose tissue*	*Liver*
Increased glucose entry	Increased glucose entry	Increased glycogen
Increased glycogen synthesis	Increased fatty acid synthesis	
Increased amino and uptake	Increased glycerol phosphate synthesis	Decreased gluconeogenesis
Increased protein synthesis	Increased triglyceride deposition	Increased protein synthesis
	Inhibition of hormone sensitive lipase in cells	Increased lipid synthesis
Increased K^+ uptake	Increased K^+ uptake	

GLUCAGON

It is a single chain peptide hormone. The amino acid sequence of glucagon in mammalian species has remained the same; both structure and function of glucagon appear to have remained the same.

Glucagon is synthesized by islets "A" cells (Fig. 13.21).

Regulation of Secretion

The stimulus for glucagon secretion is to maintain normoglycemia. Exactly opposite to insulin, glucagon is secreted in response to fall in circulating glucose level and; it acts to increase circulating glucose level.

Hypoglycemia causes an increase in plasma glucagon level whereas hyperglycemia lowers it.

Fasting increases plasma glucagon level.

Other stimuli for its secretion are **stress**; including **infection, burns** and **major surgery;** all increase glucagon secretion rapidly; probably mediated via sympathetic nervous system (on pancreatic Islets cells) by output from hypothalamus.

The excess secretion of glucagon usually results in hyperglycemia. **Somatostatin** inhibits the secretion of glucagon.

Mechanism of Action of Glucagon

The actions of glucagon are exactly opposite to those of insulin. Both hormones act at similar point in the liver but in the opposite directions. The major effect of glucagon is on the liver. Its actions on adipose tissue and muscle are minor. Glucagon exerts an immediate and intense **glycogenolytic** effect. Glucagon also stimulates **gluconeogenesis.**

Another action of glucagons on liver is to **promote β oxidation** of incoming free fatty acids rather than their synthesis to triglycerides.

Glucagon also **activates adipose tissue lipase,** stimulating lipolysis (breakdown of triglycerides), and release of free fatty acids to the liver and **ketogenesis** is also stimulated.

There is another action of glucagon; it produces some increase in cardiac output. This effect is beneficial for use in refractory heart failure; sometimes used.

Somatostatin

It inhibits the secretion of insulin, glucagon, and pancreatic polypeptide probably by paracrine route; insulin inhibits the secretion of glucagon; and glucagon stimulates the secretion of insulin and somatostatin.

Plasma Glucose Levels

Basal plasma glucose levels are maintained and regulated around an average of concentration of 80 mg/dL (4.5 mmol/L) with range of 70–110 mg/dL (fasting). When the plasma glucose level falls below 60 mg/dL, uptake of sugar and utilization of oxygen by the brain is reduced. Central nervous system function becomes progressively impaired and may result in death when it falls still more (Fig. 13.25).

Glucose Tolerance Test

The oral glucose tolerance test is used for diagnosis of diabetes.

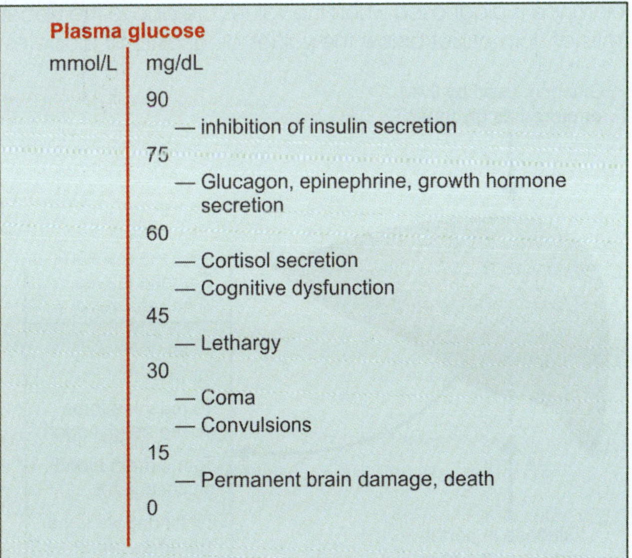

Fig. 13.25: Plasma glucose levels in blood at which various effects of hypoglycemia appear

The response to a standard oral test dose of glucose in a diabetic person is that plasma glucose level rises higher and returns to the basal level more slowly than it does in normal individuals (Fig. 13.26).

Most of the **glucose use in the basal state is independent of insulin** (Figs 13.24 and 13.27); though **insulin has important regulating effects** on glucose metabolism.

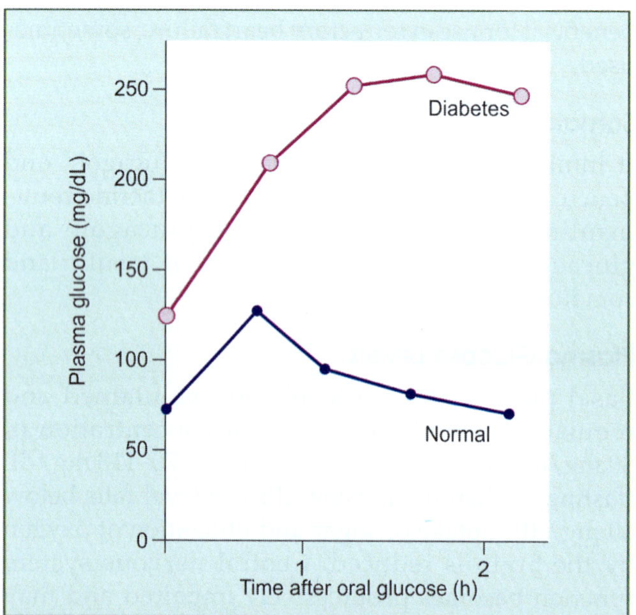

Fig. 13.26: Oral glucose tolerance test. Adults are given 75 g of glucose in 300 mL of water. In normal individuals, the fasting venous plasma glucose is less than 115 mg/dL, the 2-hour value is less than 140 mg/ dL and not greater than 200 mg/ dL. Diabetes mellitus is present if the 2-hour value and one other value are greater than 200 mg/dL. Impaired glucose tolerance is diagnosed when the values are above the upper limits of normal but below the values diagnostic of diabetes

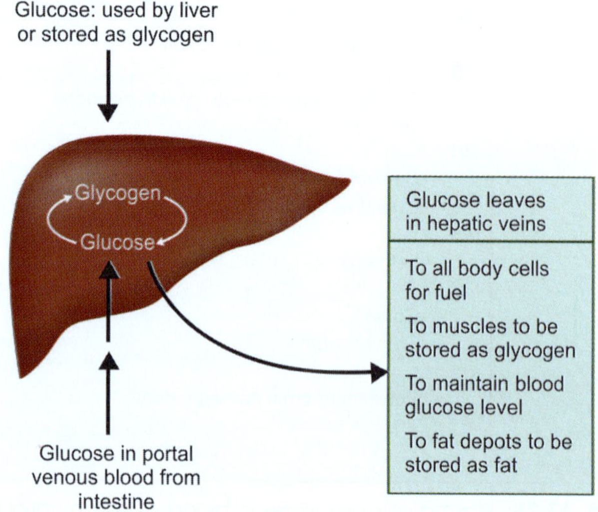

Fig. 13.27: Summary of use of glucose distribution and sources

Effects of Other Hormones on Carbohydrate Metabolism

Many hormones in addition to insulin and glucagon have important role in regulation of carbohydrate metabolism. They include epinephrine, thyroid hormones, glucocorticoids and growth hormone (Fig. 13.25).

Catecholamines

These hormones increase hepatic glucose output. Hypoglycemia stimulates their release.

Thyroid Hormones

Hyperthyroidism worsens clinical diabetes. The main effect of the hormones is to increase absorption of glucose from the intestine.

Adrenal Glucocorticoids

Glucocorticoids from adrenal cortex elevate blood glucose and produce diabetic type of glucose tolerance curve. This effect may occur only in individuals with a genetic predisposition to diabetes. In adrenal insufficiency, the blood glucose level is normal as long as food intake is maintained but fasting precipitates hypoglycemia and collapse.

Growth Hormone

Growth hormone excess makes clinical diabetes worse, and 25% of the patients with growth hormone secreting tumors of the anterior pituitary have diabetes.

Growth hormone mobilizes FFA from adipose tissue, favoring ketogenesis. It has anti-insulin action; decreases glucose uptake by muscle and adipose tissues and increases hepatic glucose output.

Clinical Significance

Glucose is the major source of energy for the brain and normal function depends upon continuous supply of glucose. Glucose enters the brain via transporter GLUT-I in cerebral capillaries. Other glucose transporters then distribute it to neurons and glial cells. Glucose uptake by the brain does not depend upon insulin. Hypoglycemia seriously affects brain function. When the plasma glucose level falls, the first symptoms are due to stimulation of the sympathetic nervous system. There is palpitation, sweating, and nervousness; as the level of sugar decreases further, disturbed central nervous system function results in defects in cerebration, cognitive dysfunction; still lower level causes loss of consciousness or convulsions and even death (Fig. 13.25).

Hypoglycemia

Insulin reactions are common in diabetics and occasional hypoglycemic episodes even when there is good diabetic control.

Severe exercise can precipitate hypoglycemia in diabetics; because of increased uptake of glucose by muscles; also due to absorption of injected insulin at more rapid rate during exercise. Patients with diabetes should take extra calories or reduce their insulin dosage when they exercise.

Symptomatic **hypoglycemia** also occurs in **non-diabetics.**

Chronic mild hypoglycemia can cause incoordination and slurred speech. (When the level of insulin secretion is chronically elevated by an **insulinoma,** a rare insulin secreting tumor, symptoms are most common in the morning, but symptoms may develop at anytime).

Before the symptoms of cognitive dysfunction occur (Fig. 13.25), sympathetic autonomic discharge due to hypoglycemia (sweating, anxiety and hunger) serve as warning to ingest sugar or glucose containing drinks before more severe symptoms appear.

But in some individuals, these warning signals fail to appear and this becomes dangerous.

Infants with GLUT-I deficiency have defective transport of glucose across the blood brain barrier. They have low cerebrospinal fluid (CSF) glucose in the presence of normal plasma glucose, leading to seizures and delay in development.

Insulin Dependent or Type 1 Diabetes Mellitus

There is deficiency of insulin due to "B" cell destruction in the islets of pancreas. The cause is some genetic abnormality with superimposition of some other cause. An autoimmune process contributes to "B" cell damage.

As a consequence of ***insulin lack*** (and ***relative glucagon excess***), glucose production is increased and peripheral glucose uptake reduced. Gluconeogenesis is increased and there is increased break down of proteins that supply amino acids (Fig. 13.28) for the same. It produces negative nitrogen balance. There is increased lipolysis in adipose tissues (fat cells) that elevates plasma free fatty acids and body fat decreases. Ketogenesis is increased, but peripheral ketoacid use is decreased. This greatly elevates plasma levels of ketone bodies (acetoacetate and β-hydroxybutyrate and acetone), i.e. **ketonemia** (Fig. 13.29) that produces **ketonuria** (excretion in urine). As they are neutralized by sodium bicarbonate, carbonic acid is formed which

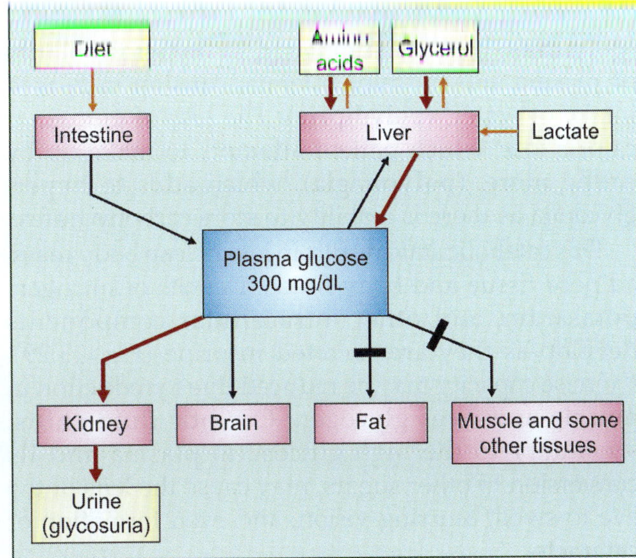

Fig. 13.28: Disordered plasma glucose homeostasis in insulin deficiency. The heavy arrows indicate increased reactions and blocked reactions are also indicated

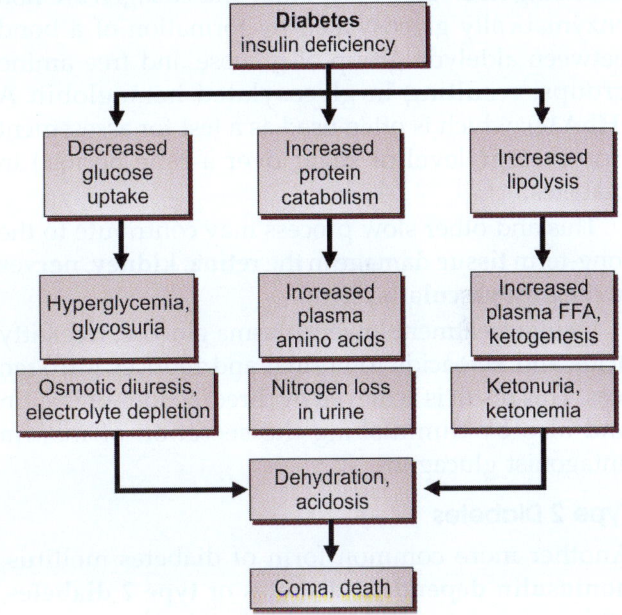

Fig. 13.29: Effects of insulin deficiency

dissociates into carbon dioxide and water. Pulmonary ventilation is stimulated as a result PCO_2 is lowered. Despite this blood pH falls to less than 6.8 and death from diabetic ketosis may result. Before the terminal point classic collection of symptoms is observed.

Symptoms of Diabetes Mellitus

Because of high plasma glucose level, the filtered load of glucose exceeds the tubular capacity for reabsorption; glucose therefore is excreted in urine in large quantities, (**glycosuria**); produces increased excretion of water and salt and frequent urination, (**polyuria**). Thirst is stimulated by hyperosmolarity of plasma and by hypovolemia, causing increased intake of water, (**polydipsia**). The loss of glucose is caloric loss, which patient attempts to make-up by eating more, (**polyphagia**), which adds to hyperglycemia as there is inability to store carbohydrates.

This catabolic state results in loss of lean body mass, adipose tissue and body fluids. Deficits of nitrogen, potassium, and other intracellular components develop as they are excreted in urine (Fig. 13.29). Exercise capacity may be reduced due to reduction in muscle and liver glycogen. Osmotic fluid shifts, secondary to the high glucose in plasma and its conversion to other sugars, may cause the lens of the eye to swell, blurring vision, and even formation of **cataracts**.

Other manifestations whose pathogenesis is not clear include ***slowed transmission of nerve impulses*** and **decreased resistance to infections.** Many proteins including hemoglobin, albumin and collagen are non enzymatically glycosylated by formation of a bond between aldelyde group of glucose and free amino groups; resulting in glycosylated hemoglobin A (**HbA1c**); which is often used as a test for assessment (for average level of sugar over a time period) in diabetes.

This and other slow process may contribute to the long-term **tissue damage** in the **retina**, **kidney**, **nerves** and **cardiovascular system**.

Insulin treatment lowers plasma glucose, free fatty acids and ketoacids to normal and reduces nitrogen loss. This result is achieved by direct actions of insulin and also by diminishing the secretion of insulin antagonist glucagons.

Type 2 Diabetes

Another more common form of diabetes mellitus, **noninsulin dependent diabetes** or **type 2 diabetes**, often is associated with ***obesity***. In this disease, major target tissues are resistant to the action of insulin. In addition there is derangement in "B" cell for recognition of glucose as a stimulus for insulin secretion; so that first phase insulin secretion is lost though delayed release does occur.

Fasting plasma glucose levels are **elevated** because of excess hepatic glucose production; ***postprandial glucose levels*** are further ***elevated, particularly after carbohydrate intake***. But, accelerated lipolysis and ketogenesis are rarely seen if there is no added illness.

Treatment of type 2 diabetes does not ordinarily require insulin; caloric regulation, weight reduction if excessive and use of drugs simultaneously improve tissue responsiveness to endogenous insulin and "B" cells responsiveness to glucose which would enhance insulin secretion (as the stimulus for insulin secretion from "B" cells is blood sugar level that directly affects the cells).

In late state, insulin administration may be required.

Obesity, the Metabolic Syndrome Relation to type 2 Diabetes

When there is increase in body weight there is increase in resistance to insulin, i.e. decreased ability of insulin to shift glucose into fat and muscle cells and to inhibit glucose release from liver. With the obesity there is hyperinsulinemia; high circulating triglyceride; and low HDL; with increased tendency for atherosclerosis. Weight reduction improves the condition and reduces insulin resistance. This combination of findings is called metabolic syndrome or syndrome X. Some of the patients are prediabetic, whereas others have type 2 diabetes.

Glucagon Excess or Deficiency

Primary glucagon excess is produced by "A" cell tumors. Catabolic action of hormone produces loss of weight and destructive skin lesion. Plasma levels of glucose and ketoacids are elevated.

There is marked increase in gluconeogenesis causing generalized reduction in plasma amino acids and increase in urinary nitrogen. Severe diabetes mellitus is uncommon because of compensatory increase in insulin secretion.

The deficiency of glucagon results in hypoglycemia. The causes are rarely recognized as other hormones; epinephrine, cortisol and growth hormones are stimulated with hypoglycemia and cover up the deficiency of glucagon.

Somatostatin Excess

Tumors of "D" cells produce somatostatin excess. This manifests as inhibition of nutrient absorption and weight loss. Plasma insulin and glucagon are low with moderate hyperglycemia due to low insulin.

ADRENAL GLANDS

The adrenal glands are essential for life. Severe illness results from their atrophy and death follows their complete removal. Although if carbohydrates and a mineralocorticoid (or sodium chloride) are provided, death can be postponed but human beings cannot survive total adrenalectomy for long without glucocorticoid replacement as are unable to tolerate any stress, to which they succumb.

Each adrenal gland consists of two endocrine organs (Fig. 13.30).

The outer zone is **adrenal cortex**, comprises 80–90% of the gland, it is source of **corticosteroid hormones.**

The inner zone or **adrenal medulla**, comprises the other 10–20% is the source of **catecholamines.** The adrenal medulla functions like sympathetic ganglions the neurons that have no axons and the cells secrete catecholamines.

Anatomy

The adrenal glands are retroperitoneal, just above each kidney (Fig. 13.30). They receive arterial blood supply from branches of aorta, the renal arteries, and the phrenic arteries. They have one of the body's highest rates of blood flow per gram of tissue.

Arterial blood enters sinusoidal capillaries in the cortex. The blood then drains into medullary venules; this exposes the medulla to high concentration of corticosteroids from the cortex.

The adrenal can be visualized by computed tomography (CT) or magnetic resonance imaging (MRI).

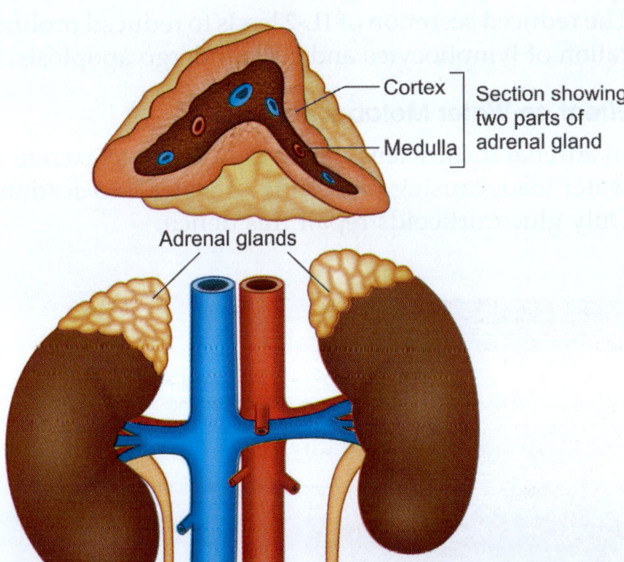

Fig. 13.30: The adrenal glands, showing their internal structure and their position over the pole of each kidney. The adrenal cortex secretes steroid hormones involved in sugar metabolism, responds to stress, control of salt balance and sexual development. The adrenal medulla produces adrenaline and noradrenaline

The Adrenal Cortex

The important hormones of adrenal cortex are grouped into three headings (Table 13.6).

1. **Glucocorticoids,** i.e. *cortisol* and *corticosterone* which are critical to life. They have widespread effects on carbohydrate and protein metabolism.
2. **Mineralocorticoids,** of which the important hormone is **aldosterone** which is vital for maintaining sodium and potassium balance, and extracellular fluid (ECF) volume.
3. **Sex steroids,** androgens and estrogens and have reproductive function. Contribute to development and maintenance of secondary sex characters.

Glucocorticoids, mineralocorticoids and sex hormones are synthesized from cholesterol.

The mineralocorticoids and glucocorticoids both have mineralocorticoid and glucocorticoid activity but each has its predominent function regulation of Na^+, K^+ excretion for mineralocorticoids and carbohydrate and protein metabolism for glucocorticoids.

Adrenal cortical hormones are under control of adrenocorticotropic hormone ACTH) but mineralocorticoids also have independent control by ciarculating factors most important of which is aldosterone.

Histology of Adrenal Cortex

The adrenal cortex has three zones, each of which secretes one of the three groups of corticosteroids (Fig. 13.31). The histological appearance of three mature zones differs (Fig. 13.32). The outermost is **zona glomerulosa** which is very thin, secretes hormone **aldosterone**. The middle zone is **zona fasciculata**, it is the widest zone and the cells form long cords, secrete **glucocorticoids**. Innermost zone, **zona reticularis** contains network of interconnecting cells that secrete **sex hormones.**

Table 13.6: Major adrenocortical hormones

Class	*Steroid*
Glucocorticoids	Cortisol
	Corticosterone
Mineralocorticoids	Aldosterone
	Deoxycorticosterone
Sex steroids	DHEA
	DHEA-S
	Androstenedione
	(Converted in fat and other tissues to estrogen and testosterone)

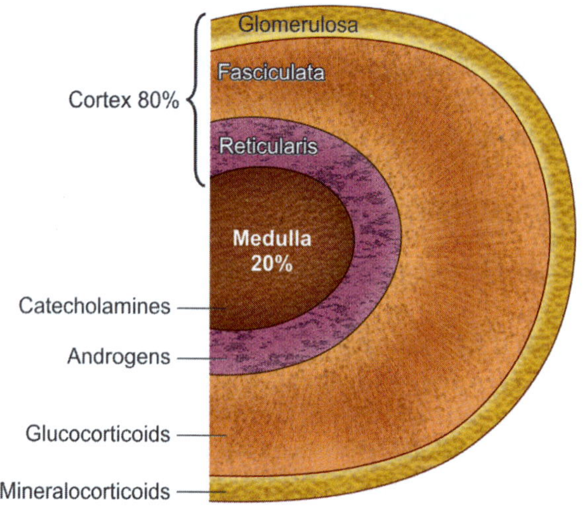

Fig. 13.31: Representation of the zones of the adrenal gland and their main secretory product

Under stimulation of ACTH, the size and the number of cells in the fasciculata and reticularis increase.

Functions of Glucocorticoids

The main corticoids are cortisol and corticosterone.

They are steroids with widespread effects on **metabolism of carbohydrates** and **proteins.**

The functions of the hormones are:

- Maintain glucose production from protein, increase protein catabolism and increase hepatic glycogenesins and gluconeogenesins
- Facilitate fat metabolism (lipolytic in action)
- Support vascular responsiveness
- Modulate CNS function
- Affect immune responses
- Affect inflammatory responses
- Provide resistance to stress
- During fetal life, glucocorticoids accelerate the maturation of surfactant in the lungs.

The net effect of the hormones is **catabolic**. They have **permissive role** for the action of **catecholamines** on arterioles; help to maintain blood volume by decreasing the permeability of the vascular endothelium.

Cortisol plays an important role in defense against hypoglycemia that is produced by insulin.

Although it is weakly lipolytic itself, the presence of cortisol is necessary for maximal stimulation of fat mobilization by epinephrine and growth hormone.

Overall it is diabetogenic, anti-insulin hormone. Hyperglycemic, lipolytic and ketogenic actions are usually exhibited only when secretion is stimulated by stress. Then cortisone potentiates and extends the duration of hyperglycemia evoked by glucagons, epinephrine and growth hormone and increases loss of body protein.

Effects on Blood Cells and Lymphatic Organs

Glucocorticoids decrease the number of circulating eosinophilis by increasing their sequestration in the spleen and lungs. Also lower basophilis in the circulatory blood but increase neutrophils, platelets and RBC. Decrease the circulating lymphocyte count by inhibiting lymphocyte mitotic activity. **Decrease cytokines** by inhibiting effect of **NF–kB** on nucleus. The reduced secretion of **IL-2** leads to reduced proliferalion of lymphocytes and cells undergo apoptosis.

Effect on Water Metabolism

In adrenal insufficiency there is inability to excrete a water load, causing possibility of water intoxication. Only glucocorticoids repair this deficit.

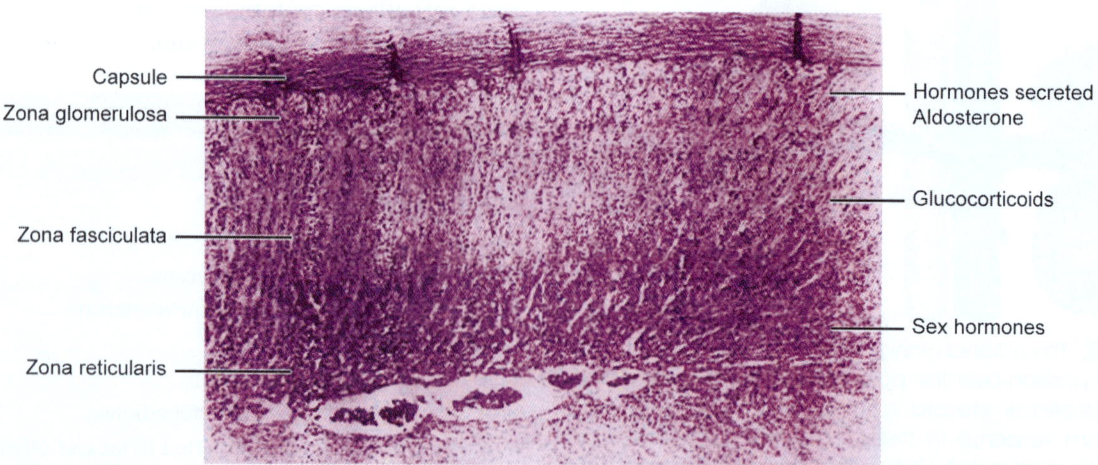

Fig. 13.32: Microscopic anatomy of the adrenal gland showing hormones secreted by different zones

Permissive Action

Small amounts of glucocorticoids must be present for a number of metabolic reactions to occur although the glucocorticoids do not produce the reactions by themselves. This is their role in permissive actions.

Permissive actions include the requirement for glucocorticoids to be present for catecholamines to exert their calorigenic effect; for catecholamines to exert their lipolytic effects; and for catecholamines to produce pressor responses on blood vessels and bronchodilation.

Effect on ACTH Secretion

Glucocorticoids inhibit ACTH secretion and hence, exert a negative feedback effect on their own secretion (Fig. 13.33). The negative feedback effect is ***also*** exerted at hypothalamus (on CRH).

Effects on CNS

There are mild personality effects which may appear during treatment with them; include irritability, apprehension and inability to concentrate.

Effects on Surfactant

During fetal life glucocorticoids accelerate the maturation of surfactant in the lungs.

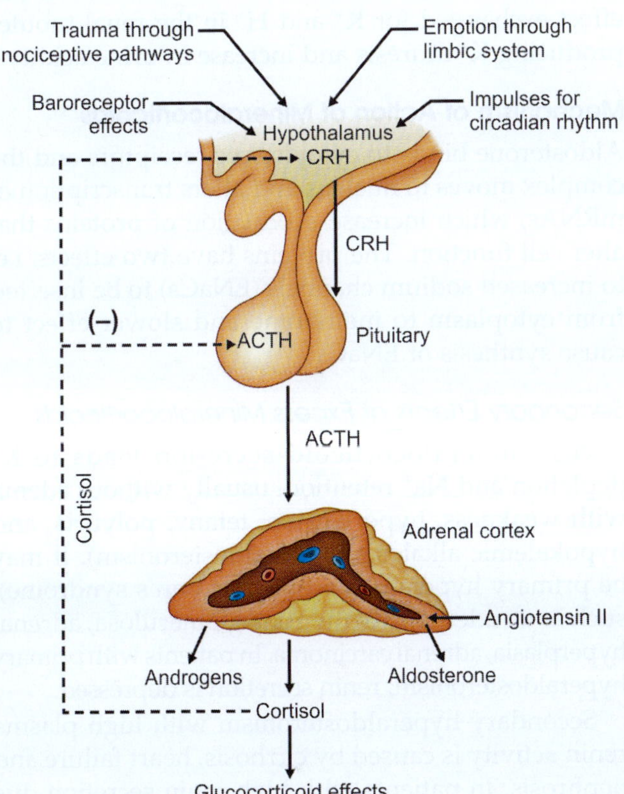

Fig. 13.33: Hypothalamic-pituitary-adrenocortical axis and negative feedback effects

Resistance to Stress

When a person is exposed to stress of any variety of noxious or potentially noxious stimuli, there is increased secretion of ACTH that results in the rise of the circulating glucocorticoid level. This rise is essential for survival.

Selye defined noxious stimuli that increase ACTH secretion as "stressors" and these stimuli are grouped together under the term "stress". The reason for the elevated glucocorticoid level that is necessary for resisting stress remains unknown.

Most of the stressful stimuli that increase ACTH secretion also activate the sympathetic nervous system and some of the functioning of circulating glucocorticoids may be the maintenance of vascular reactivity to catecholamines.

Glucocorticoids are also necessary for catecholamines to exert their full FFA mobilizing action and FFA is an important energy fuel.

It is said that stress causes increase in plasma glucocorticoids to high "pharmacologic" levels that in the short run are life-saving but in the long run are harmful and disruptive.

Other Effects

Large doses of glucocorticoids inhibit growth, decrease growth hormone secretion, decrease TSH secretion.

Glucocorticoids in doses that are higher than physiological doses have ***antiinflammatory*** and ***immunosuppressive*** actions which are used in treating nonendocrine diseases as:

- The glucocorticoids **suppress manifestations of allergic diseases** that are because of release of histamine from tissues. But, the treatment involves high level of glucocorticoids.
- When the effects of tissue injury resulting from diseases are harmful, glucocorticoids are beneficial; glucocorticoids do not cure infection; they prevent the effects of inflammation on the tissues. But, glucocorticoids are administered for long periods, they may increase susceptibility to infection allow their dissemination; and they may prevent normal wound healing after injury.
- When rejection of transplanted organs or tissues has to be prevented, they are useful.

But long use produces ***adverse reactions*** **like diabetes, osteoporosis** and **psychiatric disorders.** This may prevent their use for long peroids. But this does not apply to the individuals who are receiving replacement therapy if adrenals function is lost.

Mechanism of Action of Glucocorticoids

The hormones bind to their receptors and the complex acts as a transcription factor for certain DNA segments to synthesize mesenger RNA for synthesis of enzymes that after cell function. In addition the glucocorticoids have nongenemic functions.

Mineralocorticoids

Aldosterone is the major mineralocorticoid and its main action is to **maintain extracellular fluid volume** by **conserving body sodium**. Hence, aldosterone is largely secreted in response to signals from the kidneys when a reduction in circulating fluid volume is sensed. There is then release of renin from the JGA; which acts on angiotensinogen, a protein present in the blood this results in the formation of angiotensin I which is inactive; on which the converting enzyme mainly present in the lungs acts to convert it to **angiotensin II** which stimulates the secretion of aldosterone (Fig. 13.34).

A low sodium and **high K$^+$** in the plasma also stimulate aldosterone secretion. **ACTH** has weak stimulatory action on aldosterone secretion.

Regulation of Aldosterone Secretion

Table 13.7 lists conditions that stimulate aldosterone.

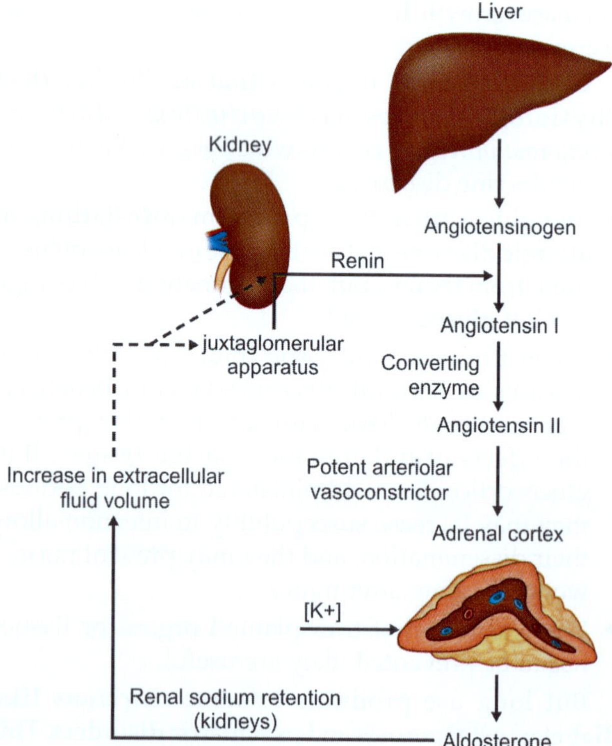

Fig. 13.34: Renin-angiotensin-aldosterone system for secretion of aldosterone and the negative feedback effects shown by dashed line

Table 13.7: Conditions that increase aldosterone secretion

Glucocorticoid secretion also increased
Surgery
Anxiety
Physical trauma
Hemorrhage
Glucocorticoid secretion also increased
High potassium intake
Low sodium intake
Constriction of inferior vena cava in thorax
Standing
Secondary hyperaldosteronism (in some cases of congestive heart failure, cirrhosis, and nephrosis)

Functions

Aldosterone and other adrenal steroids with mineralocorticoid activity increase the reabsorption of Na$^+$ from the kidney, also from sweat, saliva, and the contents of the colon. The mineralocorticoids cause retention of Na$^+$ in the ECF. This expands ECF volume. In the kidney, they act primarily on the collecting ducts on principal cells (P cells); under the influence of aldosterone increased amounts of Na$^+$ are reabsorbed and in effect exchanged for K$^+$ and H$^+$ in the renal tubules producing K$^+$ diuresis and increase in urine acidity.

Mechanism of Action of Mineralocorticoids

Aldosterone binds to cytoplasmic receiptors and the complex moves to nucleus and alters transcription of mRNAs, which increase production of proteins that alter cell function. The proteins have two effects, i.e. to increased sodium channels (ENaCs) to be inserted from cytoplasm to membrane and slower effect to cause synthesis of ENaCs.

Secondary Effects of Excess Mineralocorticoids

Excess mineralocorticoid secretion leads to K$^+$ depletion and Na$^+$ retention, usually without edema with weakness, hypertension, tetany, polyuria, and hypokalemic alkalosis (hyperaldosteronism). It may be primary hyperaldosteronism (Conn's syndrome), such as an adenoma of the zona glomerulosa, adrenal hyperplasia, adrenal carcinoma. In patients with primary hyperaldosteronism, renin secretion is depressed.

Secondary hyperaldosteronism with high plasma renin activity is caused by cirrhosis, heart failure and nephrosis. In patients with high renin secretion due to renal artery constriction, aldosterone secretion is increased.

Effects of Adrenalectomy

In adrenal insufficiency Na^+ is lost in the urine, K^+ is retained and plasma K^+ rises when adrenal insufficiency develops rapidly, the amount of Na^+ lost from ECF exceeds the amount excreted in the urine, indicating Na^+ is entering cells. But the plasma volume is also reduced, resulting in hypotension, circulating insufficiency and eventually fatal shock. These changes can be prevented to a large degree by increasing the dietary NaCl intake but most in humans the amount of supplementary salt needed is so large that it is impossible to prevent eventual collapse and death, unless mineralocorticoid treatment in started.

Primary adrenal insufficiency due to disease processes that destroy the adrenal cortex and called Addison's disease; it used to be common complication of tuberculosis. Now, it is usually due to autoimmune inflammation of the adrenal. Patients lose weight, feel tired, become chronically hypotensive and have small hearts.

Pharmacological and Pathological Effects of Glucocorticoid

The clinical picture produced by excess of plasma glucocorticoids was described by Harvey Cushing and is called Cushing's syndrome. It may be ACTH independent or ACTH dependent.

ACTH independent **Cushing syndrome** is produced by: glucocorticoid secreting adrenal tumor; adrenal hyperplasia; prolonged administration of exogenous glucocorticoids for diseases, such as rheumatoid arthritis.

The causes of the ACTH dependent Cushing syndrome include: ACTH secreting tumors of anterior pituitary gland; tumors of the lungs that secrete ACTH or CRH.

Patients of Cushing's syndrome (Fig. 13.35) are **protein depleted** as a result of protein catabolism. The skin and the subcutaneous tissue are thin and the muscles are poorly developed. Wounds heal poorly and minor injuries cause bruises. The hair is thin. Many patients with this disease have some increase in **facial hair** and acne, but this is caused by increased secretion of adrenal androgens that often accompanies the increase in glucocorticoid secretion. Body fat is redistributed in a characteristic way. The extremities are thin but fat collects in the abdominal wall, face and upper back, where it produces a "**buffalo hump**". Hyperglycemia may precipitate insulin-resistant diabetes mellitus especially in patients genetically predisposed to diabetes. The glucocorticoids are present in such large amounts in Cushing syndrome

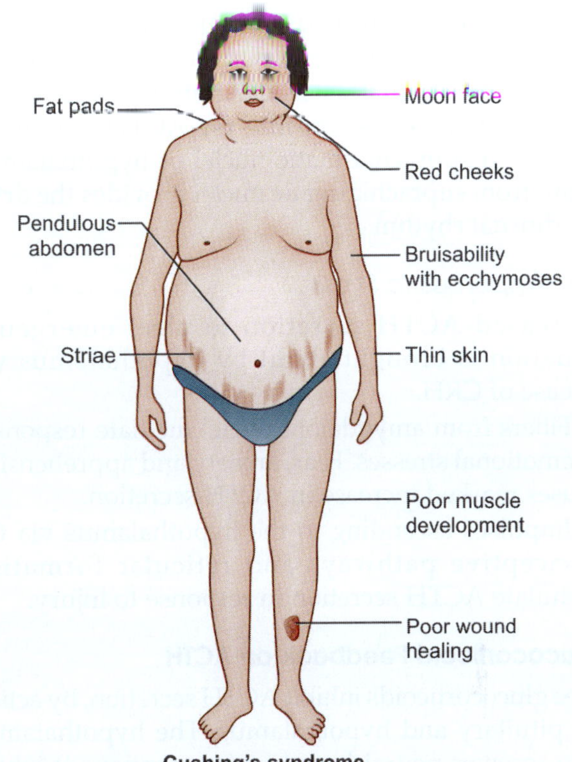

Fig. 13.35: Typical findings in Cushing's syndrome

that they may exert significant mineralocorticoid action also. The salt and water retention plus facial obesity results in the characteristic rounded "**moon faced**" appearance. There may be K^+ depletion and weakness. Patients may become hypertensive. Glucocorticoid excess leads to bone dissolution by decreasing bone formation and increasing bone resorption. This leads to **osteoporosis**, a loss of bone mass that may gradually leads to collapse of vertebral bodies or other fractures. Glucocorticoids in excess produce mental aberrations; there may be increased appetite, **insomnia** or euphoria, or even frank toxic psychoses.

Regulation of Glucocorticoid Secretion

Both basal secretion of glucocorticoid and the increased secretion produced by stress are dependent on **ACTH**. ACTH stimulates the secretion of glucocorticoids and mineralocorticoids but the effect on mineralocorticoids is less. It stimulates sex steroids also. Angiotensin II also stimulates adrenal cortex but its effect is mainly on aldosterone.

Circadian Rhythm

ACTH is secreted in irregular bursts throughout the day and plasma cortisol tends to rise and fall in response to these bursts. In humans, the bursts are more frequent in the early morning with about 75% of the daily cortisol secretion from 4 am to 10 am.

These bursts are least frequent in the evening. The biological clock responsible for ACTH rhythm is located in suprachiasmatic nuclei of hypothalamus. Input from suprachiasmatic nuclei provides the drive for diurnal rhythm.

The Responses to Stress

Increased ACTH secretion to meet emergency situation is brought about by hypothalamus via release of CRH.

Fibers from amygdaloid nuclei mediate responses to emotional stresses. Fear, anxiety and apprehension causes marked increase in ACTH secretion.

Impulses ascending to the hypothalamus via the nociceptive pathways and reticular formation stimulate ACTH secretion in response to injury.

Glucocorticoid Feedback on ACTH

Free glucocorticoids inhibit ACTH secretion, by action on pituitary and hypothalamus. The hypothalamus also receives neural impulses (as mentioned) which increase ACTH secretion. The rate of ACTH secretion is influenced by these factors.

The dangers involved after prolonged treatment with high doses of glucocorticoids when they are **stopped** are that not only adrenal becomes atrophic and unresponsive pituitary may take long time to recover for function of ACTH secretion. The complication of sudden cessation of steroid therapy can be usually avoided by slowly decreasing steroid dose over peroid of time.

Regulation of Salt Balance in the Body

The following hormones/factors regulate salt balance in the body and are described in appropriate sections.

- Aldosterone secretion
- Glomerular filtration rate (GFR)
- Atrial natriuretic peptide (ANP)
- Osmotic diuresis
- Na^+ reabsorption in tubules independent of aldosterone.

Secretion of Sex Hormones

The synthesis of sex steroids occurs in the zona reticularis of adrenal cortex. The sex steroids, secreted are weak androgens. They are converted to potent androgen, testosterone in the peripheral tissues. In males, they have no important role; but in females, they are the responsible for pubic and axillary hair growth. ACTH stimulates their secretion. Weak androgens secreted are even converted to estrogen in the peripheral and adipose tissues. This is the source of estrogen in males and postmenopausal females.

Excess of Androgen Secretion

Excess secretion of androgens results in masculinization (Fig. 13.36) (adrenogenital syndrome); produces precocious puberty or female pseudohermaphroditism.

ADRENAL MEDULLA

The adrenal medulla secretes circulating catecholamines; epinephrine and norepinephrine (also dopamine in small amounts). These hormones have effects on metabolism as well as on many organs in the body. The adrenal medulla is a specialized sympathetic ganglion which contains cell bodies of the neurons with no axons; the neurons release the hormones directly into the blood circulation; functioning as endocrine gland.

The adrenal medulla is activated along with the sympathetic nervous system; and has similar effects. During hypoglycemia adrenal medulla is activated specifically to secrete epinephrine.

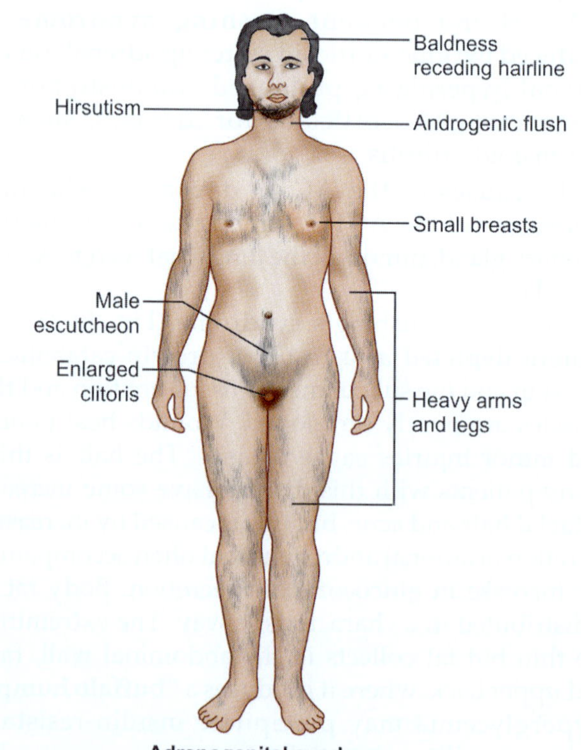

Fig. 13.36: Typical findings in the adrenogenital syndrome in a postpubertal woman

The receptors for catecholamines are situated on the cell membranes. Receptors are called alpha 1, alpha 2, beta 1 and beta 2.

Actions of Catecholamines

Both hormones increase glucose production; by stimulating glycogenolysis in the liver.

During hypoglycemia the immediate response is the secretion of catecholamines and glucagon, so that glucose is made available to the CNS.

Epinephrine also increases the basal metabolic rate; this is an important response to cold exposure; it also produces constriction of skin blood vessels to conserve heat.

The cardiac rate and force of contraction is increased by epinephrine, alertness is increased by both hormones although epinephrine produces more fear and anxiety. These and other effects are the similar to those of sympathetic stimulation.

Dopamine is also secreted by adrenal medulla. Its physiological function in circulation is not known. If injected it produces renal vasodilation, and also in mesentery; at other sites it produces vasoconstriction, probably by releasing norepinephrine and it has a positive inotropic action on the heart by an action on beta adrenergic receptors. The net affect of dopamine is moderate increase in systolic BP and no change in diastolic pressure; hence, it is useful in treatment of cardiogenic and traumatic shock.

Dopamine is also made in renal cortex. It causes natriuresis and is excreted in urine.

Pathological Secretion of Catecholamines

Pheochromocytomas are tumors of adrenal medulla; that produce hypersecretion of epinephrine or norepinephrine or both; and produce sustained hypertension; but some of the tumors that secrete epinephrine secrete it episodically, producing symptoms of sudden severe headache, palpitations, glycosuria and severe hypertension; any stress or change of posture may produce the symptoms. Extreme anxiety, cold perspiration, pallor of the skin, blurred vision may also be the symptoms produced. Blood pressure may be extremely high up to 250/150 mmHg.

The diagnosis is established by detecting high levels of plasma epinephrine and norepinephrine; increased urinary excretion of catecholamines or their degradation products which includes vanillylmandelic acid (VMA).

THYMUS

During fetal life the lymphocytes that come from bone marrow and are processed in the thymus become "T" lymphocytes which are responsible for cellular immunity. After birth lymphocytes are formed mainly in the lymphoid organs including thymus though some lymphocytes are still formed in the bone marrow.

PINEAL GLAND

The gland arises from the roof of the third ventricle under the posterior end of the corpus callosum (Fig. 13.37A and B) and is connected by a stalk to the posterior commissure and habenular commissure. There are nerve fibers in the stalk but do not reach the gland. The gland contains neuroglia and parenchymal cells. In young infants, pineal is large and cells are arranged somewhat in alveoli. Pineal gland begins to involute before puberty and small secretions of calcium phosphate and carbonate appear in the tissue, hence, it appears in X-rays films in the skulls of the adults.

The pineal gland secretes hormone **melatonin**. The hormone is synthesized by parenchymal cells and secreted into the blood and CSF. It is also synthesized in other organs. The hormone serves as a timing device that keeps internal organs synchronized with the light and dark cycle in the environment.

Regulation of Secretion

The synthesis and secretion are increased during dark period of the day and maintained at low level during the daylight time (Fig. 13.37B). The regulation is brought about by the sympathetic nerve fibers that innervate the gland; the fibers receive connections from the hypothalamic nucleus responsible for circadian rhythm. The role of pineal in gonad development and puberty is not clear. It has been said that pineal inhibits the onset of puberty, as pineal tumors were found to be associated with precocity, but that occurs only when the tumors produce hypothalamic damage which may be responsible for it.

HORMONES FROM KIDNEY

The kidneys produce three hormones:

1. 1, 25-dihydroxycholecalciferol.
2. Renin
3. Erythropoietin.

The functions of all three have been described in relevant sections.

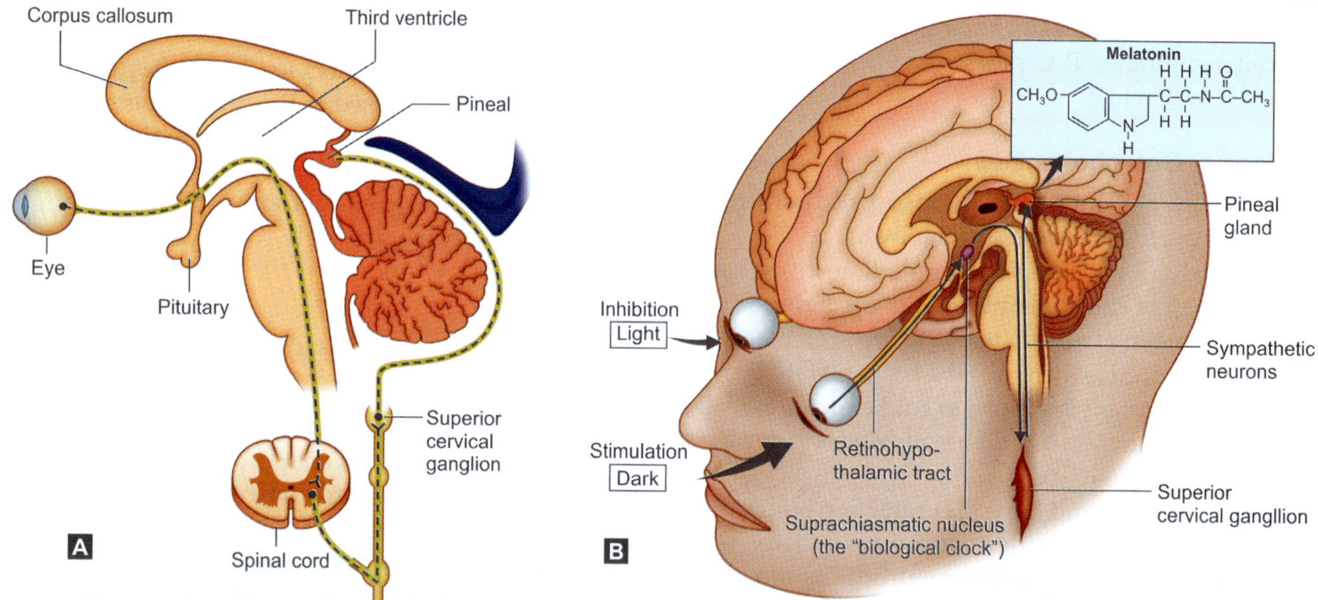

Figs 13.37A and B: (A) Left: sagittal section human brainstem showing the pineal and its innervation (dashed line), (B) Metalonin secretion stimulated in the dark

HORMONES OF THE HEART AND OTHER NATRIURETIC FACTORS

Two natriuretic hormones are secreted by the heart. Atrial natriuretic peptide (ANP), and brain natriuretic peptide (BNP). The latter though produced by the brain but more is present in the human heart including ventricles.

Functions

ANP and BNP in circulation act on the kidneys to increase sodium excretion. They perhaps act by dilating afferent arteriole and relaxing mesangial cells, both effects increase GFR. In addition, they act on the renal tubules to inhibit sodium reabsorption. They relax vascular smooth muscle in arterioles and venules. They inhibit renin secretion and counteract the pressure effects of catecholamines and angiotensin II.

Regulation of Secretion

The concentration of ANP increases in plasma when extracellular volume is increased by ingestion of high sodium diet. It appears that atria respond directly to stretch and the rate of ANP secretion is proportionate to the degree to which atria are stretched by increase in central venous pressure.

Plasma contains a number of substances with insulin like activity (Fig. 13.38). Activity is not suppressed by ant.-insulin antibodies and has been termed as non suppressable insulinable activity (NSILA) and is due to IGF-I and IGF-II. The insulin like activities of IGF-I and IGF-II are weak. These IGFs are polypeptides. Small amount free in plasma, but large amounts bound to proteins.

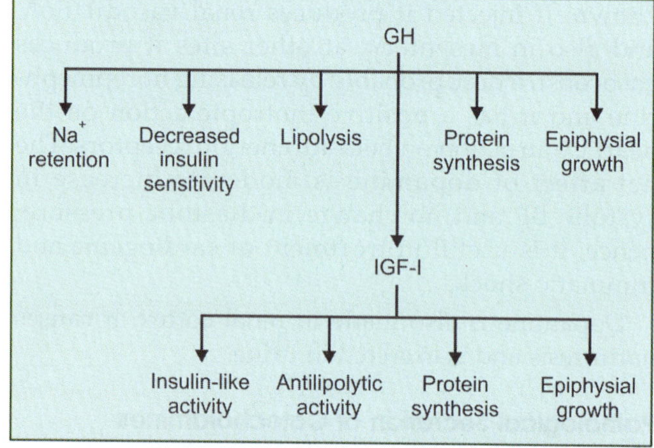

Fig. 13.38: Actions of IGF-I and growth hormone

PHYSIOLOGY OF GROWTH

Growth hormone is unimportant for fetal development, is the most important hormone for postnatal growth. Growth overall is a complex phenomenon that is affected by growth hormone and somatomedins, but also by thyroid hormones, androgens, estrogens, glucocorticoids, and insulin. It is also affected by genetic factors, and it depends on adequate nutrition. It is normally accompanied by an orderly sequence of maturational changes, involves accretion of protein and an increase in length and size, no just

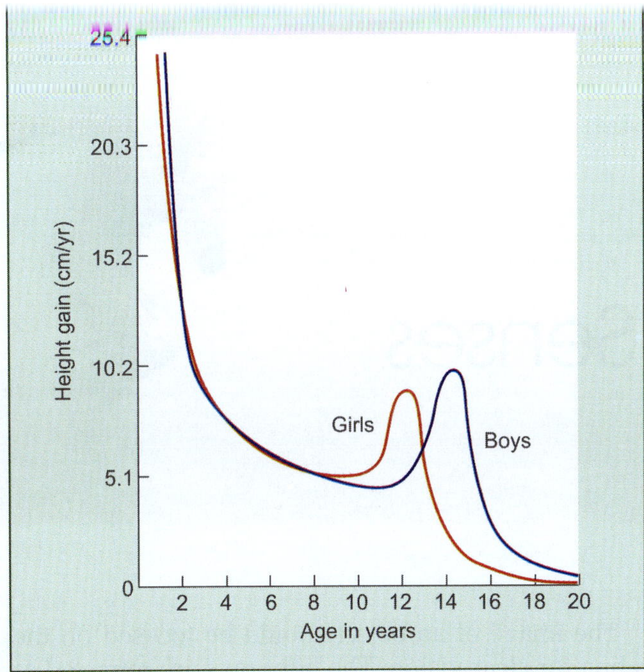

Fig. 13.39: Growth spurts in boys and girls

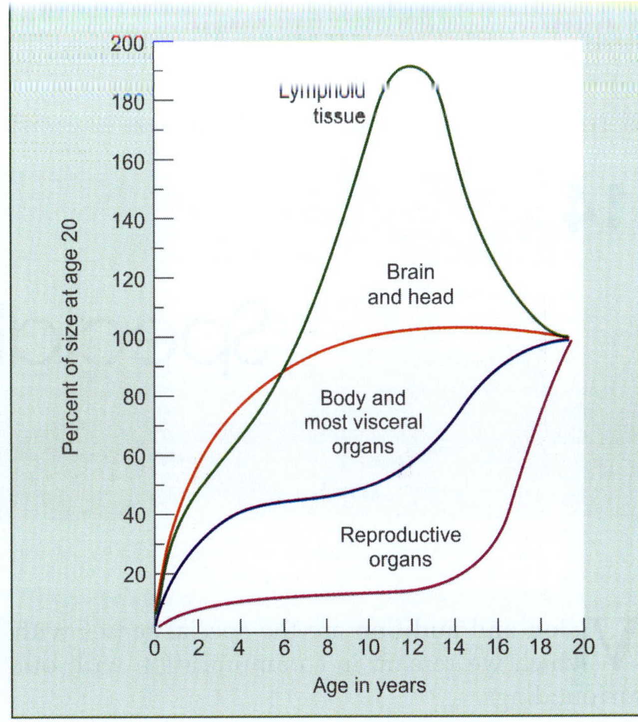

Fig. 13.40: Growth of individual tissues

an increase in weight (which could also be the formation of fat or retention of salt and water rather than growth per se).

Role of Nutrition

The food supply is the most important extrinsic factor affecting growth. The diet must be adequate not only in protein but also in essential vitamins and minerals and in calories, so that ingested protein is not burned for energy. The age at which a dietary deficiency occurs is an important consideration. For example, once the pubertal growth spurt has commenced, considerable linear growth continues even if caloric intake is reduced. Injury and disease, stunt growth because they increase protein catabolism.

Growth Periods

These are two periods of rapid growth (Fig. 13.39) one in infancy and the second in late puberty just before growth stops. The first period of accelerated growth is partly a continuation of the fetal growth period. The second growth spurt, at the time of puberty, is due to growth hormone, androgens, and estrogens, and the subsequent cessation of growth is due to closure of the epiphyses in the long bones by estrogens. After this time further increases in height are not possible. This growth spurt appears earlier in girl. In both sexes the rate of growth of individual tissues varies (Fig. 13.40).

IMPLICATIONS AND APPLICATIONS

- See any nonpitting oedema of feet.
- See the readings of blood sugar (both fasting and post prandial) and urine to be tested for sugar.
- To be able to regulate the dose of insulin.

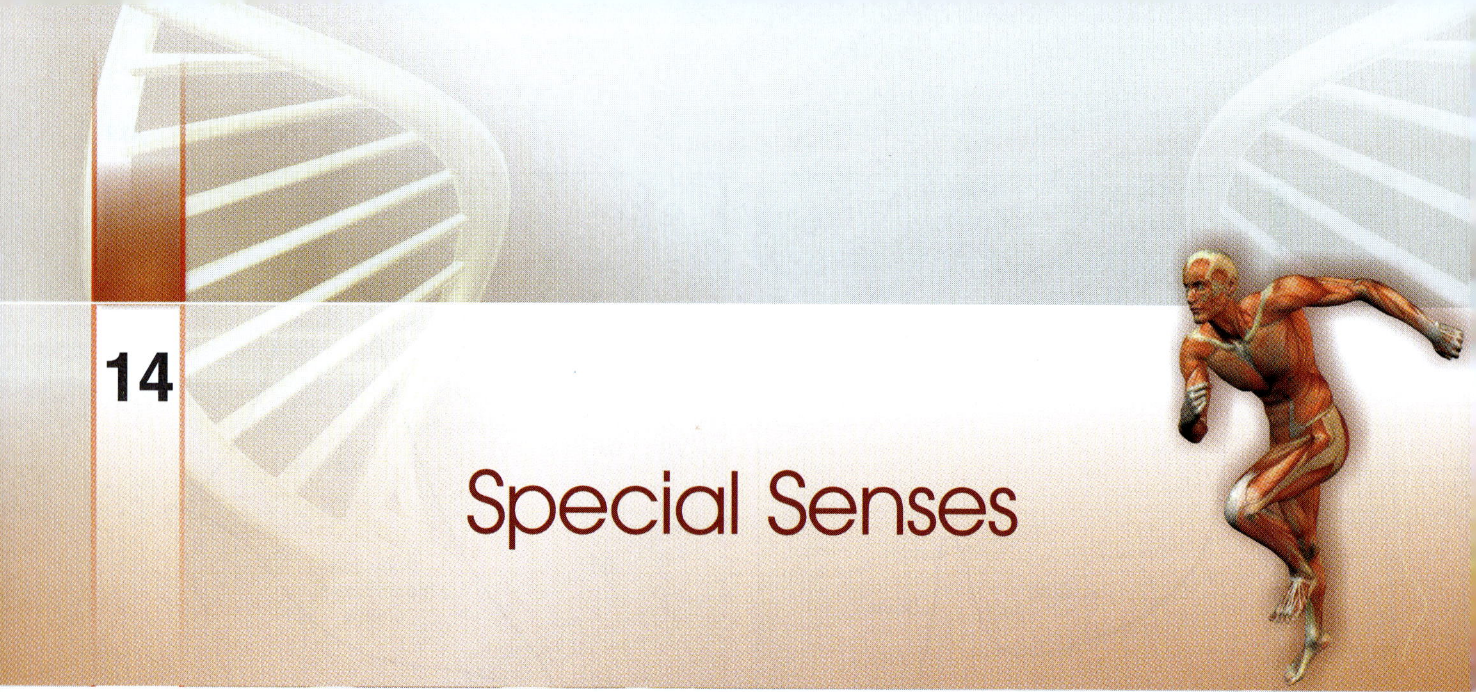

14 Special Senses

Vision and audition are the special senses with which we remain in communication with our surroundings.

VISION

BRIEF OVERVIEW

The eye is the organ for vision. It has visual receptors, (Fig. 14.1) rods and cones in the retina, which respond to light stimulus. **Rods** function in dim light and **cones** function when there is bright light. The vision in dim light is called **scotopic vision**; with this vision clear boundaries and color, cannot be perceived whereas during daylight when the cones function, the vision is known as **photopic vision** which provides acuity of vision and color vision, i.e. fine details of objects and colors can be made out. There is pigment contained in the visual receptors which is sensitive to light and is essential for visual perception; it is a derivative of vitamin A; and is called retinal which is aldehyde of vitamin A (retinol). Retinal is present in combination with a protein opsin, the two together is the photosensitive pigment. In the rods, it is called **rhodopsin** or **visual purple** and its opsin is called scotopsin. The cones also contain retinal and a protein opsin but the opsin differs in three types of cones. There are three different types of cones, each type responding maximally to a different wavelength of light (Fig. 14.2); the property is due to different structure of opsin in these three different types of cones. They are responsible for color perception. Light of different wavelengths stimulates the different cones in different proportions which produces the sensation of color.

The image of an object should be focused on the retina for clear vision. The light rays are refracted at corneal surface, cornea has a refractive power of 43D (D = diopters); and further at the anterior and posterior surfaces of the lens. An object situated at a distance of 6 meters or more, the rays of light are considered to be parallel and are converged by the cornea and lens to focus in a normal eye (emmetropic eye) on the retina. The rays of light from an object nearer than 6 meters are divergent but should again be focused

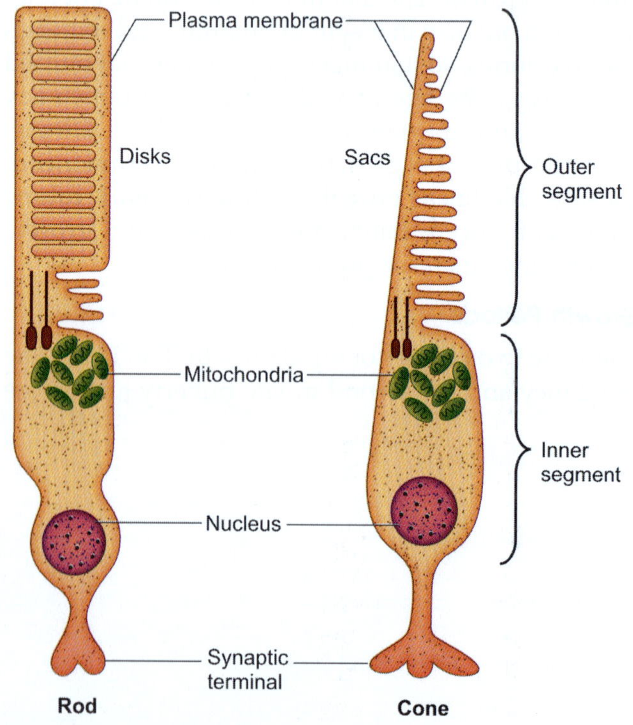

Fig. 14.1: Retinal photoreceptors as seen under the microscope

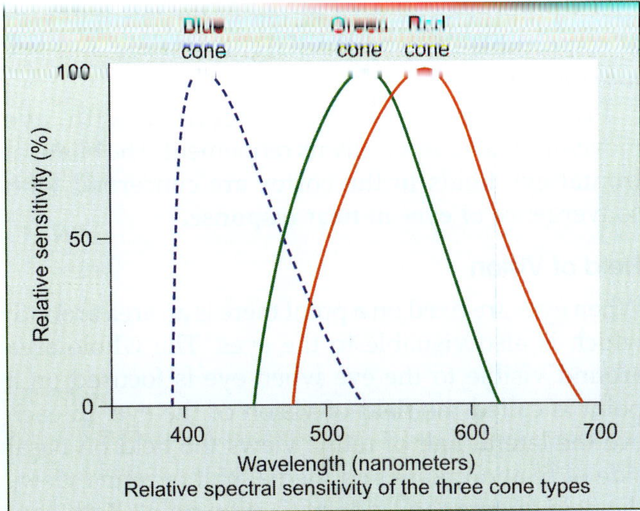

Fig. 14.2: The spectral sensitivity of the three types of cones in the retina. The curves overlap

on the retina, for clear vision, and this is brought about by increasing the refractive power of the eye. This is essential as the distance of the retina in the eye remains fixed and so the change must take place in the refractive power of the eye for divergent rays to focus again on the retina. The refractive power of the cornea remains unchanged but that of lens is increased to focus the rays on the retina. This increase in the refractive power of the eyes for near vision is called **accommodation**. This increase in the refractive power of the lens is brought about by contraction of ciliary muscles in the eye that decrease the distance between the edges of ciliary body and hence, the lens ligaments relax decreasing the tension on lens capsule that becomes lax permitting the lens to become more convex to increase its refractive power (Fig. 14.3). This phenomenon is accompanied by constriction of pupils and medial convergence of both eyes and three responses together are called **near response**.

The greater the curvature of the lens, the greater its refractive power. The refractive power of the lens is

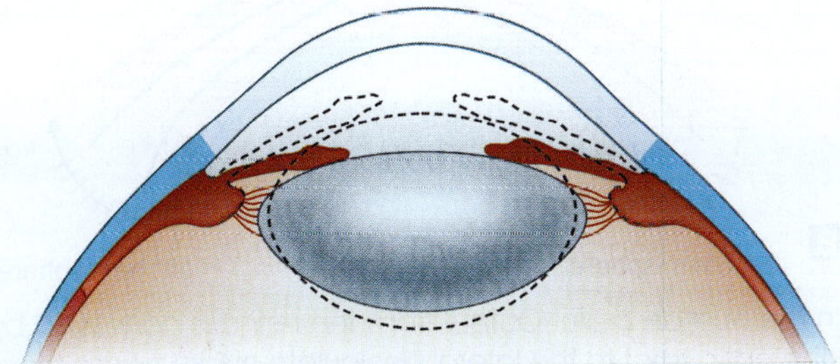

Fig. 14.3: Accommodation. The solid lines represent the shape of the lens, iris, and ciliary body at rest, and the dashed lines represent the shape during accommodation

expressed in *diopters*, the number of diopters being the reciprocal of principal focal distance in meters. (D = 1 ÷ focal distance in meters).

The human eye has a refractive power of approximately 60 diopters at rest.

The light stimulus that reaches the retina is transmitted through the different layers of the retina (Fig. 14.4). The image formed on the retina is perceived by photoreceptors which convert the light energy into electrical energy, i.e. electrical potentials which are conducted through different neurons in the layers of retina finally to the ganglion cells, and via their nerve fibers, which form optic nerve, the IInd cranial nerve, the impulses pass through optic chiasm, optic tracts to reach the lateral geniculate body and after relay of impulses there, nerve fibers of these neurons conduct impulses to the occipital lobe in the cerebral cortex (Fig. 14.5) where the image is perceived and interpreted.

Optic Pathways

The ganglion cell axons travel in the optic nerve, some cross to the opposite side of the brain in **optic chiasm** while others remain on the same side. There is a definite pattern of crossing; those from the medial halves of retina on each side cross to the opposite side; fibers from the lateral half of retina remain on the same side. From the optic chiasm (Fig. 14.6A) the

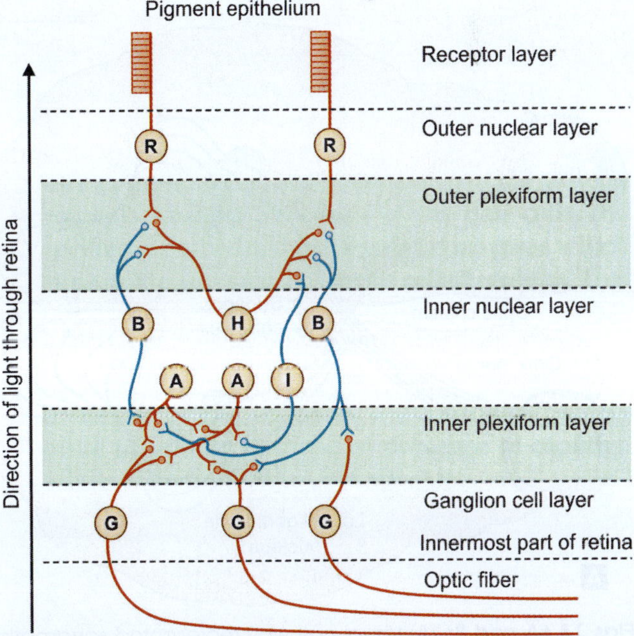

Fig. 14.4: Basic retinal circuitry. R-photoreceptors; B-bipolar cells; H-horizontal cells; A-amacrine cells; I-interplexiform cells; G-ganglion cells. Light stimulus on rods and cones stimulates ganglion cells

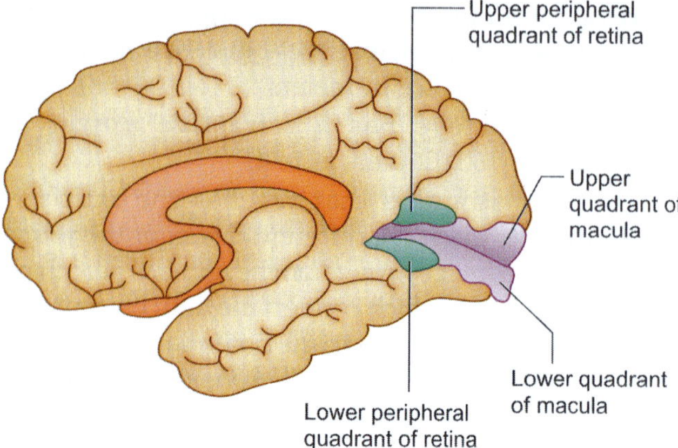

Fig. 14.5: Medial view of cerebrum showing visual area and representation of retina in the area

optic tract on each side carries fibers from the lateral half of retina (temporal half) from the eye on the same side and fibers from the medial half of retina (nasal half) from the eye of the opposite side; the fibers of the tract relay in the **lateral geniculate body** and geniculocalcarine tract fibers from there travel to the occipital cortex. Some fibers of the optic tract pass to the *midbrain* for control of *visual reflexes* and some also to the *hypothalamus* for control of *circadian rhythms*, the day and night rhythms of hormone secretions, body temperature, etc. As some axons bypass the lateral geniculate nucleus (LGN) to project directly to pretectal area in midbrain this pathway is responsible for **pupillary light reflexes** and **eye movements.**

Frontal cortex is also concerned with eye movements and especially its refinement. The bilateral frontal eye fields in the cortex are concerned with convergence of eyes in **near response.**

Field of Vision

When eyes are fixed on a point there is an area around; which is also visuable to the eyes. The whole area around visible to the eye when eye is focused on a point is called the field of vision of the eye. In each eye the lateral half of retina views the field on nasal side of fixation point and medial half of retina views the field on temporal side of fixation point. Both eyes together view a common field with binocular vision. But the nasal field of each eye seen by lateral part of retina is resticted by the nose and hence, there are areas of monocular vision on either side of binocular field these are as are seen by one eye only, by the medial parts of retina of either eye (Fig. 14.6B).

The image of an object on which eyes are focused is seen with both eyes and it falls on the corresponding points of retina in each eye; as it falls on corresponding points, it is synthesized in the brain for three dimensional perceptions by the **binocular vision.** The binocular vision helps in *depth and distance perception,*

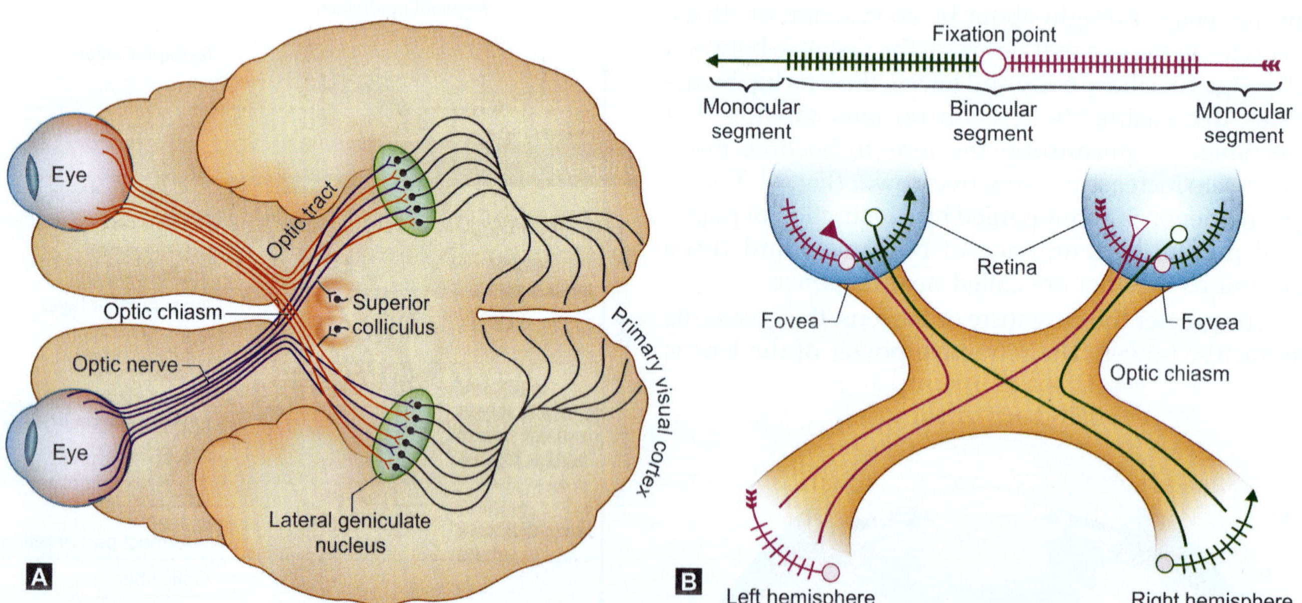

Figs 14.6A and B: (A) Visual pathway represented schematically in the human brain. Output from the retina is conveyed by ganglion cell axons via the optic, nerve and after partial crossing, the optic tract to the lateral geniculate nucleus from there to cerebral cortex and (B) Illustrating the principle of field of vision, visual object images on the retinas of the two eyes, and the projections of the ganglion cells carrying visual information about these images. Note with the eye fixed on the fixation point in the retina see parts of opposite field of vision. The image is large and extends to monocular segment of each eye

as each eye sees slightly different picture of the object, this forms the clue for it.

There are six extraocular muscles attached to each eye and their movements are coordinated as required for binocular vision. The motor nuclei of nerves for the eye movement are present in the midbrain and interconnections between the nuclei are responsible for coordination of movements of both the eyes.

Hence, there are adaptive mechanisms in the eye for vision, for:

- Twilight and day light conditions.
- Objects situated at a distance and those for near work.
- Regulation of the amount of light entering the eye (pupillary constriction or dilation).
- Binocular vision as image falls on corresponding points in two eyes for depth and distance perception.
- Fusion of stationary images, moved at a rapid rate, above the critical fusion frequency, in motion pictures (movies).

Structure of the Eye (Fig. 14.7)

The eyeball is formed of three layers:

1. Outer layer is **sclera** which is the white covering of the eye. It is fibrous and gives support to the eye and it is replaced anteriorly by the **cornea** which is transparent for the passage of light through it.
2. Middle layer is the **choroid** which is *rich in blood vessels* that supply the *outer layer of retina* and also *contains pigment* which absorbs the extra light so that there is no blurring of vision. Anteriorly, the choroid is thickened to form **ciliary body** which contains *muscle fibers* that attach near the corneoscleral junction. **Lens ligaments** are attached to the ciliary body and to the capsule of the lens. The choroid is replaced by **iris** above the lens. Iris gives color to the eye and has a central aperture, the **pupil** through which the light enters into the eye. The diameter of pupillary aperture is adjusted by contraction of radial and circular smooth muscle fibers present in the iris, which respectively make-up the pupillary dilator and constrictor (sphincter) muscles (Fig. 14A in Anatomy section) for the pupil; which regulate the amount of light entering the eye.

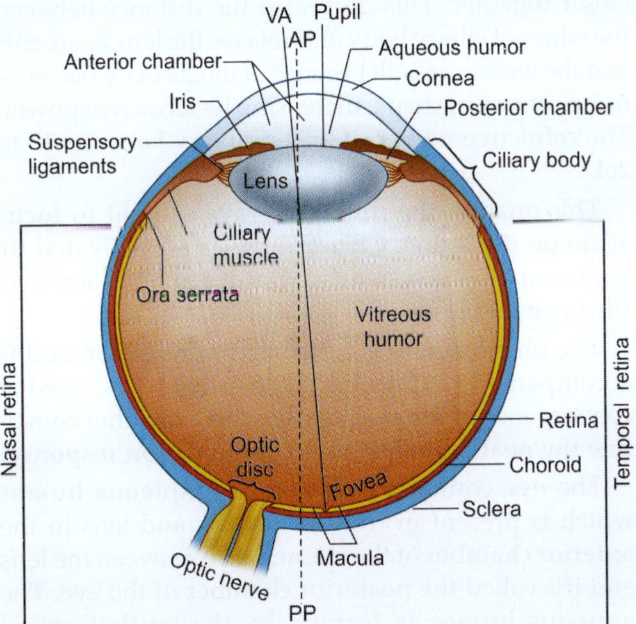

Fig. 14.7: Horizontal section of the right eye. AP-anterior pole; PP-posterior pole; VA-visual axis

The contraction of the radial fibers (dilation of pupil, mydriasis) is brought by stimulation of sympathetic nerves and contraction of the sphincter, i.e. the circular muscle fibers (constriction of pupil miosis) is by stimulation of parasympathetic nerves (IIIrd cranial nerves).

Bright light reflexly constricts the pupil (light reflex) to limit the light entering the eye while dim light dilates the pupil to allow adequate light to pass through into the eye. When light is shown in one eye, pupil of other eye also constricts even if it has been shielded from that light. This is known as ***consensual light reflex*** and is due to interconnections between nuclei of nerves responsible for ***light reflex***.

The ciliary body is the anterior continuation of the choroid; consists of ciliary muscle and secretory epithelium. It gives attachment to suspensory ligaments which at the other end attach to the capsule enclosing the lens. The ciliary body is supplied by IIIrd cranial nerve. The epithelial cells secrete aqueous fluid into the anterior segment of the eye which is present in anterior and posterior chambers (Fig. 14.8).

The inner most layer of the eyeball is retina which is many layered, containing photoreceptors, rods and cones, interneurons the neural elements and innermost layer containing the ganglion cells, which transmit the visual image via their nerve fibers which join to form optic nerve (IInd cranial nerve) in each eye to carrying impulses to the brain.

The point where optic nerve leaves the eye there are no visual receptors (rods or cones) in the retina and hence, it is called **blind spot**. There is no vision in this area. The area is medial to and slightly above the posterior pole of the eye. In the centre of the retina there is yellow pigmented spot, the **macula** where visual acuity is highest and in the centre of it there is a depression called **fovea** where there are only cones,

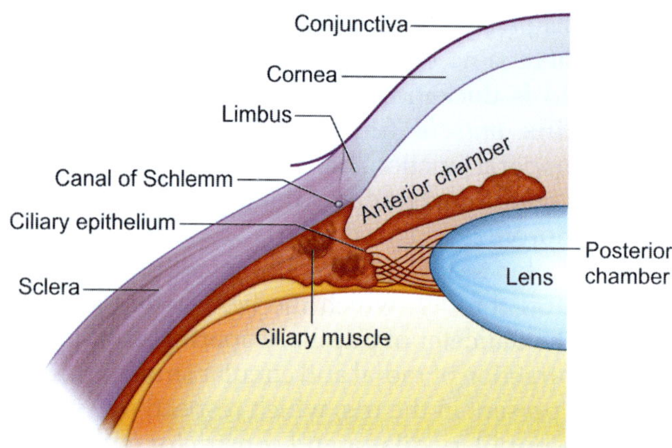

Fig. 14.8: Structures in the anterior part of the eye. The limbus (junction of the cornea and sclera), ciliary body, and lens

no rods and the vision is most accurate at this point. When eye is focused at an object the image falls on this point.

In the extrafoveal region of retina, the rods predominate. The outer layer of retina (containing rods and cones) is nourished by the capillary plexus of the blood vessels in the choroid; hence, retinal detachment can damage the photoreceptors. But, the inner layers are nourished by retinal artery which along with the retinal vein enter and leave the eye with optic nerve and travel in its sheath. The retinal artery and vein avoid macula in the retina. The artery and its branches can be seen with ophthalmoscopic examination and it is the only site in the body where the vessels, the arteries, arterioles and veins can be seen (Fig. 14.9) and this is used to view the vessels in diseased conditions like hypertension and diabetes to assess the state of vessels in the rest of the body.

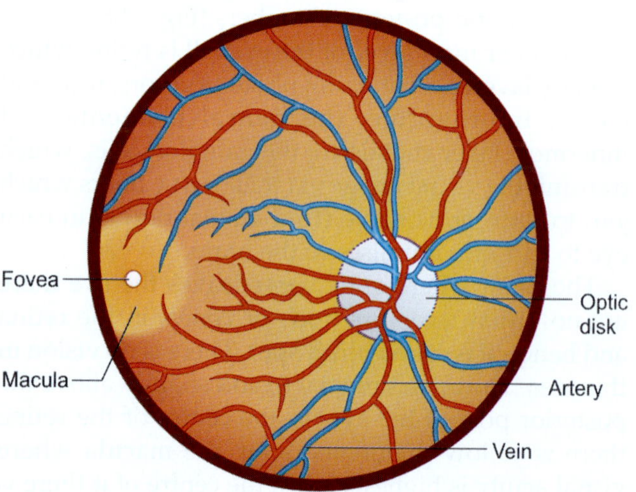

Fig. 14.9: Retina as seen through the ophthalmoscope

Physiology of light absorption by the eye. Light enters through cornea and passes through fluids and structures. Normally light from a target is focused sharply on retina by the cornea and the lens which refract (bend) the light rays. Cornea has a refractive power of 43 D and is major refractive element.

The eye contains the crystalline **lens** which is circular biconvex structure lying behind the pupil. It is enclosed in a capsule and suspended from ciliary body by suspensory ligaments. Lens is to focus the light rays on retina for clear vision for both distant and near vision. The parallel rays of light from distance focus on the retina in the optically normal (emmetropic) eye with the ciliary muscle relaxed. (At rest, the lens is held under tension by the lens ligaments, lens substance is malleable and the lens capsule has considered elasticity and lens is pulled into flattened shape).

ACCOMMODATION

When the object is at a near point the rays of light are divergent but also focus on the retina due to increase in the convexity of the lens. (If the relaxation of ciliary muscle is maintained rays from objects closer than 6 in distance would focus behind the retina and the image would appear blurred).

When vision is focused at a near object, there is contraction of ciliary muscle; they pull the whole ciliary body forward and inward, thus bring the edges of the ciliary body in the posterior chamber of the eye closer together. This decreases the distance between the edges of ciliary body and relaxes the lens ligaments and the lens as a result because of its elasticity becomes more convex in shape, increasing its refractive power. The refractive power of lens can vary between 13 to 26D.

This enables the divergent rays of light to focus again on the retina. Ciliary muscles are activated by parasympathetic system by way of oculomotor nerve, IIIrd cranial nerve.

The phenomenon is called **accommodation** and is accompanied by pupillary constriction and medial convergence of the eyeballs, the three together constitute the **near response or accommodation response.**

The eye contains fluids, called **aqueous humor** which is present in front of the iris and lens in the **anterior chamber** of the eye and also between the lens and iris called the **posterior chamber** of the eye. The aqueous humor is formed by the epithelium of the ciliary body in the posterior chamber of the eye; passes in the space between the lens and iris and through pupil into the anterior chamber (Fig. 14.10A) where it is absorbed in the canal of Schlemm, a venous channel present at the junction of sclera and cornea; hence, into venous system. Aqueous humor is constantly secreted and absorbed and its pressure remains between 10 and 20 mmHg. Aqueous fluid supplies nutrients and removes wastes from the transparent structures in front of the eye that have no blood supply, i.e. cornea, lens and lens capsule.

The space behind the lens is occupied by **vitreous humor** which is thick jelly like fluid, soft, colorless and transparent. It contains collagen and hyaluronic acid. It maintains intraocular pressure to support the retina against choroid and prevents walls of the eye ball from collapsing. It has slow rate of turnover. The eye keeps its shape because of the intraocular pressure exerted by the vitreous body and aqueous fluid.

Glaucoma is the disease when the pressure of the aqueous humor becomes high due to failure of absorption (Fig. 14.10B). Increased pressure results in increased pressure on retina which may gradually cause blindness by restricting blood flow to retina. It is treated by carbonic anhydrase inhibitors which decrease production of aqueous humor or by cholinergic agonists which increase outflow.

THE PHOTORECEPTORS

Light absorbed by the photopigments in the photoreceptors is responsible for the vision.

Rods and **cones** contain photosensitive compounds made-up of a protein called opsin and retinal, which is aldehyde of vitamin A. The photosensitive pigment in the rods is called rhodopsin or visual purple. Its opsin is called scotopsin. The rods are highly sensitive to light and hence, responsible for vision in the dim light. With the scotopic vision the details of objects are not made out and there is **no color perception.**

Cones have a much **higher threshold for light** hence, function in bright light, but the cone system has a much **greater acuity** and is the system responsible for vision in bright light (**photopic vision**) and **for color vision**. Cones are of three different types and this helps to perceive color. Each type of cone contains retinal but different opsin; the opsin is different in structure in each of these cones; as a result, each cone contains a different photopigment which is maximally sensitive to one of the primary colors (blue or green or red). As a result, the sensation of any color is determined by the relative frequency of the impulses from each of these cone systems (Fig. 14.2).

One pigment (blue sensitive or short wave pigment) absorbs light maximally in the blue violet portion of the spectrum; another green-sensitive pigment absorbs maximally in the green portion. The third red sensitive pigment absorbs maximally in the yellow portion. Blue, green and red are the primary colors. But, the cones with their maximal sensitivity in the yellow portion of the spectrum are sensitive to respond to red light at lower threshold than green.

The theory of color vision based on three types of cones in the retina is ***trichromacy theory***, called ***Young-Helmholtz theory***. Neural elements of retina also participate in color perception.

Diplopia

When the images in two eyes do not fall on corresponding points on the retina, then the images sent to the brain do not collaborate and this leads to double vision, i.e. diplopia.

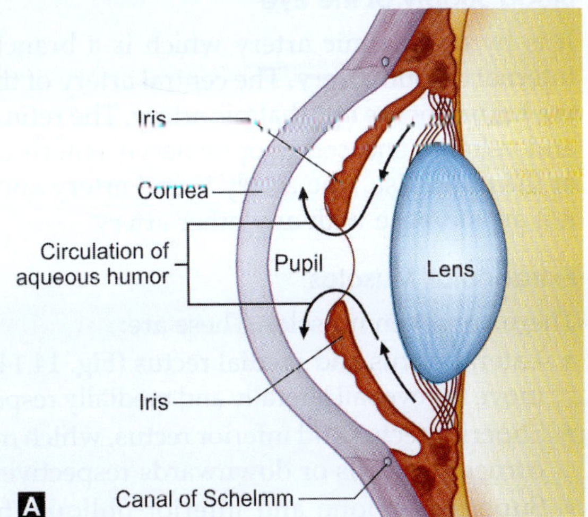

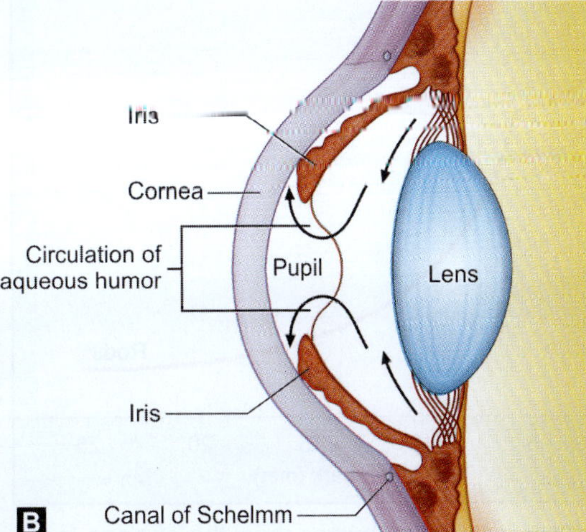

Figs 14.10A and B: Cross-section of an eye (A) Normal circulation of the equeous humor. (B) Eye affected with glaucoma in which fluid in the eye aqueous humour cannot drain away normally

Dark Adaptation

If a person spends sometime in bright environment and then moves into a dim lighted room, the individual may not be able to see for a short time till the person gets adapted to dark, i.e. till the visual threshold is declined to be able to perceive in dim light (the eyes become more sensitive to light). This is called dark adaptation and it takes about 20 minutes with some further adaptation over longer period. There are two components of the dark adaptation response. This first drop in visual threshold is rapid but small in magnitude is due to dark adaptation of cones. The subsequent drop is slower but much more and is due to adaptation of rods (Fig. 14.11).

Critical Fusion Frequency (CFF)

CFF is the maximum rate at which the stimuli when presented are still perceived as separate stimuli. Stimuli presented at higher rate than CFF are perceived as continuous stimuli. Motion pictures make use of this fact.

Protection of the Eye

The eye is protected from injury by the bony orbit. Eye is situated in the anterior part of the bony orbit. The space between the eye and the orbital cavity is occupied by adipose tissue. In the posterior part of the orbit are the various muscles, their associated blood vessels and nerves to move the eyeball in various directions.

The cornea is kept moistened by tears from **lacrimal gland** in the upper portion and laterally in each orbit (Fig. 14.12). Its ducts open into conjunctival sac. Tears flow over the surface of the eye, provide lubrication between the eyelids and the eyeball. On the medial side of conjunctival sac, there are two lacrimal canaliculi which join to open into the **nasolacrimal duct** (Fig. 14.12) which opens into the inferior meatus of the nose. The secretion flows in the sac and is drained into the nasal cavity. If excessive amount is secreted it is called tears. Blinking helps in the movement of tears to keep the cornea free of irritants like dust. Tears nourish the cornea and enzyme lysozyme is present that prevents microbial infection.

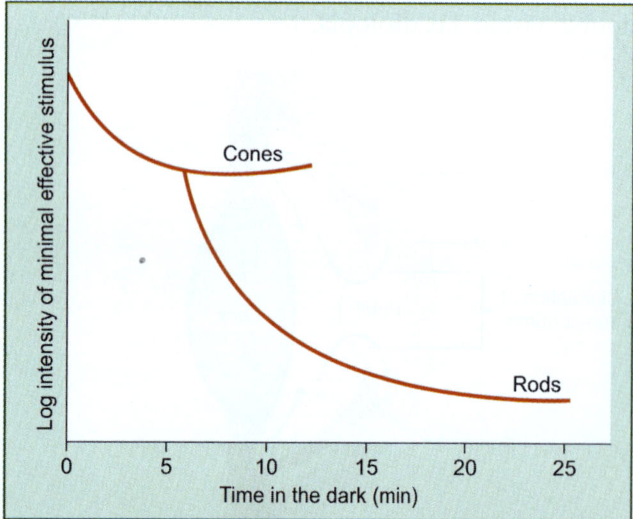

Fig. 14.11: Dark adaptation curves show the change in the intensity of the stimulus with time, necessary to just excite the retina in the dim light

Conjunctiva

It is a transparent membrane which lines the eyelids and the front of the eyeball (Fig. 14.13). It consists of vascular stratified epithelium. Corneal conjunctiva consists of less vascular stratified epithelium. When the eyelids are closed the conjunctiva becomes a closed sac. It protects the delicate cornea and the front of the eye. The fluid of lacrimal secretion fills the conjunctival sac.

Eyelids and Eyebrows

Protecting the eyeball are the upper and lower eyelids (Fig. 14.13) and eyelashes. The medial and the lateral angles of the eye where the upper and lower eyelids come together are called the medial canthus and the lateral canthus, respectively. Eyelids are moved by two muscles, orbicularis oculi and levator palpebrae superioris. Eyelid margin also has opening of several glands. Eyebrows prevent sweat of the head from entering the eyes and protect the anterior aspect of eyeball from injuries by foreign objects.

Blood Supply of the Eye

It is by ophthalmic artery which is a branch of the internal carotid artery. The central artery of the retina is a branch of the ophthalmic artery. The retinal artery and vein are encased in optic nerve, entering the eye at the optic disc. The artery is end artery and it does not anastomose with any other artery.

Extraocular Muscles

There are seven muscles. These are:

- Lateral rectus and medial rectus (Fig. 14.14) which move the eyeball laterally and medially respectively.
- Superior rectus and inferior rectus, which move the cornea upwards or downwards respectively.
- Superior oblique and inferior oblique, function mainly to rotate the eye ball to keep visual fields in upright positions.

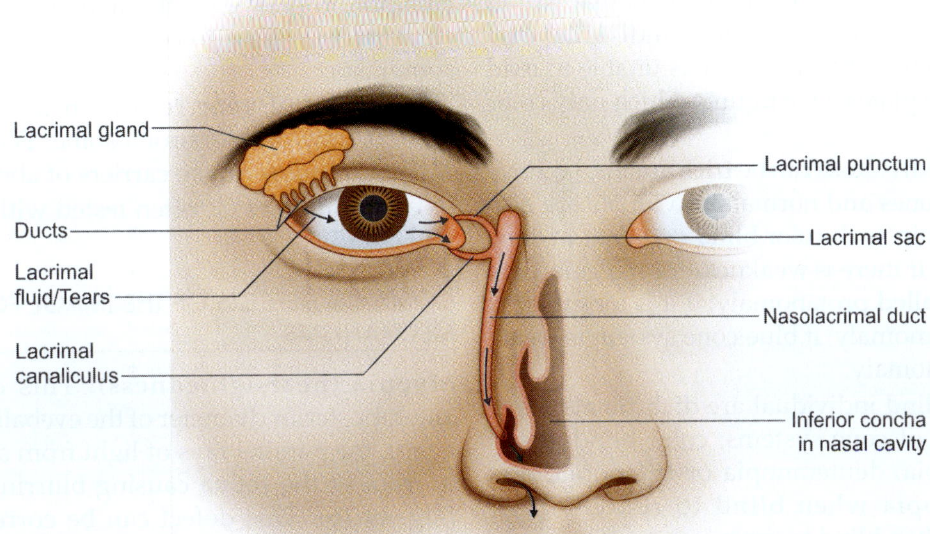

Fig. 14.12: Lacrimal apparatus

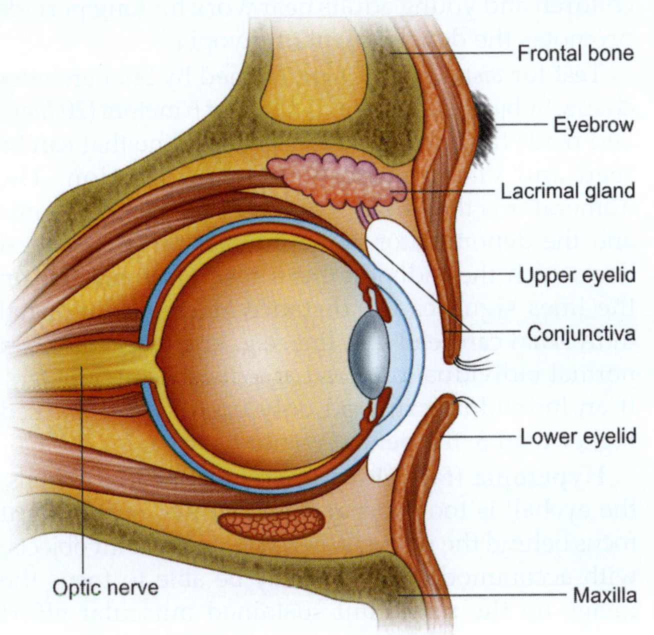

Fig. 14.13: Section of the eye and its accessory structures

- Lavetor palpebrae superioris lifts the upper eyelid to open the eye.

Muscles of the two eyes move in coordination. To look to one side lateral rectus of that side and medial rectus of the other eye would contract.

Lateral rectus is supplied by VI cranial nerve; superior oblique is by IV cranial nerve; rest of the muscles, i.e. medial rectus, inferior oblique, superior rectus, inferior rectus, levator palpebrae superioris are supplied by IIIrd cranial nerve.

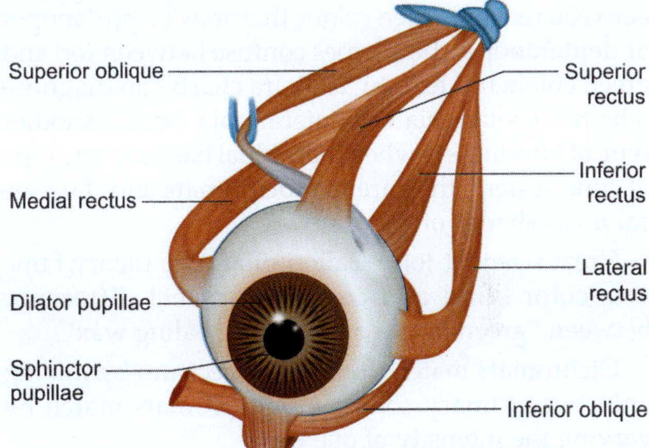

Fig. 14.14: Muscles of the eyeball

The eye movements are influenced by areas of the brain in frontal, parietal and occipital lobes.

Strabismus

When the visual images do not fall on the corresponding parts of the retina in each eye squint (strabismus) is present. Some defects can be corrected by eye exercises or use of glass prisms that bend the light rays or in some cases surgical shortening of some eye muscles can be done.

COLOR BLINDNESS

There are numerous tests for detecting color blindness. The most commonly used routine tests are Ishihara charts. The charts are printed figures of colored spots on a background of similarly shaped spots of different colors. The figures are made-up of colors that would look the same as the background to an individual who is color blind so that the individual is unable to read the figure. Some plates have figures which only color blind can read.

Color blind individuals can be **trichromats,** i.e. have three types of cones and normal individuals are also trichromats; but in such color blind one type of cone system is weak. If there is weakness for red color, the color defect is called protanomaly; if it is for green, it is called deuteranomaly; if blue cone system is weak, it is called tritanomaly.

Some color blind individual are **dichromats;** have only two types of cone systems; color blindness is called protanopia, deuteranopia or tritanopia; it is called protanopia when blind to red color, or deuteranopia when blind to green color or tritanopia blind to blue color; and so confuse colors.

The most common of color blindness is red and green blindness. When the individual confuses between red and green colors; they may be protanopes or deuteranopes; both types confuse between red and green colors but tests by Ishihara charts can diagnose whether protanopia or deuteranopia exists. Another type of blindness is when individual has only one type of cone system, they are **monochromats** and they see colors as shades of grey only.

Great scientist John Dalton of atomic theory fame was color blind and could not detect difference between "green leaf or stick of red sealing wax".

Dichromats match their color spectrum by mixing only two primary colors, monochromats match by varying the intensity of one only.

Color blindness is most usually inherited (but it can occur with lesions in the visual cortex). It affects males more commonly than females. Blue color weakness or blindness does not show sex selectivity. Gene is in autosomal chromosomes. Red green blindness is more common in males, is inherited as recessive X-linked characteristic (due to abnormal gene on X chromosome).

Mutation of gene results in defect in males as there is only one X chromosome. Females with two X chromosomes can be carriers of abnormal gene.

Color blindness is often tested with Ishihara chart (Fig. 14.15).

COMMON DEFECTS OF THE IMAGE FORMING MECHANISMS

Myopia (nearsightedness): This condition, the anteroposterior diameter of the eyeball is too long and hence, the parallel rays of light from a distance focus in front of the retina causing blurring of the image (Fig. 14.16). This defect can be corrected by using biconcave lenses which make the parallel rays diverge slightly before striking the eye (Fig. 14.16).

Myopia is believed to have genetic origin. In children and young adults near work for long periods promotes the development of myopia.

Test for *visual acuity* is performed by Snellen letter charts. Subject stands at a distance of 6 meters (20 feet), and reads the lines up to the smallest line that can be read and vision is expressed as a fraction. The numerator is the distance at which the subject stands and the denominator is the number on the smallest line which the individual can read. The number on the lines signifies the distance at which a normal individual can read that line, e.g. line marked as 5, a normal individual can read at a distance of 5 meters. If an individual can read only up to a line marked higher than 6, the person would be myopic.

Hyperopia (farsightedness): In these individuals, the eyeball is too short and the parallel rays of light focus behind the retina. When viewing distant objects, with accommodation they may be able to focus the image on the retina but sustained muscular effort

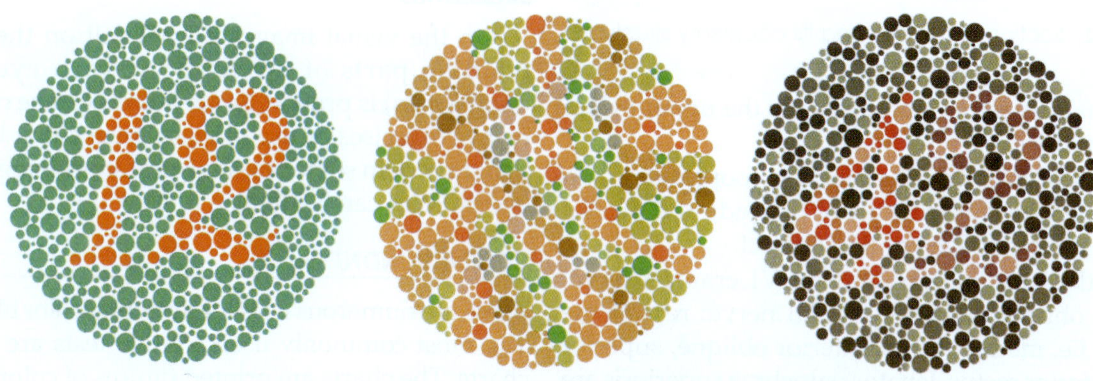

Fig. 14.15: Ishihara charts

becomes tiring and may cause headache and blurring of vision. The defect can be corrected by using biconvex lenses (Fig. 14.16).

Astigmatism: It is a condition when curvature of the cornea is not uniform. The curvature in one meridian is different from that in others and light rays in that meridian are brought to focus at a different point in the eye and retinal image is blurred. Similarly, the lens can have the same defect though this is less common. The defect can be corrected by cylindrical lenses.

Presbyopia

In old age, the lens gradually becomes hard due to loss of elasticity, resulting in loss of accommodation for near work. By the age of 40–45 years, a normal individual requires reading glasses (with biconvex lens) and the defect tends to increase with age. The near point of vision (the nearest point to the eye where vision is clear with accommodation) recedes throughout life from 9 cm in a young child to 83 cm in a person of 60 years.

Cataract

There is gradual loss of lens transparency that may occur in old people which is exaggerated by trauma, radiation (ultraviolet light and high energy photons, such as gamma-rays and X-rays) and by metabolic problems, such as uncontrolled diabetes. An eye with opacity in the lens is said to have cataract. In early stages, some of the lens proteins in the fibers become denatured. Later, these same proteins coagulate to form opaque areas. An opaque lens may have to be removed, and be replaced by implanted lens or else by use of convex glasses.

Other Defects in Eyes

Night Blindness

Severe deficiency of vitamin A produces night blindness (nyctalopia) due to defective rod function where rhodopsin requires vitamin A, if deficiency is prolonged cone function is also affected; and if still prolonged leads to degeneration of neural elements of the retina.

Other vitamins especially of the vitamin B group are necessary for visual functions of the retina.

Blindness

Loss of useful sight can be temporary or permanent. Damage to any portion of the eye the optic nerve or the area of the brain responsible for vision can lead to blindness. The current correct terms for blindness include visually handicapped and visually challenged.

Lesions in the Optic Pathways (Fig. 14.17)

Field of vision is the field which the eye sees all around a fixation point though the eye is fixed on a point (Fig. 14.17). Lesion of the optic nerve causes blindness of that eye (Fig. 14.17A). Lesion of the optic tract, causes blindness in one field of vision, i.e. when there is lesion of the left optic tract which is carrying fibers from the lateral half of the left retina and medial half of the right retina (Fig. 14.6B) that are for viewing the right field of vision that vision is lost (Fig. 14.17B), right hemianopia results (hemianopia, i.e. half field of vision is blind); and left field of vision is lost if there is lesion of the right optic tract; the nerve fibers for light reflex leave the optic tract before it relays in the lateral geniculate body; hence, if light

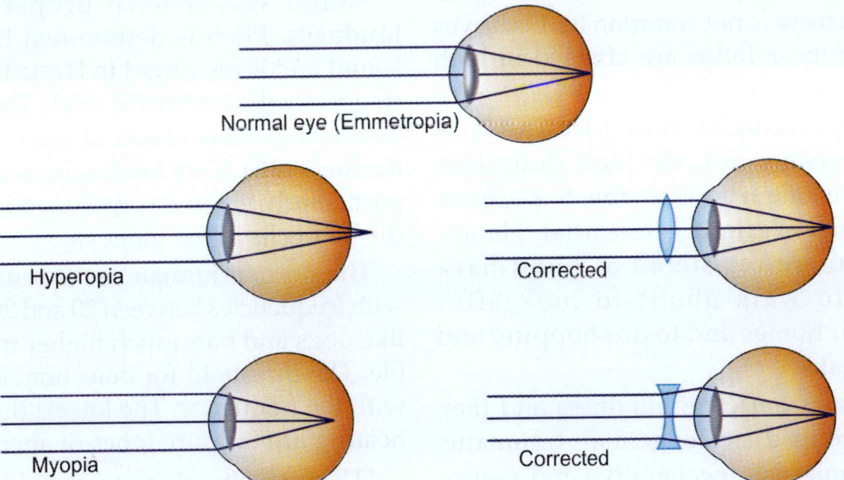

Fig. 14.16: Common defects of the optical system of the eye. A biconvex lens corrects hyperopia: biconcave lens corrects myopia

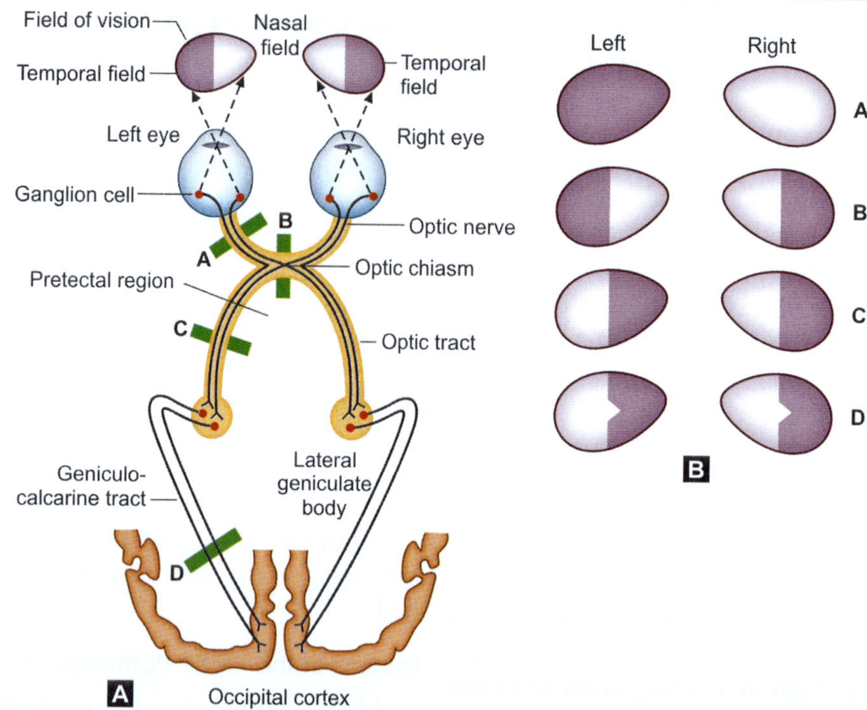

Figs 14.17A and B: Visual pathways. Occipital lesions may spare the fibers from the macula (as in D) because of the separation in the brain of these fibers from the others subserving vision (as in Fig. 14.5). The lesions at various sites indicated by letters A B C D, cause visual defects in the fields indicated. Color area indicate blind field

reflex is present the lesion is in the optic tract after the fibers of light reflex have left and if absent the lesion is before the fibers of light reflex leave. Hemianopia is half field blindness; if the blindness is in the **same field of vision** for both eyes it is called homonymous hemianopia, as in optic tract lesions; if there is lesion in optic chiasma as with pituitary tumor, the medial fibers from both the retina are affected the hemianopia (Fig. 14.17B) is heteronymous and bitemporal. Heteronymous as field affected in each eye is not common for both eyes and bitemporal as those fields are affected in both eyes.

It is generally thought that blindness is complete loss of vision. But, the legal definition of a blind person is one who is unable to perform any work for which eyesight is essential. Hence, some people who are registered as blind have enough vision to walk about to look after themselves in their homes and to do shopping and other domestic tasks.

There can be many causes of blindness and they can be roughly grouped as: congenital, traumatic, inflammatory, neoplastic, degenerative and neurological due to glaucoma or diabetes. **Macular degeneration** is sometimes a result of diabetes.

HEARING

The auditory system is important for communication with others and provides environmental cues. It is important for language functions. There is problem with speech when a child is born deaf.

Sound is produced by waves of compression and decompression transmitted in air or in other elastic material like water.

Sound waves have properties of **pitch** and **loudness**. Pitch is determined by the frequency of sound and is measured in **Hertz (Hz).** The greater the frequency the higher the pitch. The loudness depends on the amplitude of sound waves and is measured in **decibels (dB)**. Very loud noise is damaging to the ear, particularly when it is prolonged because it damages the hair cells in the inner ear.

The normal human ear is sensitive to pure tones with frequencies between 20 and 20,000 Hz. In animals like dogs and bats much higher frequencies are audible. The threshold for detection of a pure tone varies with the frequency. The lowest thresholds for human hearing are for pure tones of about 1000 to 4000 Hz.

[The intensity of sound in Bel is the logarithm of a ratio of the intensity of that sound to a standard reference sound. A decibel is 0.1 bel].

Number of dB = 10 log of intensity of sound/intensity of standard sound.

Sound intensity is proportional to the square of sound pressure.

Number of dB = 20 log pressure of sound/pressure of standard sound.

[Standard reference level taken corresponds to 0 dB at a pressure level of 0.00020 dyne/cm^2 which is a value just audible to average person. The 0 decibel does not mean the absence of sound but a sound level of intensity equal to that of the standard.]

Sounds that exceed 140 dB can damage the organ of Corti, those above 120 dB can cause discomfort and pain (Fig. 14.18). Speech has an intensity of about 65 dB. The main frequencies used in speech are in the range of 300–3,500 Hz. With age as people get old the ability to hear high frequency declines. This condition is called presbycusis.

Masking

Presence of one sound decreases the ability to hear other sounds. This phenomenon is called masking. The degree to which a tone can mask another tone is related to its pitch. Due to absence of masking effect in the sound proof room the auditory threshold is lowered.

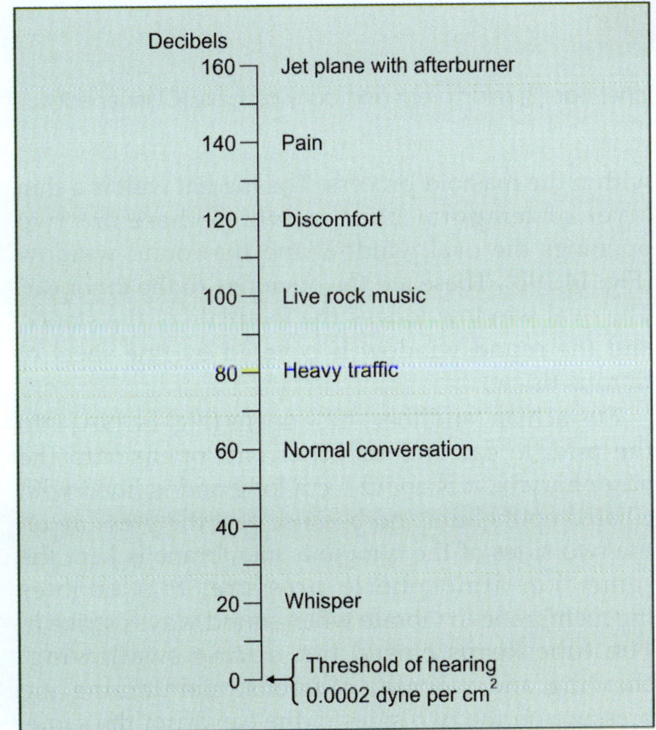

Fig. 14.18: A decibel (dB) scale showing approximate acoustic power in the presence of various sound sources

Auditory and Vestibular Systems

The main parts of both systems share parts in the inner ear. The hair cells in each of these systems act as transducers, and convert the information from either system into nerve impulses which are conducted to the CNS via the VIIIth cranial nerve; the cochlear portion of the eighth cranial nerve conducts from the hearing parts whereas the vestibular portion of the nerve from the vestibular areas.

But further pathways in the CNS are different, as the functions of the two sensory systems are also different. The **vestibular system** is *involved in the detection of position and movement of the head in space, which has the role in adjustment of body posture to enable the maintenance of balance and to control of eye movements.*

The **cochlear portion** of the VIIIth cranial nerve is involved in ***hearing functions.***

OVERVIEW OF THE AUDITORY SYSTEM

The ear converts sound waves into action potentials in the auditory nerves. The waves first impinge on the ear drum in the external ear; are transmitted to auditory ossicles in the middle ear, which results in the movements of the foot plate of stapes; the movements of which set-up waves in the fluid of inner ear. The action of waves on the organ of Corti generates action potentials in the nerve fibers of VIIIth cranial nerves.

Ear the organ of hearing is divided into three parts (Figs 14.19A to C):

1. External ear
2. Middle ear
3. Inner ear

The External Ear

It consists of auricle, external auditory meatus or external auditory canal which passes inwards to the tympanic membrane (eardrum). The auricle funnels sound waves to the external auditory meatus. In some animals, the auricle can be moved to catch sounds.

The auricle is composed of fibroelastic cartilage covered with skin. The lobule (earlobe) is soft pliable part composed of fibrous and adipose tissue.

The external auditory canal is slightly "S" shaped tube about 2.5 cm long. Its outer third is cartilaginous and the remainder is a canal in the temporal bone. The lining skin contains hairs and numerous glands that secrete cerumen, a waxy substance which is sticky and contains lysozyme and immunoglobulins, in the skin of outer third. The glands are modified sweat glands. Foreign materials like dust, insects are

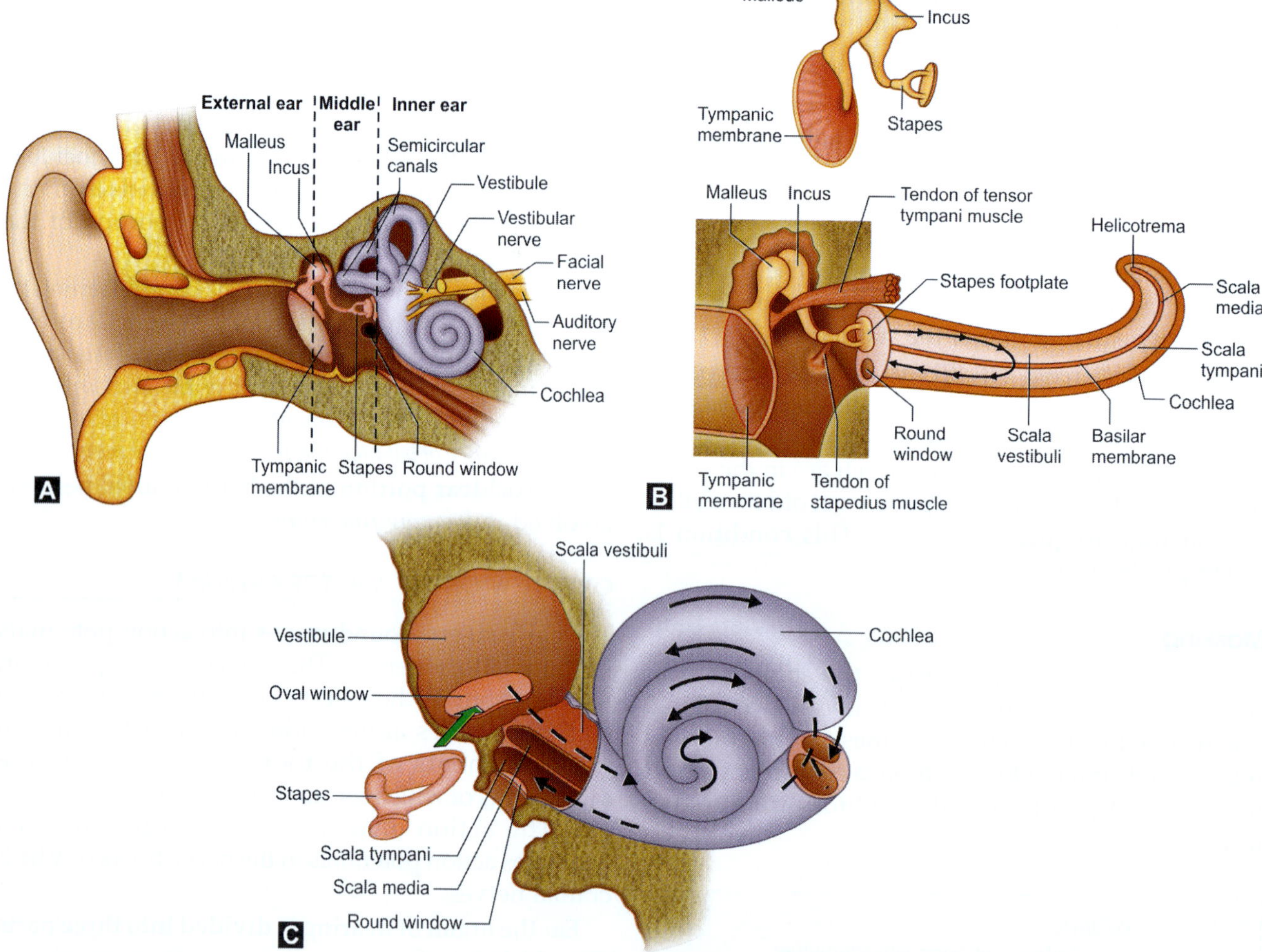

Figs 14.19A to C: (A) Structure of the external, middle and inner ear, (B) middle ear and bony ossicles, (C) inner ear

prevented from reaching the tympanic membrane by wax and hairs. Movements of the temporomandibular joint which occur during chewing and speaking massage the cartilaginous canal, thus the wax moves out.

The tympanic membrane at the other end of the external auditory canal separates it from middle ear. The membrane is made-up of three layers: (1) the outer hairless skin, (2) the middle is fibrous tissue and (3) the inner is mucous membrane which is continuous with the mucous membrane covering of the middle ear.

Middle Ear (Tympanic Cavity)

This is a cavity within the petrous portion of the temporal bone and filled with air. Roof and floor are made by temporal bone. The posterior wall is formed by the temporal bone with openings to the mastoid antrum through which the air passes to the air cells within the mastoid process. The medial wall is a thin layer of temporal bone in which there are two openings the oval window and the round window (Fig. 14.19B). These are the openings to the inner ear. The oval window lodges the footplate of the stapes, and the round window is covered by fine sheet of fibrous tissue.

Eustachian (auditory) tube opens (Fig. 14.19A) into the middle ear and its other end opens into the nasopharynx, it is about 4 cm long and is lined with ciliated epithelium and because of it the pressure on the two sides of the tympanic membrane is kept the same, i.e. atmospheric pressure, that enables the membrane to vibrate when sound waves strike it. The tube keeps closed but during swallowing, chewing and yawning it opens, maintaining the pressure on the two sides of the ear drum the same. When the pressure is unequal on two sides as during take off or landing in air flight or during diving, it may cause pain. If the Eustachian tube is blocked, e.g. due to collection of fluid during middle ear infection, the resulting difference in pressure between external and middle ears can produce pain by displacement of tympanic membrane; rupture of membrane may occur in extreme cases.

Auditory Ossicles

There are three small bones in the middle ear (Fig. 14.19B) which form a link between the tympanic membrane and the oval window and the sound waves are transmitted along this path. The bones are called, the malleus, the incus and the stapes. They form a series of movable joints with each other.

The handle of the **malleus** is attached to the back of the tympanic membrane and head forms a movable joint with the incus. The body of **incus** articulates with malleus and its long process with the stapes. The **stapes** is like a stirrup and its foot plate is attached by an annular ligament to the walls of the oval window.

There are two small skeletal muscles in the middle ear (Fig. 14.19B) called the **tensor tympani** with nerve supply by trigeminal nerve and the **stapedius** with nerve supply by facial nerve. Contraction of tensor tympani pulls the handle of the malleus medially thereby decreasing the amplitude of vibrations of the tympanic membrane; contraction of **stapedius** pulls the foot plate of stapes outward.

The loud sounds cause reflex contraction of these muscles, and reflex is called **tympanic reflex**. The contractions of the muscles provide protection during loud sound as they dampen movements of the bony ossicles preventing excessive stimulation of auditory receptors in the inner ear. But, sudden explosion can still damage the hearing apparatus as the contractions cannot occur that fast, it being a reflex. This action can be protective for sounds that can be anticipated, such as vocalization. This mechanism is unable to protect against sudden brief intense stimulation that is produced by gunshots.

Function of Auditory Ossicles

The auditory ossicles function as a lever system that transmits the vibrations of the tympanic membrane into movements of stapes against the perilymph which fills scala vestibuli of the cochlea, in the inner ear. The movements of head of stapes swing its foot plate to and fro like a door hinged at the posterior edge of the oval window. The lever system increases the sound pressure that arrives at the oval window, because the lever action of malleus and incus multiplies the force; and the area of the tympanic membrane is much greater than the area of the foot plate of the stapes which also increases the force of the sound. This is important as the sound waves incident on tympanic membrane arrive through air and are transmitted to the fluid in the internal ear which has much higher impedance for sound. Hence, the lever action of ossicles along with the greater area of the tympanic membrane serve as impedance matching device enabling transmission of sound energy from air over tympanic membrane to fluid medium in the inner ear.

Adjacent to the oval window is the round window, another membrane covered opening between the middle and the inner ears.

On the other side of the oval window is the fluid filled component of cochlea, called the vestibule. The vestibule is continuous with tubular structure called scala vestibuli (Fig. 14.19C).

Inward movement of the tympanic membrane by sound pressure causes the chain of the ossicles to push the foot plate of stapes into the oval window. This in turn displaces the fluid in the scala vestibuli in the inner ear. The pressure wave is transmitted through the basilar membrane of the cochlea to the scala tympani and causes the round window to bulge in the middle ear (Fig. 14.19B).

The Inner Ear

The inner ear includes **bony** and **membranous labyrinths**. The **cochlea** and the **vestibular apparatus** are formed from these (Fig. 14.20).

The bony labyrinth is series of cavities within the petrous portion of the temporal bone. It encloses the membranous labyrinth of the same shape that fits into it, like a tube within a tube (Fig. 14.20). Between the bony and the membranous labyrinth is watery fluid called perilymph which resembles CSF and within the membranous labyrinth is also watery fluid, the endolymph which is different in composition.

The bony labyrinth (Fig. 14.20) consists of:

- Vestibule
- Cochlea: It is apparatus for hearing
- Semicircular canals: They are parts of vestibular apparatus for balance.

The Hearing Apparatus

The vestibule is the expanded part nearest the middle ear (Figs 14.19C and 14.20). It contains oval and round windows in its lateral wall.

The cochlea is spiral shaped organ. The spiral in humans consists of 2¾ turns (Fig. 14.19C) around a central bony column modiolus, and it starts from

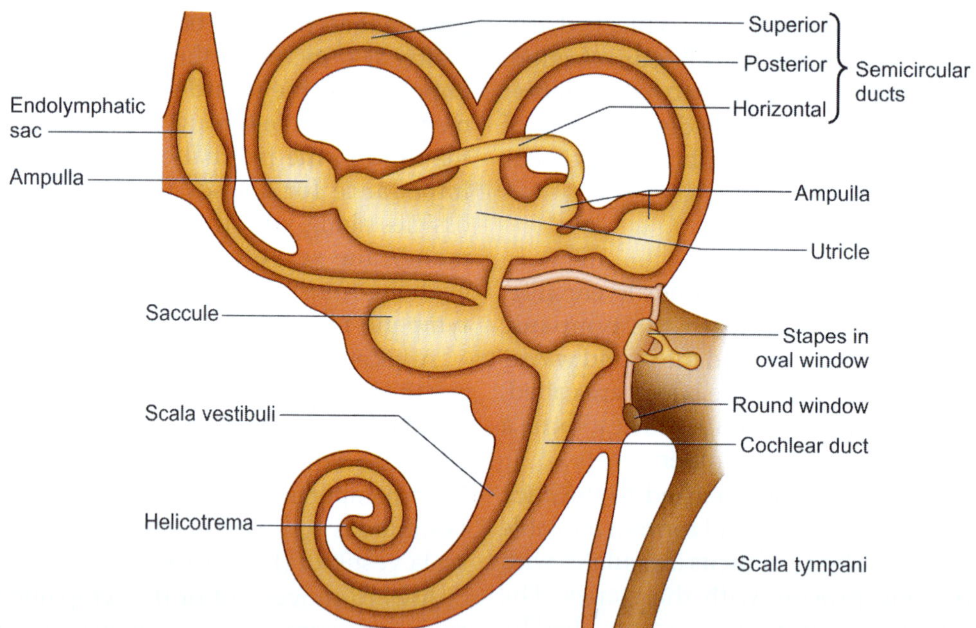

Fig. 14.20: Vestibular apparatus

broad base from vestibule and extends to a narrow apex (Fig. 14.20). It encloses membranous component, the cochlear duct (Fig. 14.20) which forms scala media and contains endolymph. The cochlea contains two more chambers around the scala media. The scala vestibuli which starts at the oval window and scala tympani which ends at round window that is closed by the flexible secondary tympanic membrane; both wind along with the cochlea, contain perilymph, communicate with each other at apex of cochlea through an aperture called helicotrema.

There is no communication between endolymph and perilymph.

The wall of the scala media are formed by the basilar membrane, below which is scala tympani, another wall is by Reissner's membrane, above which is scala vestibule, and the third, the outer wall is by stria vascularis (Fig. 14.21). Endolymph is secreted by stria vascularis and is drained through the endolymphatic duct into the dural venous sinuses (Fig. 14.20). Endolymph contains a high concentration of K^+, low concentration of Na^+ hence, it resembles intracellular fluid.

The neural apparatus responsible for transmission of sound is organ of corti. The **organ of corti** (Fig. 14.21) is positioned within the cochlear duct. It

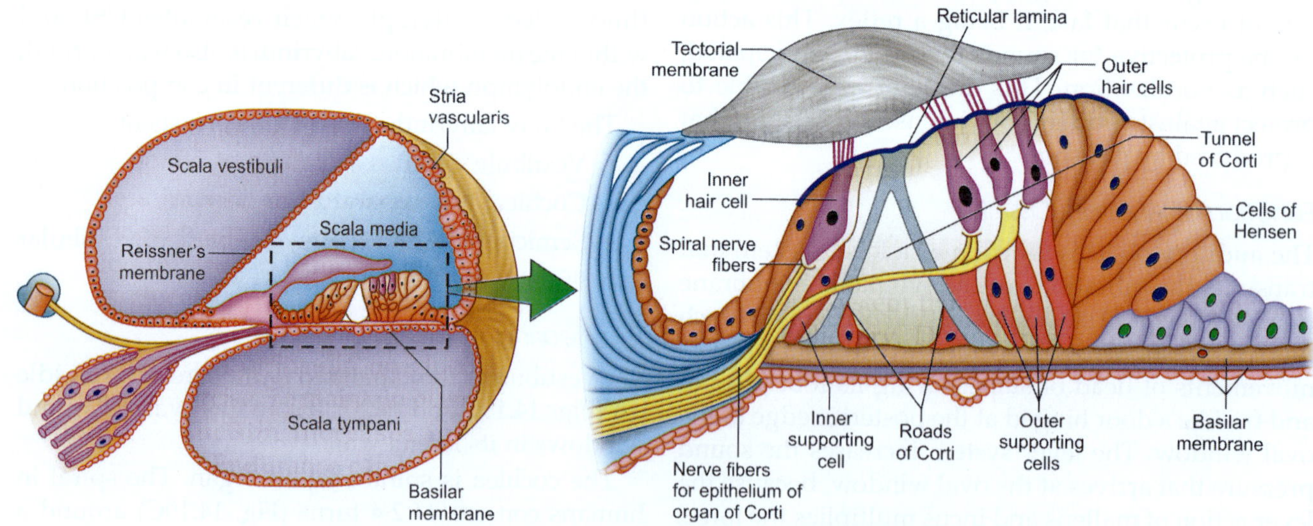

Fig. 14.21: Cross-section through cochlea details of organ of corti

lies on the basilar membrane and consists of rows of hair cells, and a number of supporting cells. A rigid support is formed by the rods of corti and hair cells are around it in outer and inner rows. The processes of hair cells, the stereocilia pass through the tough reticular lamina and are embedded in a gelatinous tectorial membrane.

The nerve to the organ of corti is the cochlear division of the eighth cranial nerve. Sound waves affecting the organ of corti are transmitted as nerve impulses in the cochlear part VIIIth cranial nerve, the fibers of which are present at the base of hair cells (Fig. 14.21) and take origin in sensory neurons in the spiral ganglion, located in the modiolus.

On being stimulated at the base of the hair cells; the central processes of these neurons carry impulses via the VIIIth cranial nerve to the nuclei in brainstem. The auditory pathways in the brainstem relay in several nuclei and from there relay in the medial geniculate body of the thalamus, from there to the auditory area in the temporal lobe of cerebrum in the superior temporal gyrus where sound is perceived. The pathway in passing through the brainstem relays in the nuclei on both sides so that the cerebral area on each side of the brain receives impulses from both the ears.

Summary of Sound Transmission

Sound waves cause the tympanic membrane to vibrate. The tympanic membrane vibrations are amplified and transmitted by the ossicles in the middle ear and the foot plate of the stapes moves to and fro in the oval window, causing vibrations in the perilymph in the scala vestibuli.

As the waves are transmitted along the length of the scala vestibuli and the fluid waves travel back to scala tympani then to the membrane of the round window; at the same time, the pressure is transmitted to the cochlear duct. This causes movement of basilar membrane between scala media and scala tympani that results in the stimulation of the hair cells of the organ of Corti; hence, nerve impulses are initiated; that are transmitted in the afferent fibers of the VIIIth cranial nerve.

The structure of the inner ear allows analysis of the pitch and volume of sound. The pitch analysis depends upon the site of the basilar membrane that is maximally affected by the sound. High frequencies cause maximal vibration of the basilar membrane at the base of the cochlea while lower frequencies cause maximal vibrations at the tip of the cochlea. Therefore, the sound waves produce distortion of the basilar membrane and the site at which this distortion is maximal is determined by the frequency of the sound. The basilar membrane is widest at the tip of the cochlea although the cochlea is narrowest; at the base of cochlea, the basilar membrane is narrowest and is stiff. High frequency causes maximum stimulation at the base of cochlear and low frequency maximum at the apex of cochlear though whole of basilar membrane vibrates.

The volume analysis is by the *number* of fibers of the cochlear nerve that get stimulated and the *frequency* of nerve impulses transmitted by these fibers.

Bone and Air Conduction

In the normal hearing, the sound waves are conducted from the tympanic membrane and the auditory ossicles to the fluid of the inner ear. This is the main pathways and is called ossicular conduction. Another type of conduction is bone conduction, it is the transmission of sound through the bones of the skull to the fluid of the inner ear. This route has a role with very loud sounds.

Considerable bone conduction occurs when tuning fork or other vibrating bodies are applied directly to the skull.

Tests for Deafness (Table 14.1)

Clinical deafness may be due to impaired sound transmission in the external or middle ear (conduction deafness); or due to damage of the hair cells, or neural pathways (sensorineural deafness). The distinction between the two can be made by using a tuning fork (usually with vibrating frequency of 256 Hz). There are two simple tests to distinguish between the conduction deafness and the sensorineural loss called nerve deafness.

The **Rinne test** is performed for each ear; the base of a vibrating tuning fork is placed on the mastoid process and the subject is asked to indicate when sound is no longer heard. The tuning fork is then held near the external auditory meatus. In normal persons, sound is still heard, i.e. air conduction is better than bone conduction. If the conduction system is damaged sound is not heard, the bone conduction becomes better than air conduction.

Weber test: Base of the tuning fork is kept in the middle of the forehead, and the subject is asked if the sound is better heard in one ear. Normally, it is equally heard on both sides, i.e. it is not lateralized. If the person has conductive hearing loss, the sound is localized to the deaf ear as the *masking effect* of air

Table 14.1: Common tests with a tuning fork to distinguish between nerve and conduction deafness

	Weber	*Rinne*	*Schwabach*
Method	Base of vibrating tuning fork placed on vertex of skull	Base of vibrating tuning fork placed on mastoid process until subject no longer hears it, then held in air next to ear	Bone conduction of patient compared with that of normal subject
Normal	Hears equally on both sides	Hears vibration in air after bone conduction is over	
Conduction deafness (one ear)	Sound louder in diseased ear because masking effect of environmental noise is absent on diseased side	Vibrations in air not heard after bone conduction is over	Bone conduction better than normal (conduction defect excludes masking noise)
Nerve deafness (one ear)	Sound louder in normal ear	Vibration heard in air after bone conduction is over when nerve deafness is partial	Bone conduction worse than normal

Clinical Significance

Irritation of the auricular branch of the vagal nerve in the external ear by wax or syringing may reflexly produce persistent cough called ear cough, vomiting or even death due to sudden cardiac inhibition.

Deafness

Conduction deafness can be due to wax or foreign body in the external auditory canal or punctured tympanic membrane, thickening of the ear drum after repeated middle ear infections, fluid in the middle ear, destruction of auditory ossicles, or abnormal rigidity of the attachment of the stapes to the oval window.

Antibiotics, such as streptomycin and gentamicin (aminoglycoside antibiotics) can be toxic to the hair cells, to produce nerve deafness and abnormal vestibular function. Other causes include tumors of the vestibulocochlear nerve or vascular damage to medulla.

Presbycusis is gradual hearing loss occurring in older people and is usually due to gradual loss of hair cells and neurons. It affects higher frequencies. Deafness can also be due to **genetic mutations**, which can present, in a newborn or appear in adults.

A common cause of deafness is the destruction of hair cells by **loud sounds.** Hair cells can be destroyed by exposure to industrial noice or by listening to high intensity rock music. Hair cells in certain parts of Cochles are selectively damaged and so hearing loss in discrete frequency range, which can be diagnosed by audiometry.

An important, although relatively uncommon, condition that can interrupt the function of cochlear nerve fibers is an **acoustic neurinoma,** a tumor of the Schwann cells of the eighth nerve. As the tumor grows, irritation of cochlear nerve fibers may cause a ringing sound in the affected ear (**tinnitus**). Eventually, the ear becomes deaf. The tumor may be operable while small; therefore, early diagnosis is important. If the tumor is allowed to enlarge it could not interrupt the entire eighth nerve and cause vestibular as well as auditory difficulities, it could also impinge on neighbouring cranial nerves V, VII, XI and X and it could also produce cerebellar signs by compressing the cerebellar peduncles.

conduction is absent on that side. If the subject has sensorineural hearing loss due to damage of the organ of corti, cochlear nerve or cochlear nuclei, the sound is localized to the normal side.

Audiometry

Auditory acuity is measured with an audiometer. It provides objective measurement of the degree of deafness in the different tones that are affected. The subject is presented with pure tones of various frequencies through earphones. At each frequency the threshold intensity is determined and plotted as percentage of the normal.

VESTIBULAR APPARATUS

The vestibular apparatus also consists of bony labyrinth in which is located the membranous labyrinth (Fig. 14.22). On each side, it is composed of three **semicircular canals** containing membranous canals inside; and bony vestibule containing two membranous structures called the **otolith organs** which are the **utricle** and the **saccule** (Fig. 14.20). The utricle is oriented almost horizontal and saccule is vertical. The membranous structures contain endolymph and are surrounded by perilymph. The three semicircular canals are horizontal, superior and posterior. The semicircular canals have no auditory

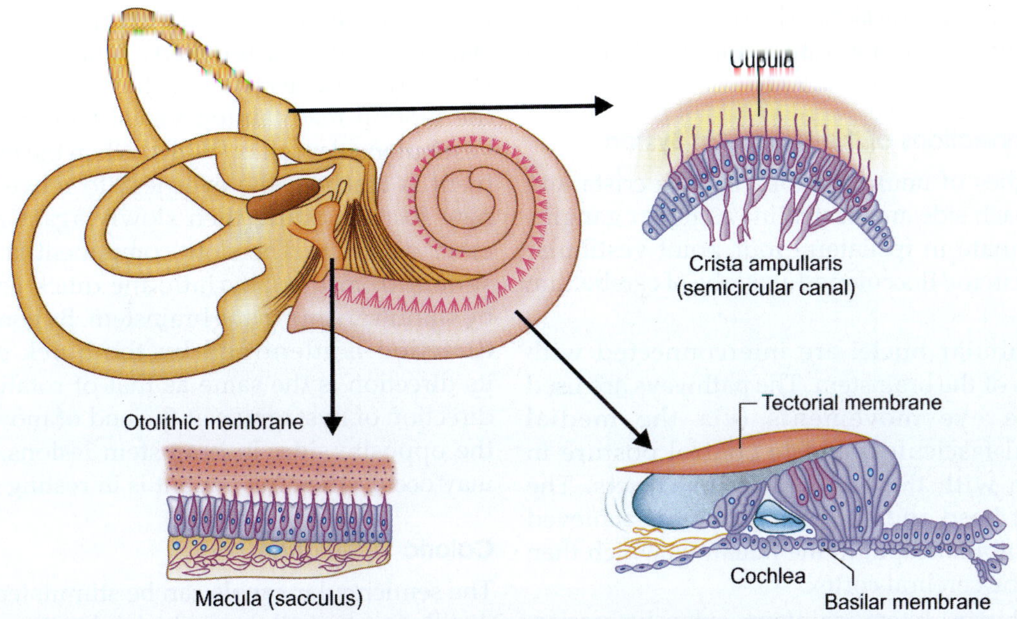

Fig. 14.22: Human membranous labyrinth with enlargements of the structures in which hair cells are embedded

function although they are closely associated with cochlea. They are continuous with vestibule (Fig. 14.19A). The horizontal canal can be placed in horizontal position if the head is tilted down by 30°.

The vestibular apparatus provides information about: the rotational movements of the head provided by semicircular canals. The position of the head in space and its linear acceleration in horizontal and vertical directions provided by otolith organs in utricle and saccule respectively. Signals from the vestibular system affect head and eye movements and enable adjustments in posture to maintain balance.

The Semicircular Canals and the Vestibule

The semicircular canals, like cochlea are composed of outer bony wall and inner membranous ducts. The membranous ducts contain endolymph and are separated from bony canal by perilymph. Three membranous ducts open at their dilated ends, the ampullae into utricle (Fig. 14.20). The dilatation, ampulla is present in each semicircular canal at one end. The sensory epithelium is present in the membranous portion of ampulla and is called **crista ampullaris**; on it are located vestibular hair cells. The cilia of these cells are embedded in gelatinous partition called cupula (Fig. 14.22). The afferent nerve fibers are of the vestibular portion of the VIII cranial nerve. The semicircular canals detect angular (rotational) acceleration of the head. The two horizontal canals detect motion in their plane. Superior canal on one side along with posterior on the other side form another pair to detect motion in their plane, and the posterior on that side with superior on the other side form the third pair for detection of motion in their plane. The canals are arranged to detect rotational motion in each of the three planes of space. *Angular head movements resulting in angular acceleration and deacceleration displace the endolymph and distort the cupula, resulting in the stimulation of hair cells and discharge of impulses in the nerves.* The stimulation does not occur during constant movement.

Balance and Vestibular Apparatus

In the otolith organs, the utricle and the saccule, the sensory epithelium is called **macula** (macula utriculi and macula sacculi). Processes of the hair cells, the stereocilia are embedded in the gelatinous mass which contains numerous small particles called otoliths. This membrane is called otolithic membrane. Otoliths increase the specific gravity of the membrane greater than that of endolymph. Linear acceleration of the head displaces the otolithic membrane which is sensitive to gravity because of presence of otoliths. Angular acceleration does not affect it.

The afferent impulses from the vestibular apparatus travel via the vestibular nerve which joins the cochlear nerve to form the VIIIth cranial nerve. The vestibular branch makes connection with the vestibular nuclei in the brainstem and with cerebellum. Vestibular nuclei project (Fig. 14.23) to the oculomotor nuclei (to control eye position) to maintain the eyes on a target when head orientation changes and project to the motor neurons of postural muscles (to control balance) and to the motor neurons of neck muscles (to control head position).

Central Connections of the Vestibular System

The cell bodies of neurons supplying the crista and macula on each side are located in vestibular ganglia. Fibers terminate in ipsilateral four point vestibular nucleus and in the flocculonodular lobe of cerebellum (Fig. 14.23).

The vestibular nuclei are interconnected with components of the brainstem. The pathways are used to regulate eye movements (via the medial longitudinal fasciculus) and to control posture in conjunction with the vestibulospinal tracts. The *perception* of head and body movement is achieved through vestibular input to the thalamus which then projects to the cerebral cortex.

The vestibular system maintains extensive projections to and receives projections from, the cerebellum. The cerebellar flocculonodular lobe is related to semicircular canal function and when affected by lesions causes a loss of equilibrium during rapid changes of the head motion. The uvula of the cerebellum plays a similar role in regard to static equilibrium.

Vertigo is the sensation of rotation when the actual rotation is not present. It is produced when **one labyrinth** is inflamed.

Nystagmus: Jerky eye movements are seen at the start and end of rotational movement. This is called nystagmus. It is a reflex that keeps visual fixation on stationary points while body rotates. When rotation starts, eyes move slowly in the opposite direction to the motion maintaining visual fixation. It is called vestibuloocular reflex (VOR). When the limit of movement is reached, the eyes jerk to move back to the new fixation point, then slowly again move in the other direction. The slow component is initiated by stimuli from the labyrinth; the quick component is by stimuli arising in the brainstem. By convention, the direction is identified by the quick component; its direction is the same as that of rotation. But, the direction of nystagmus at the end of movement is on the opposite side. In brainstem lesions, nystagmus may occur when the patient is in resting condition.

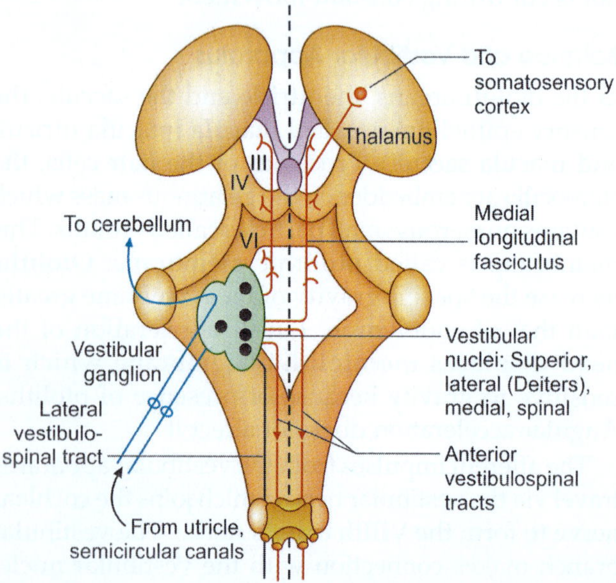

Fig. 14.23: Vestibular system controls eye movements postural muscles via connections with vestibular nuclei and their connections with nuclei of the eye muscles and lower motor neurons of postural muscles

Caloric Stimulation

The semicircular canals can be stimulated by putting distilled water in the ear which is hotter or colder than body temperature. The difference in temperature sets up convection currents in endolymph which causes nystagmus, vertigo and nausea. This is the technique of caloric stimulation which is used diagnostically to test for the function of semicircular canals.

Hence, in cases of treatment of ear infections while irrigating the ear canal it is important to be sure that the fluid used is at body temperature to avoid the irritating symptoms.

Motion Sickness

The nausea, blood pressure changes, sweating, pallor and vomiting are symptoms of motion sickness and are produced by excessive vestibular stimulation. They are probably due to reflexes mediated via vestibular connections in the brainstem and the flocculonodular lobe of cerebellum.

CHEMICAL SENSES

Smell and taste are chemical senses as the stimuli are chemical in nature present in the air for smell and in food and liquids for taste. The functions of the senses are related to each other as they both have role in digestion. The flavors of foods are due to smell and taste. Both sensations are produced when molecules are dissolved, for smell in the mucus in the upper part of the nose; and for taste in the saliva in the mouth. The receptor cells of both sensations are being constantly replaced.

The pathways for sensations and the brain regions where they are perceived are different for the two sensations.

SMELL

The **receptors** are present in the **upper part of the nose** in the yellowish pigmented olfactory epithelium (Fig. 14.24). There are supporting cells and receptor cells (Fig. 14.25) and basal stem cells. The new receptor cells are generated from these basal stem cells. The receptor cells are neurons. This is the only place in the body where neurons are exposed to external environment. Each neuron has a short thick dendrite, the olfactory rod with an expanded end from where immobile cilia project in the overlying mucus. The axons of the olfactory receptor neurons, **Ist cranial nerve (olfactory nerve)**, pierce the cribriform plate of the ethmoid bone and make connections with the olfactory bulb cells (Fig. 14.26). The olfactory bulb is a structure at the base of the cranial cavity, below the frontal lobe.

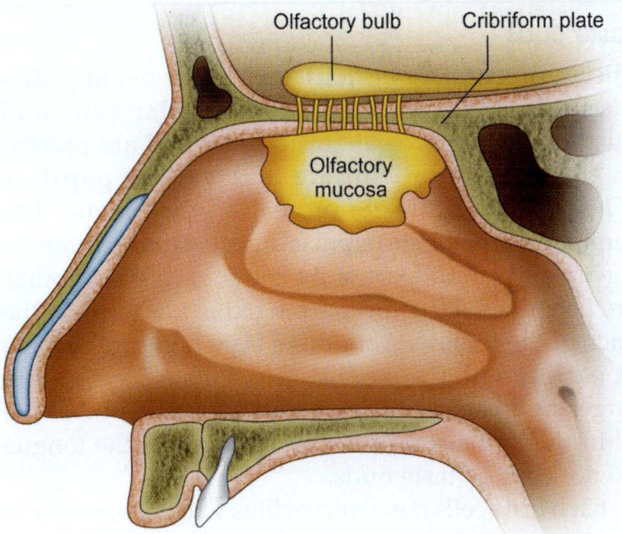

Fig. 14.24: Location of the olfactory mucosa. Overlying the olfactory mucosa is the cribriform plate of the ethmoid bond

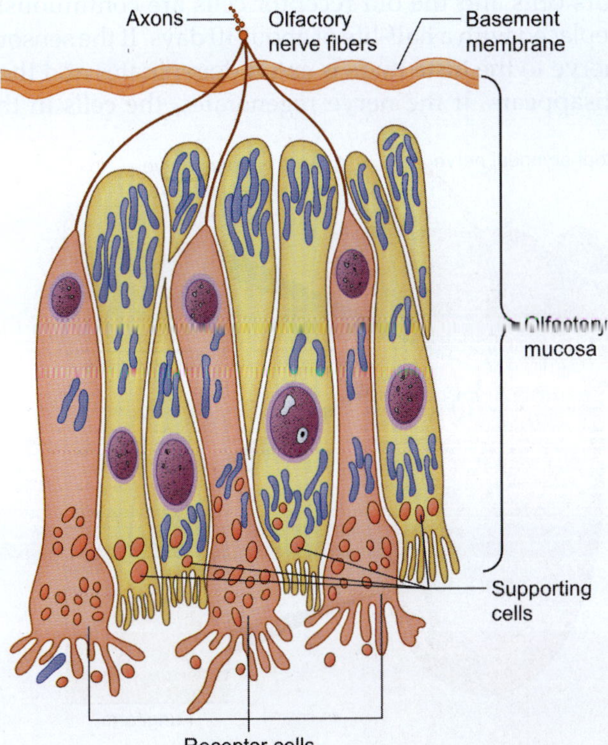

Fig. 14.25: Olfactory receptors in mucosa with supporting cells

The olfactory neurons are constantly replaced with a half-life of few weeks unlike the other neurons in the body. The covering mucus is produced by the Bowman's glands under the basal lamina and the mucus is constantly present over the olfactory membrane.

The axons of the cells in the olfactory bulb leave to form olfactory tract to pass to the **olfactory cortex**.

The primary receiving area includes **prepyriform cortex** and **cortex of the basal forebrain**. Cortical representation of olfaction is asymmetric as there is greater activation on the right side than the left.

Some fibers also project to the **amygdala** and are believed to be involved in emotional responses to olfactory stimuli. Some other fibers project to **entorhinal cortex** which is concerned with olfactory memories.

The olfaction is the only sense which does not relay in the thalamus. In dogs and in some other animals, the sense of smell is highly developed and they are

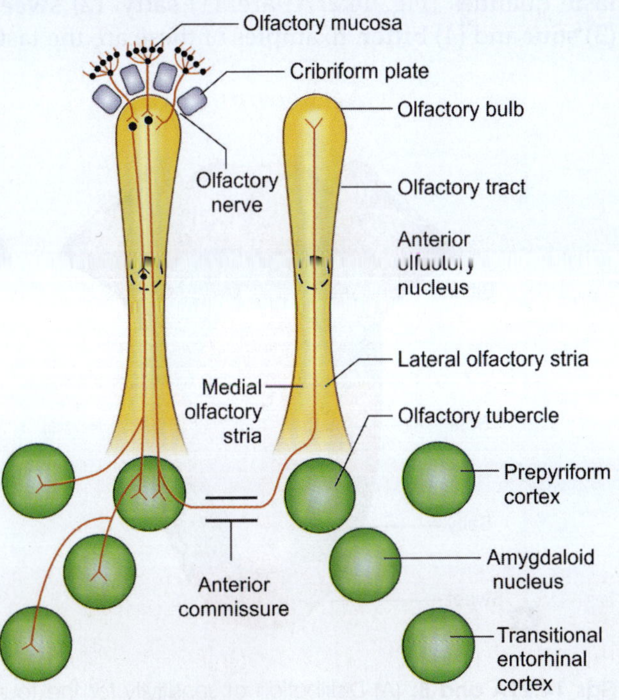

Fig. 14.26: Olfactory pathway

called macrosomatic animals against humans which are microsmatic.

In human, olfaction contributes to emotional life and odors can recall memories.

The absence of olfaction in disease is called **anosmia**; **hyposmia** is decreased olfactory sensitivity. The odorant receptor deficiencies can be diagnosed based on the symptoms. Olfactory thresholds increase with advancing age and humans over the age of 80 have impaired ability to identify odors.

Olfactory hallucinations are observed in people with temporal lobe epilepsy.

There are many qualities of odors unlike taste and at **least 6 of the odors** are: (1) floral (e.g. roses), (2) ethereal (pears), (3) musky (musk), (4) camphor (eucalyptus), (5) putrid (rotten eggs) and (6) pungent (vinegar). The olfactory mucosa also contains pain receptors which are endings of the trigeminal nerve. They are stimulated by irritating substances and thus form a part of the odor of substances like peppermint. They are also responsible for sneezing, and other reflex responses to irritants in the nasal cavity. Chemical testing of olfaction must avoid activating these somatosensory receptors with noxious or thermal stimuli.

TASTE

Taste consists of **four basic sensations** or a mixture of these sensations that are perceived. The four basic taste qualities (Fig. 14.27A) are: (1) **salty**, (2) **sweet**, (3) **sour** and (4) **bitter**. Examples of these are the taste of common salt, sucrose, hydrochloric acid and quinine. Recently a **fifth taste** sensation has been added called **umami**, the taste which has been known for long. It has now become established as its receptor has been identified. It is triggered by glutamate more so by monosodium glutamate. The taste is pleasant and sweet but differs from standard sweet taste.

RECEPTOR ORGANS AND PATHWAYS

Taste Buds

These are sense organs for taste and are ovoid bodies made-up of basal cells, sustentacular cells and gustatory receptor cells (**taste cells**) and are present in the **fungiform, foliate** and **vallate papillae** (Figs 14.27B and 14.28) present on the tongue. The fungiform and foliate papillae are most numerous near the tip and lateral part of the tongue; vallate papillae are prominent structures arranged in a V form on the back of the tongue. About five taste buds are present in each fungiform papilla. The vallate papillae are larger and each contains about 100 taste buds. The filiform papillae that cover the dorsum of the tongue do not contain taste buds.

Each taste cells has a microvillus which projects into the taste pore an opening to the oral cavity.

The basal cells arise from epithelial cells surrounding the taste bud, they differentiate into new receptors cells and the old receptor cells are continuously replaced with a half-life of about 10 days. If the sensory nerve to the taste buds is cut, it degenerates and then disappears. If the nerve regenerates, the cells in the

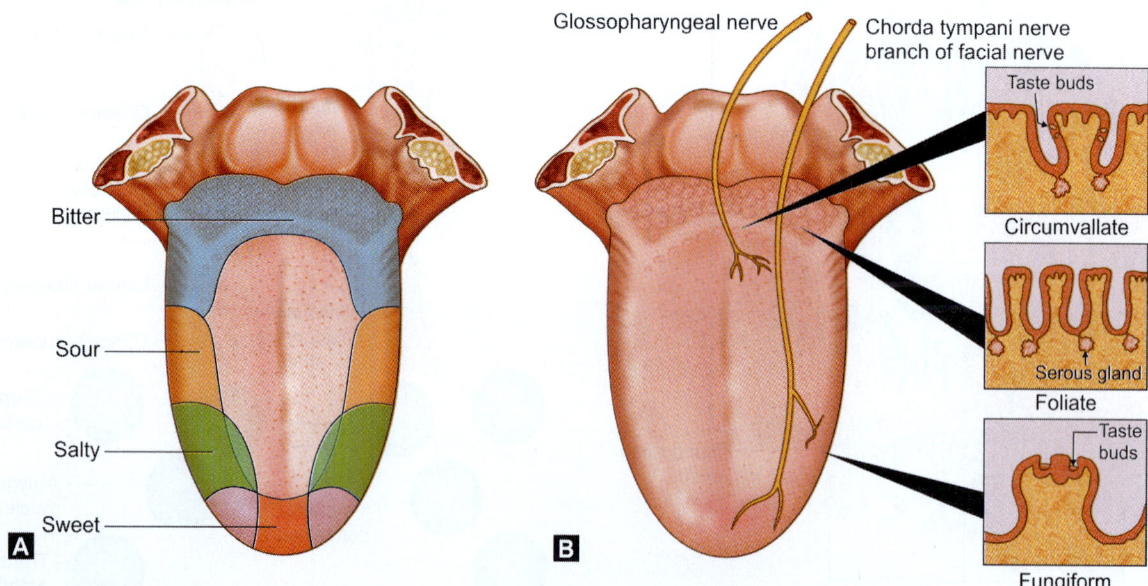

Figs 14.27A and B: (A) Distribution of sensitivity for the four taste qualities, (B) the innervation of the anterior two-thirds and posterior one-third of the tongue by the facial and glossopharyngeal nerves, respectively

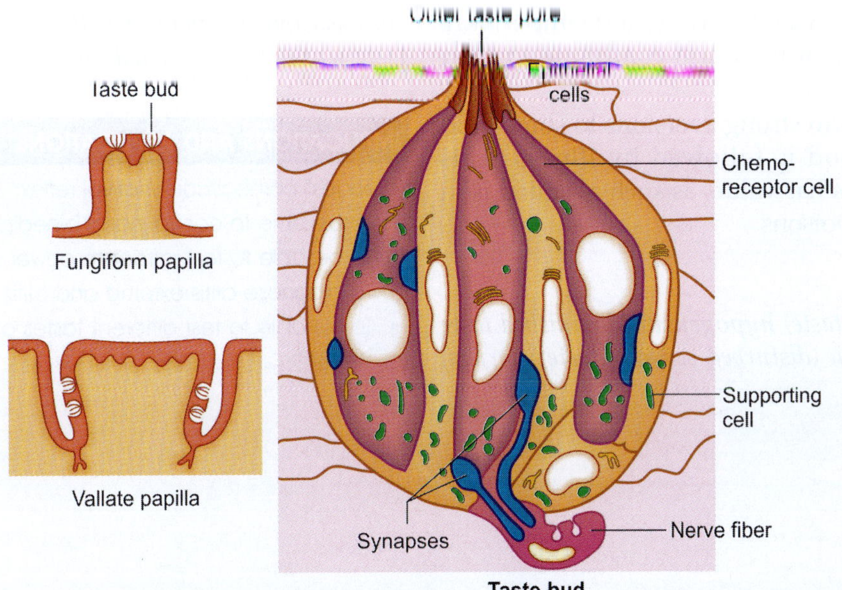

Fig. 14.28: Taste bud. The locations of taste buds on fungiform and vallate papillae. Taste bud on the right side with taste pore above and innervation below, chemoreceptor cells are shown in dark color and uncolored are supporting cells

neighborhood become organized into new taste buds due to some sort of chemical influence from the regenerating nerve fiber.

The taste buds are also located on the mucosa of epiglottis, palate and pharynx besides being present in the papillae on the tongue.

Taste Pathways

Sensory nerve fibers from taste buds on the anterior two-thirds of the tongue are carried by the **VIIth cranial nerve** (**facial nerve**) though the general sensations from this area are carried by Vth cranial nerve; and those from the posterior third of the tongue are carried by **glossopharyngeal nerve (IXth cranial nerve)**.

The fibers from epiglottis, palate, and posterior most part of the tongue are carried by the **vagal nerves**. On each side the **myelinated** slowly conducting fibers in the these nerves unite in the medulla oblongata and relay in the nucleus tractus solitarius and the axons of these neurons (Fig. 14.29) travel in the same side (unlike other general sensory pathways where second-order neurons cross over to the opposite side) and ascend joining the general sensations and relay in the thalamus from where the third-order neurons carry impulses to the cerebral cortex in the face area of the sensory cortex (S1) and also pass to the anterior part of insula.

The relevant insular cortex is anterior to the face area of the postcentral gyrus and is probably the area that mediates conscious perception of taste and taste discrimination.

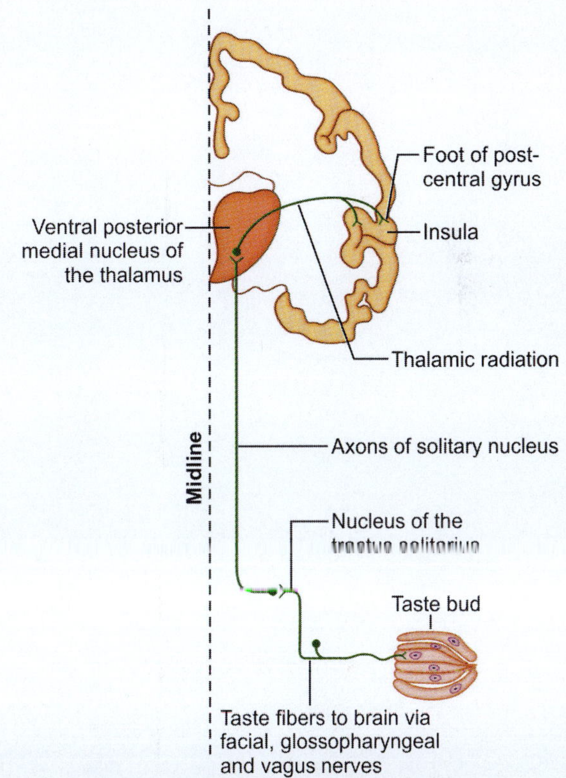

Fig. 14.29: Diagram of taste pathways

Flavor

The tastes are mostly synthesized from five basic taste sensations. In some cases, a component of taste includes an element of pain stimulation, e.g. hot sauces. In addition, smell plays an important role in overall sensation produced by taste, and temperature and the consistency of food also contribute to their flavors.

A person may form strong aversions to some food if eating of the food is followed by illness. This mechanism perhaps has value, as such aversion is in terms of avoiding poisons.

Abnormalities

Ageusia *(absence of taste)* ***hypogeusia*** *(diminished taste sensitivity) dysgeusia (disturbed sense of taste). Drugs, such as captopril and some others cause temporary loss of taste sensations (cause not known).*

IMPLICATIONS AND APPLICATIONS

- To test corneal/conjunctival reflex.
- To be able to control nasal bleeding or epistaxis.
- To be able to test refractive power of eye.
- To diagnose otitis externa and otitis media.
- To be able to test different tastes on various parts of the tongue.

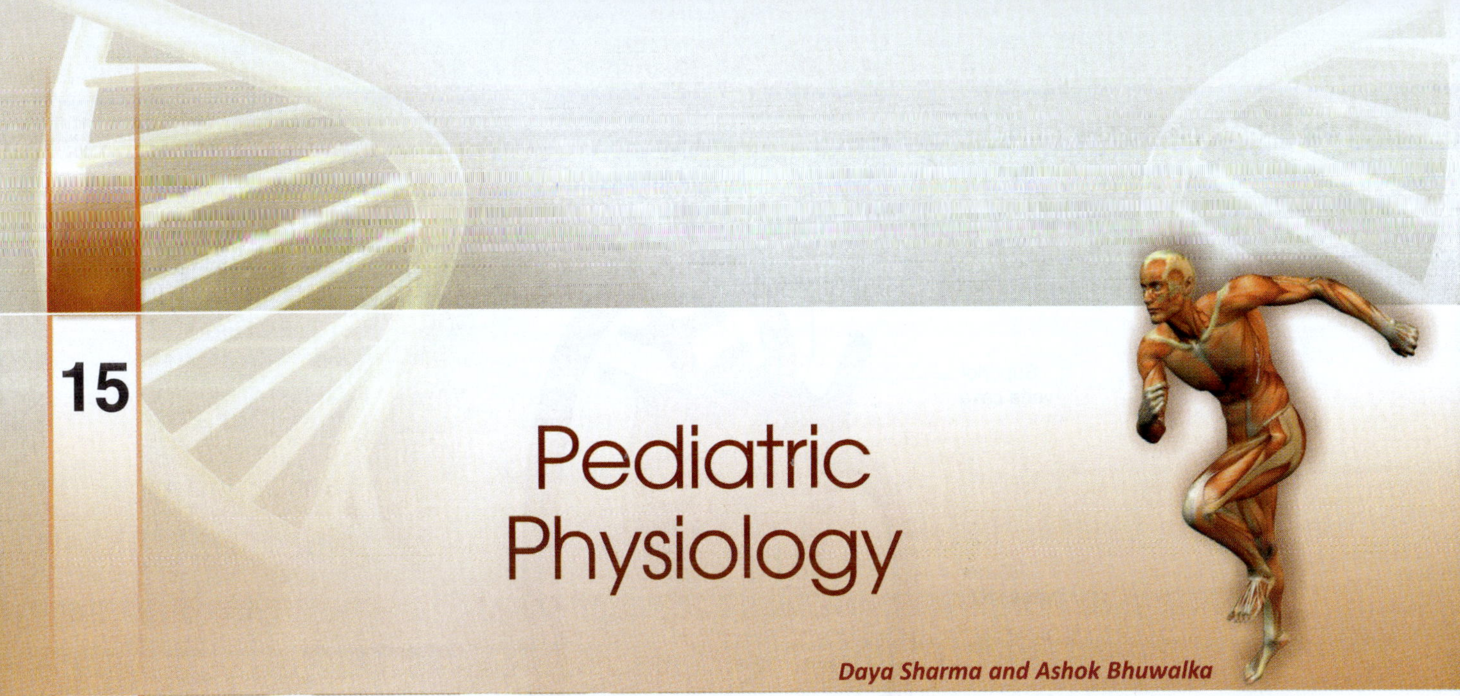

15 Pediatric Physiology

Daya Sharma and Ashok Bhuwalka

FETAL CIRCULATION AND CARDIORESPIRATORY CHANGES AT BIRTH

It is important to understand that there is a basic difference in the circulatory system during intrauterine and extrauterine life. During fetal life, lungs do not play any role in the exchange of gases. The placenta supplies oxygen and nutrition to the fetus during intrauterine life.

Fetal Circulation

The first few moments of an infant's life can be critical as the infant is making an abrupt transition from the mother's womb into the extrauterine environment. A major problem that can arise during this period is asphyxia.

During fetal life, the alveoli or the lungs do not contain air but contain a fluid produced by the lungs. Due to this fluid blood flowing through the lungs cannot pick-up oxygen to supply to the body tissues. Also, the blood flow to the lungs is markedly diminished due to partial closure of the arterioles. As a result most of the blood is diverted away from the lungs through **ductus arteriosis**.

During fetal life, oxygenated blood in the placenta is returned to the fetus (Fig. 15.1) through the umbilical vein which joins the portal vein and forms the ductus venosus. Most of the blood from ductus venosus passes into the inferior vena cava which has higher oxygen concentration it also receives blood from hepatic veins, kidneys, liver, and extremities. Blood from inferior vena cava (IVC) enters the right atrium (RA). Here, blood is divided into two streams by the septum secundum.

About one-third of the blood of IVC with higher oxygen saturation enters the left atrium (LA) through foramen ovale. Rest two-third of the blood mixes with the blood entering the RA through superior vena cava (SVC). This blood enters the right ventricle.

The blood reaching the LA from RA mixes with some blood coming through pulmonary veins into the LA, passes into the left ventricle (LV). LV pushes the blood into the ascending aorta to supply oxygenated blood to the coronary arteries, head and upper extremities. The blood returning from head and neck, upper extremities passes almost directly into the right ventricle (RV). The RV pushes this blood into the pulmonary trunk. A small amount of this blood enters the pulmonary circulation, the rest passes through the ductus arteriosus (Fig. 15.2) into the descending aorta from where blood is supplied to the rest of the body and then through umbilical arteries to the placenta for oxygenation.

CIRCULATORY ADJUSTMENTS AT BIRTH

- Clamping of the umbilical cord leads to increased systemic vascular resistance due to removal of low resistance placental circulation.
- Ductus venosus closes down as there is no blood flowing from the placenta.
- At birth as the infant cries and takes first few breaths, the lungs expand and take the function of supplying oxygen to the body.
- Lungs expand as they get filled with air, the fetal fluid is cleared from the alveoli. The arterioles begin to open allowing a considerable increase in the

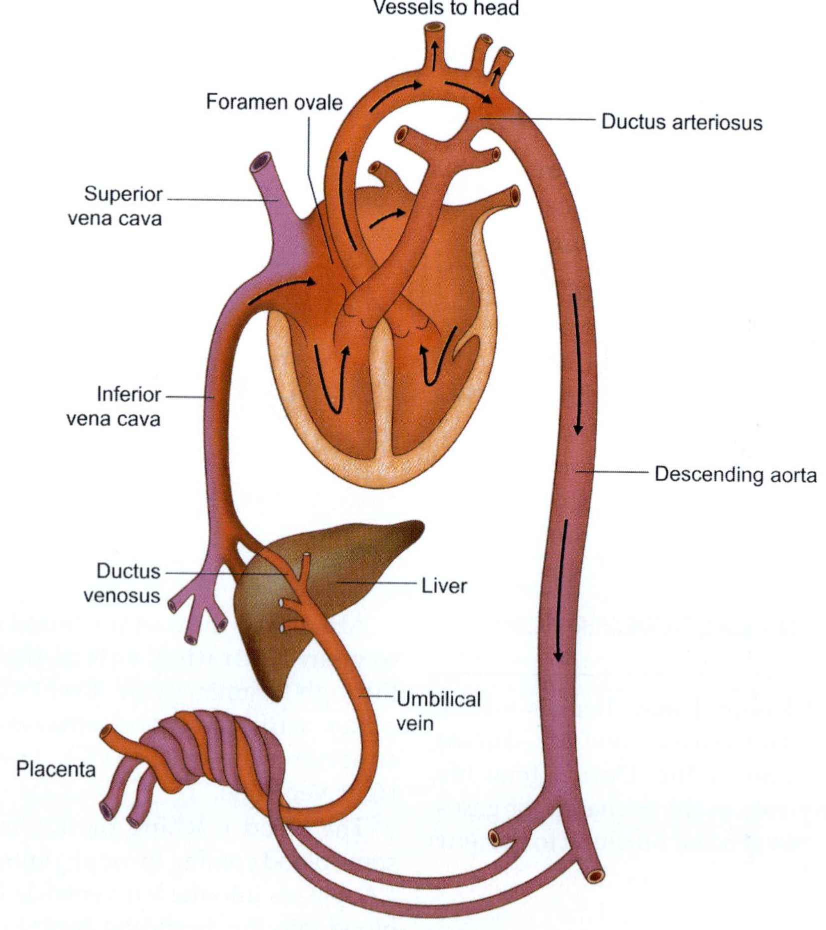

Fig. 15.1: Fetal circulation

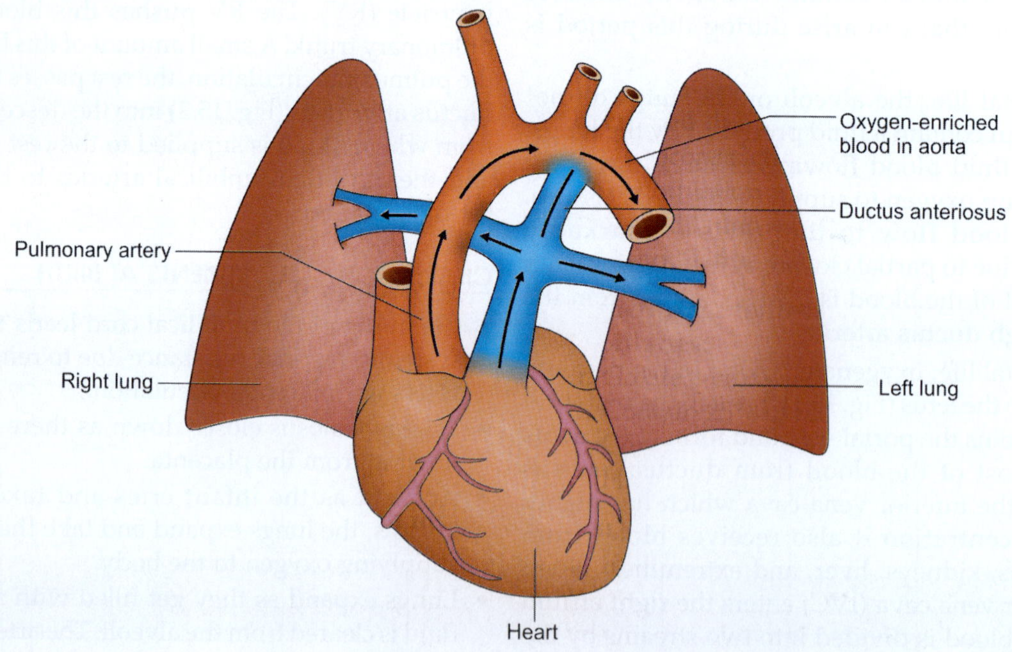

Fig. 15.2: Ductus arteriosus

amount of blood flowing through the lungs leading to a fall in pulmonary artery pressure (Fig. 15.3).

- There is functional closure of foramen ovale due to increased in left atrial pressure which is now higher than right atrial pressure. This is because of increased blood flow from the lungs into the LA through pulmonary veins. Also right atrial pressure falls due to closure of ductus venosus.
- As the blood level of oxygen increase and the pulmonary blood vessels relax the ductus arteriosis closes. The blood which was previously flowing through the ductus arteriosus now flows through the lungs where it takes up more oxygen to transport to the body tissues (Fig. 15.4).

Once this, transition is complete, the baby is breathing air and is using the lungs to get oxygen. Normally a strong cry and deep breaths are enough to drive fluid out of the airway. Oxygen and expansion of the lungs stimulate the pulmonary vessels to relax so that adequate oxygen enters the blood and the baby becomes pink.

If the baby does not cry or breathe at birth there is lack of oxygen leading to sustained constriction of pulmonary arterioles thus preventing oxygen reaching the body tissues. This is called persistent pulmonary artery hypertension which is a serious condition and requires prompt attention of a specialist (Fig. 15.5).

During neonatal period and early infancy the heart rate is rapid and comes to the adult level by about adolescence. Similarly BP is lower in neonates and infants. It also reaches the adult level by adolescence.

Heart rate (HR) in a neonate is double that of an adult and BP is half of that of an adult.

Adult HR–70 beats/min. Newborn HR–140/min

BP–120/80 min Hg Newborn BP 60/40 mmHg (Table 15.1).

If an infant or a young child presents with cough you should count the respiratory rate per minute and also look for chest indrawing.

WHO recommends certain clinical criteria for diagnosing pneumonia in children at primary health care level. These are:

i. Rapid respiration (RR). If RR/min is
   a. Age < 2 months 60 or more
   b. 2–12 months 50 or more
   c. 12–60 months 40 or more

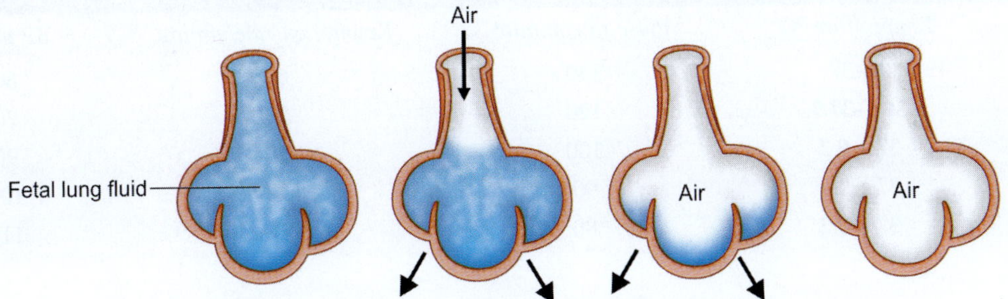

Fig. 15.3: Effect of pulmonary artery pressure

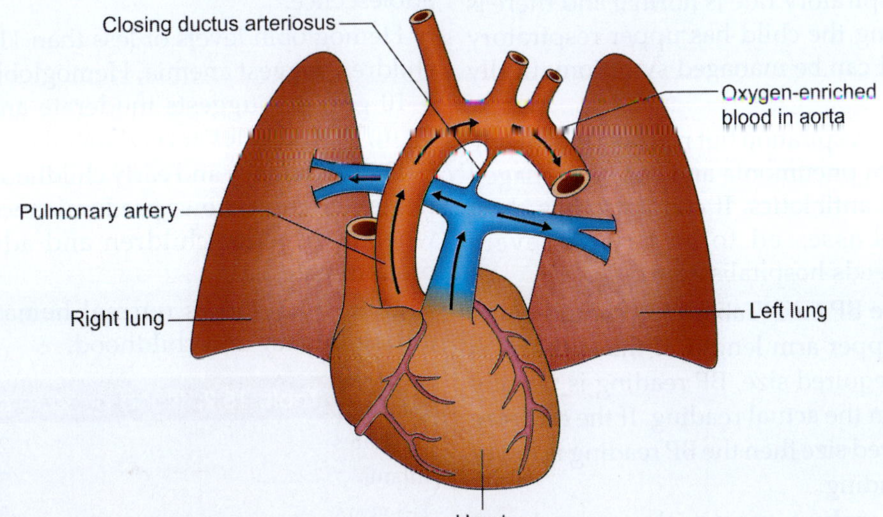

Fig. 15.4: Circulation after birth

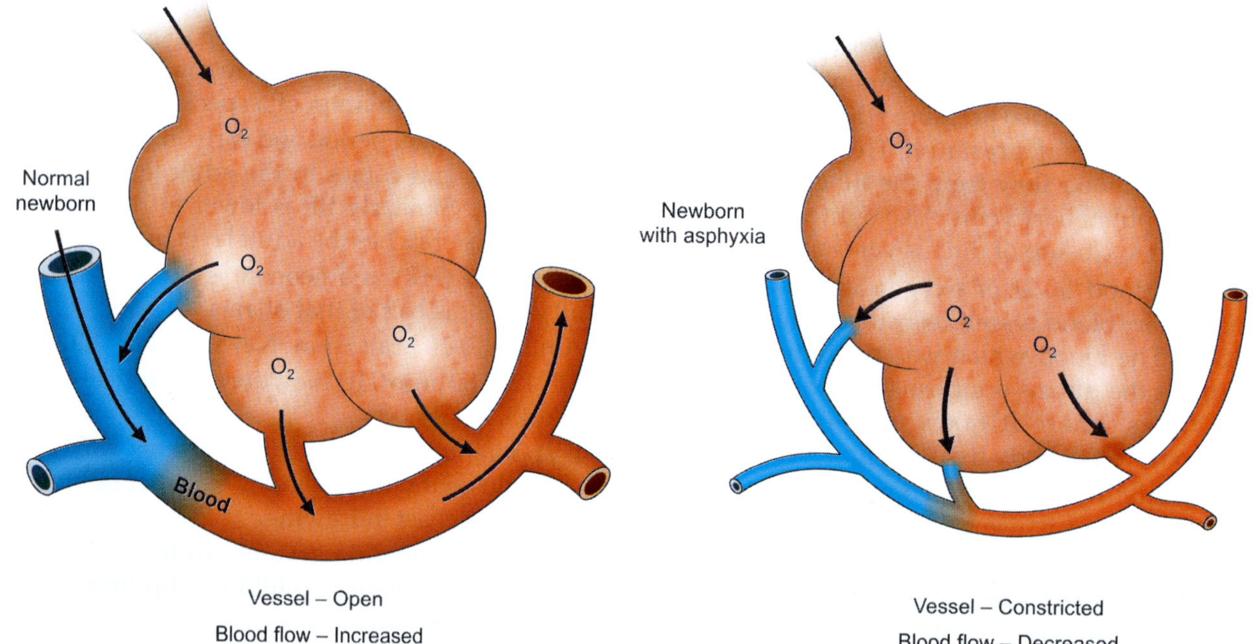

Fig. 15.5: Effect of pulmonary hypertension

Table 15.1: Average values for body temperature, heart rate, respiratory rate and blood pressure during infancy and childhood

Age	*Temperature °C*	*Pulse rate/minute*	*Respiration rate/minute*	*BP in mmHg*
Newborn	36–37	140	40	60/40
1 year	36.5–37.5	120	30	70/50
5 years	37 ± 0.2	100	20	90/50
10 years	37 ± 0.2	90	18	100/70
> 10 years	37 ± 0.2	80	18	110/80

ii. Chest in-drawing or difficulty in breathing.

If the child's respiratory rate is normal and there is no chest in-drawing the child has upper respiratory tract infection and can be managed symptomatically at home.

If child has rapid respiration but no chest indrawing he is suffering from pneumonia and can be managed at home with oral antibiotics. If child also has chest in-drawing he is assessed to be having severe pneumonia and needs hospitalisation.

The width of the BP cuff (Table 15.2) should cover two-third of the upper arm length. If the cuff size is smaller than the required size, BP reading is usually slightly higher than the actual reading. If the cuff size is more than required size then the BP reading is lower than the actual reading.

Hematological values vary with age and sex. Hemoglobin levels and WBC count are higher at birth and gradually come to normal adult levels during adolescence.

Hemoglobin levels of less than 11 gm/dL in older children suggest anemia. Hemoglobin levels between 5–10 gm/dL suggests moderate anemia and below 5 gm/dL indicates severe anemia.

During infancy and early childhood, the differential white cell count shows predominance of lymphocytes whereas in older children and adults neutrophils predominate.

Table 15.3 shows normal hematological values during infancy and childhood.

Table 15.2: Blood pressure cuff size

Neonates	...	2.5 cm
Infants	...	5.0 cm
1–8 years	...	9.0 cm
> 9 years	...	12.5 cm

Table 15.3: Hematologic values during infancy and childhood

Age	Hemoglobin gm%	WBC/mL	Neutrophils	Lymphocytes WBC percentage of total	Eosinophils	Monocytes
Cord blood	16.8	18,000	61	31	2	6
3 months	12.0	12,000	32	62	2	5
6 months to 6 years	12.0	10,000	45	48	2	5
7–12 years	13.0	8,000	55	38	2	5
Adult (female and male)	14.16	7,500	55	35	3	7

IMPLICATIONS AND APPLICATIONS

Appreciate that the parameters for RR, HR and BP are changing to adult level during growing period. The cuff for the measurement of BP has to be different sizes for children of different age groups.

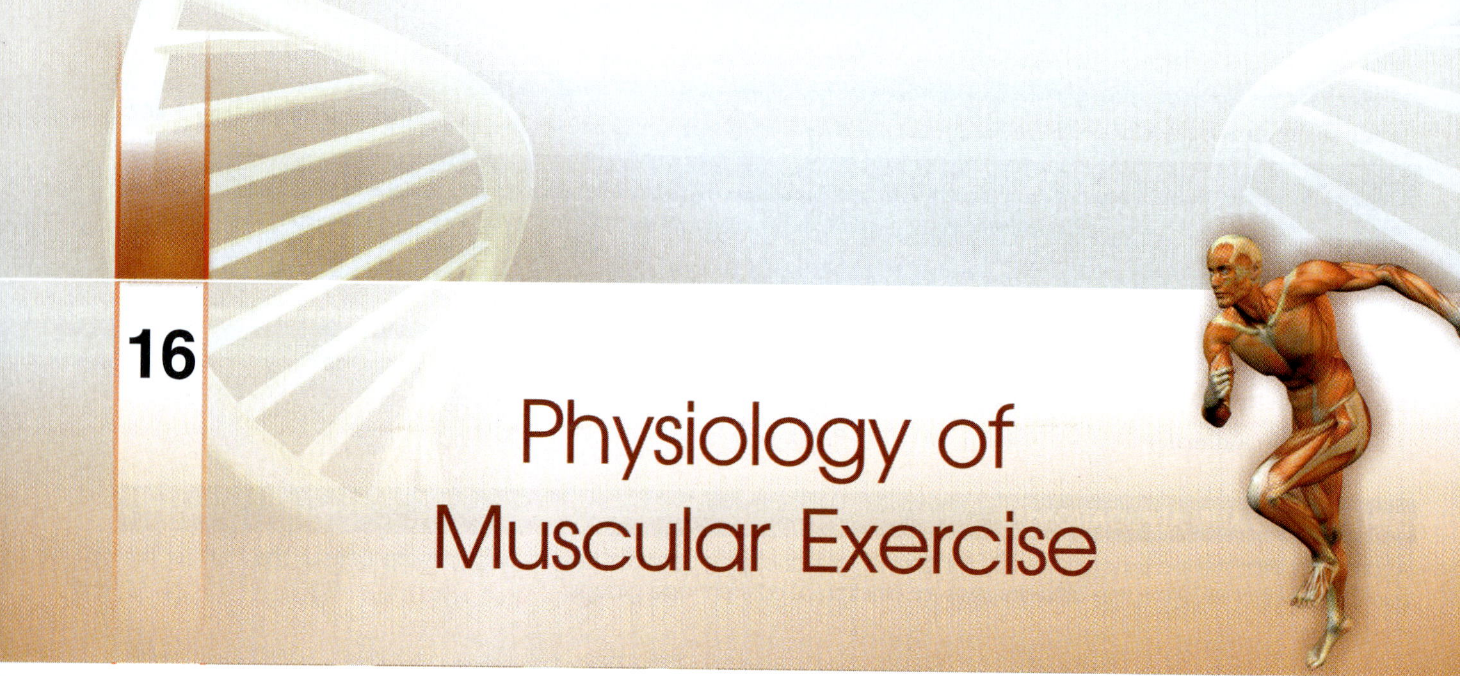

16 Physiology of Muscular Exercise

RESPIRATORY, CARDIOVASCULAR, METABOLIC RESPONSES AND EFFECTS OF TRAINING

Introduction: Regular Physical exercise has many beneficial effects on health. The description shows the responses occurring in the body with exercise.

Breif review: Many **cardiovascular** and **respiratory mechanisms** operate in an integrative manner during exercise. Circulatory changes increase **blood flow** to the active muscles but at the same time maintain adequate circulation in the rest of the body. There is increase in the **extraction of oxygen** from each unit of the blood flow in the active muscles with blood flow also increased. There is **increase in ventilation** to provide extra oxygen to the body and to remove extra carbon dioxide and heat. The increase occurs to provide each unit of pulmonary blood flow with more oxygen and blood flow increases as well.

The ability of exercise depends on the capacity of cardiac and respiratory systems to increase oxygen delivery to the tissues and removal of CO_2. **Ventilation increases** immediately as exercise begins and is linearly related to the CO_2 production and O_2 consumption. ***Arterial*** PO_2 and PCO_2 remain at normal level except at the maximal exercise level. Arterial pH remains at a normal level in moderate exercise but in heavy exercise begins to fall because of lactic acid during anaerobic metabolism.

The level of exercise at which sustained metabolic acidosis begins is called anaerobic threshold, which is different in fit and unfit individuals.

The *actual **cause of increase in ventilation is unknown***. Hypoxia or hypercapnia do not play a role. *Neural input from the motor cortex to the medullary respiratory centre, afferents from muscles, tendons and joints or unknown mediators released from working muscles are believed to contribute.*

Cardiovascular responses: Neural and chemical factors have a role. Cerebrocortical ***activation of sympathetic nervous system*** produces centrally an *increase in cardiac output* due to increase in heart rate and force of contraction and *peripherally produces vasoconstriction*. Reflexes are activated intramuscularly due to activation of stretch and tension receptors and chemoreceptors (due to metabolic products), the central connections are unknown but the efferent limb consists of sympathetic fibers to the heart and blood vessels The **local factors** in the active muscles (i.e. changes in pH, PCO_2 and PO_2) are vasodilators. *Potassium* is one of the dilator metabolites responsible for **vasodilatation in active muscles.** Other factors may be *release of adenosine* and *decrease of pH during sustained exercise.* The ***decrease in total peripheral resistance*** (TPR) enables the heart to pump more blood at a lesser load and so pumps more efficiently. ***Peripheral resistance increases in skin, kidney, splanchnic and inactive muscles*** due to *sympathetic mediated vasoconstriction* diverting blood away from these areas. It persists throughout the period of exercise. As cardiac output and blood flow to active muscles increases with progressive increase in intensity of exercise visceral blood flow (splanchnic and renal circulations) decreases. ***Blood flow to myocardium increases,*** to the ***brain remains unchanged,*** *skin blood flow initially decreases and then increases as body temperature rises* with intensity or duration of exercise. *Skin blood flow decreases when total body O_2 consumption is maximal.*

Mild to Moderate Exercise

Anticipation of physical activity increases sympathetic impulses and inhibits vagal impulses to the heart. This produces *increase in* ***cardiac output*** due to increase in heart rate and the force of contraction of the myocardium. Increase in peripheral resistance occurs in inactive tissues *and in skin, kidney, splanchnic tissues, diverts blood from these areas.* The major circulatory adjustments to prolonged exercise occur in the vasculature of active muscles. Local formation of vasodilator metabolites dilates the resistance vessels. Dilatation progresses with increase in intensity of exercise. *Potassium is released by contracting muscles and partly responsible for initial decrease in the vascular resistance.* Other factors may be *release of adenosine* and *decrease of tissue pH during sustained exercise. The local accumulation of metabolites dilates the terminal arterioles. May increase the blood flow in muscles by 15–20 fold. The metabolic dilatation of the precapillary vessesls occurs very early on the onset of exercise.* Marked *changes occur in the* ***capillary circulation***. At rest only a small percentage of capillary circulation are perfused but in actively contracting muscles *nearly all capillaries are open.* Surface area for exchange is increased. The **release of oxygen** *from the blood is facilitated by drop in tissue PO_2 in the active muscle. The oxyhemoglobin dissociation curve is steep below 60 mm of mercury* and with each mm drop in oxygen pressure relatively larger amounts of oxygen are supplied by *the release from the blood, this is further* facilitated by *the shift of oxyhemoglobin dissociation* curve with *high concentration of CO_2 and lactic acid*, and *increase in temperature in* the active tissue, the oxygen consumption *increases much more than the blood flow to the muscle. A–V difference in oxygen content increases* and more oxygen per unit of blood flow is delivered to the tissues. With that venous blood PO_2 from exercising muscles may fall to almost zero.

The arteriolar dilatation increases the *hydrostatic pressure in capillaries.* Exudation of fluid in tissues increases, carried back by lymphatics (where flow increase) aided by muscle contraction.

Limits of exercise performance: Two main factors limit performance. The rate of oxygen utilization and the oxygen supply to the muscles depending on pumping capacity of the heart.

Muscle pain and ***feeling of exhaustion*** and loss of will to continue determine the tolerance to exercise.

Cardiac output (CO): Tachycardia persists during exercise. If the workload is moderate and constant, heart rate will reach a level and remain there throughout the period of exercise. If the workload increases heart rate increases until a plateau of about 180 beats per minute reached during strenuous exercise. The increase in stroke volume is about 10–35%, the larger are in trained persons. In well trained persons where the cardiac output reaches six to seven times the resting level stroke volume reaches about twice the resting value. *Circulating catecholamines also have* a role to increase cardiac output.

The ***venous return increases*** due to sympathetic venoconstriction, the pumping action of skeletal muscles and activity of respiratory muscles. The deeper and more frequent respirations increase pressure gradient for blood flow to the thoracic veins. The venous reservoirs do not contribute much to the circulating volume.

Arterial Pressure *If the exercise involves a* **large portion of the body,** such as running or swimming the reduction in total vascular resistance may be considerable. *BP starts to rise and parallels the severity of exercise.* So the increase in CO is proportionally greater than decrease in TPR. The vasoconstriction produced in inactive tissues by the sympathetic nervous system including release of catecholamines from adrenal medulla is important in maintenance of normal or increased BP. In general the mean BP rises during exercise due to increase in cardiac output. But the effect of enhanced cardiac output is offset by decrease in TPR and so the **mean BP** *increases only slightly. Systolic BP* increases more than diastolic BP.

Physical conditioning and training: The response of CVS is to increase the capacity to deliver O_2 to the active muscles and to improve the ability of muscles to utilize oxygen. VO_{2max}, the maximal oxygen consumption varies with the level of physical training. ***Training increases*** VO_{2max}, which reaches at a plateau at the highest level of conditioning. *Highly trained individuals have lower HR, greater stroke volume and lower peripheral resistance than they had before training.* They have higher vagal tone and lower sympathetic tone at rest. During exercise the maximal HR of trained individual is the same as that of untrained but at a higher level of exercise. Physical training is also associated with greater extraction of oxygen from blood in the muscles. *With long-term training capillary density in the muscles increases* and may be the number of arterioles that cause decrease in the vascular resistance. The number of *mitochondria and its oxidative enzymes* *increase*, the level of ATPase activity, myoglobin and enzymes of lipid metabolism increase. Uptake during exercise is limited by the maximum rate at which O_2 is transported to the mitochondria in the exercising muscles. Limitation is not due to deficient O_2 intake in the lungs.

Severe Exercise

During exhaustive exercise the compensatory mechanisms begin to fail. Heart rate reaches maximal value of 180 beats/min and stroke volume reaches a plateau. The heart rate *may* then decrease to result in fall of BP and subjects may become dehydrated. Sympathetic vasoconstriction overcomes vasodilation influence on the skin, decreases the rate of heat loss due to vasoconstriction, leading to high body temperature and may also to distress. The tissue and blood pH decrease as a result of increased lactic acid and CO_2 production. The reduced pH is believed to be the key factor responsible for the maximal amount of exercise an individual can tolerate.

Metabolic responses: Involve utilisation and generation of fuel. The type and amount of substrate used depends on the duration and intensity of exercise. For very intense short term excercise (sprint run), stored creatine phosphate and ATP provide the energy. When the stores get deleted exercise can be sustained for 2 minutes by breakdown of muscle glycogen. The anaerobic phase is not limited by depletion of glycogen but rather by rapid accumulation of lactic acid in the muscle and blood.

After several minutes of exhaustive anaerobic exercise an oxygen debt is built up. This must be repaid before exercise can be repeated. Oxygen is required to rebuild lactic acid back into glucose in the liver or to oxidize it to CO_2.

Oxygen is required to replenish normal muscle ATP and creatine phosphate content; to replenish the oxygen present normally in the lungs and body fluids and that bound to myoglobin and haemoglobin.

For less intense and prolonged exercise aerobic oxidation, is required to produce energy. Substrates from blood are added to muscle glycogen. After a few minutes glucose uptake from plasma increases. The major intake in exercise becomes insulin independent though the effect of insulin on glucose uptake also increases in exercise. To maintain plasma glucose level hepatic production increases initially by high glycogenolysis. Endurance can be improved by high carbohydrate feeding for several days prior to prolonged exercise (marathon run) to increase muscle and liver glycogen. When the exercise is of longer duration gluconeogenesis becomes important and to support this amino acids are increasingly released from muscles and their uptake by the liver is increased. The effects are coordinated by sympathetic neural activity and relative effects of glucagon and insulin.

Eventually fatty acids are liberated from adipose tissue, triglycerides form important source of energy and supply two thirds of needs during sustained exercise.

During recovery from exercise muscle and liver glycogen stores must be re-built and re-synthesis of unused fatty acids into triglycerides, the processes require energy.

Post Exercise Recovery

When exercise stops heart rate and cardiac output abruptly decrease the sympathetic drive to heart is reduced, but the TPR remains low for sometime after exercise is stopped due to the vasodilator metabolites in the muscle, as a result of these the BP often falls below exercise levels for a brief period. BP then stabilizes.

Oxygen debt: If the energy demands have not been met with oxidative phosphorylation, oxygen debt is incurred. Respiration remains above resting value after exercise to repay the debt; during recovery phase oxygen is used to restore creatine phosphate and ATP and metabolize lactic acid. Some oxygen debt occurs even in low level of exercise because of slow oxidative motor units consume ATP derived from creatine phosphate and glycolysis before oxidative metabolism can increase ATP production to restore steady state requirements. O_2 debt is much more in strenuous exercise.

Fatigue: The ability of muscle to met energy requirements is the major determinant of duration of exercise. Fatigue is not a result of depletion of energy, metabolic by-products are important factors. Fatigue may occur at any point involving muscle contraction, from brain to muscle cells as well as cardiovascular and respiratory system that maintain energy supply and oxygen delievery. During intense exercise accumulation of inorganic phosphate and lactic acid in the myoplasm causes muscle fatigue. The decrease in pH alters Ca^{2+} binding to trponin. General Physical fatigue, the factors involved may be many, decrease in plasma glucose level and accumulation of metabolites. Motivational factors may be involved.

During exercise of small group of muscles, such as hand, limiting factors are unknown but could be muscle itself.

Limits of Exercise Performance

Two main factors limit skeletal muscle performance, the rate of oxygen utilization by muscle and oxygen supply to the muscle. Oxygen usage is probably not the critical factor. Limitation of oxygen supply could be caused by inadequate oxygenation of blood in the lungs or limitation of the supply of oxygenated blood to the muscles, the delivery to the active muscles appears to be the limiting factor. The limitation could be caused by inability to increase cardiac output beyond a critical level. Hence, the major factor perhaps is the pumping capacity of the heart.

Training Regimes

There are three types of training regimes.

1. *Learning:* Adaptive response is increase in rate and accuracy of motor skills, e.g. in typing. Involves CNS. Learning aspect of training also involves motivational and neuromuscular coordination, does not involve adaptive changes in muscle fibres.
2. *Endurance* (submaximal sustained effort), e.g. marathon running. Produces increase oxidative capacity of all muscles with limited cellular hypertrophy.
3. *Strength* (maximal efforts), e.g. weight lifting. Hypertrophy and enhanced glycolytic capacity of motor units employed.

Weight lifting induces synthesis of more myofibrils and hypertrophy of muscle cells and also growth of tendons. Regular maximal strength exercise, the muscle strength can be increased by regular massive efforts that involve most motor units. The effort involves fast glycolytic motor units and oxidative motor units. The blood supply may be interrupted as tissue pressure rises.

Healthy persons can maintain continuous muscular activity supplied by oxidative metabolism. The level increases by regular exercise that induces adaptive changes due to increase in the oxidative capacity of motor units. The demand places increased load on CVS and respiratory system and increases the capacity of heart and respiratory system.

Endurance training, such as running or swimming increases left ventricular volume without increasing left ventricular wall thickness. Strength exercises, such as weight lifting increase left ventricular wall thickening (not as such as in hypertension) with little effect on ventricular volume.

Delayed Muscle Soreness

Activities like hiking or downhill running where the muscles are stretched and lengthened, later cause more pain and stiffness as compared to activities like cycling where activity is not vigorous. The cause of pain and swelling is injury to the muscle cells commonly near myotendinous junction.

YOGA PRACTICE

Yoga practice has been shown to benefit patients of hypertension, diabetes, asthma and some other diseases. It is claimed their regular practice of Yoga improves both Physical and Mental Health. It is believed that the beneficial effects are due to shift of body balance from sympathetic mode to parasympathetic mode.

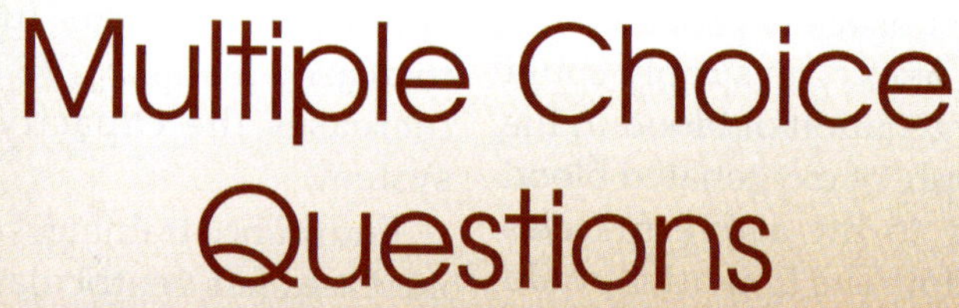

Multiple Choice Questions

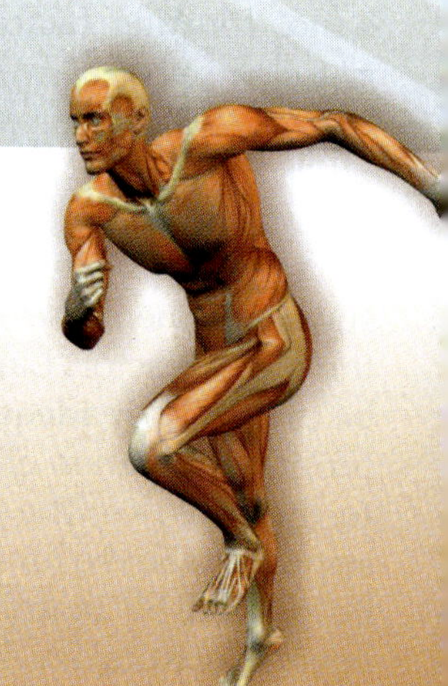

1. Introduction to Physiology

1. True statement regarding extracellular fluid to intracellular fluid is:

a. ECF is rich K^+
b. ECF is more than ICF
c. ECF is rich in organic anion
d. High Na^+ K^+ ratio is seen

2. Function of lysosome is:

a. Breakdown of peroxides
b. Intracellular digestion by hydrolytic enzymes
c. Oxidative phosphorylation
d. Concentration and processing of secretory granules

3. Percentage of body weight constituted by intracellular water is:

a. 20% b. 40%
c. 60% d. 80%

4. Which of the following organelle has phagocytic functions?

a. Lysosome b. Golgi apparatus
c. Mitochondria d. Nucleus

5. Protein synthesis occurs in:

a. Smooth ER b. Rough ER
c. Golgi apparatus d. Lysosomes

6. In a man weighing 60 kg, water content of body is:

a. 30 L b. 35 L
c. 60 L d. 100 L

Answers

1. d 2. b 3. b 4. a 5. b 6. b

2. Introduction to Chemistry of Life

1. Most diffusible ion in resting excitable tissue is:

a. Na^+ b. K^+
c. PO_4^{3-} d. Ca^{2+}

2. True regarding transport across a cell membrane is:

a. Cl^- with glucose symport
b. Na^+ with glucose antiport
c. Na^+ with glucose symport
d. K^+ with glucose symport

3. Receptor-induce endocytosis is mediated by:

a. Perforin b. Vimentin
c. Cytosin d. Clarithrin

4. Most abundant intracellular ion is:

a. Na^+ b. K^+
c. Cl^- d. HCO^-

5. The most important buffer in extracellular fluid space is:

a. Hemoglobinate-hemoglobin
b. Bicarbonate-carbonic acid

c. Phosphate
d. Protein

6. Normal serum osmolality is:
a. 180 mos/l b. 280 mos/l
c. 230 mos/l d. 330 mos/l

7. Which of the following contribute maximally to osmolality of plasma:
a. Na^+ b. K^+
c. Inorganic phosphate d. Proteins

8. Major buffer of the interstitial fluid is:
a. Carbonic acid bicarbonate
b. Hemoglobin
c. Minor proteins d. Phosphates

9. True about facilitated diffusion is:
a. Concentration gradient
b. Does not require energy
c. In their chemical electrical gradient
d. All of the above

10. Exocytosis:
a. Extrusion of cell bound vesicles
b. Intrusion of liquid particles
c. Intrusion of solid particles
d. All of the above

11. Nernst equations deals with:
a. Cl shift b. O_2 uptake
c. CO_2 transfer
d. Equilibrium potential of permeable ion

Answers

1. b	2. c	3. d	4. b	5. b	6. b
7. a	8. a	9. d	10. a	11. d	

3. Muscles

1. Tropomyosin:
a. Helps in the fusion of action and myosin
b. Covers actin and prevents attachments of actin and myosin
c. Slides over myosin
d. Causes Ca^{2+} release

2. Which protein prevents contraction by covering binding sites on actin and myosin:
a. Troponin b. Calmodulin
c. Thymosin d. Tropomyosin

3. Force generating proteins are:
a. Myosin and myglobin
b. Dynein and kinesin
c. Calmodulin and G protein
d. Troponin

4. In excitation contraction coupling in smooth muscle true is:
a. The presence of intracellular calcium is essential to cause contraction
b. Presence of troponin is essential
c. Phosphorylation of myosin occurs
d. Increased calcium in sarcoplasmic reticulum causes sustained contraction

5. Muscle relaxation after contraction is due to:
a. Reuptake of Ca ions into sarcoplasmic reticulum
b. Inhibition of reuptake of Ca ions
c. ATP hydrolysis to ADP
d. Formation of actin-troponin complex

6. Relaxation of a skeletal muscle is due to:
a. Release of acetylcholine
b. ATP consumption
c. Reuptake of calcium
d. Not known

7. The motor unit includes:
a. Motor nerve and the muscle fibers it supplies
b. All the muscle fibers in a muscle
c. Afferent neuron, center and efferent neuron
d. Single muscle fibre and all neurons that innervate it

8. Which statement about skeletal muscle structure is not true:
a. The area between 2.adjacent Z lines is sarcomers
b. During muscle contraction, width of I band decreases
c. T system is present at Z lines
d. Both contraction and relaxation of muscle requires ATP

9. Which of the following statement about 'red muscles' is true:
a. Extraocular muscles are type of red muscles
b. They are specialized for fine, skilled movements

c. They have little mitochondrial ATPase
d. They are also called slow muscles

10. Nerve fibre most susceptible to hypoxia is:
a. a
b. b
c. c
d. All are equally sensitive

11. The band which disappears on muscle contraction is:
a. I
b. A
c. H
d. Z

12. Action potential at motor end plate in skeletal muscle is initiated by:
a. Release of acetylcholine
b. Release of epinephrine
c. Summation potentials
d. Temporal potentials

13. Smooth muscle contraction due to release of calcium occurs because of:
a. Increased cAMP
b. Troponin C
c. Increased ATP
d. Calmodulin dependent

14. During skeletal muscle contraction:
a. A band shortens
b. Both H and I band shorten
c. Both A and I band shorten
d. Both A and H band shorten

15. Which of the following is not true about action potential in skeletal muscle:
a. Duration of action potential and muscle twitch is same
b. Action potential spreads along T tubules which releases Ca^{2+}
c. Is shorter than the action potential of cardiac muscle
d. Ca^{2+} in response to action potential is released form terminal cisterns

16. Length of the muscle at which the active tension is maximal is:
a. Optimal length
b. Resting length
c. Maximal length
d. Minimal length

17. Beta cell activation cause Ca^+ influx in:
a. Cardiac muscle
b. Smooth muscle
c. Skeltal muscle
d. Renal tubular epithelium

18. Rheobase is a magnitude of:
a. Current
b. Time
c. Velocity
d. Radiation

Answers

1. b	2. d	3. b	4. c	5. a	6. c
7. a	8. c	9. d	10. b	11. c	12. a
13. d	14. b	15. a	16. b	17. a	18. a

4. Respiratory System

1. CO_2 is transported in blood mainly as:
a. Bicarbonate
b. Carbamino-compounds
c. Free CO_2
d. Plasma-protein combination

2. In upper airway obstruction all of the following changes are seen except:
a. Decreased maximum breathing capacity
b. RV decreased
c. Decreased FEV
d. Decreased vital capacity

3. In moderate exercise respiratory rate increase is due to response of:
a. Proprioceptor receptor in the joints
b. PCO_2 in arterial blood
c. CO_2 in arterial blood
d. J-receptors stimulation

4. Spirometry can demonstrate and measure all of the following except:
a. Tidal volume
b. Residual volume
c. Vital capacity
d. Inspiratory reserve capacity

5. Surfacant is made-up of:
a. Fibrin
b. Mucoprotein
c. Phospholipids
d. Fibrinogen

6. Tidal volume is calculated by:
a. Inspiratory capacity minus the inspiratory reserve volume

b. Total lung capacity minus the reserve volume
c. Functional residual capacity minus residual volume
d. Vital capacity minus expiratory reserve volumes

7. Surfactant production in lungs starts at:
a. 28 weeks
b. 31 weeks
c. 34 weeks
d. 36 weeks

8. Surfactant is produced by:
a. Type II pneumocytes
b. Type I pneumocytes
c. Macrophages
d. Endothelial cells

9. True statement regarding pulmonary ventilation is:
a. PaO_2 is maximum at the apex
b. $\dot{V}/\dot{Q}$ is minimum at the base
c. Ventilation per unit lung volume is maximum at the apex
d. Blood circulation is minimum at the base

10. Oxygen dissociation curve is shifted to the left by following except:
a. Increase in temperature
b. Increase in pH
c. Decrease in CO_2
d. Increase in carboxy Hb

11. Which of the following is false:
a. FEV1 is the fraction of VC volume in one second
b. PEFR is maximum expiratory flow of lung capacity
c. Respiratory minute volume is the amount of the air inspired per minute
d. MBC is the largest volume of gas can be moved into and out of lungs in one second by effort

12. Normal PO_2 in an 85 year healthy male in his room air breath is:
a. 80
b. 60
c. 45
d. 110

13. Flow during last stage of expiration decreases because of:
a. Breaking by inspiratory muscles
b. Dynamic compression of airways
c. Collapse of alveoli
d. All of the above

14. Inspiratory flow curve:
a. Can be used to evaluate efficacy of broncho-dilator therapy
b. Can be used to differentiate emphysema bronchitis
c. Indicates small airway disease
d. Can diagnose upper airway obstruction

15. Hypoxia causes tachycardia by stimulating:
a. Reflex (peripheral chemoreceptors)
b. Stimulation of central receptors
c. Stimulation of vasomotor nucleus
d. Direct sympathetic stimulation

16. Which gas is not responsible for green house effect:
a. Carbondioxide
b. Ozone
c. Nitrogen
d. Nitrous oxide

17. FEV1/FVC is reduced in:
a. Asthma
b. Pleural effusion
c. Fibrosis
d. All of the above

18. All of the following are measured by spirometry except:
a. TLC
b. VC
c. FEV1
d. Inspiratory capacity

19. What is the mechanism by which hyperventilation may cause muscle spasm:
a. Decreased calcium ion concentration
b. Decreased carbon dioxide
c. Decreased potassium
d. Decreased sodium

20. After hyperventilating for some time, holding the breath is dangerous since:
a. It can lead on to CO_2 narcosis
b. Due to the lack of stimulation by CO_2 anoxia can go into dangerous levels
c. Decreased CO_2 shift the ODC to the left
d. Alkalosis can lead on to tetany

21. A patient is having normal lung compliance and increased airway resistance. What is the most economical way of breathing for him?
a. Slow and deep
b. Slow and shallow
c. Rapid and deep
d. Rapid and shallow

22. Spirometer cannot measure:
a. Tidal volume
b. Vital capacity
c. Expiratory reserve volume
d. Residul volume

23. Oxygen dissociation curve is shifted to the right in all except:
a. Fall in pH
b. Rise in temperature and pCO_2
c. Increase in 2, 3 DPG
d. Increased HbF

24. Surfactants acts by decreasing:
a. Pleural pressure
b. Intrathoracic pressure
c. Surface tension
d. Pleural fluid secretion

25. Apneustic centre is located in:
a. Ventromedial part of medulla
b. Dorsolateral part of medulla
c. Lower part of pons
d. Upper part of pons

26. If at sea level alveolar O_2 pressure is one then at 20 m depth, pressure will be:
a. 1 b. 3
c. 2 d. 4

27. J receptor stimulation causes:
a. Tachycardia b. Tachypnoea
c. Hypertension d. Bronchodilation

28. Lung compliance is decreased in all except:
a. Emphysema
b. Interstitial lung disease
c. Kyphosis
d. Pulmonary congestion
e. Pneumothorax

29. Haldane effect is:
a. Effect of pCO_2 on oxygen carriage in blood
b. Effect of pO_2 on carbon dioxide carriage in blood
c. Effect of pCO_2 on carbon dioxide carriage in blood
d. Effect of pH oxygen carriage of blood

30. Which of the following tends to decrease with increasing age:
a. Vital capacity
b. Systolic blood pressure
c. Pulse pressure
d. Residunal volume

31. Apnoea is:
a. Slowing of respiration
b. Cessation of respiration
c. Type I respiratory failure
d. Difficulty in breathing

32. Normal PaO_2 is:
a. 100 mmHg b. 96 mmHg
c. 90 mmHg d. 80 mmHg

33. Intrapleural pressure at end of normal inspiration is:
a. – 6 mmHg b. – 18 mmHg
c. + 4 mmHg d. + 18 mmHg

34. CO_2 enters the capillaries by:
a. Diffusion b. Permeation
c. Osmosis d. Active transport

35. Hypoxic stimulation of receptors occurs at an altitude of:
a. 3000 m b. 3000 ft
c. 10,400 m d. 10,400 ft

36. Which of the following statement about 'myoglobin' is not true:
a. It is found in skeletal muscle
b. It binds 4 mols of O_2 per mol
c. Its disociation curve is a rectangular hyperbole
d. It releases O_2 only at low pO_2

37. Respiratory centre controlled by pons is:
a. Pneumotaxic b. Gasping
c. Inspiratory d. Expiratory

38. FEV1/FVC less than 60% is seen in:
a. Emphysema
b. Pectus excavatum
c. Interstitial lung disease
d. Pulmonary oedema

39. In Interstitial lung disease, not seen is:
a. Raised PaO_2 in blood
b. Normal $PaCO_2$ in blood
c. Responds to oral prednisone
d. FEV1 and FVC are decreased in same proportions

40. In respiratory acidosis buffering occurs:
a. Mainly extracellular b. Mainly intracellular
c. Both equally d. None of the above

41. Which statement about 'surfactant' is not true:
a. It is synthesized by type II pneumocyte
b. It has surface tension lowering property
c. It is decreased in hyaline membrane disease
d. Its synthesis is increased by 100% oxygen in premature infants

42. Oxygen-hemoglobin dissociation curve is:
a. Sigmoid b. Hyperbolic
c. Parabolic d. None of the above

43. If minute volume is 6,000 ml/min, respiratory rate 15/min, dead space is 150 ml and pulmonary flow is 5.000 ml/min. The ventilation perfusion ratio is:
a. 1.25 b. 1.00
c. 0.75 d. 0.50

44. 'Cl-shift' during carbon dioxide transport is seen in:
a. Lungs b. RBCs
c. Kidney d. Skeletal muscle

45. At high/altitude one will develop:
a. Respiratory acidosis b. Respiratory alkalosis
c. Metabolic acidosis d. Metabolic alkalosis

46. Vital capacity is:
a. Inspiratory capacity and expiratory reserve volume
b. Tidal volume and inspiratory reserve volume
c. Inspiratory reserve volume and expiratory reserve volume
d. Inspiratory capacity and residual volume

47. Average vital capacity in young men is:
a. 3 L b. 4.5 L
c. 6 L d. 7.5 L

48. Most potent respiratory stimulant is:
a. Oxygen b. Carbon dioxide
c. H^+ d. K^+

49. Type II pulmonary epithelial cells secrete:
a. Surfactant b. Mucus
c. Heparin d. Polypeptides

50. Hyperpnea during exercise is because of:
a. Hypercapnia
b. Hypoxemia
c. Reflex stimulation of proprioceptors and cerebral cortex
d. None of the above

51. At rest, the stimuli for ventilation if derived from:
a. O_2 b. CO_2
c. pH d. HCO_3

52. Alveolar hyperventilation causes:
a. Respiratory alkalosis
b. Respiratory acidosis
c. Metabolic alkalosis
d. Metabolic acidosis

53. Major factor regulating alveolar ventilation during rest is:
a. Arterial pO_2
b. Arterial pCO_2
c. Arterial pH
d. Nervous output from propriceptors

54. A patient is respiring 2 lit./min (pulmonary ventilation) and has respiratory rate of 20 per minute. Which of the following is true:
a. Doing exercise
b. Has respiratory acidosis
c. Cheyne- Stokes breathing
d. Respiring in dead space

55. Which of the following substance has respiratory quotient more than I:
a. Glycerol b. Fat
c. Protein d. Pyruvic acid

56. Resting total body oxygen consumption is:
a. 100 ml/min b. 150 ml/min
c. 200 ml/min d. 250 ml/min

57. 1 gm of hemoglobin combines with:
a. 1.34 ml of O_2 b. 0.34 ml of O_2
c. 13.4 ml of O_2 d. 0.034 ml of O_2

58. Diffusing capacity of O_2 at rest is:
a. 25 ml/min/mmHg b. 10 ml/min/mmHg
c. 50 ml/min/mmHg d. 100 ml/min/mmHg

59. True statement about FEV1/FVC ratio is:
a. Most sensitive test to differentiate between restrictive and obstructive lung disease
b. Is normally above 0.6
c. Decreased in emphysema
d. All of the above

60. The pulmonary alveoli are normally kept dry because of the:
a. Macrophages
b. Negative intrapleural pressure
c. Surfactant
d. High pO_2 in alveoli

61. N2 washout test is used to measure:
a. Residual volume
b. Inspiratory reserve volume
c. Expiratory reserve volume
d. Vital capacity

62. In high altitude mountain sickness, feature of pulmonary edema is:
a. Decreased pulmonary capillary permeability
b. Increased pulmonary capillary pressure
c. Normal left atrial pressure
d. Increased left ventricular back-pressure

63. The ODC is shifted to the left by:
a. Acidosis
b. Raised pH
c. Raised CO_2
d. Raised temperature

64. Toxicity of hyperbaric oxygen is due to:
a. Displacement of O_2 from Hb
b. Respiratory drive
c. Enzymatic damage
d. Superooxide

65. Volume of air taken in and given out during normal respiration is referred to as:
a. Inspiratory reserve volume
b. Tidal volume
c. Expiratory reserve volume
d. Vital capacity
e. Inspiratory capacity

66. True regarding idiopathic pulmonary fibrosis is:
a. Decreased FEV1
b. Decreased FEV/FVC
c. Decreased DLCO
d. Decreased residual volume

67. Hypoxia causes vasoconstriction in:
a. Muscle
b. Lungs
c. Liver
d. Spleen

68. Which of the following receptors is activated in pulmonary embolism:
a. J receptors
b. Stretch receptors
c. Rapidly adapting receptors
d. Slow adapting receptors

69. All the following occur in high altitude acclimatization except:
a. Respiratory alkalosis
b. Increased mitochondria
c. Increased erythropoietin
d. Increased blood glucose

70. FEV_1% is:
a. 50 percent
b. 65 percent
c. 83 percent
d. 95 percent

71. Work of breathing in quiet respiration is:
a. Maximum for elastic work
b. Maximum for non elastic work
c. Equal for both

72. Weightlessness result in:
a. Increased plasma volume
b. Loss of bone mineral
c. RBC mass
d. Decreased Ca^{2+} exeretion

73. Respiratory minute volume is:
a. 4 2 L
b. 5 L
c. 4.8 L
d. 6 L

74. Apneustic breathing results due to transection at:
a. Between pons and medulla
b. Between pons and midbrain
c. Mid pons with vagi cut
d. Mid pons

75. Pulmonary compliance is increased in case of:
a. Pulmonary congestion
b. Asthma
c. Emphysema
d. All of the above

76. Which is true about chloride shift
a. Cl^- content of RBC in venous blood is higher
b. Chloride shift is complete in 1 sec
c. Both of the above
d. None of the above

Answers

1. a	2. b	3. a	4. b	5. c	6. a
7. a	8. a	9. b	10. a	11 d	12. a
13. b	14. a	15. a	16. c	17. a	18. a
19. a	20. b	21. a	22. d	23. d	24. c
25. c	26. b	27. b	28. a	29. b	30. a
31. b	32. a	33. a	34. a	35. a	36. b
37. a	38. a	39. a	40. c	41. d	42. a
43. c	44. b	45. b	46. a	47. b	48. b
49. a	50. c	51. b	52. a	53. b	54. d
55. d	56. d	57. a	58. a	59. d	60. c
61. a	62. b	63. b	64. d	65. b	66. c
67. b	68. a	69. d	70. c	71. a	72. b
73. d	74. c	75. c	76. c		

5. Blood

1. Erythropoietin level are increased by:
a. PO_2 b. PCO_2
c. Hb d. pH

2. Albumin contributes the maximum to oncotic pressure because it has:
a. High mol wt, low concentration
b. Low mol wt, high concentration
c. High mol wt, high concentration
d. Low mol wt, high concentration

3. Best anticoagulant for Wintrobe's tube for measuring ESR is:
a. Double oxalate b. DTA
c. Heparin d. Citrate

4. Which of the following is responsible for maintaining the structure of the RBC membrane:
a. Spectrin b. Fibrin
c. Integrin d. Alpha glycoprotein

5. *In vitro* coagulation is initiated by factor:
a. XII b. XI
c. X d. VII

6. When fully saturated Ig of Hb contains:
a. 1 ml of O_2 b. 1.34 ml of O_2
c. 2.94 ml of O_2 d. 2.4ml of O_2

7. B and T cells are:
a. Bone marrow and thymus derived lymphocytes
b. Type of cells in lists of Langerhans
c. Calcitonin secreting cells of thyroid
d. Thymus and bursa derived lymphocytes

8. The conversion of fibrinogen to fibrin is caused by:
a. Thrombin b. Calcium ions
c. Factor XIII d. Thromboplastin

9. Platelet adhesion is stimulated by all except:
a. Prostaglandin E2 b. Thromboxane
c. cAMP d. Thrombin

10. Basic stimulus for eythropoiesis is:
a. Decreased PO_2 b. Erythropoietin
c. Increased PCO_2 d. Thyroxine

11. Which of the following is true about capillaries:
a. Contain about 5% of total blood volume
b. Contain about 25% of total blood volume
c. Offer more peripheral resistance than arterioles
d. Endothelial cells form thight junctions which allow passage by diffusion only

12. Which of the following is not a vitamin K dependent coagulation factor:
a. Factor VIII b. Prothrombin
c. Factor VII d. Factor X

13. All of the following are true about lymphocytes except:
a. Enter the bloodstream via lymphatics
b. Most lymphocytes are formed in lymph nodes, thymus and spleen
c. No change in number throughout life
d. Glucocorticoids decrease the circulating lymphocyte count

14. All of the following factors contribute to increased interstitial pressure except:
a. Increased capillary hydrostatic pressure
b. Decreased capillary permeability
c. Increased interstitial fluid colloid osmotic pressure
d. Decreased plasma colloid osmotic pressure

15. Endothedial cells synthesize:
a. Fibrinogen b. Factor VII
c. Factor X d. Factor XII

16. Osmotic pressure of plasma is mainly maintained by:
a. Albumin b. γ-globulin
c. β-globulin d. α-globulin

17. Life span of RBC is:
a. 120 days b. 90 days
c. 60 days d. 30 days

18. Carbon monoxide is released in lungs from:
a. Iron of heme molecule
b. Plasma
c. Transferrin
d. Plasma protein

19. Histamine is released by:
a. Mast cells b. Lymphocyte
c. Neutrophils d. Eosinophils

20. Earlier site of hemopoiesis in fetus is:
a. Yolk sac b. Spleen
c. Bone marrow d. GIT

21. **At what age fetal hemoglobin is complete replaced by adult hemoglobin:**
    a. Immediately after birth
    b. One month
    c. Three months
    d. Six months

22. **Both parents are of blood group A, children will be of:**
    a. A group
    b. A or O group
    c. A or B group
    d. AB group

23. **Maximum number of O_2 combining with each molecule of hemoglobin is:**
    a. 1 b. 2
    c. 4 d. 8

24. **Erythropoietin secretion is increased by all except:**
    a. Hypoxia b. Exercise
    c. High altitude d. Androgens

25. **The following are synthesized in liver except:**
    a. Albumin b. Gamma globulin
    c. Fibrinogen d. Prothrombin

26. **First precursor of RBC's is:**
    a. Proerythroblast b. Erythroblast
    c. Reticulocyte d. Thromboplast

27. **Individuals with DU antigen are frequently typed as:**
    a. Rh negative b. Rh positive
    c. Both of the above d. None of the above

28. **Macrophages are the mature form of:**
    a. Basophils b. Neutrophils
    c. Monocytes d. Lymphocytes

29. **Which of the following is true about hemoglobin as compared to myoglobin:**
    a. Hemoglobin oxygen dissociation curve is hyperbolic
    b. Myoglobin oxygen dissociation curve is sigmoid shaped
    c. Myolglobin dissociation curve is left to that of hemoglobin curve
    d. Myoglobin binds 4 mol of O_2 per mole

30. **Which of the following coagulation factor is not involved in the intrinsic pathway of coagulation:**
    a. VII b. VIII
    c. IX d. X

Answers

1. a	2. b	3. a	4. a	5. a	6. b
7. a	8. a	9. c	10. b	11. a	12. a
13. c	14. b	15. d	16. a	17. a	18. a
19. a	20. a	21. d	22. b	23. c	24. b
25. b	26. a	27. b	28. c	29. c	30. a

6. Cardiovascular System

1. **QRS complex indicates:**
    a. Atrial repolarization
    b. Atrial depolarization
    c. Ventricular repolarization
    d. Ventricular depolarization

2. **Isovolumic relaxation phase of the cardiac cycle ends with:**
    a. Peak of 'C' waves
    b. Opening of A.V. valve
    c. Closure of semilunar valve
    d. Beginning 'T' wave

3. **Plateau phase of action potential is seen in:**
    a. SA node
    b. AV node
    c. Skeletal muscle
    d. Ventricular fibers

4. **Blood in splanchnic area during exercise is decreased due to:**
    a. Venoconstriction with decreased blood flow
    b. Venodilation with decreased blood flow
    c. Venodilation with increased blood flow
    d. Venodilation with normal blood flow

5. **Which of the following is NOT correct regarding capillaries:**
    a. Greatest cross sectional area
    b. Contain 25% of blood
    c. Contain less blood than veins
    d. Have single layer of cells bounding

6. **A 0.5 litre blood loss in 30 minutes will lead to:**
    a. Increase in HR, decrease in BP
    b. Slight increase in HR, normal BP
    c. Decrease in HR and BP
    d. Prominent increase in HR

7. Most important factor in control of contractility of heart is:

a. Myocardial wall thickness
b. Right atrial volume
c. SA node pacemaker potential
d. Sympathetic stimulation

8. 'Flare' in triple response is mediated by:

a. Axon reflex b. Capillary dilation
c. Histamine release d. Local hormones

9. During exercise increase in O_2 delivery to muscles is because of all except:

a. Oxygen dissociation curve shifts to left
b. Increased stroke volume
c. Increased extraction of oxygen from the blood
d. Increased blood flow to muscles

10. At the end of isometric relaxation phase:

a. Atrioventricular valves open
b. Atrioventricular valves close
c. Corresponds to peak of 'C' wave in JVP
d. Corresponds to T wave in ECG

11. Which of the following statement is true about capillaries:

a. Contain 5% of total blood volume
b. Contain 10% of total blood volume
c. Velocity of blood flow is maximum
d. Offer maximum resistance to blood flow

12. True about changes in exercise are following except:

a. Increased venous return by muscle pumping action
b. CO_2 production increases
c. Circulating catecholamines inhibited
d. Increased syst BP

13. In Isovolumetric contraction of ventricles:

a. Both aortic and AV valves closed
b. Both aortic and AV valves open
c. Aortic open, AV closed
d. AV open, aortic closed

14. Which of the following feature is common to all forms of shock:

a. Decreased cardiac output
b. Decreased heart rate
c. Decreased right atrial pressure
d. Decreased tissue perfusion

15. Mixed venous O_2 pressure is:

a. 100 mmHg b. 80 mmHg
c. 60 mmHg d. 40 mmHg

16. Sodium enters the cardiac cell in:

a. Repolarization phase
b. Depolarization phase
c. Phase of relaxation
d. End of cardiac cycle

17. Swan-Ganz catheter is used to measure:

a. Central venous pressure
b. Pulmonary artery wedge pressure
c. Right atrial pressure
d. Right ventricular pressure

18. In athletes, bradycardia is because of:

a. Decreased sympathetic tone
b. Increased vagal tone
c. Low cardiac output
d. Low venous return

19. At the time of AV valve closure there is:

a. Isometric contraction
b. Isotonic contraction
c. Isometric relaxation
d. Isotonic relaxation

20. Arteriovenous junction regulate the:

a. Temperature b. Pressure
c. Proprioception d. Touch

21. Stimulation of stretch receptors present in the left ventricle causes hypertension and bradycardia. This phenomenon is known as:

a. Bainbridge reflex
b. Bezold-Jarish
c. Cushing reflex
d. Hering-Breurer reflex

22. In a person who stands suddenly from lying posture there is:

a. Increased afferent discharge from IX (glossopharyngeal) nerve
b. Increased tone of capacitance veins
c. Decreased heart rate
d. None of the above

23. Venous return is increased in:

a. Inspiration
b. Expiration
c. Not affected by respiration
d. None of the above

24. Wenckeback phenomenon is:
a. Progressive prolongation of PR interval followed by absent QRS complex
b. Same as R on T phenomenon
c. Shortened PR interval with prolonged QRS interval
d. None of the above

25. Capillaries with tight functions allowing the passage of only small molecules are found in:
a. Brain b. Skin
c. Kidney d. Muscle

26. In pacemaker of heart, after the impulse action potential comes back to firing level due to:
a. Increased permeability to sodium ions
b. Decreased permeability to potassium ions
c. Cessation of sodium influx
d. Increased permeability to chloride ions

27. Vessels least under sympathetic control are:
a. Cerebral b. Splanchnic
c. Cardiac d. Cutaneous

28. 'C' wave in jugular venous pulse is due to:
a. Ventricular filling
b. Atrial filling
c. Ventricular contraction
d. Atrial contraction

29. Left artery coronary blood flow is minimum during:
a. End of diastole b. Protodiastole
c. Isometric contraction d. Isometric relaxation

30. According to Starling's law, cardiac output is increased by:
a. Increased end diastolic volume
b. Increased end systolic volume
c. Increased heart rate
d. Decrease in blood pressure

31. Blood pressure is decreased if stimulation occurs in all except:
a. Sympathetic system b. Carotid sinus
c. Ventricular receptors d. Aortic sinus

32. Conduction velocity is maximum in:
a. SA node b. AV node
c. Bundle of His d. Purkinje fibers

33. Vagal stimulation can cause all except:
a. Delayed A-V conduction
b. Increased ventricular contraction
c. Decreased atrial contraction
d. Decreased heart rate

34. Which of the following component of peripheral vascular system is not supplied by sympathetic system: (DU 86)
a. Arteries b. Arterioles
c. Capillaries d. Venules

35. Parasympathetic nerve supply affects the cardiovascular system mainly by altering:
a. Vascular resistance b. Heart rate
c. Contractility of heart d. Venous return

36. Pacemaker of the heart is:
a. SA node
b. AV node
c. Bundle of His
d. Purkinje fibers

37. Stimulation of baroreceptors results in:
a. Decreased cardiac contractility and heart rate
b. Increased blood pressure and heart rate
c. Decreased heart rate and increased blood pressure
d. Increased heart rate and increased cardiac output

38. Which of the following statement about first heart sound is not true:
a. Results from closure of A-V valves
b. Results from closure of semilunar valves
c. Best heard at apex of heart
d. Occurs at the beginning of ventricular contraction

39. Delay in cardiac impulses maximally occurs at:
a. SA node b. AV node
c. Bundle of His d. Left bundle branch

40. Which of the following about cardiac output is correct:
a. Not necessarily increases with heart rate
b. Increases to 50 L/min. during exercise
c. Proportionately falls with increase in heart rate
d. Proportional to blood pressure

41. Which of the following statement about 'baroreceptors' is not true:
a. Present in the carotid sinus and aortic arch
b. From these afferent fibers pass to the medulla
c. Impulses generated by these inhibit the vagal innervation of heart
d. Responds both to sustained pressure and pulse pressure

42. In arteriolar constriction, capillaries are filled by:
a. Pulsatile flow b. Nonpulsatile flow
c. Newtonian flow d. None of the above

43. Which of the following regulates the fine control of blood pressure:
a. Medulla b. Hypothalamus
c. Midbrain d. Median eminence

44. Increased radius of resistance vessels lead to:
a. Increased systolic blood pressure
b. Increased diastolic blood pressure
c. Increased rate of blood flow
d. None of the above

45. True statement about 'Purkinje fibers' is:
a. Forms conducting tissue between skeletal and smooth muscle
b. Forms neural tissue of the smooth muscle
c. Forms conducting tissue of the cardiac muscle
d. Are fibers of vagus nerve which regulate the heart rate

46. An increase in the cross section of the capillary will lead to a decrease in the :
a. Rate of blood flow
b. Diastolic blood pressure
c. Systolic blood pressure
d. Peripheral resistance

47. Basal cardiac output per min in adults is:
a. 10 L b. 5.0 L
c. 6.5 L d. 7.5 L

48. Pressure on carotic sinus causes:
a. Reflex bradycardia b. Tachycardia
c. Bainbridge reflex d. Increase in BP

49. Cardiac Index is:
a. Stroke volume per BSA
b. COP per unit body surface area
c. Syst press/BSA
d. None

50. Determines preload of heart:
a. End diastolic volume of ventricles
b. End systolic volume
c. End ventricular pressure
d. All of the above

51. In Isovolumetric contraction of ventricles:
a. Both aortic and AV valves closed
b. Both aortic and AV valves open
c. Aortic open, AV closed
d. AV open, aortic closed

52. The cardiac output can be determined by all except:
a. Fick's principle
b. Dye dilution technique
c. Angiocardiography
d. Thermodillution

53. True about blood flow in various organs:
a. Liver > kidney > brain > heart
b. Liver > brain > kidney > heart
c. Kidney > brain > heart > liver
d. Liver > heart > brain > kidney

54. Least conduction velocity is seen in:
a. AV node
b. Purkinje fibers
c. Bundles of His
d. Ventricular myocardial fibers

55. Cardiac index is determined by:
a. CO and surface area
b. SV and surface area
c. Surface area only
d. Peripheral resistance

56. Normal portal venous pressure is ____ cms saline
a. 5–10 b. 10–15
c. 1–5 d. 20–25

57. Blood flow changes are least during exercise in:
a. Brain b. Heart
c. Skin d. Kidney

58. Endothelium derived relaxation factor is supposed to be:
a. Nitric oxide b. Adenosine
c. ANP d. Histamine

59. Carotid sinus nerve is:
a. Glossopharyngeal b. Vagus
c. Phrenic d. C^7

60. Cardiac index is:
a. Cardiac output/min/m^2
b. Stroke volume X HR
c. 3.2 L
d. a and c

61. True about S2 is:
a. Due to opening of semilunar valves
b. Higher frequency than S1
c. Longer duration than S1
d. Due to AV valves

62. Average coronary blood flow at rest as percentage of cardiac output is:
a. 5
b. 10
c. 25
d. 15

Answers

1. d 2. b 3. d 4. a 5. b 6. b
7. d 8. a 9. a 10. a 11. a 12. c
13. a 14. d 15. d 16. b 17. b 18. b
19. a 20. a 21. b 22. b 23 a 24 a
25. a 26. b 27. a 28. c 29. c 30. a
31. a 32. d 33. b 34. c 35. b 36. a
37. a 38. b 39. b 40. a 41. c 42. b
43. a 44. c 45. c 46. a 47. b 48. a
49. b 50. a 51. a 52. c 53. a 54. a
55. a 56. b 57. a 58. a 59. a 60. a
61. b 62. a

7. Digestive System and 8. Metabolism and Nutrition

1. CCK-PZ causes all of the following except:
a. Gallbladder contraction
b. Pancreatic enzyme secretion
c. Increased gastrin secretion
d. Relaxes sphincter of Oddi

2. Gallbladder contraction is stimulation by:
a. Gastrin
b. Secretin
c. Vagus
d. Cholycystokinin

3. Most important stimulate for bile secretion is:
a. Cholecystokinin
b. Secretin
c. Bile acid
d. Bile salt

4. Fat in the duodenum lumen:
a. Stimulates gallbladder contraction
b. Inhibits gallbladder contraction
c. Inhibits CCK secretion
d. Releases secretion

5. Salivation by dog seen when food is given along with ringing of a bell is:
a. Conditional reflex
b. Innate reflex
c. Reinforcement
d. Habituation

6. True about high roughage in diet is:
a. Decreases stool transit time
b. Increase stool transit time
c. Normalize stool transit
d. No effect on stool transit time

7. True about small intestinal peristalsis is:
a. Inhibited by gastrin
b. Stimulated by CCK
c. Stimulated by secretin
d. Inhibited by insulin

8. In distal ileum resection, following are seen except:
a. B_{12} deficiency
b. Fe deficiency
c. Absorption of bile salts
d. None

9. Fe absorption decreases by following except:
a. Phytates
b. Vit. C
c. Phosphate
d. Taurine

10. False about pancreatic secretion is:
a. 1 L/day
b. Osmolality ½ of plasma
c. Secretin-produces HCO_3 rich
d. Pancreozymin-enzyme rich

11. Propulsion of chyme in small intestine is because of:
a. Peristaltic movements
b. Gravitational forces
c. Segmentation movements
d. Pendular movements

12. Basal migrating motor complex in gut originate in the:
a. Pyloric end of stomach
b. Longitudinal muscle layer of small intestine
c. Circular muscle layer in small intestine
d. Oesophagus

13. Maximum absorption of fluid and electrolytes occur in the:
a. Stomach
b. Proximal small intestine
c. Colon
d. Distal small intestine

14. Function of bile salts is to:
a. Facilitate absorption of proteins
b. Regulate cholesterol synthesis
c. Emulsification of fats
d. All of the above

15. Which of the following does not have a proenzyme
    a. Pepsin
    b. Phospholipase A
    c. Chymotrypsin
    d. Ribonuclease

16. End product of ingested sugar in gastrointestinal tract is:
    a. Fructose and glucose
    b. Glucose and galactose
    c. Xylose and mannose
    d. Ribose and mannose

17. Pancreatic juice rich in water and electrolytes in response to:
    a. Pancreozymin b. Cholecystokinin
    c. Secretin d. Proteins

18. The following hormones are secreted locally in gut except:
    a. Gastrin b. Enterogastrone
    c. Secretin d. Dopamine

19. Which of the following is the fastest to be absorbed from the stomach:
    a. Carbohydrate b. Protein
    c. Fats d. Water

20. True about secretin is:
    a. Increased gallbladder contraction and HCO_3 rich pancreatic fluid
    b. Increased gastrin secretion
    c. Gastric hypermotility
    d. Increased HCO_3 rich pancreatic fluid

21. In dog, increased salivation on hearing bell is:
    a. Gastric phase b. Intestinal phase
    c. Conditional reflex d. Unconditional reflex

22. Maximum absorption of bile occurs at:
    a. Duodenum b. Jejunum
    c. Ileum d. Colon

23. Function of gallbladder is:
    a. Increases alkalinity of bile
    b. Increases concentration of bile
    c. Increases intrabiliary pressure
    d. Increases phosphate level

24. Water absorbed by human gut in a day is:
    a. 1L b. 2L
    c. 5L d. 10L

25. Chemoreceptor trigger zone initiating vomiting:
    a. Medial mammilary nucleus
    b. Area postrema
    c. Vomiting centre
    d. Periventricular nucleus

26. Gastric seceration is stimulated by all of the following except:
    a. Secretin b. Gastric distension
    c. Gastrin d. Vagal stimulus

27. Dietary fat is mainly absorbed in:
    a. Duodenum and jejunum
    b. Ileum
    c. Colon
    d. Cecum

28. Following enzymes are activated by trypsin except:
    a. Chymotrypsinogen b. Prophospholipase A
    c. Pepsinogen d. Proelastase

29. Brush border of intestine is formed by:
    a. Vili b. Cilia
    c. Microvili d. Mucosal folds

30. Vitamin B_{12} is absorbed in:
    a. Duodenum b. Jejunum
    c. Ileum d. Stomach

31. Maximum contraction of gallbladder is seen with:
    a. CCK b. Secretion
    c. Gastrin d. Enterogastrone

32. The cephalic phase of gastric secretion is brought about by:
    a. Sympathetic fibers b. Parasympathetic fibers
    c. Hormonal factors d. None of the above

33. Enterogastric reflex results in:
    a. Gastric motility increase
    b. Gastric motility decrease
    c. No change in gastric motility
    d. Any of the above

Answers

1. c	2. d	3. d.	4. a	5. a	6. a
7. b	8. b	9. b	10. b	11. a	12. a
13. b	14. c	15. d	16. a	17. c	18. d
19. d	20. d	21. c	22. c	23. b	24. d
25. b	26. a	27. a	28. c	29. c	30. c
31. a	32. b	33. c			

9. Urinary System

1. **Which of the following is true about nephron function:**
   a. Ascending thick limb is permeable to water
   b. Descending thin limb impermeable to water
   c. Osmolality of intratubular content in DCT is more than surrounding interstitution
   d. Osmolality of intratubular content in PCT is isotonic to surrounding interstitium.

2. **Maximum absorption of water takes place in:**
   a. Proximal convoluted tubule
   b. Distal convoluted tubule
   c. Collecting duct
   d. Loop of Henle

3. **Maximum site of absorption of sodium is:**
   a. Proximal convoluted tubule
   b. Distal convoluted tubule
   c. Loop of Henle (thick portion)
   d. Collecting duct

4. **The site of acidification of urine is:**
   a. Distal convoluted tubule
   b. Proximal convoluted tubule
   c. Loop of Henle
   d. Collecting duct

5. **Most sensitive test for renal functional:**
   a. GFR
   b. Water deprivation with SG
   c. Creatine clearance
   d. Blood urea

6. **The first even to occur in the micturition reflex:**
   a. Relaxation of sphincter
   b. Detrusor contraction
   c. Fall in urethral pressure
   d. Activity of EMG stops at Ext. sphincter

7. **Concentration of urine by ADH, absorption of water occurs in:**
   a. PCT
   b. CT
   c. Ascending limb of Henle
   d. Descending limb of Henle

8. **In DCT, following are absorbed except:**
   a. Na^+ b. K^+
   c. Water d. Cl

9. **Renin secretion is increased by following except:**
   a. Hypovolemia
   b. Hyponatremia in PCT
   c. Hyponatremia in DCT
   d. Sympathetic

10. **Creatinine clearance indicates:**
    a. Renal blood flow
    b. Glomerular filtration rate
    c. Tubular reabsorption
    d. All of above

11. **Antidiuretic hormone acts on:**
    a. Proximal convoluted tubule
    b. Distal convoluted tubule
    c. Loop of Henle
    d. Collecting duct

12. **Normal GFR is:**
    a. 5 lit/hr b. 7.5 lit/hr
    c. 10 lit/hr d. 15 lit/hr

13. **Minimum amount of urine to excrete solute load is:**
    a. 300 ml/day b. 400 ml/day
    c. 500 ml/day d. 600 ml/day

14. **GFR indicates:**
    a. Total plasma filtered through both kidneys
    b. Total plasma filtered through each kidney
    c. Urine formed in ml/minute/kidney
    d. Urine formed in ml/minute in both kidneys

15. **Water is not freely permeable but sodium and potassium are, in which portion of nephron:**
    a. Thick ascending limb
    b. Descending limb
    c. Distal convoluted tubule
    d. Collecting duct

16. **Juxtamedullary nephrones in kidney are what percentage of total nephrones:**
    a. 15 b. 50
    c. 70 d. 85

17. **Inulin clearance closely resembles:**
    a. GFR
    b. Renal plasma flow
    c. Creatinine clearance
    d. Prostatic fluid

18. **The renal threshold for glucose excretion corresponds to arterial glucose level of:**
   a. 150 mg/dl b. 180 ml/dl
   c. 200 mg/dl d. 220 mg/dl

19. **Renin is secreted by:**
   a. Aldosterone b. Angiotensin II
   c. Angiotensin I d. Juxtaglomerular cells

20. **Normal urinary protein excretion is:**
   a. 1 gm/day b. < 150 mg/day
   c. 2 gm/day d. < 500 mg/day

21. **High threshold substance is:**
   a. Urea b. Uric acid
   c. Glucose d. Creatinine

22. **Active reabsorption of sodium occurs in which part of nephron:**
   a. Collecting duct
   b. Ascending limb of Henle
   c. Distal tutbule
   d. All of the above

23. **Normal GFR is:**
   a. 50 ml/min b. 75 ml/min
   c. 100 ml/min d. 125 ml/min

24. **First urge to micturate occurs at:**
   a. 150 ml b. 50 ml
   c. 300 ml d. 400 ml

25. **Normal filtration fraction is:**
   a. 0.16–0.2 b. 1–2.2
   c. 0.6–1 d. 5

26. **Which is counter current exchanger:**
   a. Vasa recta b. Loop of Henle
   c. Both of the above d. None of the above

Answers

1. d	2. a	3. a	4. d	5. a	6. d
7. b	8. b	9. b	10. b	11. d	12. b
13. c	14. a	15. a	16. a	17. a	18. c
19. d	20. b	21. c	22. d	23. d	24. a
25. a	26. a				

10. Reproductive System

1. **Sperm acquires motility in:**
   a. Seminal vesicle b. Testes
   c. Epidydimis d. Ejaculatory duct

2. **Antibodies against sperms may develop after:**
   a. Trauma b. Infection
   c. Vasectomy d. Orchidectomy

3. **The role of prolactin:**
   a. Growth of fetus b. Estrogen secretion
   c. Milk production d. Milk secretion

4. **Corpus luteum is maintained by:**
   a. Progesterone b. LH
   c. FSH d. Estrogen

5. **All of the following hormones have a role in maturation of spermatozoa except:**
   a. Testosterone
   b. Follicle stimulating hormone
   c. Leutinising hormones
   d. Estrogens

6. **FSH and LH synthesis and secretion is regulated by which part of hypothalamus:**
   a. Supraoptic nuclei
   b. Paraventricular nuclei
   c. Mammillary body
   d. Arcuate nucelus

7. **Spermatozoa are stored and mature in which of the following organ:**
   a. Epididymis b. Vas deferens
   c. Rete testes d. Prostate

8. **FSH and LH are secreted by:**
   a. Adenohypophysis b. Hypothalamus
   c. Ovaries d. Placenta

9. **Which of the following changes in iron metabolism does not occur in pregnancy:**
   a. Total iron binding capacity increased
   b. Increased iron absorption
   c. Normal or decreased plasma iron
   d. Increased plasma iron

10. **Growth of the ductal system of breast is stimulated by:**
   a. Estrogen b. Progesterone
   c. Oxytocin d. Prolactin

11. **Lack of which of the following hormone causes osteoporosis:**
   a. Estrogen b. Progesterone
   c. Thyroxine d. Prolactin

12. **Which of the following statement is not true about spermatogenesis:**
   a. Spermatozoa acquire motility in the epididymis
   b. Complete maturation takes about 74 days
   c. Daily sperm production is 10–20 million
   d. Each spermatogonium gives rise to 512 spermatids

13. **Germ cells in the testes give rise to all of the following cell types except:**
   a. Spermatogonia b. Primary spermatocyte
   c. Spermatiols d. Leydig cells

14. **True about testosterotone:**
   a. C19 steroid
   b. Synthesised by Leydig cells
   c. Under control of LH
   d. All are true

Answers

1. c 2. c 3. c 4. b 5. d 6. d 7. a 8. a 9. d 10. a 11. a 12. c 13. d 14. d

11. Skin and Temperature Regulation

1. **In an unacclimatised person suddenly exposed to cold, the physiological effect seen is:**
   a. Hypertension
   b. Tachycardia
   c. Shift of blood from shell to core
   d. Nonthermogenic shivering

2. **Dilatation of capillaries may result from:**
   a. Norepinephrine b. 5-HT
   c. Low temperature d. Axon reflex

3. **The insensible water loss per day is normally:**
   a. 200 ml b. 400 ml
   c. 800 ml d. 2000 ml

4. **Normal body temperature can be raised by:**
   a. Androgen b. Gonadotrophin
   c. Oestrogen d. Progesterone

5. **Neurohormone responsible for axon reflex is:**
   a. Norepinephrine b. Histamine
   c. Glycine d. Substance P

6. **Endogenous pyrogen is:**
   a. TNF alpha b. IL-1
   c. IL-6 d. All of the above

Answers

1. d 2. d 3. c 4. d 5. d 6. d

12. Nervous System

1. **Sympathetic stimulation causes all of the following except:**
   a. Increase in heart rate
   b. Increase in blood pressure
   c. Increase in total peripheral resistance
   d. Increase in venous capacitance

2. **Pain-sensitive intracranial structure is:**
   a. Pia mater b. Pial vassels
   c. Dura mater d. Brain matter

3. **Parasympathetic stimulation causes:**
   a. Decrease GI secretion b. Bronchodilation
   c. Sweat-secretion d. Pupillary constriction

4. **Blood brain barrier is present at all of the following sites except:**
   a. Hebenular nucleus b. Subfornical organ
   c. Cerebellum d. Pontine nucleus

5. **CSF/plasma glucose ratio is:**
   a. 0.2–0.4 b. 0.6–0.8
   c. 1.2–1.6 d. 1.6–2.2

6. **Features of pyramidal tract lesion are all except:**
   a. Clasp knife rigidity
   b. Involuntary movements
   c. Positive Babinski sign
   d. Exaggerated reflexes

7. **Motor aphasia refers to defect in:**
   a. Peripheral speech apparatus
   b. Verbal expression
   c. Auditory comprehension
   d. Verbal comprehension

8. **In hippocampus EEG wave are:**
   a. A wave b. B wave
   c. Theta wave d. Delta wave

9. **Flocculo nodular lobe has direct connection with:**
   a. Red nucleus
   b. Inferior olivary nucleus
   c. Vestibular nucleus
   d. Dentate nucleus

10. **Modality that is lost on the ipsilateral side in brown sequard syndrome is:**
    a. Pain b. Temperature
    c. Crude touch d. Proprioception

11. **Amyotrophic lateral sclerosis involves:**
    a. Motor neuron
    b. Posterior column only
    c. Spinothalamic tract
    d. Raphae nucleus

12. **All of the following are known functions of hypothalamus except:**
    a. Temperature regulation
    b. Increased in heart rate with exercise
    c. Food intake
    d. Hypophyseal control

13. **Ablation of the 'somatosensory area 1' of the cerebral cortex leads to:**
    a. Total loss of pain sensation
    b. Total loss of touch sensation
    c. Loss of tactile localization but not of two point discrimination.
    d. Loss of tactle localization and two point discrimination.

14. **Initiation of nerve impulse occurs at the axon hillock because:**
    a. It has a lower threshold than the rest of the axon
    b. It is unmyelinated
    c. Neurotransmitter release occurs here
    d. None of the above

15. **During flight or fight reaction, which of the following is responsible for increase in local blood flow:**
    a. Sympathetic system mediated cholinergic release
    b. Local hormones
    c. Parasympathetic cholinergic
    d. Endocrine factors only

16. **Nightmare is seen in:**
    a. REM sleep b. Stage II NREM sleep
    c. Stage IV NREM sleep d. Stage I NREM sleep

17. **Conscious proprioception is carried by:**
    a. Dorsal column fibers
    b. Anterior spinothalamic tract
    c. Lateral spinothalamic tract
    d. Vestibular tract

18. **Renshaw cell inhibition is an example of:**
    a. Feedback inhibition
    b. Oscillating motor activity
    c. Circuitry forward
    d. All of the above

19. **Afferent for segmental stretch reflex is:**
    a. Secondary muscle spindle
    b. Golgi tendon organ
    c. 1a
    d. 1b

20. **In frontal lobe lesion following are true except:**
    a. Right-left dissociation
    b. Urinary incontinence
    c. Personality change
    d. Monoparesis

21. **Muscle is stimulated by following except:**
    a. α-motor neurone b. γ-motor neurone
    c. Ia fibers d. Type IV afferent

22. **Blood brain barrier is not in:**
    a. Area postrema b. Corpus striatum
    c. Corpus callosum d. Cerebral cortex

23. **Type B fibers are seen in:**
    a. Preganglionic autonomic
    b. Motor
    c. Extrafusal
    d. Spindle fibre

24. **Which of the following statement about EEG is not true:**
    a. Normal pattern at rest with eyes closed is alpha rhythm
    b. Alpha rhythm is most marked over frontal region
    c. Activity recorded in EEG is mostly that of superficial layers of cortical gray substance
    d. Psychomotor seizures are not associated with any typical EEG changes

25. **CSF sugar is which proportion of blood sugar:**
    a. One-third b. One-half
    c. Two-third d. Three-fourth

26. **First relay station of pain is:**
    a. Spinal cord b. Medulla
    c. Pons d. Thalamus

27. **First synapse for peripheral sensation is:**
    a. Cerebellum
    b. Anterior horn cells
    c. Posterior horn cells
    d. Midbrain

28. **Highest concentration of serotonin is found in:**
    a. Liver b. Brain
    c. Platelets d. Retina

29. **Head ganglion of the autonomic system is:**
    a. Hypothalamus
    b. Medulla oblongata
    c. Superior cervical ganglion
    d. Stellate ganglia

30. **Osmoreceptors are present in:**
    a. JG cells of kidney
    b. Anterior hypothalamus
    c. Internal carotid artery
    d. Left atrium

31. **Cross extension refelx originates in:**
    a. Spinal cord b. Brainstem
    c. Cerebral cortex d. Dentate nuclei

32. **Itching is produced by the stimulation of all except:**
    a. C fibers b. Naked nerve endings
    c. Histamine d. Pacinian corpuscles

33. **Sleep spindles occurs in which phase of sleep cycle:**
    a. NREM1 b. NREM2
    c. NREM3 d. REM

34. **Normal CSF pressure is:**
    a. 80–100 mmHg b. 80–100 mm H_2O
    c. 70–180 mmHg d. 70–180 mm H_2O

35. **Parkinson's disease results from a lesion in the:**
    a. Hypothalamus b. Thalamus
    c. Striatum d. Pituitary

36. **Basic function of basal ganglia is:**
    a. Voluntary movements
    b. Emotions
    c. Sexual behaviour
    d. Regulation of circadian rhythm

37. **Proprioception is mediated by:**
    a. Lateral spinothalamic tract
    b. Ventral spinothalamic tract
    c. Dorsal column
    d. Corticospinal tract

38. **Representational hemisphere is more than categorical hemisphere for:**
    a. Language
    b. Form sense
    c. Mathematical calculations
    d. Sequential thought process

39. **Which of the following sensation is not relayed by thalamus:**
    a. Proprioception b. Smell
    c. Taste d. Pain

40. **Rate of a wave on EEG is:**
    a. 8–13 per second
    b. Below 3.5 per second
    c. 14–80 per second
    d. 4–7 per second

41. **EEG rhythm when the eyes are closed and mind wandering in a resting person is:**
    a. Alpha b. Beta
    c. Delta d. Theta

42. **Skilled motor acticity is due to**
    a. Motor cortex
    b. Basal ganglia
    c. Cerebellum
    d. All of the above

43. **Excitatory neurotransmitter among following is:**
    a. Glycine
    b. Glutamate
    c. Gamma aminobutyric acid
    d. Adenosine

44. **The fine movements of voluntary muscles are controlled by:**
    a. Anterior corticospinal tract
    b. Lateral corticospinal tract
    c. Tectospinal
    d. Vestibulospinal

45. **In EEG, highest frequency is for:**
    a. a waves b. b waves
    c. q waves d. d waves

46. **Purkinje cell is:**
   a. Output cell b. Input
   c. Connector d. Interneuron

47. **Frequency of Parkinsonian tremor is:**
   a. 5 Hz b. 8 Hz
   c. 10 Hz d. 15 Hz

48. **Which of the following nerve fibre has maximum conduction velocity:**
   a. Aα b. Aβ
   c. B d. C

Answers

1. d	2. b	3. d	4. b	5. b	6. b
7. b	8. c	9. c	10. d	11. a	12. b
13. d	14. a	15. a	16. a	17. a	18. a
19. c	20. d	21. d	22. a	23. a	24. b
25. c	26. a	27. c	28. c	29. a	30. b
31. a	32. d	33. b	34. d	35. c	36. a
37. c	38. b	39. b	40. a	41. a	42 d
43. b	44. b	45. b	46. a	47. b	48. a

13. Endocrine System

1. **Delta cells of pancreas secretes:**
   a. Glucagon b. Insulin
   c. Somatostatin d. Pancreatic polypeptide

2. **Glucose mediated insulin release is mediated through:**
   a. ATP dependent K^+ channels
   b. cAMP
   c. Carrier modulators
   d. Receptor phosphorylation

3. **Sudden decrease in serum calcium is associated with:**
   a. Increased thyroxine and PTH secretion
   b. Increased phosphate
   c. Increased excitability of muscle and nerve
   d. Cardiac conduction abnormalities

4. **TRH stimulation testing is useful in diagnosis of disorders of following hormones:**
   a. Insulin b. ACTH
   c. T_3, T_4 hormones d. PTH

5. **Regarding thyroid hormone all are true except:**
   a. T_3 is more avidly bound to nuclear receptors than T_4
   b. T_4 has the maximum plasma concentration
   c. T_3 is more active than T_4
   d. T_4 has shorter half-life thatn T_3

6. **A polypeptide causing decrease is plasma calcium is:**
   a. Vitamin D b. Parathyroid hormone
   c. Calcitonin d. Steroid

7. **Which of the following hormone is responsible for skeletal maturation?**
   a. Calcitonin
   b. Cortisol
   c. Testosterone/estrogen ratio
   d. Thyroxine

8. **Insulin promotes glucose metabolism by all of the following except:**
   a. Decrease renal resorption of glucose
   b. Stimulates glycogenesis
   c. Inhibits gluconeogenesis
   d. Increase peripheral utilization of glucose

9. **Insulin causes all except:**
   a. Glucose metabolism b. Gluconeogenesis
   c. Glycogen synthesis d. Hypopotassemia

10. **The following hormones are not produced by 'acidophil cells' of pituitary except:**
    a. ACTH b. Growth hormone
    c. FSH d. TSH

11. **cAMP serves as a second messenger in the secretion of all except:**
    a. FSH b. Glucagon
    c. Epinephrine d. Estrogen

12. **In hypoglycemia, hormone to be decreased is:**
    a. Insulin b. Glucagon
    c. Growth hormone d. Adrenaline

13. **In which of the following organ, glucose uptake depends on insulin:**
    a. Renal epithelium b. Heart
    c. Brain d. Intestinal epithelium

14. **Vitamin D deficiency leads to:**
    a. Decreased calcium absorption by renal tubules
    b. Decreased calcium absorption by intestine
    c. Increased phosphate excretion by renal tubules
    d. None of the above

15. Growth hormone secretion by anterior pituitary is stimulated by:

a. Somatostatin b. Somatomedin
c. IGF-1 d. Glucagon

16. Calcium metabolism is mainly dependent on:

a. Calcitonin b. Parathormone
c. Thyroxine d. Growth hormone

17. Which of the following is not true about calcium metabolism:

a. Phytates in diet increase absorption
b. Dihydroxycholecalciferol increases absorption
c. High protein diet increases absorption
d. 40% of total calcium is in inonized form

18. Somatostatin is secreted by:

a. F cells in pancreatic islets
b. Acidophil cells of pituitary
c. D cells in pancreatic islets
d. Mucosa of the duodenum

19. Thyroxine binding globulin is increased in:

a. Pregnancy
b. Nephrotic syndrome
c. Glucocorticoid treatment
d. Cancer chemotherapy

20. Decreased hypothalamic function causes depressed levels of all the following hormones except:

a. Growth b. Prolactin
c. TSH d. ACTH

21. Aldosterone is secreted by:

a. Zona glomerulosa b. Zona fasciculata
c. Zona reticularis d. Adrenal medulla

22. All of the following increase cAMP except:

a. Glucagon
b. Parathormone
c. Growth hormone
d. Luteinizing hormone

23. Aldosterone causes:

a. Increased sodium reabsorption
b. Decreased potassium secretion
c. Water reabsorption
d. All of the above

24. Neuroendrocrine control is by:

a. Hypothalamus b. Hippocampus
c. Pituitary d. Internal capsule

25. Which of the following is required for milk synthesis:

a. Prolactin b. Growth hormone
c. Insulin d. All of the above

26. 'Milk let down reflex' is initiated by hormone:

a. Oxytocin b. Oestrogen
c. Prolactin d. Progesterone

27. Calcitonin is produced by:

a. C-cells of thyroid b. Parathyroid
c. Thymus d. Kidney

28. Growth hormone has diabetogenic effect because of:

a. Increase in gluconeogenesis
b. Blocking of beta cells of pancreas
c. Glycogenolysis
d. Glucose absorption

29. Thyroid binding globulins are decreased in:

a. Pregnancy b. Nephrotic syndrome
c. Kidney failure d. Anaemia

30. Which of the following has analgesic effects:

a. MSH b. Corticotrophin
c. Growth hormone d. Endorphins

31. Hormone secreted by hypothalamus is:

a. Somatostatin b. Somatotrophin
c. Gonadotrophin d. Luteotrophin

32. Decrease in ADH secretion is caused by:

a. Thiazides b. Caffeine
c. Alcohol d. Vitamin C

33. ADH is secreted from:

a. Posterior hypophysis b. Anterior hypophysis
c. Median eminence d. Adrenal gland

34. Aldosterone acts on:

a. PCT
b. DCT and collecting duct
c. PCT and DCT
d. Collecting duct

35. All are effects of thyroid hormone except:

a. Increased rate of carbohydrate absorption from GIT
b. Decreased cholesterol level
c. Decreased dissociation of oxygen from hemoglobin
d. Increased number and affinity of β receptors in heart

36. Stimulation of both glucocorticoids and mineralocorticoids is seen in:
a. Exercise b. Anxiety
c. Hyperkalemia d. Low sodium diet

37. High levels of parathormone are found in all except:
a. Chronic renal failure
b. Pseudohypoparathyroidism
c. Parathyroid hyperplasia
d. Hypoparathyroidism

38. Major pathway of excretion of calcium is:
a. Kidney b. Gut
c. Kidney and gut d. None of the above

39. The secretion of alodosterone is controlled by:
a. Angiotensin II b. ADH
c. Epinephrine d. Insulin

40. Calcium absorption from duodenum and jejunum is increased by all except:
a. Cortisol b. Parathormone
c. Growth hormone d. Hypocalcemia

41. Which of the following does not acts at the membrane receptors:
a. TRH b. Thyroxine
c. Insulin d. Epinephrine

42. Normal levels of creatinine in serum is:
a. 0.6 to 1.2 mg% b. 1 to 2 mg%
c. 0.01 to 0.04 mg% d. 0.04 to 0.1 mg%

43. The metabolic action of 'T_3' is all except:
a. Increase O_2 consumption of tissues
b. Increases absorption of carbohydrate from gut
c. Inhibit growth
d. Increases dissociation of O_2 from hemoglobin

44. Longest acting hormone is:
a. Glucagon b. Insulin
c. Epinerphrine d. FSH

45. B cells of pancreas secrete:
a. Glucagon b. Insulin
c. Somatostatin d. Calcitonin

46. Which of the following feature is not seen in hypopituitary state:
a. Cachexia
b. Growth failure
c. Infertility
d. Increased sensitivity to insulin

47. Insulin like growth factor is synthesized in all except:
a. Brain b. Liver
c. Pancreas b cells d. Cartilage

48. Daily amount of insulin secreted normally is:
a. 10 units b. 20 units
c. 40 units d. 80 units

49. Vasopressin act's by:
a. Water transport across collecting duct
b. Water absorption at medullary ducts
c. Water at loop of Henle
d. Water at PCT

50. All can cause hyperglycemia except:
a. Growth hormone b. Cortisol
c. Epinephrine d. Insulin

51. Hormones secreted by adrenal medulla are:
a. Glucagon b. Epinephrine
c. Cortisol d. Insulin

52. Which of the following hormones are increased after major trauma:
a. Calcitonin b. GH
c. Glucocorticoids d. Thyroxine

53. Following hormones are produced by endocrinal part of pancreas except:
a. Insulin b. Somatostatin
c. Glucagon d. Secretin

54. cAMP action mediates all except:
a. Glucagon b. FSH
c. LH d. Estrogen

55. FSH is produced by:
a. Hypothalamus b. Ovary
c. Anterior pituitary d. All of the above

56. ADH is stimulated by all except:
a. Hyperosmolarity
b. Increased ECF volume
c. Standing
d. Angiotensin II

57. Which of the following hormones is not required for growth:
a. Insulin b. Aldosterone
c. Growth hormone d. Thyroxine

58. Exocrine pancreas is stimulated by:
a. Fat in chyme
b. Increased alkanity of intestinal secretion

c. Bile salts
d. Hyperglycemia

59. Which of the following hormones does show rise of serum levels nocturnally:
a. Epinephrine
b. Growth hormone
c. Melatonin
d. Corticosteriods

60. Prolactin is secreted by:
a. Anterior lobe pituitary
b. Intermediate lobe
c. Posterior lobe
d. None of the above

61. GH is secreted by:
a. Acidophils
b. Basophils
c. Chromophobes
d. Theca cells

62. All are true about insulin except:
a. Glycopeptide
b. Lipogenetic
c. Glycogenetic
d. Secreted by B cells

63. TSH is:
a. Acidophil
b. Polypeptide
c. Glycoprotein
d. C and A

64. All the following are choleretics except:
a. Vagus
b. Secretin
c. Bile salt
d. CCK

Answers

1. c	2. a	3. c	4. c	5. d	6. c
7. d	8. a	9. b	10. b	11. d	12. a
13. b	14. b	15. d	16. b	17. a	18. c
19. a	20. b	21. a	22. c	23. a	24. a
25. d	26. a	27. a	28. a	29. b	30. d
31. a	32. c	33. a	34. b	35. c	36. b
37. d	38. c	39. a	40. a	41. b	42. a
43. c	44. d	45. b	46. a	47. c	48. c
49. a	50. d	51. b	52. c	53. d	54. d
55. c	56. b	57. b	58. a	59. c	60. a
61. a	62. a	63. c	64. d		

14. Special Senses

1. Function of stapedius is:
a. Protects the ear from loud frequency sound
b. Helps in hearing sounds of low frequency
c. Helps in hearing sounds of high frequency
d. Helps in hearing whispered words

2. The light rays come to focus in front of the retina because of the increased length of the eyeball in:
a. Myopia
b. Hypermetropia
c. Astigmatism
d. Presbyopia

3. Visual accommodation is by:
a. Contraction of ciliary muscle
b. Relaxation of ciliary muscle
c. Contraction of sphincter pupillae muscle
d. Contraction of lens ligament

4. Most sensitive hearing range (Hz) is:
a. 1,000–4,000
b. 4,000–6,000
c. 6,000–10,000
d. 10,000–20,000

5. At rest, the refractive power of human eye is:
a. 22.5 diopters
b. 40.3 diopters
c. 60 diopters
d. 56.6 diopters

6. Which of the following is not true about rods:
a. Pigment is rhodopsin
b. Useful for the color vision
c. Least number is present in fovea centralis
d. More number than cones

7. Brodmanns area 17 is:
a. Auditory cortex
b. Visual cortex
c. Brocas
d. Frontal eye field

8. According to Young-Helmholtz theory:
a. There are three kinds of cones
b. There are two kinds of cones
c. There are seven kinds of cones
d. Rods are of two types

9. Tympanic reflex is due to:
a. Contraction of stapedius
b. Contraction of tensor tympani
c. A and b
d. None of the above

Answers

1. a	2. a	3. a	4. a	5. c.	6. b
7. b	8. a	9. c			

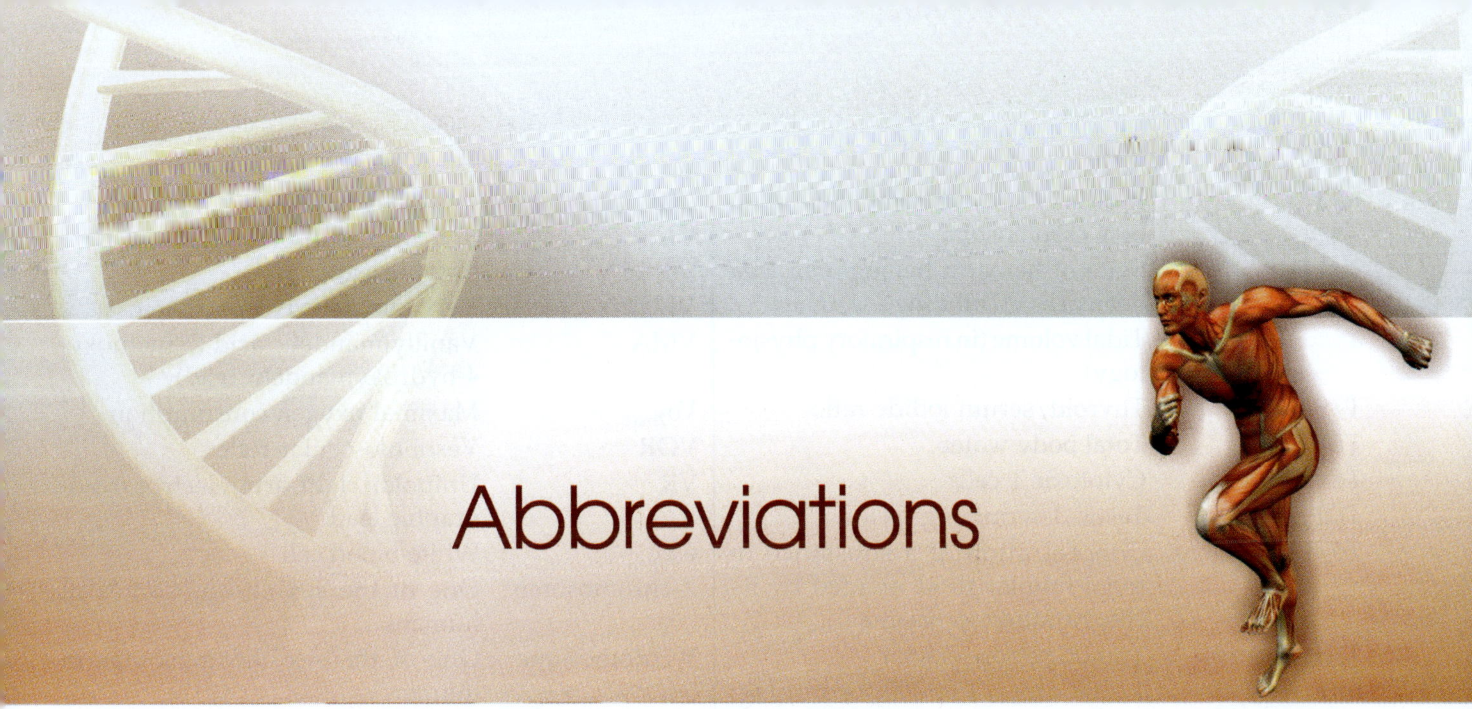

Abbreviations

BASIC UNITS

Length	meter	m
Mass	kilogram	kg
Time	second	s
Electric current	ampere	A
Amount of substance	mole	mol

SOME DERIVED SI UNITS AND STANDARD PREFIXES

Area	Square meter	m^2
Centi	c	10^{-2}
Concentration		
Mass	Kilogram/liter	kg/L
Substance	mole/liter	mol/L
deca	da	10^1
deci	d	10^{-1}
femto	f	10^{-15}
Frequency	Hertz	Hz
Kilo	K	10^3
milli	m	10^{-3}
micro	μ	10^{-6}
nano	n, mμ	10^{-9}
picro	p, mμ	10^{-12}
Temperature	degree celsius	°C
Volume	Cubic meter	m^3
	liter	L

ABBREVIATION AND SYMBOLS USED IN PHYSIOLOGY

Δ	Change
[ ]	Concentration
μ	micro, 10^{-6}
A^-	General symbol for anion
ACE	Angiotensin converting enzyme
Acetyl CoA	Acetyl coenzyme A
ANP	Atrial natriuretic peptide
AUPD	Amine precursor uptake and decarboxylation cells that secrete homone
COPD	Chronic obstructive pulmonary disease
dl, dL	deciliter - 100 mL
ECF	Extracellular fluid
g, gm	Gram
GLUT	Glucose transporter
hCG	Human chorionic gonadotropin
Hct	Hematocrit
ICF	Intracelluar fluid
L, l	liter
LES	Lower esophageal sphincter
m	meter min minute
O	Absence of chromosome
P	Gas pressure
$\bar{P}$	Mean gas pressure
PAM	Pulmonary alveolar macrophages
PDGF	Platelet derived growth factor
PET	Positron emission tomography
Q	Volume of blood
Rh factor	Rhesus group of red cell agglutinogen
RQ	Respiratory quotient
s	Second
SGLT	Sodium dependent glucose transporter

SRY	Product of sex determining region of Y chromosome
T state	State of heme in hemoglobin that decreases O_2 binding
T	Tidal volume (in respiratory physiology)
T/S ratio	Thyroid/serum iodide ratio
TBW	Total body water
Tc cells	Cytotoxic T cells
TDF	Testis-determining factor
TF/P	Concentration of a substance in renal tubular fluid divided by its concentration in plasma
TNF	Tumor necroses factor
torr	1/760 atm = 1.00000014 mmHg; unit for various pressures in the body
t-PA	Tissue type plasminogen activator
TR	Thyroid hormone receptor
TRH, TRF	Thyrotropin-releasing hormone or factor
tRNA	Transfer RNA
TSF	Thrombopoietic-stimulating factor, thrombopoietin
TSH	Thyroid-stimulating hormone
TSH-R (block) Ab	TSH receptor-blocking antibodies
TSH-R (stim) Ab	TSH receptor-stimulating antibodies
TSI	Thyroid-stimulating immunoglobulins
TTX	Tetrodotoxin
U	Unit
U followed by subscript	Urine concentration, e.g. UCr = urine creatinine concentration
UFA	Unesterified free fatty acid, same as FFA
UL	Unstirred layer
u-PA	Urokinase-type plasminogen activator
URF	Uterine-relaxing factor; relaxin
US	Unconditioned stimulus
V	Gas volume; volt; also valine
$\dot{V}/\dot{v}$	Volume per unit time (dot over symbol indicates rate)
V_1, V_2, etc.	Unipolar chest electrocardiographic leads
V_D	Dead space gas volume
VEGF	Vascular endothelial growth factor
VF	Unipolar left leg electrocardiographic lead
VIP	Vasoactive intestinal peptide
VL	Left arm unipolar electrocardiographic lead
VLDL	Very low density lipoprotein
VMA	Vanillylmandelic acid (3-methoxy-4-hydroxymandelic acid)
$\dot{V}o_{2max}$	Maximal oxygen consumption
VOR	Vestibulo-ocular reflex
VR	Unipolar right arm electrocardiographic lead
wbc	White blood cell
X-chromosome	One of the sex chromosomes in humans
Y chromosome	One of the sex chromosomes in humans

ABBREVIATIONS AND SYMBOLS FOR PULMONARY FUNCTION

General Variables

D	Diffusing capacity
f	Respiratory frequency (breaths/unit of time)
P	Gas pressure
$\bar{P}$	Mean gas pressure
Q	Volume of blood
R	Respiratory exchange ratio = V_{CO_2}/V_{O_2}

Localization (Subscript Letters)

a	Arterial blood
A	Alveolar gas
ATPD	Ambient temperature and pressure dry
ATPS	Ambient temperature and pressure saturated with water vapor
B	Barometric
BTPS	Body temperature and pressure saturated with water vapor
c	Capillary blood
P_{IO_2}	Pressure of oxygen in inspired air
T	Tidal gas
v	Venous blood
V_D	Dead space gas volume

Some other Abbreviations

C	Compliance
Ca_{O_2}	Concentration of oxygen in arterial blood
Cv_{O_2}	Concentration of oxygen in mixed venous blood
DL_{O_2}	Diffusing capacity of the lung for oxygen
D_{LCO}	Diffusing capacity of the lung for carbon monoxide

PB Atmospheric pressure
Palv Alveolar pressure
Ppl Pleural pressure
PO_2 Partial pressure of oxygen
PCO_2 Partial pressure of carbon dioxide
PN_2 Partial pressure of nitrogen
Q Cardiac output
QS Shunt flow
R Respiratory exchange ratio
Raw Resistance of tracheobronchial tree to flow of air into the lung
So_2 Percentage saturation of hemoglobin with oxygen
Sa_{O_2} Percentage saturation of hemoglobin with oxygen in arterial blood
TLC Total lung capacity
VC Vital capacity
$\dot{V}A$ Alveolar ventilation per minute

SYMBOLS

α	alpha	η	eta
β	beta	θ	theta
γ	gamma	ι	iota
Δ, δ	delta	κ	kappa
ε	epsilon	λ	lambda
ζ	zeta	μ	mu

EQUIVALENTS OF METRIC

Length

1 mile = 5280 feet = 1.61 kilometers
1 inch = 1/12 foot = 2.54 centimeters

Temperature

To convert **C**elsius degrees into **F**ahrenheit: multiply by 9/5 and add 32

To convert **F**ahrenheitt degrees into **C**elsius: subtract 32 and multiply by 5/9

Volume

1 milliliter = 0.03 fluid ounce
1 fluid ounce = 29.57 milliliters

Weight

1 kilogram = 2.20 pounds (avoirdupois) = 2.68 pounds (apothecaries)
1 pound (avoirdupois) = 16 ounces = 453.60 grams
1 grain = 65 milligrams

Energy

1 kilogram-meter = 7.25 feet-pounds
1 feet-pound = 0.14 kilogram-meter

LABORATORY REFERENCE VALUES

Hematological, Coagulation and Chemical Chemistry

	Specimen		
Bleeding time (adult)	(WB)		2–9.5 min
ESR	(WB)	Females	1–25 mm/hr
		Males	0–17 mm/hr
Fibrinogen	(P)		150–400 mg/dL
Hematocrit	(WB)	Adult male	41.0–53.0
		Adult female	36.0–46.0
Hemoglobin	(WB)	Adult males	13.5–17.5 g/dL
		Adult female	12.0–16.0 g/dL
Platelet count	(WB)		1,50,000–3,50,000 mm^3
Prothrombin time	(P)		11.1–13.1 s
Glucose	(P)		
Fasting			75–115 mg/dL
Diabetes			> 125 mg/dL
Glucose 2 hr (Post prandial)			< 120 mg/dL
Iron	(S)		50–150 μg/dL
Osmolality	(P)		275–295 mosmol/kg serum water

Potassium	(S)		3.5–5.0 meq/L
Protein total	(S)		6–8 g/dL
Albumin	(S)		3.5–5.5
Globulin	(S)		2.0–3.5
Prostate specific antigen	(PSA)	Males < 40 yrs	0.0–2.0 ng/mL
		> 40 yrs	0.0–4.0 ng/mL
		45–75 yrs	> 25% associated with benign prostatic hyperplasia
Sodium	(S)		136–145 meq/L
Triglycerides	(S)		< 160 mg/dL
Troponin I	(S)		0–0.4 ng/mL
Troponin T	(S)		0–0.1 ng/mL
Urea nitrogen	(S)		10–20 mg/dL
Uric acid	(S)	Male	2.5–8 mg/dL
		Female	3.0–5.9 mg/dL

Note: (S) stands for serum sample; **(P)** for plasma sample; **(WB)** for whole blood sample.

Scanning Procedures

CT or CAT = Computerized axial tomography
(X-ray beam rotates round the body while detectors measure how much the X-ray pass through the tissue and organs indicating density)

MRI scan = Magnetic resonance imaging
(Uses strong magnetic fields and radiowaves to produce detailed images of the inside of the body)

fMRI = Functional magnetic resonance imaging
(A form of MRI blood oxygen level dependent)

PET = Positron emission tomography
(is a nuclear medicine, functional imaging technique that is used to observe metabolic process in the body)

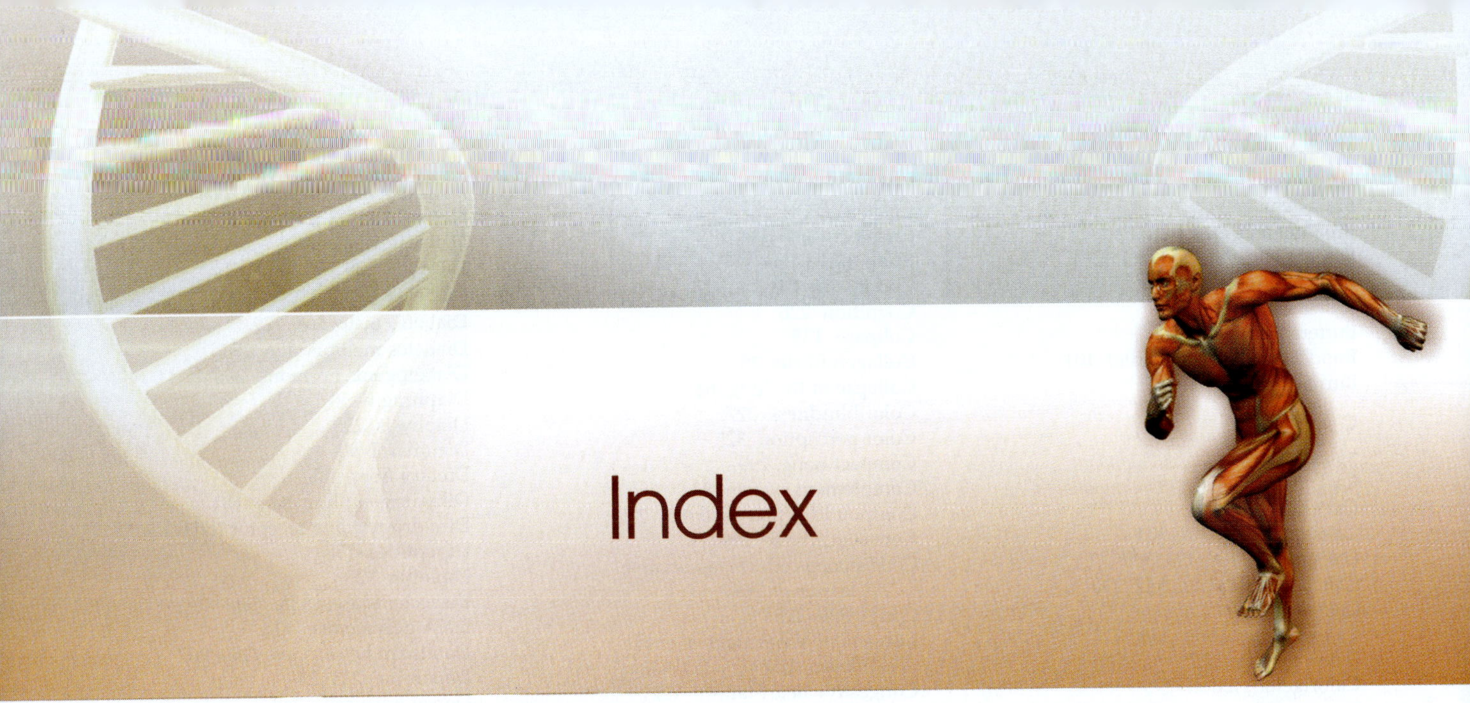

Index

J

K

L

M

N

O

T

U

V

W

X

Y

Z